CLINICAL
NEUROSURGERY

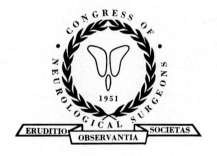

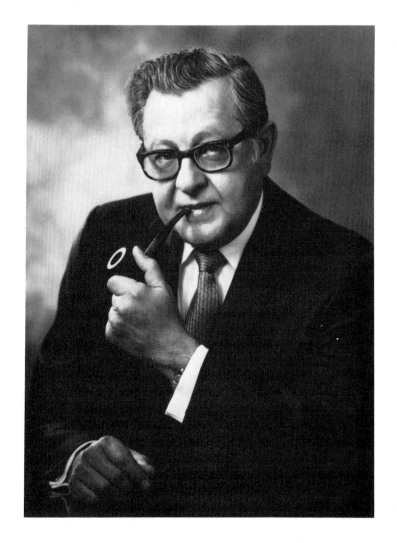

HUGO V. RIZZOLI, M.D.

CLINICAL NEUROSURGERY

Proceedings

OF THE

CONGRESS OF NEUROLOGICAL SURGEONS

New York, New York

1984

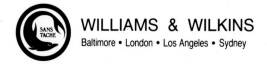

WILLIAMS & WILKINS

Baltimore • London • Los Angeles • Sydney

Made in the United States of America

Library of Congress
Catalog Card Number
S4-12666
ISBN 0-683-02027-7

The Library of Congress cataloged this serial as follows:
Congress of Neurological Surgeons.
    Clinical neurosurgery.   v. 1- 1953-
Baltimore, Williams & Wilkins.
        v.   ill.   24 cm.
    Annual.
    "Proceedings of the Congress of Neurological Surgeons."
    Issues for 1954–70 include the Membership roster of the Congress
of Neurological Surgeons.
    Each vol. honors an individual scientist and presents a biograph-
ical sketch, bibliography, and some of his original papers.
    Indexes:
        Vols. 1–19, 1953–72, in v. 19.
    Key title: Clinical neurosurgery, ISSN 0069-4827.
    1. Nervous system—Surgery.   I. Congress of Neurosurgical Sur-
geons. Proceedings. II. Congress of Neurological Surgeons. Mem-
bership roster. III. Title.
    [DNLM: W1 CL732]
RD593.A1C63   617.48   54-12666
                                                     MARC-S

Composed and printed at the   85 86 87 88 89
Waverly Press, Inc.   10 9 8 7 6 5 4 3 2 1

Preface

The 34th Annual Meeting of the American Congress of Neurological Surgeons was dedicated to Dr. Walter E. Dandy and his contributions to neurosurgery. During the course of the meeting, the remarkable influence of Dr. Dandy upon present day neurosurgery was widely evident.

Dr. Hugo V. Rizzoli was the Honored Guest of the American Congress of Neurological Surgeons. As a former resident of Dr. Dandy, he recounted a number of his memories about the "Chief." The personal recollections are included in Dr. Rizzoli's chapters entitled, "Walter Dandy—An Historical Perspective," and "Dandy's Brain Team."

The American Congress of Neurological Surgeons also was honored to have Dr. Edward R. Laws as President for 1983–1984. Under the able direction of Dr. Laws, Dr. Fremont P. Wirth (General Chairman, Annual Meeting Committee), and Dr. J. Michael McWhorter (Chairman, Scientific Sessions), an outstanding scientific program was organized. The main topics of the program and this volume include aneurysm surgery, cerebellopontine angle tumors, trigeminal neuralgia, pineal tumors, orbital tumors, and hydrocephalus. The material contained in chapters dealing with these topics provides an update and important new insights into these important clinical problems.

I would like to express my appreciation to the members of the Editorial Board for their superb effort in putting together this volume. My secretary, Ms. Joyce Orban, is also to be congratulated for her help in this endeavor. A special thanks to Ms. Carol-Lynn Brown, Williams & Wilkins, for her guidance and support.

JOHN R. LITTLE, M.D.
Editor-In-Chief
Associate Editors
MICHAEL L. J. APUZZO, M.D.
JOHN ANTUNES, M.D.
JANET W. BAY, M.D.
ARTHUR L. DAY, M.D.
MICHAEL EBERSOLD, M.D.
TAKANORI FUKUSHIMA, M.D.
HOWARD H. KAUFMAN, M.D.
HAROLD L. REKATE, M.D.
JON H. ROBERTSON, M.D.
MICHAEL SALCMAN, M.D.
JAMES WOODS, M.D.

Honored Guests

1952—Professor Herbert Olivecrona, Stockholm, Sweden
1953—Sir Geoffrey Jefferson, Manchester, England
1954—Dr. Kenneth G. McKenzie, Toronto, Canada
1955—Dr. Carl W. Rand, Los Angeles, California
1956—Dr. Wilder G. Penfield, Montreal, Canada
1957—Dr. Francis C. Grant, Philadelphia, Pennsylvania
1958—Dr. A. Earl Walker, Baltimore, Maryland
1959—Dr. William J. German, New Haven, Connecticut
1960—Dr. Paul C. Bucy, Chicago, Illinois
1961—Professor Eduard A. V. Busch, Copenhagen, Denmark
1962—Dr. Bronson S. Ray, New York, New York
1963—Dr. James L. Poppen, Boston, Massachusetts
1964—Dr. Edgar A. Kahn, Ann Arbor, Michigan
1965—Dr. James C. White, Boston, Massachusetts
1966—Dr. Hugo A. Krayenbühl, Zurich, Switzerland
1967—Dr. W. James Gardner, Cleveland, Ohio
1968—Professor Norman M. Dott, Edinburgh, Scotland
1969—Dr. Wallace B. Hamby, Cleveland, Ohio
1970—Dr. Barnes Woodhall, Durham, North Carolina
1971—Dr. Elisha S. Gurdjian, Detroit, Michigan
1972—Dr. Francis Murphey, Memphis, Tennessee
1973—Dr. Henry G. Schwartz, St. Louis, Missouri
1974—Dr. Guy L. Odom, Durham, North Carolina
1975—Dr. William H. Sweet, Boston, Massachusetts
1976—Dr. Lyle A. French, Minneapolis, Minnesota
1977—Dr. Richard C. Schneider, Ann Arbor, Michigan
1978—Dr. Charles G. Drake, London, Ontario, Canada
1979—Dr. Frank H. Mayfield, Cincinnati, Ohio
1980—Dr. Eben Alexander, Jr., Winston-Salem, North Carolina
1981—Dr. J. Garber Galbraith, Birmingham, Alabama
1982—Dr. Keiji Sano, Tokyo, Japan
1983—Dr. C. Miller Fisher, Boston, Massachusetts
1984—Dr. Hugo V. Rizzoli
   Dr. Walter E. Dandy (posthumously)

Officers of the Congress
of
Neurological Surgeons
1984

Contributors

GEORGE S. ALLEN, M.D., PH.D., Department of Neurological Surgery, Vanderbilt University, School of Medicine, Nashville, Tennessee (*Chapter 5*)

RONALD I. APFELBAUM, M.D., The Albert Einstein College of Medicine, and Montefiore Medical Center, Bronx, New York, (*Chapter 16*)

HILLIER L. BAKER, JR., M.D., Department of Diagnostic Radiology, Mayo Clinic and Mayo Foundation, Rochester, Minnesota (*Chapter 27*)

DAVID J. BISSONETTE, P.A.-C., Instructor in Neurosurgery, University of Pittsburgh, School of Medicine, Pittsburgh, Pennsylvania (*Chapter 17*)

PETER McL. BLACK, M.D., PH.D., Neurosurgical Service, Massachusetts General Hospital, Department of Surgery, Harvard Medical School, Boston, Massachusetts (*Chapter 31*)

LAWRENCE F. BORGES, M.D., Division of Neurosurgery, Massachusetts General Hospital, Boston, Massachusetts (*Chapter 32*)

L. PHILIP CARTER, M.D., Barrow Neurological Institute, Phoenix, Arizona, (*Chapter 6*)

PAUL H. CHAPMAN, M.D., Division of Neurosurgery, Massachusetts General Hospital, Boston, Massachusetts (*Chapter 32*)

KENNETH R. DAVIS, M.D., Associate Professor of Radiology, Harvard Medical School, Director of Neuroradiology, Massachusetts General Hospital, Boston, Massachusetts (*Chapter 10*)

CHARLES G. DRAKE, M.D., F.R.C.S.(C), Professor of Neurosurgery, The University of Western Ontario, London, Ontario, Canada, (*Chapter 3*)

FRANKLIN EARNEST, IV, M.D., Department of Diagnostic Radiology, Mayo Clinic and Mayo Foundation, Rochester, Minnesota (*Chapter 27*)

FRED EPSTEIN, M.D., Professor of Neurosurgery, New York University Medical Center, New York, New York (*Chapter 30*)

MICHAEL R. FETELL, M.D., Assistant Professor of Clinical Neurology, Director of Neuro-Oncology Service, Columbia Presbyterian Medical Center, The Neurological Institute, New York, New York (*Chapter 22*)

GLENN FORBES, M.D., Consultant, Neuroradiologist, Department of Diagnostic Radiology, Mayo Clinic and Mayo Foundation, Associate Professor of Radiology, Mayo Medical School, Rochester, Minnesota (*Chapter 24*)

ix

JEREMY M. GIBBS, M.B., M.R.C.P., Registrar in Neurology, The National Hospital, Queen Square, London, WC1E 3BG, England (*Chapter 4*)

C. R. HAMPF, M.D., Department of Clinical Neurological Sciences, Division of Neurosurgery, The University of Western Ontario, London, Ontario, Canada (*Chapter 8*)

WILLIAM E. HITSELBERGER, M.D., Neurosurgical Consultant, House Ear Institute, Los Angeles, California (*Chapter 11*)

WILLIAM F. HOUSE, M.D., Director, House Ear Institute, Los Angeles, California (*Chapter 11*)

PETER J. JANNETTA, M.D., Professor and Chairman, Department of Neurosurgery, University of Pittsburgh, School of Medicine, Pittsburgh, Pennsylvania (*Chapter 17*)

JEFFREY T. KELLER, PH.D., Department of Neurosurgery, The Christ Hospital; Department of Neurosurgery, University of Cincinnati, Member Mayfield Neurological Institute, Cincinnati, Ohio (*Chapter 14*)

DAVID B. KISPERT, M.D., Department of Diagnostic Radiology, Mayo Clinic and Mayo Foundation, Rochester, Minnesota (*Chapter 27*)

EDWARD R. LAWS, JR., M.D., Department of Neurologic Surgery, Mayo Clinic and Mayo Foundation, Rochester, Minnesota (*Chapters 19 and 27*)

DONLIN M. LONG, M.D., Professor and Chairman, Department of Neurological Surgery, The Johns Hopkins School of Medicine, Baltimore, Maryland (*Chapter 25*)

L. DADE LUNSFORD, M.D., Department of Neurological Surgery, University of Pittsburgh, School of Medicine, Pittsburgh, Pennsylvania (*Chapter 16*)

MICHAEL L. MANCO-JOHNSON, M.D., University of Colorado Health Sciences Center, Division of Diagnostic Ultrasound, Denver, Colorado (*Chapter 28*)

W. RICHARD MARSH, M.D., Consultant, Mayo Clinic, Department of Neurosurgery, Instructor, Mayo Medical School, Rochester, Minnesota (*Chapter 19*)

NEIL A. MARTIN, M.D., Barrow Neurological Institute, Phoenix, Arizona, (*Chapter 6*)

ROBERT L. MARTUZA, M.D., Assistant Professor of Surgery, Harvard Medical School, Assisting Visiting Neurosurgeon, Massachusetts General Hospital, Boston, Massachusetts (*Chapter 10*)

DAVID G. MCLONE, M.D., PH.D., Professor of Neurological Surgery, Department of Surgery, The Children's Memorial Hospital, Northwestern University Medical School, Chicago, Illinois (*Chapter 26*)

FREDRIC B. MEYER, M.D., Department of Neurosurgery, Mayo Clinic and Mayo Graduate School of Medicine, Rochester, Minnesota (*Chapter 9*)

JOHN D. MICHENFELDER, M.D., Professor of Anesthesiology, Mayo Medical School and Mayo Clinic, Rochester, Minnesota (*Chapter 7*)

NEIL R. MILLER, M.D., Associate Professor of Ophthalmology, Neurology, and Neurosurgery, Neuro-Ophthalmology Unit, The Departments of Ophthalmology, Neurology, and Neurosurgery, The Johns Hopkins Medical Institutions, Baltimore, Maryland (*Chapter 23*)

JOSEPH B. NADOL, JR., M.D., Associate Professor of Otolaryngology, Harvard Medical School, and Massachusetts Eye and Ear Infirmary, Boston, Massachusetts (*Chapter 10*)

THOMAS P. NAIDICH, M.D., Professor of Radiology, Section of Neuroradiology, Children's Memorial Hospital, Northwestern University Medical School, Chicago, Illinois (*Chapter 26*)

DANIEL G. NEHLS, M.D., CPT MC USA, Division of Neurological Surgery, Barrow Neurological Institute, Phoenix, Arizona (*Chapter 12*)

EDWARD A. NEUWELT, M.D., Associate Professor of Neurosurgery, Oregon Health Sciences University, Portland, Oregon (*Chapter 20*)

ROBERT G. OJEMANN, M.D., Professor of Surgery, Harvard Medical School, Visiting Neurosurgeon, Massachusetts General Hospital, Boston Massachusetts (*Chapters 10, 31*)

STEPHEN W. PARKER, M.D., Assistant Professor of Neurology, Harvard Medical School, Associate Neurologist and Director of the Otoneurology Unit of the Neurophysiology Laboratory, Massachusetts General Hospital, Boston, Massachusetts (*Chapter 10*)

SIDNEY (SKIP) J. PEERLESS, M.D., F.R.C.S.(C), Department of Clinical Neurological Sciences, Division of Neurosurgery, The University of Western Ontario, London, Ontario, Canada (*Chapter 8*)

GOTZ PENKERT, M.D., Neurosurgical Clinic, Nordstadt Hospital, Hannover, West Germany (*Chapter 13*)

DAVID G. PIEPGRAS, M.D., Department of Neurosurgery, Mayo Clinic and Mayo Graduate School of Medicine, Rochester, Minnesota (*Chapter 9*)

DOLORES H. PRETORIUS, M.D., Assistant Professor of Radiology, University of Colorado Health Sciences Center, Denver, Colorado (*Chapter 28*)

HAROLD L. REKATE, M.D., Division of Neurological Surgery, Barrow Neurological Institute, Phoenix, Arizona (*Chapter 29*)

HUGO V. RIZZOLI, M.D., Professor and Chairman, Department of Neurological Surgery, George Washington University, Washington, D.C. (*Chapters 1 and 2*)

MADJID SAMII, M.D., Professor and Chairman Neurosurgical Clinic,

Nordstadt Hospital, Hannover, West Germany (*Chapter 13*)

BERND W. SCHEITHAUER, M.D., Department of Pathology, Mayo Clinic and Mayo Graduate School of Medicine, Rochester, Minnesota (*Chapter 18*)

ANDREW G. SHETTER, M.D., Division of Neurological Surgery, Barrow Neurological Institute, Phoenix, Arizona (*Chapter 12*)

VOLKER K. H. SONNTAG, M.D. Division of Neurological Surgery, Barrow Neurological Institute, Phoenix, Arizona (*Chapter 12*)

ROBERT F. SPETZLER, M.D., Division of Neurological Surgery, Barrow Neurological Institute, Phoenix, Arizona (*Chapters 6, 12*)

BENNETT M. STEIN, M.D., Byron S. Stookey Professor of Neurological Surgery, Columbia Presbyterian Medical Center, The Neurological Institute, New York, New York (*Chapter 22*)

THORALF M. SUNDT, M.D., Department of Neurosurgery, Mayo Clinic and Mayo Graduate School of Medicine, Rochester, Minnesota (*Chapter 9*)

WILLIAM H. SWEET, M.D., D.SC., D.H.C., Professor Emeritus, Department of Surgery, Harvard Medical School, Boston, Massachusetts (*Chapter 15*)

KINTOMO TAKAKURA, M.D., D.M.SC., Professor and Chairman, Department of Neurosurgery, University of Tokyo Hospital, Tokyo, Japan (*Chapter 21*)

DAVID G. T. THOMAS, M.A., M.B., M.R.C.P., F.R.C.S., Consultant Neurosurgeon and Senior Lecturer, The National Hospital, Queen Square, London, WC1E 3BG; Maida Vale Hospital, London W.9, England (*Chapter 4*)

KEKI E. TUREL, M.D., M.S. (NEUROSURGERY), F.I.C.S., Neurosurgical Clinic, Nordstadt Hospital, Hannover, West Germany (*Chapter 13*)

ARGYRIS TZOURAS, M.D., Neurosurgical Service, Massachusetts General Hospital, Department of Surgery, Harvard Medical School, Boston, Massachusetts (*Chapter 31*)

HARRY VAN LOVEREN, M.D., Department of Neurosurgery, University of Cincinnati, Member Mayfield Neurological Institute, Cincinnati, Ohio (*Chapter 14*)

RICHARD J. S. WISE, M.B., M.R.C.P., Senior Registrar in Neurology, The National Hospital, Queen Square, London WC1E 3BG, England (*Chapter 4*)

TAKEHIKO YANAGIHARA, M.D., Department of Neurology, Mayo Clinic and Mayo Graduate School of Medicine, Rochester, Minnesota (*Chapter 9*)

Biography of Hugo V. Rizzoli, M.D.

Hugo Victor Rizzoli was born in Newark, New Jersey, on August 20, 1916. He received his A.B. degree in Chemistry from the Johns Hopkins University in Baltimore, Maryland, in 1936. Doctor Rizzoli then went on to receive his M.D. from Johns Hopkins in 1940. He interned in Medicine in 1940–41, and then entered the Surgery program at Johns Hopkins. He became a Harvey Cushing Fellow in 1942–43 and then served as neurosurgical resident with Walter E. Dandy as Chief of Service.

Doctor Rizzoli completed his residency during World War II and immediately entered the U.S. Army, serving as neurosurgeon at Halloran General Hospital and later at Walter Reed Army Hospital. Major Rizzoli served as Chief of the Neurosurgical Section at Walter Reed for the year prior to his discharge from the Army in October 1946.

After leaving the Army, Doctor Rizzoli stayed in Washington, D.C., to practice neurosurgery. In addition to his private practice, he became Chief of the Department of Neurosurgery at Emergency Hospital. Always a respected teacher, Doctor Rizzoli then became formally involved with the residency training program at the George Washington University. He had been Chairman of the Department of Neurological Surgery and a Member of the Board of Directors of the Washington Hospital Center, and was Director of Training and Education there from 1964 to 1973. He has been Professor and Chairman of the Department of Neurological Surgery at the George Washington University since 1969.

Doctor Rizzoli's career has exemplified neurosurgery in the nation's service. He has been deeply involved with the Veterans Administration and has made numerous site visits to their spinal cord injury centers. He has continued to serve as Consultant in Neurological Surgery to Walter Reed Army Medical Center, Bethesda Naval Hospital, Malcolm Grow Air Force Hospital, the Washington Veterans Administration Hospital, Andrews Air Force Base Hospital, and the National Institutes of Health. He was a member of the health exchange team of the Department of Health, Education and Welfare on a trip to the Soviet Union to study medical services for the treatment of spinal cord-injured patients. In 1979 he received the Department of the Army Commander's Award for Civilian Service which was presented by Walter Reed Army Hospital.

Many Societies have had the benefit of Hugo Rizzoli's active participation. In the American Association of Neurological Surgeons he has served as Vice President (1982), member of the Board of Directors and its Executive Committee, and Chairman of the Graduate Education Subcommittee on Recertification of the Joint Committee on Education.

He has been a member of the American Board of Neurological Surgery, has served as its Vice Chairman, and has served as Residency Review Committee member representing the American Medical Association. He represents the Society of Neurological Surgeons in the Association of Specialty Societies and Service Delegates and on the American Registry of Pathology. He is a member of the American Academy of Neurological Surgeons, the Neurosurgical Society of America (Vice President in 1976–77), the American College of Surgeons, the Osler Society, the Clinical Pathological Society, and the Society of Medical Consultants to the Armed Forces. He has been a Member of the Congress of Neurological Surgeons since 1955.

Contributions to the medical literature have included his book on postoperative complications in neurosurgical practice, co-authored with Norman Horwitz and now in its second edition, numerous articles on investigative work in spinal cord injury, earlier important papers on lumbar and cervical disc disease, peripheral nerve surgery, and the surgical management of aneurysms. His most recent contributions on the management of radiation necrosis of the brain continue to be both scientifically provocative and clinically useful.

Doctor Rizzoli and his wife, Helen Vargo Rizzoli, have four children, and they live in Chevy Chase, Maryland. Few neurosurgical educators have been as respected and beloved as Hugo Rizzoli. To the superb background in investigative and clinical neurosurgery he received from Walter Dandy, he has added his own brand of quiet and thoughtful excellence in practice, research, and education, and the Congress of Neurological Surgeons is privileged to honor him.

Bibliography of C. Hugo V. Rizzoli, M.D.

1. KING, J. T., JR., RIZZOLI, H. V., and BELL, J. P. Chronic valvular disease. In: *Geriatric Medicine*, edited by E. J. Stieglitz. W.B. Saunders, Philadelphia, 1943, pp. 405–415.
2. RIZZOLI, H. V., McCUNE, W. S., and SHERMAN, I. J. Surgical management of metastatic brain abscess. *J. Neurosurg.*, 5: 372–384, 1948.
3. PRICE, P. B., and RIZZOLI, H. V. The crush syndrome. West. J. Surg. Obstet. Gynecol., 57: 569, 1949.
4. RIZZOLI, H. V., WANNAMAKER, G., and HAYES, G. J. Lateral rupture of cervical intervertebral discs. A review of fourteen surgically treated cases. Med. Ann. D.C., 19: 6, 1950.
5. RIZZOLI, H. V. Autonomic nervous system. In: *Nash's Surgical Physiology*, edited by B. B. Blades. Charles C Thomas. Springfield, Ill., 1953, pp. 575–622.
6. RIZZOLI, H. V., and HAYES, G. J. Congenital berry aneurysm of the posterior fossa. J. Neurosurg., 10: 550–551, 1953.
7. STEELMAN, H. F., HAYES, G. J., and RIZZOLI, H. V. Surgical treatment of saccular intracranial aneurysms. A report of 56 consecutively treated patients. J. Neurosurg., 10: 564–567, 1953.
8. BERSACK, S. R., and RIZZOLI, H. V. Malignant sympathetic neurorectodermal tumor. Am. J. Surg.: 568–574, 1953.
9. RIZZOLI, H. V., HAYES, G. J., and STEELMAN, H. F. Rhinorrhea and pneumocephalus-surgical treatment. J. Neurosurg., 11: 227–283, 1954.
10. FEFFER, H. L., and RIZZOLI, H. V. The negative myelogram. Postgrad. Med., 19: 4, 1956.
11. ADAMS, J. P., and RIZZOLI, H. V. Tardy radial and ulnar nerve palsy: Case report. J. Neurosurg., 16: 342–344, 1959.
12. RIZZOLI, H. V. Fracture, concussion, contusion and laceration. Trauma, 2: 1, 1960.
13. RIZZOLI, H. V. Peripheral Nerve Injury. In: *Current Therapy*, edited by H. Conn. W.B. Saunders, Philadelphia, 1960, pp. 553–563.
14. WISE, C., and RIZZOLI, H. V. Herniation of the lumbar intervertebral disc. Bull. Rheum. Dis., 10: 219–222, 1960.
15. RIZZOLI, H. V. Trauma of peripheral nerves. In: *Neurological Surgery of Trauma*. Department of Army Publishers, Washington, D.C., 1965.
16. SMYTH, N. P. D., RIZZOLI, H. V., ORDMAN, C. W., KHOURY, J. N.,

and CHIOCCA, J. C. Gluteal aneurysms. Arch. Surg., *91:* 1014–1020, 1965.

17. RIZZOLI, H. V. Neuralgia, trigeminal and glossopharyngeal. Curr. Ther.: 1966.

18. HORWITZ, N. H., and RIZZOLI, H. V. Complications following the surgical treatment of head injuries. Clin. Neurosurg., *12:* 277–292, 1966.

19. HORWITZ, N. H., and RIZZOLI, H. V. *Postoperative Complications of Neurosurgical Practice: Recognition, Prevention, and Management.* Williams & Wilkins, Baltimore, 1967.

20. TREADGILL, F. D., KNEIPP, J. A., RIZZOLI, H. V., and ENGH, O. A. Conversion reaction following injury. The New Physician, *15:* 201–204, 1966.

21. RESTAK, R. M., and RIZZOLI, H. V. Tuberculoid leprosy: A neurological case report. Med. Ann. D.C., *41:* 359–360, 1972.

22. RIZZOLI, H. V. Trigeminal and glossopharyngeal neuralgia. Curr. Ther.: 699–701, 1973.

23. RIZZOLI, H. V. The back. In: *Ferguson's Surgery of the Ambulatory Patient,* Chap. 19, edited by Mark W. Wolcott, pp. 267–279. J.B. Lippincott, Philadelphia, 1974.

24. FOX, J. L., and RIZZOLI, H. V. Identification of radiologic coordinates for the posterior articular nerve of Luschka in the lumbar spine. Surg. Neurol., *1:* 343–346, 1973.

25. RIZZOLI, H. V. Walter Dandy, 1886–1946. Surg. Neurol., *2:* 293–294, 1974.

26. SMITH, D. R., PRESSMAN, B. D., LAWRENCE, W. H., DAVIS, D. O., and RIZZOLI, H. V. Computerized tomography: A new clinical modality. VA Med. Monthly, *102:* 827–834, 1975.

27. KOBRINE, A. I., DOYLE, T. F., and RIZZOLI, H. V. Spinal cord blood flow as effected by changes in systemic arterial blood pressure. J. Neurosurg., *44:* 12–15, 1976.

28. KOBRINE, A. I., DOYLE, T. F., and RIZZOLI, H. V. Further studies on histamine in spinal cord injury and post-traumatic hypermia. Surg. Neurol., *5:* 101–103, 1976.

29. KOBRINE, A. I., DOYLE, T. F., NEWBY, N., AND RIZZOLI, H. V. Preserved autoregulation in the rhesus spinal cord after high cervical cord section. J. Neurosurg., *44:* 425–428, 1976.

30. KOBRINE, A. I., DOYLE, T. F., and RIZZOLI, H. V. The effect of antihistamine on experimental post-traumatic edema of the spinal cord. Surg. Neurol., *5:* 307–309, 1976.

31. KOBRINE, A. I., DOYLE, T. F., and RIZZOLI, H. V. A method of estimating edema in experimental traumatic spinal cord injury. Exp. Neurol., *50:* 240–245, 1976.

32. KOBRINE, A. I., EVANS, D. E., and RIZZOLI, H. V. The mechanisms of autoregulation in the spinal cord. Surg. Forum, 27: 468–469, 1976.
33. KOBRINE, A. I., TIMINS, E., RAJJOUB, R. K., RIZZOLI, H. V., and DAVIS, D. O. Demonstration of massive traumatic brain swelling within 20 minutes after injury: Case report. J. Neurosurg., 46: 356–358, 1977.
34. SMITH, D. R., JACOBSON, J., KOBRINE, A. I., and RIZZOLI, H. V. Regional cerebral blood flow with intracranial mass lesions. Part I. Local alterations in cerebral blood flow. Surg. Neurol., 7: 233–237, 1977.
35. SMITH, D. R., JACOBSON, J., KOBRINE, A. I., and RIZZOLI, H. V. Autoregulation in localized mass lesions. Surg. Neurol., 7: 238–240, 1977.
36. HITCHCOCK, M. H., HOLLINSHEAD, A. C., CHRETIEN, P., and RIZZOLI, H. V. Soluble membrane antigens of brain tumors. I. Controlled testing for cell-mediated immune responses in a long surviving glioblastoma multiforme patient. Cancer, 40: 660–666, 1977.
37. RIZZOLI, H. V., RANDALL, J. D., AND SMITH, D. R. Psammoma bodies in meningioma. Virchows Arch. (Pathol. Anat.), 380: 317–325, 1978.
38. KOBRINE, A. I., EVANS, D. E., and RIZZOLI, H. V. The sympathetic nervous system in spinal cord autoregulation. Acta Neurol. Scand., 56 (Suppl. 64): 54–57, 1977.
39. KOBRINE, A. I., EVANS, D. E., and RIZZOLI, H. V. Correlation of spinal cord blood flow and function in experimental compression. Surg. Neurol., 10: 54–59, 1978.
40. EVANS, D. E., KOBRINE, A. I., and RIZZOLI, H. V. Cardiac arrythmias accompanying acute experimental spinal cord compression. J. Neurosurg., 52: 52–59, 1980.
41. KOBRINE, A. I., EVANS, D. E., and RIZZOLI, H. V. Effect of sciatic nerve stimulation on spinal cord blood flow. J. Neurol. Sci., 38: 435–439, 1978.
42. KOBRINE, A. I., EVANS, D. E., and RIZZOLI, H. V. The role of the sympathetic nervous system in spinal cord autoregulation. In: Cerebral Function, Metabolism and Circulation, edited by D. H. Infvar and N. A. Lassen. Munksgaard, Copenhagen, pp. 161–118, 1977.
43. KOBRINE, A. I., EVANS, D. E., and RIZZOLI, H. V. Correlation of spinal cord blood flow, sensory evoked response and spinal cord function in subacute experimental spinal cord compression. In: Advances in Neurology, edited by J. Cervos-Navarro et al., pp. 389–394. Raven Press, New York, 1978.

44. KOBRINE, A. I., EVANS, D. E., and RIZZOLI, H. V. The effect of ischemia on long tract neural conduction in spinal cord. J. Neurosurg., *50:* 639–644, 1979.
45. KOBRINE, A. I., EVANS, D. E., and RIZZOLI, H. V. Factors affecting return of the evoked response in acute balloon compression of the spinal cord. J. Neurosurg., *51:* 841–845, 1979.
46. KOBRINE, A. I., EVANS, D. E., and RIZZOLI, H. V. Spinal cord autoregulation. In: *Neurogenic Control of Brain Circulation*, edited by C. Owman and L. Edvinson. Pergamon Press, Oxford, 1977, pp. 403–406.
47. KOBRINE, A. I., EVANS, D. E., and RIZZOLI, H. V. The acute experimental spinal cord injury. J. Neurosurg., *51:* 841–845, 1979.
48. KOBRINE, A. I., EVANS, D. E., and RIZZOLI, H. V. Effects of progressive hypoxia on long tract neural conduction in the spinal cord. Neurosurgery, *7:* 369–376, 1980.
49. RIZZOLI, H. V. Failures of lumbar disc surgery. Surg. Rounds, *4:* 34–44, 1981.
50. KOBRINE, A. I., DAVIS, D. O., and RIZZOLI, H. V. Multiple abscesses of the brain. J. Neurosurg., *54:* 93–97, 1981.
51. KOULOURIS, S., and RIZZOLI, H. V. Coexisting intracranial aneurysm and arteriovenous malformation: Case report. Neurosurgery, *8:* 2, 1981.
52. KOULOURIS, S., and RIZZOLI, H. V. Delayed traumatic intracerebral hematoma after compound depressed skull fracture: Case report. Neurosurgery, *8:* 2, 1981.
53. PAGNANELLI, D. M., NARADZY, J. F. X., PAIT, T. G., RIZZOLI, H. V., and KOBRINE, A. I. The cutting edged microvascular needle: A scanning electron microscopic study. J. Neurosurg., *59:* 510–513, 1983.
54. KOULOURIS, S., and RIZZOLI, H. V. Bilateral extradural hematoma: A case report. Neurosurgery, *7:* 608–610, 1980.
55. PATRONAS, N. J., *et al.* Work in progress: Fluorodeoxyglucose and positron emission tomography in the evaluation of radiation necrosis of the brain. Radiology, *144:* 885–889, 1982.
56. HORWITZ, N. H., and RIZZOLI, H. V. *Postoperative Complications of Intracranial Neurological Surgery.* Williams & Wilkins, Baltimore, 1982.
57. RIZZOLI, H. V., and PAGNANELLI, D. M. Treatment of delayed radiation necrosis of the brain: A clinical observation. J. Neurosurg., *60:* 589–594, 1984.

Contents

I

CHAPTER 1

CHAPTER 2

II

CEREBROVASCULAR SURGERY

CHAPTER 3

CHAPTER 4

CHAPTER 5

CHAPTER 6

CHAPTER 7

CHAPTER 8

I

1

Walter E. Dandy: An Historical Perspective

HUGO V. RIZZOLI, M.D.

It's a great pleasure for me to have this opportunity to review with you Walter Dandy's role in the history of neurological surgery (Fig. 1.1). What had Dandy contributed to medicine and humanity to justify this bold headline on the first page of the *Baltimore Evening Sun* on April 19, 1946, the day of his death (Fig. 1.2)? Intellectually, Dandy possessed several exceptional qualities: (*a*) his experience with patients led him to ask searching questions which at times he resolved in the laboratory; (*b*) he had the intuitive facility to get to the core of a problem; and (*c*) he had the capacity for astute analysis of the dynamics of a number of pathophysiological states and for the design of corrective operative procedures. In addition, his surgical skills and dexterity were unequaled. The answer to this question can best be understood by focusing on various facets of his career which had a profound effect on the development of surgery of the nervous system.

Our story begins with his graduation from the Johns Hopkins University School of Medicine in 1910, where he entered in 1907 with advanced standing in recognition of his exceptional work at the University of Missouri. He was to remain at Hopkins throughout his extraordinary professional career. In 1910 neurological surgery was in its infancy. Three advancements—the introduction of ether anesthesia, Lister's report on antiseptic principles, and cerebral localization—were important to the birth of modern neurological surgery. Successful intracranial operations had been reported since the 1880s. Some of the well-publicized cases include intracranial operations for brain tumor by Macewen, Godlee, Durrante, Horsley, Weir, and Keen. In fact, between 1889 and 1905, there was a 10-fold increase in the number of intracranial operations. However, there was no real gain in accuracy of diagnosis or outcome. Many of these operations were done by general surgeons who had no special interest or expertise in brain surgery. They soon became discouraged. Although more than 500 general surgeons reported the results of their intracranial transgressions from 1886 to 1896, this number decreased to 80 in the next decade. In 1910 only a handful of surgeons were regularly doing neurosurgery as well as general surgery. Overseas, Ma-

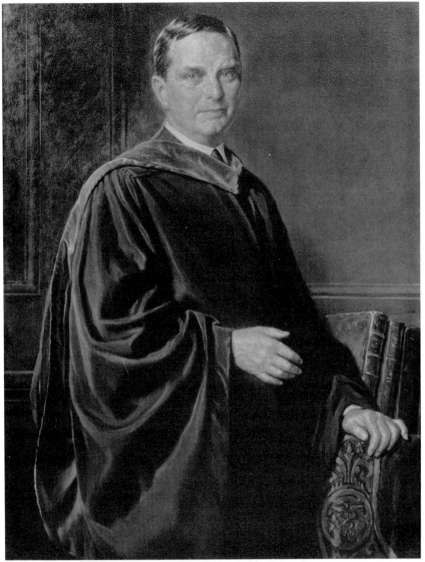

FIG. 1.1. Portrait of Dandy painted by Julian Lamar.

cewen, Horsley, and Krause were probably the most important. In the United States, Cushing and Frazier were to emerge as the most productive early pioneers.

Sir William Macewen (1848–1924) studied under Lister at the University of Glasgow and subsequently became Regius Professor of Surgery in 1892, 3 years after he rejected the Chair of Surgery at Johns Hopkins.

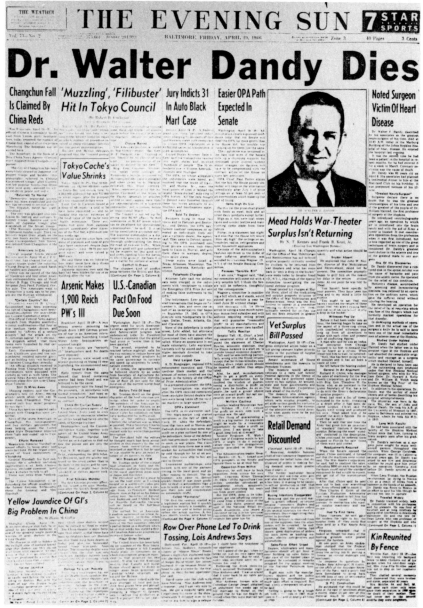

FIG. 1.2. Front page, *Baltimore Evening Sun*, April 19, 1946.

His classic monograph, *Pyogenic Diseases of the Brain and Spinal Cord*, was published in 1893 (23). His case mortality of 5% following the surgical treatment of brain abscess has never been equaled.

Sir Victor Horsley (1857–1916) was probably the greatest of the early neurosurgeons with many firsts to his credit. Research and clinical endeavors resulted in fundamental contributions to neuroanatomy, neurophysiology, and neurosurgery. In addition, he was a great teacher and a bold, skillful surgeon.

Professor Fedor Krause (1856–1937), from Berlin, was the pioneer of neurological surgery in Germany. Although meticulous and slow, he was a superb technician. His 3-volume treatise, *Surgery of the Brain and Spinal Cord* (1908–1911), was translated into English (20).

Charles H. Frazier (1870–1936) was one of the renowned American pioneers of neurosurgery. After a year of study in Europe, he returned to the University of Pennsylvania Hospital in 1896. He was appointed clinical professor in 1901. His association with Spiller and the other neurologists at the University of Pennsylvania was very fruitful. The Frazier-Spiller collaboration resulted in his introduction of the subtotal retrogasserian section of the fifth nerve via the subtemporal route, which he performed with an excellent score (0.5% mortality in over 700 cases).

Harvey Cushing (1869–1939) received his M.D. from Harvard in 1895. After a surgical internship at the Massachusetts General Hospital, he completed his surgical training at Hopkins under Halsted in 1900. Shortly thereafter he went overseas for a period of observation, study, and laboratory research. When he returned to Baltimore in September 1901, he became Assistant in Surgery with the responsibility for the Hunterian Laboratory of Experimental Medicine and for the neurosurgical patients. In 1912 he left Hopkins and moved to the Peter Bent Brigham Hospital in Boston as the Moseley Professor of Surgery. He was a perfectionist who improved the technical aspects of neurological surgery by applying the Halstedian principles of meticulous and delicate surgery. His article on the use of silver clips which appeared in 1911 and his subsequent publication on the introduction of the Bovie electrosurgical unit in 1928 contributed immensely to hemostasis. Although he has been described as intolerant and domineering, he was one of the giants of neurological surgery. He trained many neurosurgeons, and he contributed greatly to the neurosurgical literature. Most of his monographs are classics (Table 1.1).

For 1 year following graduation from medical school, Dandy became Cushing's man in the Hunterian Laboratory of Experimental Medicine at Hopkins, where he worked on the vasculature and nerve supply to the pituitary gland of the dog.

From 1911 to 1912 he was Cushing's surgical assistant in the hospital. This was not a happy year for Dandy. Incidents arose which caused personality clashes between Dandy and his mentor. This was the year

TABLE 1.1

Cushing's Books and Monographs

Pituitary Body, 1912
Tumors of Nervus Acusticus, 1917
Story of Base Hospital No. 5, 1919
Life of Sir William Osler, 1925
   with P. Bailey
Classification of Gliomas, 1926
Studies in Intracranial Physiology, 1926
   with L.M. Davidoff
Pathological Findings in Acromegaly, 1927
   with P. Bailey
Tumors Arising from Blood-Vessels, 1928
Consecratio Medici, 1928
Intracranial Tumours, 1932
Pituitary Body and Hypothalamus, 1932
From a Surgeon's Journal, 1936
Meningiomas, 1938
Medical Career, 1940

prior to Cushing's departure for Boston. When he made his house staff selection, Halsted believed that Dandy was leaving Hopkins with Cushing. Cushing's change of mind deprived Dandy of a position on Halsted's house staff. When it became apparent that Dandy was not going to Boston, Halsted was away for the summer. Dr. Winford Smith, Director of the hospital, provided Dandy a room in the hospital, hoping Halsted would offer him an appointment to his staff later in the year. Almost immediately Dandy returned to the Hunterian Laboratory and began to work on the cause of hydrocephalus with a pediatric resident, Kenneth Blackfan. Understanding the origin, circulation, and absorption of cerebrospinal fluid was essential to the project. Although hydrocephalus had never been produced in experimental animals, Dandy and Blackfan were able to do so by obstructing the aqueduct of Sylvius in dogs. Experimental studies with extensive clinical and pathological correlations resulted in a thorough understanding of the circulation of the cerebrospinal fluid and the causes of hydrocephalus. He was able to reproduce experimentally the various types of hydrocephalus encountered. The first report with Blackfan, which appeared in *JAMA* in 1913, also discussed the clinical use of neutral phenolsulfonphthalein in differentiating communicating from noncommunicating hydrocephalus (Fig. 1.3) (19). He used this dye in the laboratory to study absorption from within the ventricles and from within the subarachnoid space.

Dr. Halsted was greatly impressed by this work and soon found a place for Dandy on his staff. Park, who later was to become professor of

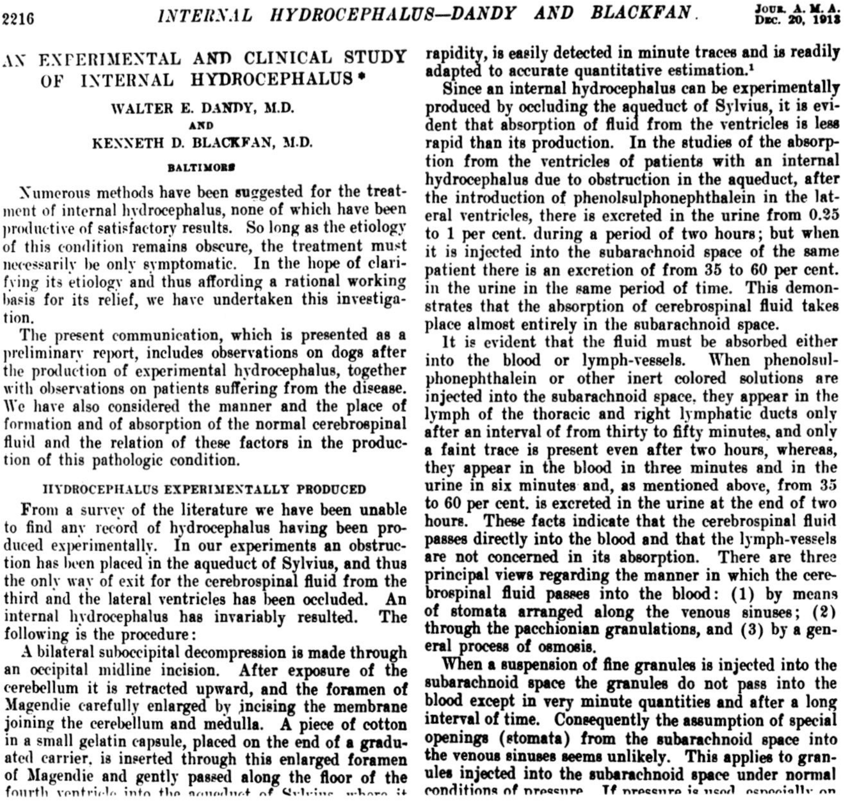

2216 *INTERNAL HYDROCEPHALUS—DANDY AND BLACKFAN.* JOUR. A. M. A. DEC. 20, 1913

AN EXPERIMENTAL AND CLINICAL STUDY OF INTERNAL HYDROCEPHALUS *

WALTER E. DANDY, M.D.
AND
KENNETH D. BLACKFAN, M.D.
BALTIMORE

Numerous methods have been suggested for the treatment of internal hydrocephalus, none of which have been productive of satisfactory results. So long as the etiology of this condition remains obscure, the treatment must necessarily be only symptomatic. In the hope of clarifying its etiology and thus affording a rational working basis for its relief, we have undertaken this investigation.

The present communication, which is presented as a preliminary report, includes observations on dogs after the production of experimental hydrocephalus, together with observations on patients suffering from the disease. We have also considered the manner and the place of formation and of absorption of the normal cerebrospinal fluid and the relation of these factors in the production of this pathologic condition.

HYDROCEPHALUS EXPERIMENTALLY PRODUCED

From a survey of the literature we have been unable to find any record of hydrocephalus having been produced experimentally. In our experiments an obstruction has been placed in the aqueduct of Sylvius, and thus the only way of exit for the cerebrospinal fluid from the third and the lateral ventricles has been occluded. An internal hydrocephalus has invariably resulted. The following is the procedure:

A bilateral suboccipital decompression is made through an occipital midline incision. After exposure of the cerebellum it is retracted upward, and the foramen of Magendie carefully enlarged by incising the membrane joining the cerebellum and medulla. A piece of cotton in a small gelatin capsule, placed on the end of a graduated carrier, is inserted through this enlarged foramen of Magendie and gently passed along the floor of the fourth ventricle into the aqueduct of Sylvius, where it

rapidity, is easily detected in minute traces and is readily adapted to accurate quantitative estimation.[1]

Since an internal hydrocephalus can be experimentally produced by occluding the aqueduct of Sylvius, it is evident that absorption of fluid from the ventricles is less rapid than its production. In the studies of the absorption from the ventricles of patients with an internal hydrocephalus due to obstruction in the aqueduct, after the introduction of phenolsulphonephthalein in the lateral ventricles, there is excreted in the urine from 0.25 to 1 per cent. during a period of two hours; but when it is injected into the subarachnoid space of the same patient there is an excretion of from 35 to 60 per cent. in the urine in the same period of time. This demonstrates that the absorption of cerebrospinal fluid takes place almost entirely in the subarachnoid space.

It is evident that the fluid must be absorbed either into the blood or lymph-vessels. When phenolsulphonephthalein or other inert colored solutions are injected into the subarachnoid space, they appear in the lymph of the thoracic and right lymphatic ducts only after an interval of from thirty to fifty minutes, and only a faint trace is present even after two hours, whereas, they appear in the blood in three minutes and in the urine in six minutes and, as mentioned above, from 35 to 60 per cent. is excreted in the urine at the end of two hours. These facts indicate that the cerebrospinal fluid passes directly into the blood and that the lymph-vessels are not concerned in its absorption. There are three principal views regarding the manner in which the cerebrospinal fluid passes into the blood: (1) by means of stomata arranged along the venous sinuses; (2) through the pacchionian granulations, and (3) by a general process of osmosis.

When a suspension of fine granules is injected into the subarachnoid space the granules do not pass into the blood except in very minute quantities and after a long interval of time. Consequently the assumption of special openings (stomata) from the subarachnoid space into the venous sinuses seems unlikely. This applies to granules injected into the subarachnoid space under normal conditions of pressure. If pressure is used, especially on

FIG. 1.3. Dandy's first article on hydrocephalus (Reproduced with permission from: W. E. Dandy and K. D. Blackfan (19)).

pediatrics at Hopkins, reports that when he and Halsted were discussing this work Halsted said, "Dandy will never do anything equal to this again. Few men make more than one great contribution to medicine (1)." How wrong he was! In addition to establishing the criteria for the accurate clinical diagnosis of the various sites of obstruction in patients with hydrocephalus, he devised the appropriate operative treatment for each. This work alone qualifies him for a place in the "Neurosurgical Hall of Fame." The fundamental physiological data resulting from these studies undoubtedly were most important in understanding the role of brain tumor in obstruction and displacement of the ventricular system. Ventriculography was the logical sequel to these studies.

While still a surgical resident in 1918, Dandy introduced pneumoventriculography and in the following year pneumoencephalography (Fig. 1.4) (4, 5). Many consider ventriculography his greatest contribution to neurosurgery. Prior to this giant step forward, only about 50% of brain

Ann. of Surg.
68: 5–11, 1918.
VENTRICULOGRAPHY FOLLOWING THE INJECTION OF AIR INTO THE CEREBRAL VENTRICLES

By Walter E. Dandy, M.D.

of Baltimore, Md.

(From the Department of Surgery, the Johns Hopkins Hospital and University)

THE value of röntgenography in the diagnosis and localization of intracranial tumors is mainly restricted to the cases in which the neoplasm has affected the skull. In an analysis of the X-ray findings in one hundred cases of brain tumor from Doctor Halsted's Clinic, Heuer and I [1] have shown that in only 6 per cent. of the cases did the tumor cast a shadow, and in these it was only the calcified areas that were differentiated by the X-rays from the normal cerebral tissues.

In those instances (9 per cent. of our cases) in which a tumor has encroached upon the sphenoid, ethmoid or frontal sinus, the invading portion casts a shadow in the röntgenogram. Such shadows are due to the displacement of the normally contained air by tissues which are less pervious to the X-ray. This group of shadows is of minor practical importance because the growth can be recognized by the destruction of the walls or bony septa of the sinuses.

Since the X-rays penetrate normal brain tissues, blood, cerebrospinal fluid and non-calcified tumor tissue almost equally, any changes in the brain produced by altered proportions of these components will not materially alter the röntgenogram.

Although skull changes are shown by the X-ray in 45 per cent. of our cases and are frequently pathognomonic, on the whole they represent late stages of the disease. As intracranial tumors come to be diagnosed and localized earlier, the value of the X-ray will be correspondingly diminished.

For some time I have considered the possibility of filling the cerebral ventricles with a medium that will produce a shadow in the radiogram. If this could be done, an accurate outline of the cerebral ventricles could be photographed with X-rays, and since most neoplasms either directly or indirectly modify the size or shape of the ventricles, we should then possess an early and accurate aid to the localization of intracranial affections. In addition to its radiographic properties, any substance injected into the ventricles must satisfy two very rigid exactions: (1) It must be absolutely non-irritating and non-toxic; and (2) it must be readily absorbed and excreted.

The various solutions and suspensions used in pyelography—thorium,

---

[1] Röntgenography in the Localization of Brain Tumor, Based Upon a Series of One Hundred Consecutive Cases. The Johns Hopkins Hosp. Bull., 1916, xxvii, 311. Also: A Report of Seventy Cases of Brain Tumor. The Johns Hopkins Hosp. Bull., 1916, xxvii, 224.

FIG. 1.4. Dandy's first article on ventriculography (Reproduced with permission from: W. E. Dandy (4)).

tumors could be localized by neurological examination and skull x-ray. The remainder had to be treated palliatively with decompression. Crowe recalled that Dandy was outspoken against that practice. His objective was the early and accurate localization with total extirpation of intracranial neoplasms. Surprisingly, many were slow to accept this great contribution. Nevertheless, with this discovery, neurosurgery came of age.

Upon completion of his surgical residency in 1918 at the age of 32, Dandy was appointed Associate Surgeon at the Johns Hopkins Hospital. In 1922, after Heuer assumed the Professorship of Surgery in Cincinnati, Dandy became Neurosurgeon to the Johns Hopkins Hospital.

Cushing's famous monograph on acoustic tumors was published in 1917 (Fig. 1.2). He was able to report his excellent score in 33 patients in whom he performed subtotal intracapsular removal—a case mortality of 18.1% and an operative mortality of 13.9%. By coincidence, in the same year, Dandy performed his first successful total excision of an acoustic tumor. His preliminary report appeared in 1922 with a more complete report on total removal in 1925 and a subsequent publication in 1934 describing the unilateral approach to this lesion (Fig. 1.5) (7, 8,

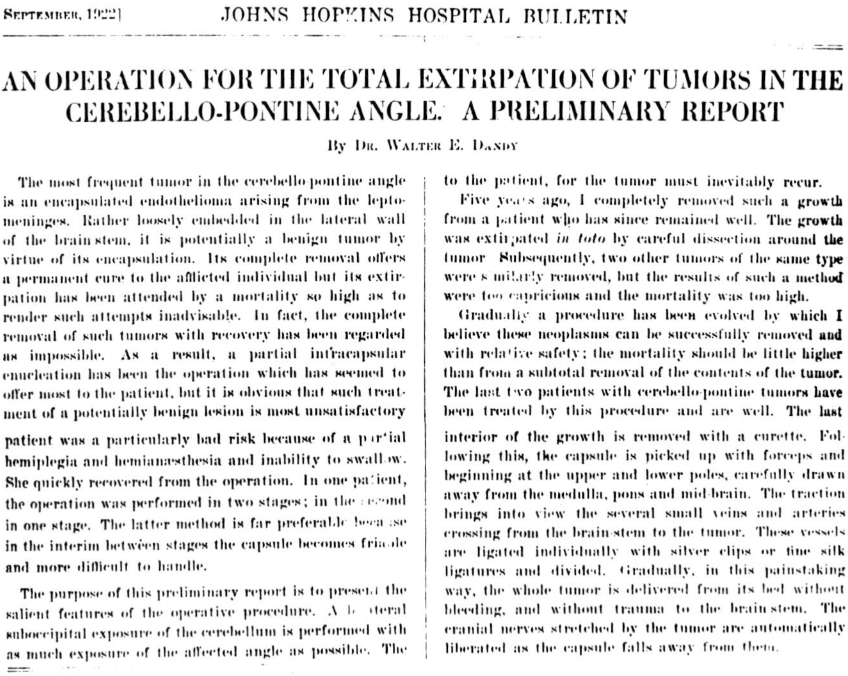

SEPTEMBER, 1922] JOHNS HOPKINS HOSPITAL BULLETIN

AN OPERATION FOR THE TOTAL EXTIRPATION OF TUMORS IN THE CEREBELLO-PONTINE ANGLE. A PRELIMINARY REPORT

By DR. WALTER E. DANDY

The most frequent tumor in the cerebello-pontine angle is an encapsulated endothelioma arising from the leptomeninges. Rather loosely embedded in the lateral wall of the brain stem, it is potentially a benign tumor by virtue of its encapsulation. Its complete removal offers a permanent cure to the afflicted individual but its extirpation has been attended by a mortality so high as to render such attempts inadvisable. In fact, the complete removal of such tumors with recovery has been regarded as impossible. As a result, a partial intracapsular enucleation has been the operation which has seemed to offer most to the patient, but it is obvious that such treatment of a potentially benign lesion is most unsatisfactory

patient was a particularly bad risk because of a partial hemiplegia and hemianæsthesia and inability to swallow. She quickly recovered from the operation. In one patient, the operation was performed in two stages; in the second in one stage. The latter method is far preferable because in the interim between stages the capsule becomes friable and more difficult to handle.

The purpose of this preliminary report is to present the salient features of the operative procedure. A lateral suboccipital exposure of the cerebellum is performed with as much exposure of the affected angle as possible. The

to the patient, for the tumor must inevitably recur.

Five years ago, I completely removed such a growth from a patient who has since remained well. The growth was extirpated in toto by careful dissection around the tumor. Subsequently, two other tumors of the same type were similarly removed, but the results of such a method were too capricious and the mortality was too high.

Gradually a procedure has been evolved by which I believe these neoplasms can be successfully removed and with relative safety; the mortality should be little higher than from a subtotal removal of the contents of the tumor. The last two patients with cerebello-pontine tumors have been treated by this procedure and are well. The last interior of the growth is removed with a curette. Following this, the capsule is picked up with forceps and beginning at the upper and lower poles, carefully drawn away from the medulla, pons and mid-brain. The traction brings into view the several small veins and arteries crossing from the brain-stem to the tumor. These vessels are ligated individually with silver clips or fine silk ligatures and divided. Gradually, in this painstaking way, the whole tumor is delivered from its bed without bleeding, and without trauma to the brain-stem. The cranial nerves stretched by the tumor are automatically liberated as the capsule falls away from them.

FIG. 1.5. Dandy's preliminary article on total extirpation of an acoustic tumor (Reproduced with permission from: W. E. Dandy (7)).

14). In his last 41 cases of total extirpation by the unilateral approach, Dandy reduced his mortality to 2.4% (25), a truly great achievement!

Cushing's capricious and acerbic attack on Dandy's preliminary report further strained their relationship. In submitting Cushing's letter to the editorial board of the Johns Hopkins Hospital Bulletin, Dandy stated that he was "absolutely at a loss to discover the point for such a letter other than personal animus" (20).

Following the advent of ventriculography, tumors of the lateral and third ventricles became precisely localized and thus were amenable to surgery. Indeed it was logical for Dandy to direct his efforts to the development of the appropriate surgical techniques and skills for the surgical attack on these heretofore undiagnosed and unoperated tumors. In 1934, he noted that the results of his struggle over the previous 15 years in the pursuit of this goal "progressively reflect the important advances that have occurred on the operative front during this period, *i.e.*, the electrocautery, avertin anesthesia and continuous suction" (13).

To Dandy belongs the credit for the first successful total enucleation of a benign lateral ventricle tumor, an ependymoma of the left lateral ventricle (Fig. 1.6). It was the first tumor localized by ventriculography and was removed in 1918.

In 1934, when he published his monograph *Benign Tumors in the Lateral Ventricles of the Brain*, the patient was alive and well 15 years later (13). In October 1921, Dandy localized and successfully removed a colloid cyst of the third ventricle (Fig. 1.7). This was another milestone in the annals of his specialty. In 1933, his monograph *Benign Tumors of the Third Ventricle of the Brain* was published, describing 21 lesions in that location with a total mortality of 33% and with only a 14.3% mortality in the last 14 cases (12).

His 1915 canine experiments with removal of the pineal body helped him devise a similar transcallosal approach for the removal of pineal tumors in humans (Fig. 1.8) (3). In his first article in 1921, he reported three cases, one of which was a patient with a tuberculoma of the pineal gland who survived for 8 months (6). In 1945 Dandy (18) stated that he had operated on 20 pineal tumors with a 20% operative mortality.

After operating on two children with orbital tumors in 1921, he was the first to recommend the transcranial approach with resection of the orbital roof for certain tumors within the orbit. In his monograph *Orbital Tumors*, published in 1941, he advocated the hypophyseal pterional approach (16). Intracranial extension of a primary orbital tumor was found in approximately 80% of 31 patients. Meningioma was the most common tumor encountered. Today, this operation is usually advocated for all orbital tumors with intracranial involvement and for tumors at the apex of the orbit, especially when situated medially.

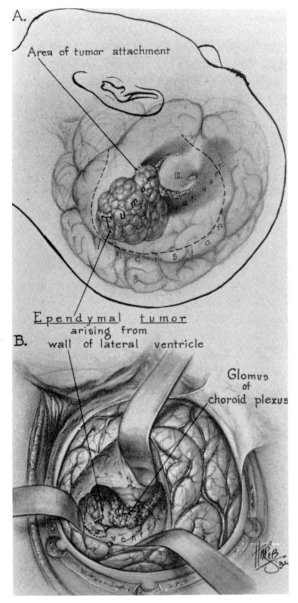

FIG. 1.6. Ependymoma of the lateral ventricle successfully removed in 1918. This was the first successful removal of an intraventricular tumor and the first patient on whom Dr. Dandy performed a ventriculogram. (Reproduced with permission from: W. E. Dandy (13)).

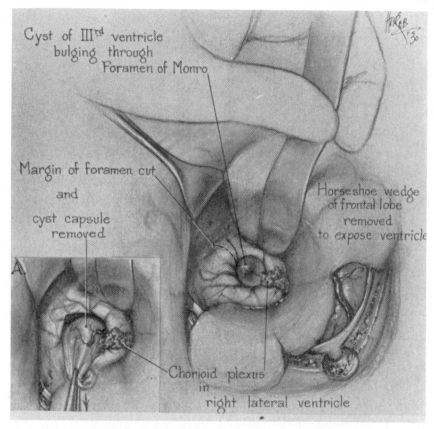

FIG. 1.7. Dandy was the first to successfully remove a colloid cyst of the third ventricle in 1921. (Reproduced with permission from: W. E. Dandy (18) (Figure 374)).

His approach to gliomas was always in keeping with his objective of radical removal. He championed lobectomies whenever possible, hoping to accomplish a total removal (Fig. 1.9). In eight cases he performed right hemispherectomy in an attempt to effect a cure.

Dandy soon became interested in cranial nerve syndromes which could be treated surgically. Several of the neurosurgical pioneers devised operative treatments for tic douloureux. To Krause in 1893 belongs credit for the first successful excision of the Gasserian ganglion for this affliction. Although a difficult operative procedure, it was more likely to produce permanent relief than the previous operations, and accordingly this operation was adopted by several surgeons, including Horsley and Cushing. In fact, for several years Cushing was reluctant to accept the next advance in the treatment of this malady. At Spiller's suggestion in

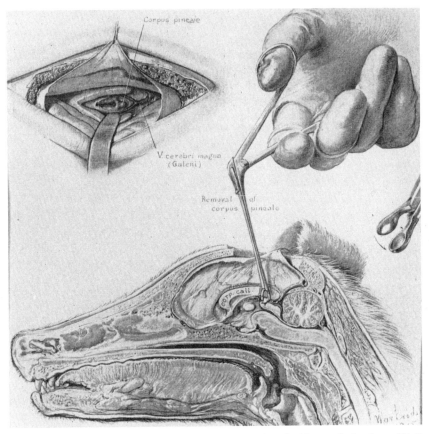

FIG. 1.8. Removal of pineal body in the dog. (Reproduced with permission from: W. E. Dandy (Ref. 3: Figure 3, Plate 32)).

1901, Frazier was successful in treating this syndrome by sectioning the sensory root behind the ganglion, using the subtemporal extradural approach. In time, it became the standard procedure for several decades throughout the world. Frazier improved the operation in 1915 when he began to spare the ophthalmic fibers and, thus, corneal sensation. This was reported in 1925. Another step forward occurred in 1918 when Peet was able to preserve the motor root.

It was Dandy who first performed section of the sensory root at the pons in 1925. Doubtless his experience in the cerebellopontine angle while operating on acoustic tumors led to this important innovation. In 1929 after having achieved excellent results in 88 cases he discussed total and partial section of this root (10). He ascribed the preservation of light touch and corneal sensation in some cases to accessory sensory nerve

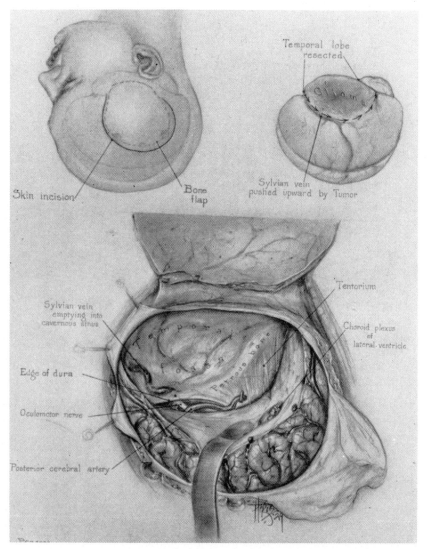

FIG. 1.9. Resection of the right temporal lobe for glioma. (Reproduced with permission from: W. E. Dandy (Ref. 18: Figure 259)).

fibers. In the 1945 revision of *Surgery of the Brain,* he stated that in 10% of his patients, tumor or aneurysm was the cause. When tumor was not present, the etiology was almost always an arterial loop compressing and at times grooving the sensory root (Fig. 1.10). Although Dandy performed this operation in more than 500 patients with less than 0.5% mortality and with excellent and permanent relief of pain, most neurosurgeons

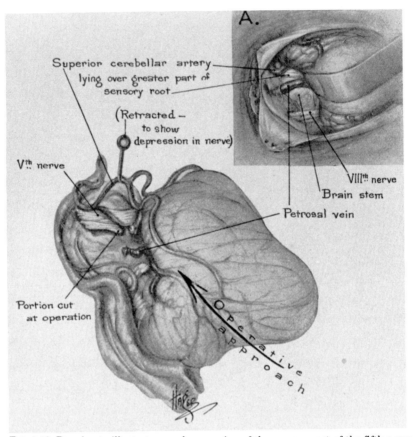

FIG. 1.10. Drawing to illustrate vascular grooving of the sensory root of the fifth nerve. (Reproduced with permission from: W. E. Dandy (Ref. 18: Figure 66)).

were reluctant to use this procedure. It obviously required more skill than the elegant Frazier operation, which was performed in the sitting position. Except for Gardner, Dandy's perceptive anatomic observations were generally ignored until Jannetta, building on these data in 1976, proposed and performed successfully microvascular decompression at the root entry zone, thus obviating, in most cases, the need for anatomic division of the portio major of the fifth nerve. In 1927 Dandy was the first to section the ninth nerve in the posterior fossa for glossopharyngeal tic.

The observation in 1874 that the attacks of vertigo in Meniere's syndrome decreased and became less frequent and less severe as deafness increased suggested to Charcot that these patients might be cured surgically. Except for some early ventures, eighth nerve section was not reported until Dandy became interested in Meniere's disease, and he became persuaded that the paroxysmal attacks of vertigo in this syndrome were analogous to the paroxysmal attacks of pain with tic douloureux. In 1928, he first reported total section of the eighth nerve for Meniere's syndrome in nine cases; the first case was operated in 1924 (9). He did a total of 692 operations for Meniere's disease with only two fatalities, both from infection. Because of this magnificent record, he was not the first to report the pathological distention of the endolymphatic system in the cochlea. At first he performed total section of the nerve. McKenzie (1932), Cairns (1933), and Dandy (1933) independently reported partial section of the nerve, *i.e.*, only the vestibular division. Dandy found tumors to be the cause in 2% of cases and reasoned that this was too great a number to be simply coincidental. Frequently (20%) there was vascular compression of the nerve.

In 1911 Goldthwaite of Boston published a remarkable paper on the anatomy of the low back based on cadaver dissections (21). He postulated that traumatic herniation of the disc could be responsible for low back pain and sciatica. Unfortunately his hypothesis did not generate any great interest. Dandy in 1929 reported two cases of L3 disc extrusion with back pain, bilateral sciatic pain, and cauda equina syndrome (Fig. 1.11) (11). A cisternal lipoidal myelogram was performed in both cases, and a block was demonstrated just above the L3 disc in each case. In both cases, free fragments of disc were found and removed. Since tumor was suspected, he elected total laminectomy and a transdural approach. Both patients experienced excellent relief of pain and of neurological deficit. Krause reported a similar case in 1908, but he mistakenly diagnosed the lesion as an enchondroma. Dandy, on the other hand, made the correct postoperative diagnosis and recognized the traumatic origin. He stated: "The trauma at onset is relatively trivial and perhaps repeated." He also noted: "The lesion offers a pathologic basis for cases of 'so called sciatica' especially bilateral sciatica." Although he could not find any similar reports of ruptured intervertebral disc in the literature, he intuitively reasoned that they must not be infrequent since two cases appeared on his service within a few months. Nonetheless he did not pursue this subject until after the famous contribution of Mixter and Barr in 1934 (24). Along with Semmes, Love, and Spurling he became very enthusiastic in performing operations on patients with herniated discs. In all he operated on 2000 discs without preoperative myelography.

The saga of intracranial aneurysm surgery is one of the more exciting chapters in the history of neurological surgery. Charles Symonds in 1923 described five patients in whom the clinical diagnosis of intracranial aneurysm was made antemortem (26). The diagnosis was confirmed at autopsy in the three patients who died. Dott in 1931 treated an internal

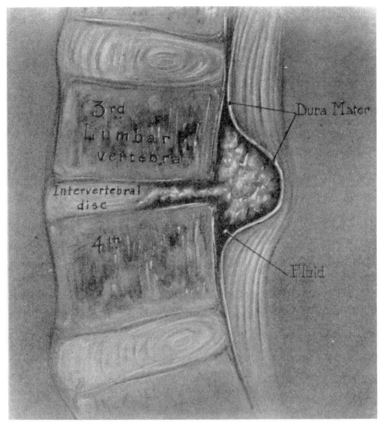

FIG. 1.11. From Dandy's 1929 article on intervertebral discs. (Reproduced with permission from: W. E. Dandy (11)).

carotid bifurcation aneurysm by covering it with muscle strips, and in 1933 he was the first to operate on an aneurysm verified by angiography. His patient was treated by cervical carotid ligation. In March 1937, Dandy was the first to cure an internal carotid-posterior communicating artery junction aneurysm by occluding the neck of the aneurysm with a silver clip (Fig. 1.12). He also reported cauterizing the sac of the aneurysm. When this case was published in 1938 he wrote: "The present effort is but a beginning or a suggestion that an aneurysm at the Circle of Willis is not entirely hopeless" (15). His classic monograph, *Intracranial Arterial Aneurysms*, which appeared in 1944 gave impetus to the surgical treatment of intracranial aneurysms (Fig. 1.13) (17). He documented 133 aneurysms verified by necropsy or operation. He noted six methods

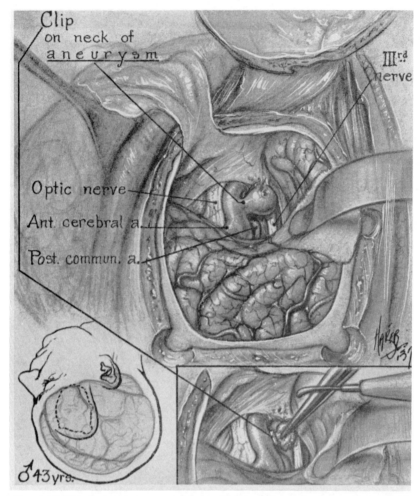

Clip
on neck of
a n e u r y s m

IIIʳᵈ
nerve

Optic nerve

Ant. cerebral a.

Post. commun. a.

♂ 43 yrs.

FIG. 1.12. The first aneurysm cured by occlusion of the neck of an aneurysm with a silver clip. (Reproduced with permission from: W. E. Dandy (Ref. 15: Figure 4)).

employed in the treatment of aneurysms. All of his cases were tabulated and many were beautifully illustrated by his medical artist, Dorcas Hager Padget. He also had her study the embryology of the circle of Willis and write the classic chapter on the embryology and anatomy of the circle of Willis. During the 6¼-year span of this study, he operated upon 36 patients; 6 patients were not definitively treated, and of the remaining 30 patients, 20 were cured, 1 was probably cured, and 9 died, an operative mortality of 25%! Amazingly only four of these patients had had arteriograms—all prior to their arrival at Hopkins. Cerebral angiography,

Intracranial Arterial
ANEURYSMS

BY

WALTER E. DANDY

Adjunct Professor of Surgery in
The Johns Hopkins University

ITHACA   NEW YORK

COMSTOCK PUBLISHING COMPANY, INC.

CORNELL UNIVERSITY

1944

FIG. 1.13. Front piece from Dandy's monograph on intracranial arterial aneurysms. (Reproduced with permission from: W. E. Dandy (17)).

Moniz's great contribution in 1927, was also a great stimulus to the surgery of these lesions. This diagnostic procedure was not frequently employed in the United States until World War II.

Much progress has been made since Dandy's death in April 1946; microsurgical technology and advances in neuroanesthesia and neuroradiology have added immeasurably to the welfare of neurosurgical patients. The future augurs well for neurological surgery. However, it seems unlikely that one man will ever again repeatedly contribute so much to the development of this specialty. This quotation from an editorial in the *Baltimore Evening Sun* says it all: "He had imaginative genius to conceive of new and startling operative techniques, courage to try them, and skill, superb skill to make them successful."

REFERENCES

1. Crowe, S. J. *Halsted of Johns Hopkins.* Charles C Thomas, Springfield, Ill., 1957.
2. Cushing, H. *Tumors of the Nervus Acusticus and the Syndrome of the Cerebellopontine Angle.* W.B. Saunders, Philadelphia, 1917.
3. Dandy, W. E. Extirpation of the pineal body. J. Exp. Med., *22:* 237–248, 1915.
4. Dandy, W. E. Ventriculography following the injection of air into the cerebral ventricles. Ann. Surg., *68:* 5–11, 1918.
5. Dandy, W. E. Roentgenography of the brain after the injection of air into the spinal canal. Ann. Surg., *70:* 397–403, 1919.
6. Dandy, W. E. An operation for the removal of pineal tumors. Surg. Gynecol. Obstet., *33:* 113–119, 1921.
7. Dandy, W. E. An operation for the total extirpation of tumors in the cerebello-pontine angle: A preliminary report. Johns Hopkins Hosp. Bull., *33:* 344, 1922.
8. Dandy, W. E. An operation for the total removal for cerebello-pontine (acoustic) tumors. Surg. Gynecol. Obstet., *41:* 129–148, 1925.
9. Dandy, W. E. Meniere's disease: It's diagnosis and a method of treatment. Arch. Surg., *16:* 1125–1152, 1928.
10. Dandy, W. E. An operation for the cure of tic douloureux. Arch. Surg., *18:* 687–734, 1929.
11. Dandy, W. E. Loose cartilage from intervertebral disk simulating tumor of the spinal cord. Arch. Surg., *19:* 660–672, 1929.
12. Dandy, W. E. *Benign Tumors in the Third Ventricle of the Brain: Diagnosis and Treatment.* Charles C Thomas, Springfield, Ill., 1933.
13. Dandy, W. E. *Benign, Encapsulated Tumors in the Lateral Ventricles of the Brain.* Williams & Wilkins, Baltimore, 1934.
14. Dandy, W. E. Removal of cerebellopontine (acoustic) tumors through a unilateral approach. Arch. Surg., *29:* 337, 1934.
15. Dandy, W. E. Intracranial aneurysm of the internal carotid artery cured by operation. Ann. Surg., *107:* 654–659, 1938.
16. Dandy, W. E. *Orbital Tumors: Results following the Transcranial Operative Attack.* Oskar Piest, New York, 1941.
17. Dandy, W. E. *Intracranial Arterial Aneurysms.* Comstock Publishing, Ithaca, N.Y., 1944.
18. Dandy, W. E. The surgery of the brain: a monograph. In: *Dean Lewis' Practice of Surgery,* Vol. 12. W.F. Prior, Hagerstown, Md., 1945.

19. Dandy, W. E., and Blackfan, K. D. An experimental and clinical study of internal hydrocephalus. J.A.M.A., *61:* 2216–2217, 1913.
20. Fox, W. L. *Dandy of Johns Hopkins.* Williams & Wilkins, Baltimore, 1984.
21. Goldthwaite, J. E. The lumbosacral articulation. An explanation of many cases of "lumbago," "sciatica," and paraplegia. Boston M. & S. J., *164:* 365–372, 1911.
22. Krause, F. *Chirurgie des Gehirns und Rueckenmarks.* Urban & Schwarzenberg, Berlin, 1908–1911. English translation: Haubold, H. and Thorek, M. *Surgery of the Brain and Spinal Cord,* 3 Vols. Rebman, New York, 1912.
23. Macewen, W. *Pyogenic Infective Diseases of the Brain and Spinal Cord. Meningitis, Abscess of the Brain, Infective Sinus Thrombosis.* J. Maclehose & Sons, Glasgow, 1893.
24. Mixter, W. J., and Barr, J. S. Rupture of the intervertebral disc with involvement of the spinal canal. N. Engl. J. Med., *211:* 210–214, 1934.
25. Revilla, A. G. Neurinomas of the cerebellopontine recess. Bull. Johns Hopkins Hosp., *80:* 254–296, 1947.
26. Symonds, C. P. Contributions to the clinical study of intercranial aneurysms. Guy's Hosp. Rep., *73:* 139–158, 1923.

2

Dandy's Brain Team

HUGO V. RIZZOLI, M.D.

In this chapter, I shall focus on Dr. Dandy's career as a teacher. The principle vehicle for his didactic role was the "Brain Team." In this environment he displayed his public persona, but it also allowed him, perhaps inadvertently, to reveal, occasionally, the private man.

Although the medical students enjoyed his lucid conferences, the curriculum did not allow much access to the confines of a specialty service like neurological surgery. Consequently, the chief beneficiaries were the house officers and nurses on the Brain Team. Dandy himself was of course a stellar product of Halsted's much admired residency program, and yet he did not in fact have a full-time assistant assigned to help him until 1922 (Fig. 2.1) (4). However, soon thereafter under Halsted's successor, Dean Lewis, the 8-year residency at Hopkins included 2 years of neurosurgery rotation. This was to change again in 1941 when the new Chairman of Surgery, Alfred Blalock, reduced this period of time to an intern rotation in an effort to shorten the overall length of training (Fig. 2.2) (5). Dandy then annually appointed one or more residents to remain on his service. Thus, during my participation on the Brain Team, it consisted of Dandy's first assistant or resident, the assistant resident, a surgical intern rotating on this service for 1 month who usually was in constant fear lest he arouse the wrath of the Chief, the anesthetist, the operating room scrub nurse, the chief ward nurse, the operating room orderly, and Dandy's secretary, Bertha Shauck (Fig. 2.3) (1).

Everybody in the hospital seemed to respect and fear Dr. Dandy. They complied with his demanding requests. An occasional x-ray technician dared question the need for x-rays of the lumbar spine at 3:30 a.m. in a patient with a routine disc. He or she was told to do it or discuss it with Dr. Dandy. Nobody dared cross swords with him. There was enough awe and respect to spill over to the rest of the Brain Team. The facilities for neurosurgery were certainly adequate. Halsted 7, the Neurosurgical Ward, was situated a few yards from the entrance to the operating suite (Figs. 2.4 and 2.5) (1). Ward, semiprivate, and a few private beds were

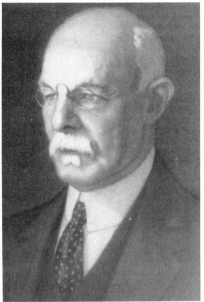 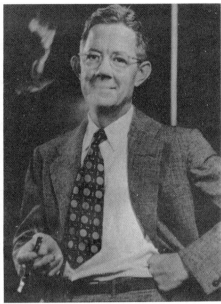

FIG. 2.1. (*Left*) Dandy's favorite portrait of Halsted (1852–1922), painted by Hermann Becker. Halsted served as the first Surgeon-in-Chief at the Hopkins from 1890 to 1922. (Reproduced with permission from: G. W. Heuer (4)).

FIG. 2.2. (*Right*) Alfred Blalock (1899–1964). Surgeon-in-Chief at Hopkins 1941–1964. (Photographed by and reproduced with permission from: Karsh (5)).

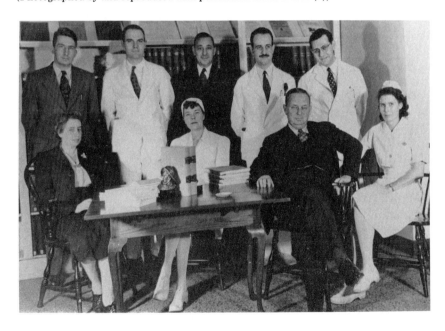

THE JOHNS HOPKINS HOSPITAL
HALSTED 7

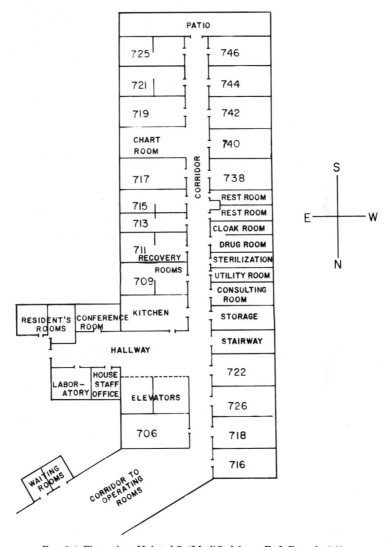

FIG. 2.4. Floor plan, Halsted 7. (Modified from: F. J. Barcala (1)).

FIG. 2.3. Staff photo taken in 1944. Standing: Drs. John Chambers, Charles Burklund, Frank Otenasek, Fermin J. Barcala, and Hugo V. Rizzoli. Seated: Mrs. Bertha Shauck (Secretary), Miss Grace Smith (Anesthetist), Dr. Walter E. Dandy, and Ms. Sarah Lambert (Scrub Nurse). (Reproduced with permission from: F. J. Barcala (1)).

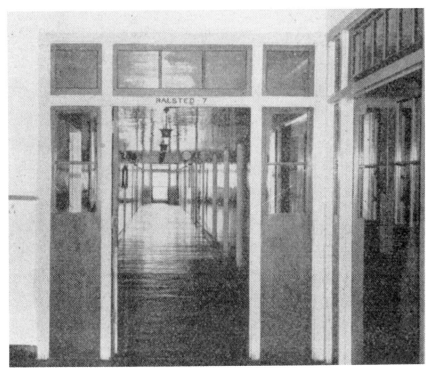

FIG. 2.5. Entrance to Halsted 7.

located on this unit. Other patients were located on the pediatric wing and in the deluxe Marburg pavilion. Dandy and Warfield Firor, his assistant in 1923, probably organized the first Recovery Room/Intensive Care Unit (ICU). After 1932, when the Halsted wing was dedicated, this concept of a Recovery Room/ICU for neurosurgical patients was continued on Halsted 7. Two adjoining large semiprivate rooms were dedicated for this use. All patients were taken to this unit after surgery to recover from anesthesia and, when conscious and alert, they were moved to their respective rooms. More seriously ill patients with craniotomies were observed in this unit 1 or more days until they became stable. There was a nurse in each of these two adjacent rooms continuously—day and night.

Dandy's Brain Team performed like an efficient, faultless machine. I am not sure whether the team was energized by fear or respect for its leader, probably both. All patients were worked up shortly after admission, whether or not they were scheduled for surgery the next day. The resident never left the hospital when Dandy was in town. The "Old Man" occasionally called at night to inquire about a patient

The resident took Dandy's office calls after 5:00 p.m. They were usually long distance calls from someone seeking an appointment with Dr. Dandy. They were told to come to his office at 12:00 noon on whichever weekday they could arrive in Baltimore. He had a large waiting room for patients two floors immediately below the operating room. He would see patients in his office between operations. Usually he had information about the patients from their referring doctors. His examination was brief. He probably completed most of it by watching the patient walk into the room toward his desk. He would arrive at a diagnosis and arrange for admission if neurosurgery was indicated.

He responded to consultations from other services by seeing the patient on rounds with the residents. The consultation included a brief examination and a concise report in the progress notes. In the case of a patient with a herniated disc the entire note was usually: "It's a disc, should be operated upon."

Rounds were made at the end of the day. Following a call from Mrs. Shauck, the residents met the "Old Man" at the elevator on Halsted 7 and immediately offered him a Chesterfield cigarette. Since he rarely learned a patient's name we had to identify them in some other way. If the patient was referred by a doctor known to Dandy, the patient was then "Dr. Smith's patient from Montgomery." But if the doctor did not refer to Dr. Dandy regularly, then the patient was identified by his diagnosis and his home city or state, for example, the "disc man from Miami." At times he seemed to have trouble differentiating the sex of children. The little girl with the cerebellar tumor from Miami might well be a "little boy from Cleveland" who was referred by a doctor in Miami.

In addition to our consultant in neurology, Frank Ford, affectionately known as "The Judge," Frank Walsh consulted in neuro-ophthalmology and Sam Crowe in neuro-otology (Figs. 2.6 and 2.7). Because of their active participation, they were indeed *ex officio* members of the Brain Team. Crowe recalled that a 35-year-old woman in coma admitted on the otolaryngological service continued to deteriorate (2). None of the consultants, including Ford, could explain her symptoms. An hour or so after Ford's careful examination, Crowe, by chance, met Dandy in the corridor and related the dilemma to him. Dandy accompanied Crowe to the patient's bedside. Except for looking at the patient's eyegrounds, counting her pulse, and observing the patient and her respirations from the foot of the bed, he made no examination. Dandy turned to Crowe and said: "She has a frontal lobe abscess." She was taken to the operating room immediately. While she was still on the stretcher, Dandy needled the right frontal lobe; out came thick yellow pus under pressure. Crowe related this to Ford on the following day when the patient was conscious

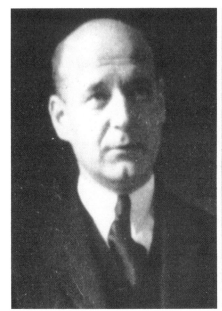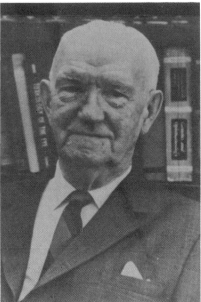

FIG. 2.6. (*Left*) Dr. Frank R. Ford (1892–1970).
FIG. 2.7. (*Right*) Dr. Frank B. Walsh (1895–1978).

and rapidly improving. Ford, shaking his head, said, "Doctor, I think God must whisper into that man's ear."

Dandy carried a heavy operative schedule estimated at over 1000 major cases per year exclusive of ventriculograms. Except when posting an eighth nerve tumor, he would schedule four or five cases 6 days per week, possibly less on Thursdays and Saturdays. Although his operating room (704) was not reserved for him on Mondays and Thursdays, his resident almost always managed to rearrange the operating room schedule by calling various surgeons on the list who graciously agreed, when possible, to move a case to an earlier or later time to accommodate Dr. Dandy.

The resident and assistant resident were awakened at 6:15 a.m., quickly dressed, and then were off to quick rounds. Sick patients were last seen at 2:00 a.m. The resident would see all of the private patients as well as the patients in the special care unit. The assistant resident would see all the ward and semiprivate patients. They would meet in the dining room for breakfast at 7:00 a.m. At 7:30 a.m. the neurosurgical house staff was on its way to the operating room.

Almost always, a patient scheduled for ventriculography under local anesthesia was the first case of the day and was positioned face down on the cerebellar headrest with a small shaved area in the occipital region.

The resident would stand above the patient, sponge stick in hand, ready to scrub the operative area at exactly 8:00 a.m. The matriarch supervising the OR apparently had the power to determine this time. However, at 8:00 a.m. we were in command, and we lost no time in making the trephine openings. The team always performed as though there were three ventriculograms posted. This kept us in training for the occasions when three were posted, since the first major case had to start at 8:45 a.m.

By a snap of his fingers, Dandy's arrival at 9:00 was announced by Wallace Lawrence, his devoted orderly. The resident would be opening the first case, often a cerebellar approach to the fifth nerve or the eighth nerve. The Chief would open the swinging door of the operating room and receive a quick report on the patients in the house. He then changed and returned to our induction room to put air into the ventricles of the first ventriculogram patient (Fig. 2.8) (3). Lawrence seemed to be the only one who could hold the head and manipulate it to his satisfaction. We also preferred this because we could instruct him as to which way to mobilize the scalp when it was apparent that the openings in the scalp and skull did not align well.

When a cerebral mass was suspected, Dandy tapped the ipsilateral ventricle with that side up and replaced the ventricular fluid with air cc for cc using a closed system. When the air injection was completed, the assistant resident dropped out of the operative procedure and took the patient to x-ray. One or two wet films were brought back to the operating room with the patient. The assistant resident announced to the resident that the patient was back from x-ray; he also stated his opinion of the findings on x-ray and then asked whether he should release the air. The resident repeated this to Dandy, and he decided whether he wanted the air evacuated. Patients with positive ventriculograms were always operated on on the day of the study.

One day, when he had difficulty cannulating a ventricle, Dandy insisted that the trephine openings I had made were too high and that he would be better off getting a 4th-year medical student to make the holes and as an afterthought he said, "Even Chambers might do better!" (referring to our assistant resident). Sometime later, in x-ray when he seemed to be in a good mood, I put that patient's x-rays on the view box and asked him where he wanted the openings. He pointed 2 inches above the holes and said that that point was too high. In fact, the holes were well placed. I decided this genius was just being contrary.

No time was lost between cases. After dropping out of a case, Dandy returned in 1 hour, expecting the next case to be opened and ready for him. During this hour the bleeding had to be controlled, the wound

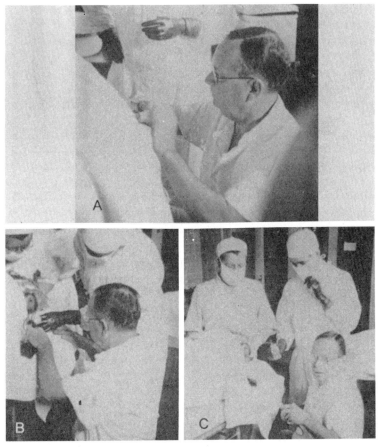

FIG. 2.8. Photographs (*A* and *B*) of Dr. Dandy replacing ventricular fluid with air for ventriculography. Wallace Lawrence, his orderly, on the left in *C* is holding the patient's head.

closed, the room cleaned, and the next patient put to sleep, draped, and opened. Accordingly, when he left, Gracie Smith, his invaluable Nurse Anesthetist, would drop out to put the next patient to sleep in the induction room (Fig. 2.9) (1). The scrub nurse would ask her assistant to be sure the sterilizers were filled and boiling. When we started to suture the wound, the instruments were stacked and put in the sterilizers. As the water returned to boiling in the sterilizers, a 10-minute countdown was started.

The intern always picked the instruments the night before surgery from the neurosurgical cabinet. He had to learn to recognize the favorite instruments from the many in the cabinet. The flaws on the handle or

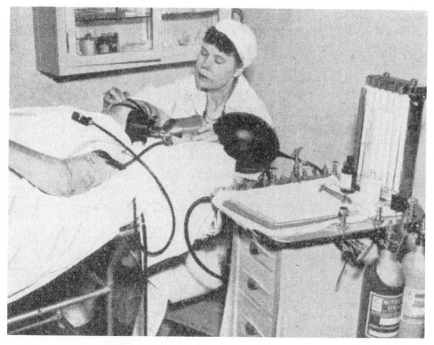

FIG. 2.9. Grace Smith anesthetizing a neurosurgical patient.

the jiggle in the handle when shaken identified the favorite joker, etc. Many instruments would be used only rarely. Nonetheless, they were called for on occasions and were expected to be in the set.

Fifth nerve tics were usually operated on by the cerebellar approach and were done first because Dandy wanted to spare these patients continued pain. Eighth nerve sections for Meniere's syndrome were done second, discs third, and craniotomies for tumor last. The Old Man was a superb, dextrous, and peerless technician and, when operating, he said very little, except to verbally lash someone who dared not perform to perfection. However, when things were going smoothly, he might ignore minor infractions. During surgery the Bovie was always hot. Dandy was too impatient to accept a foot pedal switch. When not in use, the Bovie wand and tip were in a glass test tube secured to the drapes. His delicate bayonet forceps were used to coagulate bleeders. When in the depths of the wound, the bayonet often shorted on the edge of the wound and we would say, "Short, Sir! Short, Sir!." When dealing with brisk bleeding deep in the head, he seemed to ignore Grace Smith's countdown of the dropping blood pressure. She would say, "The pressure is 80, 70, 60, 50." Somehow he heard 50 and would lament and ask "Why didn't someone tell me before?" He would then pack with cotton balls and ask for a transfusion. We were sure he wanted a few minutes of hypotension to help control the bleeding. Despite the fact that Hopkins had one of the first blood banks in this country, he would not use bottled blood in the OR—he wanted fresh blood by direct transfusion from a waiting donor. Students and house officers on other services were used as donors. The assistant resident often had difficulty cannulating a foot or ankle vein with a large bore needle when the patient was in shock. Under the drapes with the room darkened, the foot was illuminated with a gooseneck reading lamp. Before there was time to get in, Dandy would raise his head and shine his headlight on the transfusion team and ask how much blood had been given. Once the vein was cannulated with a large bore needle by a team of three and the 50 cc syringes had been rinsed in a citrate solution between injections, we could give 500 cc of blood rapidly. An edict had come from above in the past about not using IV fluids to keep a vein open. However, Chambers gradually began to do this more and more, and if Dandy noted it, he never objected.

Because a headlight was used, surgery was done in a darkened room. Dandy's light really gave acceptable illumination. It consisted of an electric light bulb and socket attached to a headband (Figs. 2.10 and 2.11) (3). Most of the upper portion of the bulb was covered with dark green paint so only the operative field was illuminated. It was important

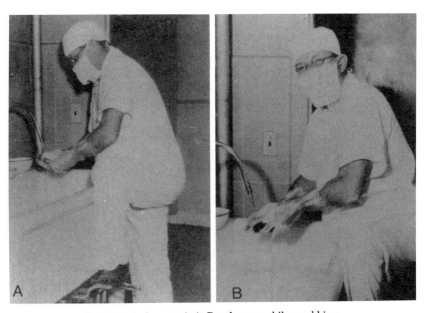

FIG. 2.10. A characteristic Dandy pose while scrubbing.

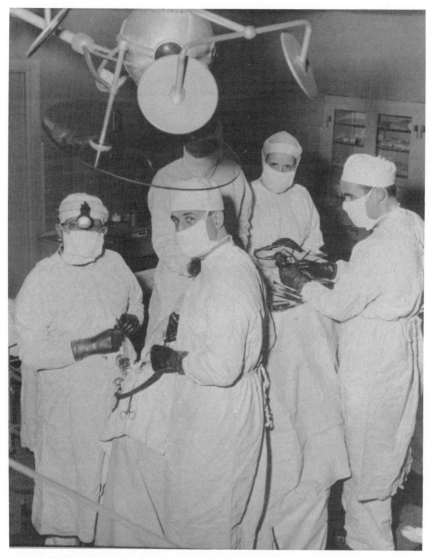

FIG. 2.11. Dr. Dandy wearing his headlight during an operation.

that Lawrence make the transfer from the resident to the Chief when he was ready to take over. A careless transfer of the hot light could result in a mild burn. At times the residents would tease Lawrence during this maneuver. As Dr. Dandy was being gowned a few feet away, the resident would often say, "Tell that so and so to get in here, we don't have all day." Lawrence, or Barney as he was known to the residents, in turn would say, "I am going to tell him what you said." This would go on until Dandy was at the table, each hoping to get the last word before Dandy could hear what was said. We all believed Dandy had some hearing defect. If he ever heard, he never commented.

We certainly developed great respect for his unrivaled surgical skill; we felt if anybody could do it, he could. Almost never in doubt, he was quick, bold, and gentle. I was somewhat surprised when he paused one day after exposing a large cerebral arteriovenous malformation. He kept repeating, "I can't take it out." Then with a bold reach of his right arm to the instrument table, he picked up his favorite bayonet forceps and signaled for the Bovie as he began to excise the lesion.

On completion of the operative schedule, the house staff returned to the wards to prepare for rounds with the Old Man sometime between 4:00 and 5:00 p.m. At times a craniotomy patient had one or two seizures postoperatively, and we had not reported this to Dr. Dandy because he would insist that the wound be reopened. Accordingly, when we felt this was not necessary, we neglected to tell him. To Dandy, every postoperative seizure was an intracranial clot until proved otherwise. If we felt the patient should be reopened, we tried to do it after Dr. Dandy left the hospital; otherwise, he was sure to come to the OR to see what was found. I guess every resident on one occasion or another palmed some extradural blood clot from under the convexity of the bone flap as he was told that there was no hematoma. Obviously, if we felt the clot was significant, we would tell him so. However, if he came into the OR before the bone flap was elevated, he would consider a small amount of clot a hemorrhage, and I suppose he did this to justify reopening the wound and to highlight the need for more meticulous hemostasis.

Shortly after rounds he would extricate his long black Packard Sedan from the long line of parked cars on Monument Street. He was not very gentle in this maneuver; he rewarded people who parked too close to him by driving back and forth to create enough room to get his car out. One day, before serving on his team, I saw the barber on Monument Street running out the door and across the street with scissors and comb in hand, yelling "Wait, Dr. Dandy! Wait Dr. Dandy! I'll move my car." I am sure no harm was ever done. Cars were built more solidly in those days.

Every day, 5 or 10 minutes before 7:00 p.m. the resident went to his quarters to prepare the list of patients he needed to discuss with Dr. Dandy. When the nearby church bells tolled 7:00, he made his telephone call. Even before I spoke, Dandy would answer, "Yes Rizzoli." Mrs. Dandy may well have set her clocks by these calls. It was rarely necessary for him to return to the hospital for emergency cases. However, on more than one occasion when he operated during the night, on completion of the emergency operation he would begin the next day's schedule. I think he thought it was great fun to be walking out at 8 or 9 a.m. with his schedule completed when everybody else was just starting the operating day. Every emergency case was used to keep the team in training. All emergencies would be posted by the resident without warning, and it was expected that the incision would be made in 15 or 20 minutes, regardless of whether there was urgency or not. This was to keep the team perpetually in training for the rare patient whose life might be saved by efficient and speedy intervention. The reins were never relaxed.

The resident was always reluctant to give Dandy disagreeable information. On one or two occasions when a patient's course was deteriorating during the night, I was hesitant to call Dandy because I didn't believe there was anything to do. On the other hand, I could not let the patient die without getting the "green light" from the Old Man. Accordingly, I paced the floor with brief and frequent interruptions to re-examine the patient, hoping that I could be persuaded that the patient would survive until morning.

By now it must be apparent to those familiar with Cushing's methods that Dandy's attitude was considerably different in some important respects. The former prided himself on doing everything himself from skin to skin. He carried over this compulsion to performing dressing changes personally. Dandy believed in delegating authority. His confidence in his assistants was characteristically all or none. In the 1940s, he usually took two vacations a year. In the summer he went to Capon Springs, West Virginia, and in the winter he liked to go to Ponte Vedra, Florida. Mrs. Shauck would often suggest a month or so before his vacation that he might not go because of the large backlog. This encouraged us to work harder to get more cases done because we enjoyed his vacation more than he did. We were allowed to do the surgery on most ward patients and on all emergency patients while he was away.

He taught by stern example. Although quick to chastise, he could be complimentary and could be very warm. A warm smile from Dandy made you feel great for a few hours. Whenever a patient who had previously had disc surgery either at Hopkins or elsewhere was admitted with persistent or recurrent symptoms, we did a lumbar puncture to rule out a spinal cord tumor. Of course he was told when we found an abnormality. One Monday morning, at student rounds a patient with a previous history of disc surgery and with persistent pain was presented (Fig. 2.12). I had told him I was unable to get any spinal fluid when I tried a spinal puncture. Without hesitation, Dandy told the students that if I could not get fluid, there wasn't any, so the patient needed a total laminectomy and an intradural exposure. He then instructed me to take the patient to the OR and start the operation while he continued with the students.

Many have recorded anecdotes, hoping to describe some facets of the

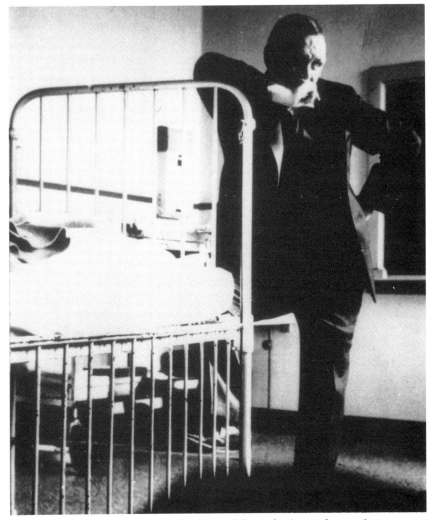

FIG. 2.12. A characteristic Dandy stance while conducting student conferences.

Old Man's colorful personality. Woodhall recalled assisting Dr. Dandy just before dawn to drain a subdural hematoma under local anesthesia on a comatose patient shortly after he had arrived in Baltimore by plane. As the patient began to waken on the operating table, Dandy discarded a hemostat and asked for another one, which apparently was no better than the first. He grumbled, "What am I going to do with this one?" The patient responded, "Throw it on the floor the way you did the first one." When Dandy asked what the patient had said, Woodhall answered, "He says he's feeling better."

The empathic side of this man is disclosed by the following incidents. Troland relates that following a postoperative death experienced by Watson after a cerebellar tic operation, Dr. Dandy sensed this resident's distress (6). That evening the resident received a call from Mrs. Dandy asking him to meet the Chief at the accident room entrance. Dandy was sitting in his car and simply had the resident sit beside him for a few moments and then said, "Don't worry, these things happen to all of us." During a similar operation, I personally experienced an intraoperative anesthetic-related death. Upon Dandy's return to Baltimore, I had to report this catastrophic experience. I was absolutely certain it would result in my dismissal. I couldn't decide whether to pack first. Instead, tearfully I went to his office to relate this occurrence and the findings at autopsy. To my amazement his reaction and verbal response were identical to that described by Troland. I sensed that he would have reacted differently had he performed the surgery.

His generosity and kindness to numerous students, residents, and patients in need of financial aid are legendary. Dandy's seemingly cold exterior was only superficial and probably resulted from his great concern over his patients. At times he was excessive in his criticism of his assistants, but this was often short lived, and soon he rewarded us with an unusually warm smile. He probably was aware of his occasionally capricious behavior, but he demanded perfection. For the residents, the Brain Team was a priceless experience.

REFERENCES

1. Barcala, F. J. *Walter E. Dandy, Su Obra en Neurocirugia.* Ferrari Hnos., Buenos Aires, Brazil, 1946.
2. Crowe, S. J. *Halsted of Johns Hopkins.* Charles C Thomas, Springfield, Ill., 1957.
3. Fox, W. L. *Dandy of Johns Hopkins.* Williams & Wilkins, Baltimore, 1984.
4. Heuer, G. W. Dr. Halsted. Bull. Johns Hopkins Hosp., *90* (Suppl.): 1–105, 1952.
5. Ravitch, M. M. *The Papers of Alfred Blalock.* The Johns Hopkins University Press, Baltimore, 1966.
6. Troland, C. E. Walter E. Dandy. Presented at the 18th Annual Meeting of The Neurosurgical Society of America, San Juan, Puerto Rico, January 1985.

II

Cerebrovascular Surgery

CHAPTER

3

Earlier Times in Aneurysm Surgery*

CHARLES G. DRAKE, M.D., F.R.C.S.(C)

My task is to relate an historical perspective on the early days of aneurysm surgery, beginning with the Dandy era and extending through the period up to the introduction of the operating microscope. My Chief, Kenneth McKenzie of Toronto, greatly admired Walter Dandy and felt he was as innovative as Cushing in many ways. In fact, I might have attended this meeting myself as an old Dandy resident, as Dr. McKenzie mentioned several times that I should spend some training time with him. Dr. Dandy's untimely end, however, precluded this possibility.

Dandy, in the mid 1920s, was surely aware of the syndrome of the cerebral aneurysm and its role in subarachnoid hemorrhage, for he frequently quoted Symond's 1924 paper (27), and he had used internal carotid ligation for carotid cavernous fistulae. His first operation for intracranial aneurysm was performed in 1928, when Fuller Albright persuaded him to ligate the carotid artery on a patient with a carotid aneurysm producing a sudden third nerve palsy. Unfortunately, the patient died a few days later from infarction (1). Even so, his relationship with that remarkable physician may have been a factor in his developing interest. Albright, in his 1929 review of the 30 cases published to that time (in addition to two of his own), wrote "It is to be hoped that, as the diagnosis becomes more exact, some surgical technique can be developed to save this unfortunate group of patients." He even postulated intracranial ligation of carotid aneurysms!

Although carotid ligation had been used occasionally in the late 18th century and throughout the 19th century for carotid injuries, carotid cavernous fistulae, and cervical aneurysms, there is only one account of its use for nonfistulous intracranial aneurysm before this century. In 1885, Sir Victor Horsley had exposed a middle fossa tumor and had found it to be an aneurysm. The carotid artery was ligated in the neck, and Keen (15) reported that the patient was in "extremely good health" 5 years later . In 1924, Magnus (17) in Copenhagen had opened a trigeminal tumor that had caused intractable trigeminal neuralgia and a sixth nerve

---

* Published in part as Gordon Murray Lecture in *Canadian Journal of Surgery*, 27:1984.

palsy. About half of the old clot could be removed before "a great gush of blood appeared that could not be stopped with tamponade." Fortunately, he had just ligated the external carotid artery because of a tear in the middle meningeal artery at the skull base. Subsequent ligation of the internal carotid promptly stopped the bleeding, and the remaining contents of the aneurysm were removed. The patient was relieved of his pain, although he developed a paresis of his left hand on the third postoperative day.

In 1940, Schorstein (26) reported on 60 cases of carotid ligature for the treatment of nontraumatic saccular intracranial aneurysms: 27 were collected from the literature, and 33 were from the British experience. There were eight deaths and eight cases of hemiplegia, a 13% incidence of each. In this article, Schorstein suggests that Wilfred Trotter, in 1924, was the first to ligate a carotid artery without having first exposed an intracranial aneurysm (a traumatic aneurysm producing severe epistaxis). In noting Grey Turner's case in 1928, Schorstein was obviously not aware that Walter Dandy, in the same year, also had occluded the internal carotid artery for a ruptured intracranial carotid aneurysm; both patients had a localizing oculomotor paresis with the hemorrhage.

Norman Dott's name, from Edinburgh, must be inseparably linked with Dandy's in the story of early aneurysm surgery. The first planned intracranial aneurysm operation was done by Dott in 1931, on the Chairman of his hospital board. After three bleeds, an aneurysm in the region of the carotid bifurcation was localized by left retroorbital pain and was wrapped in muscle (6). Following Dott's report, other surgeons described direct attack on intracranial aneurysms. In 1934, Tonnis (28) split the corpus callosum to cover the surface of an anterior communicating aneurysm with muscle, and McConnell, in 1937, opened a subchiasmal aneurysm and packed it with muscle (18).

However, it was Dandy who added so immeasurably to intracranial procedures when he first trapped a carotid cavernous aneurysm in 1936. Later, on March 22, 1937, he used a McKenzie silver clip to occlude the neck of a posterior communicating artery aneurysm which produced a third nerve palsy (5). The palsy cleared in 6 weeks. He was rightly critical, as it turned out, of the use of muscle as reinforcement for these sacs and felt that an aneurysm could only be "cured" by neck clipping, trapping, stuffing with muscle, and coagulation or excision, tenets that persist today.

In his 1944 monograph, he was able to report on 64 aneurysms found at operation. Before the 1937 clipping operation, all previous 28 aneurysms had been exposed accidentally in the search for tumors. After 1937, with 3 exceptions in 36 cases, the presence of an aneurysm had been diagnosed beforehand in spite of the fact he never used angiography! He knew about this new diagnostic test, for it had been described by Moniz (20) in 1927, but he was worried about the toxicity and the cerebral thrombosis reports related to the use of Thorotrast and Diatrast. In his series, only four aneurysms had been visualized by angiography, all of which had the studies done by the referring neurosurgeons. He said, "It is quite possible—if the freedom from accident is proved to be minimal— that I may yet come to use it."

He relied on localization by clinical means, using neighborhood compression of the IInd and IIIrd cranial nerves and, in one case, the XIth and XIIth. With the exception of the oculomotor nerve, aneurysms usually must be very large to produce signs of neighborhood compression of other cranial nerves or brain, which explains why he operated on so few of the ordinary small aneurysms (only seven or eight in all), and why all the patients in question had oculomotor palsy. In six cases he tried neck clipping, but the aneurysms ruptured in four instances and had to be trapped, usually with clips on the carotid on either side of the torn neck. He charred some of these small aneurysms with the Bovie to shrink them away from the oculomotor nerve and, on at least one occasion, stroked an intact sac with the cautery to shrink it. All six anterior cerebral, four middle cerebral, and two vertebral basilar aneurysms which Dandy exposed were for tumorous syndromes. Two large anterior communicating aneurysms were cured; one was excised and one was stuffed with muscle. All of the patients with the middle cerebral aneurysms died, and he had predicted a poor surgical future for them. He "shelled out" one vertebral aneurysm from which the patient did not survive. He ligated the vertebral artery for aneurysm three times, including his well-known and only attempt at bilateral occlusion, which immediately resulted in sudden death. As he later said, "There could be no more rapid death or one so silent." Overall he was optimistic about the future of aneurysm surgery, for he felt "with due appreciation of the errors of the past" that both his mortality rate of 25% and cure rate of 55% would be improved.

He relied heavily on carotid occlusion, with trapping above and below the aneurysm if possible, and deemed the Matas test of utmost importance. With few exceptions, he occluded the cervical internal carotid, usually partially at first using fascial or dural bands, which he felt would produce further stenosis by contracting fibrosis. He knew about thromboembolism from his teacher, Halsted, who felt it resulted from intimal injury with ligatures.

Remarkably, in his series of 51 cervical carotid occlusions, which included some for carotid cavernous fistulae and tumors, he had only 5 disabling infarctions and 3 deaths, a success which he attributed to the Matas test. Twenty-five were partial occlusions, however, and 4 of the infarctions and 1 death occurred in this group. At least 3 infarctions and 3 deaths occurred in the 21 aneurysm cases.

Dandy had no experience with acute aneurysm surgery, except for one acute carotid occlusion and another evacuation of a clot, so he was unaware of the ischemic phenomenon with vasospasm. Undoubtedly, had it not been for his reluctance to use arteriography, he would have ventured much further. Dott (6) was more prophetic when he described the first use of arteriography as a guide to surgical treatment in 1933. After performing the first carotid ligation for an aneurysm visualized with Thorotrast, he reported that "arteriography has come to our aid. By this means an intracranial aneurysm can be seen, together with the cerebral arteries."

Dott (6) continued to be innovative when he described, in 1941, the opening and stuffing of a large ruptured middle cerebral aneurysm with a chunk of muscle while using temporary occlusion of the middle cerebral artery with an artery forceps whose handles were approximated gently with an elastic band. This must have been the first use of temporary proximal cerebral artery occlusion. In 1944 (6) the Hunterian principle of proximal ligation was first used intracranially when he clipped a dominant anterior cerebral artery proximal to a ruptured anterior communicating aneurysm in a young Dutch sailor.

The further development of aneurysm surgery came to a standstill during World War II but began again in the late 1940s. Meanwhile, Richardson, and Hyland (24) of Toronto, in 1941, provided new stimulus to the recognition of the disorder with their clinical and pathological findings showing the diverse nature of cerebral aneurysms and the consequences of their rupture. At that time, they favored medical management of subarachnoid hemorrhage.

By 1955, 278 patients with an intracranial operation for aneurysm had been reported, with an overall 28.4% mortality. Within the various small series, however, mortalities varied from as low as 8 to 40%, 56%, and even 86% (25). No doubt this was the reason that most surgeons preferred to use carotid ligation, with which long-term survival, as reported by Jefferson and Poppen, was 86% and 79%, respectively. I recall Sir Geofrey Jefferson saying at that time that carotid occlusion was the sheet anchor for the surgical treatment of aneurysms.

The Cooperative Study of 1969 (25), reviewing 800 cases subjected to carotid occlusion, revealed that the technique was useful only for aneurysms arising from the carotid itself. There was still, however, a rebleed rate of 3% and a 30% risk of cerebral infarction. This risk was significantly lower with gradual common carotid occlusion or when more than a week free from bleeding had elapsed prior to the ligation. About two-thirds of the carotid aneurysms visualized after carotid occlusion had decreased in size, but we now know that carotid ligation confers protection only for about 6 months. I still feel that "simple" carotid occlusion, by whatever means and even with the protection of surgically made bypass collateral, is still one of the most dangerous operations neurosurgeons perform, not so much from hemodynamic ischemia as from thromboembolism.

Intracranial surgery early after aneurysm rupture was the mark of the 1950s, a result of anxiety to prevent the disaster of recurrent bleeding. It is important to remember the circumstances of these operations. The brain was swollen, with a red and "angry" look. Little was known about anesthesia for brain operations, and the anesthetists were all too often disinterested and were rarely dedicated. To glimpse the circle of Willis meant tapping the ventricle, and firm, even harsh, retraction of the frontal lobe was usually required. Removal of a clot made the situation a little easier. Aneurysms proved to be very fragile, often bursting with the least manipulation. Application of the small silver clip not infrequently tore the neck, often because the blunt nose of the appliers was too difficult to manipulate in the narrow confines on either side. The bleeding obscured the field, and these closed clips could not be removed. Frantic clip applications could not be accurate, and often the parent artery or an important branch was occluded, sometimes deliberately to prevent the patient from bleeding to death.

Temporary occlusion of the carotid artery, exposed in the neck at the same time or compressed with the anesthetist's thumb, was helpful in making the sac softer or in controlling hemorrhage. In 1946, Gardner (12), in Cleveland, had introduced deliberate systemic hypotension for brain procedures by withdrawing large quantities of blood into a reservoir, a form of hypovolemic shock. Fortunately, reduced blood pressure with pharmacologic ganglionic blockade became available soon after and was used for aneurysm operations in the early 1950s.

Artificial hypothermia to 28–30°C was introduced by Lougheed and Botterell (4) in Toronto in 1956. This technique reduced the surgical hazards by allowing temporary total arterial occlusion in the neck for 8–10 minutes, and its use became widespread over the next several years. However, as surgical techniques improved, it was found to be unnecessary in most situations, particularly when deeper levels of normothermic artificial hypotension (down to 40 mean arterial pressure (MAP)) were found to be safe in otherwise healthy patients.

Deep hypothermia (to 15°C or below), with arrest and exsanguination under cardiopulmonary bypass, was tried in the early 1960s (9, 23, 29) but was associated with bleeding and moderate hypothermia problems. It did not prevent the vasospasm and ischemia which so often followed early operations. Hypothermia was, therefore, abandoned in the early 1960s by most surgeons in favor of deeper levels of hypotension, and operations were delayed for a week or so after bleeding.

Gradually, in the late 1950s and early 1960s, a new phenomenon was recognized, peculiar to early direct operation on a ruptured aneurysm. It occurred even when the operation went smoothly, the brain was reasonably slack, and clip application was accurate. Initially, the patient awoke without deficit, only to deteriorate a few hours or days later. This deterioration often was signaled by confusion and the complaint of tingling or weakness in an extremity. Within a few hours, the patient would be stuporous and hemiplegic. A postoperative clot was suspected, but urgent reopening revealed only a swollen, softened brain. As a consequence, death or severe neurological deficit was commonplace. It did not take much persuading of my neuroradiological colleague, Dr. John Allcock (3), to do postoperative angiography on these cases. This puzzling sequence was shown to be associated with severe arterial narrowing. The vessels irrigating the hemisphere were often no larger than the size of threads. The brain showed swelling and infarction. This arterial spasm became dreaded and was blamed for the poor results in otherwise uncomplicated aneurysm surgery. Consequently, there was a tendency to delay operation until the acute reaction of the brain and its vessels had subsided, for few surgeons would accept the high morbidity of early operation, which in most instances equaled or exceeded the rebleeding risks.

During the 1950s, some clinical observers were appalled at the mortality and morbidity of early operations and at the disasters that occurred from rebleeding while the surgeon waited for the patient to become a good risk. Wide acceptance of the emerging intracranial operations was slow. In 1960, McKissock et al. (19) reported on the only controlled study on the surgery of aneurysms, which suggested that the surgical treatment of that time was no better than the conservative measure of bed rest for a few weeks. This study, in my view, delayed the development of intracranial techniques and experience in many centers.

Then, in 1968, Mullan and Dawley (22) introduced the concept of using an antifibrinolysin, ϵ-aminocaproic acid, to preserve the clot, sealing the rent in the aneurysm for a week or two until the patient became a good risk for surgical treatment. In initial studies, it appeared to reduce rebleeding by about 50% during this time interval. This was seen as a remarkable accomplishment, and under this presumed safety umbrella, surgeons were even more inclined to delay operation for a week or so. There were a few voices of concern about more ischemic calamities, but the real extent was not known until 1983 (14, 16).

Because of the apparent deadly nature of arterial spasm and its prohibition of lifesaving early operation, there was an extraordinary amount of research, both clinical and experimental, on its nature and relief. It is now known to occur to some degree in most patients who show CT evidence of blood in their basal cisterns. The degree of narrowing and subsequent ischemia seemed to be directly and predictively related to the thickness of the clot around the basal arteries. Cerebral blood flow (CBF) correlation between vasospasm and ischemia has only recently been established by Ferguson *et al.* (10), with one of the difficulties being that the brain tolerates reduction in blood flow to nearly half its normal value before neuronal function decays. This explained why some patients remain neurologically well in spite of severe and frightening angiographic narrowing. They are probably teetering on the brink of ischemic disaster with any insult, such as craniotomy.

Initial attempts at relief were centered on altering the vasospastic state. Every conceivable vasoactive drug, alone or in combination, was administered systemically or even locally, without credible consistent success. The use of low molecular weight Dextran in the 1960s was promising in improving perfusion but did not receive wide favor because prolonged use led to a bleeding disorder. Only recently (13) has it become known how effective the improvement of perfusion can be for this ischemia, using blood volume expansion and improved rheology with albumin and artificial hypertension if necessary. Sustained reversal of hemiplegia and aphasia are now common dramatic events.

The fragile nature of aneurysms, the problems with limited exposure, and the lack of a clear field of blood for accurate clip application following rupture engendered a healthy respect and even fear and trepidation in surgeons who exposed them. This led some to develop other containment methods which did not require the wider exposure and prolonged meticulous dissection around the aneurysm. Coating with gauze or plastic (muscle was shown to be of no use), promotion of intraluminal thrombosis by the injection of animal hair (11) or thrombogenic wire (21) into the sac, and even iron filings injected into anterior communicating aneurysms through a fine needle placed into the sac and held there by a magnet until thrombosis occurred (2) were testimonies to the great ingenuity of neurosurgeons.

Initial appeal of these methods was tempered because intraluminal thrombosis often did not include the neck, which would later expand into a new and dangerous sac. Encasement, if it were to be effective, demanded a fairly complete dissection anyway, and as such techniques improved, a clip could be applied instead. Gauze was an insecure restraint during the months required for a firm fibrous sheath to occur. Plastic coating is still used for some otherwise unmanageable complex aneurysms, but a few aneurysms have grown out of the base of the plastic encasement and reruptured.

The surgical microscope first saw neurosurgical use in the mid 1960s but was not widely used until the early 1970s. The usefulness of magnified vision, however, was perceived as early as the late 1950s. Loupes of 2.5 power with near coaxial fiber-optic light gave the first good magnified view of the intimacies of an aneurysm. Now it might be called mesosurgery, in contrast to microsurgery, although it is now generally recognized that these loupes were equivalent to the lowest setting of the original microscope. Also during that period, spring clips were introduced, requiring only the blades to cross the aneurysm neck and allowing easy removal and replacement.

Direct operation for aneurysms on the vertebrobasilar system was slower in development, both because of their lower incidence and lack of routine simple vertebral angiography via the catheter techniques. Furthermore, many thought that their hidden position in front of the brain stem precluded a direct attack. I began my adventures with them in 1958, and it wasn't long before the approaches were worked out. The final refinements awaited the microscope and finer instrumentation so vital for treatment of these lesions (8).

Although most of Dandy's aneurysm experience was with the giant variety, no concerted direct attack on these lesions began until the late 1960s and early 1970s. Gradually, it was learned that perhaps half, even on the posterior circulation, had necks small enough for clipping. Then, in 1969, extracranial-intracranial (EC-IC) bypass largely solved the hemodynamic problems associated with proximal carotid and middle cerebral artery occlusion for their giant aneurysms. Hunterian proximal ligation of the carotid artery has been extended to all other major cerebral arteries giving rise to giant aneurysms—including the anterior cerebral, the vertebrals, and the basilar artery with all its branches (except anterior inferior communicating artery (AICA) and posterior inferior communicating artery (PICA) (7).

In the last decade or so, the microscope, finer instrumentation, modern neuroanesthesia, and the temporary or permanent interruption followed by restoration and maintenance of brain blood flow have greatly enhanced the safety and accuracy of surgery for all intracranial saccular aneurysms. Such advancements have led to a return of urgent early operation. While there are still some problems to be solved, especially with certain giant aneurysms, the burden for significant further improvement in satisfactory aneurysm outcome now rests with the primary care physicians, who must improve their recognition of this disorder in their community practices.

It was Dr. Dandy who initiated these surgical treatments of this deadly disorder, and I hope that Dr. Dandy would be pleased with the accomplishments of his students, whose safe sure surgical obliteration gives the patient a whole and new *life*.

REFERENCES

1. Albright, F. The syndrome produced by aneurysm at or near the function of the internal carotid artery and the circle of Willis. Johns Hopkins Hosp. Bull., *44:* 215–245, 1929.
2. Alksne, J. F., and Rand, R. W. Current status of metallic thrombosis of intracranial aneurysms. In: *Progress in Neurological Surgery*, Vol. 3, pp. 212–229. Yearbook Medical Publisher, Chicago, 1969.
3. Allcock, J. M., and Drake, C. G. Ruptured intracranial aneurysms—The role of arterial spasm. J. Neurosurg., *21:* 21–29, 1965.
4. Botterell, E. H., Lougheed, W. M., Scott, J. W., and Vandewater, S. L. Hypothermia, and interruption of carotid, or carotid and vertebral circulation in the surgical management of intracranial aneurysms. J. Neurosurg., *13:* 1–42, 1956.
5. Dandy, W. E. *Intracranial Arterial Aneurysms*. Comstock Publishing, Ithaca, N.Y., 1945.
6. Dott, N. Intracranial aneurysmal formations. Clin. Neurosurg., *16:* 1–16, 1969.
7. Drake, C. G. Giant intracranial aneurysms. Experience with surgical treatment in 174 patients. Clin. Neurosurg., *26:* 12–95, 1979.
8. Drake, C. G. The treatment of aneurysms of the posterior circulation. Clin. Neurosurg., *26:* 96–144, 1979.
9. Drake, C. G., Barr, H. W. K., Coles, J. C., and Gergely, N. F. The use of extracorporeal circulation and profound hypothermia in treatment of ruptured intracranial aneurysm. J. Neurosurg., *21:* 575–581, 1964.
10. Ferguson, G. G., Farrar, J. K., Meguro, K., Peerless, S. J., Drake, C. G., and Barnett, H. J. M. Serial measurements of CBF as a guide to surgery in patients with ruptured intracranial aneurysms. J. Cereb. Blood Flow Metab., *1*(1): 518–519, 1981.
11. Gallagher, J. P. The closure of intracranial aneurysms by pilo injection. In: *Intracranial Aneurysms and Subarachnoid Hemorrhage*, edited by W. S. Fields and A. L. Sahs, Charles C Thomas, Springfield, Ill., 1965.
12. Gardner, W. J. The control of bleeding during operation by induced hypotension. J.A.M.A., *132:* 572–574, 1946.
13. Kassell, N. F., Peerless, S. J., Durward, Q. J., Beck, D. W., Drake, C. G., and Adams, H. P. Treatment of ischemic deficits from vasospasm with intravascular volume expansion and induced arterial hypertension. Neurosurgery, *3*(2): 337–343, 1982.
14. Kassell, N. F., Torner, J. C., and Adams, H. P. Antifibrinolytic agents in the acute period following aneurysmal subarachnoid hemorrhage: preliminary observations from the Cooperative Aneurysm Study. Presented at the American Association of Neurological Surgeons Annual Meeting, San Francisco, April 1984.
15. Keen, W. W. Intracranial lesions. Med. News, *57:* 439–449, 1890.
16. Lindsay, K. W., Vermeulen, M., Murray, G., *et al.* Antifibrinolytic therapy in subarachnoid hemorrhage: Reduction of rebleeding without benefit to outcome. Presented at

the American Association of Neurological Surgeons Annual Meeting, San Francisco, April 1984.

17. Magnus, V. Aneurysm of the internal carotid artery. J.A.M.A., *88:* 1712–1713, 1927.

18. McConnell, A. A. Subchiasmal aneurysm treated by implantation of muscle. Zentralbl. Neurochir., *2:* 269–274, 1937.

19. McKissock, W., Richardson, A., and Walsh, L. Posterior-communicating aneurysms. A controlled trial of the conservative and surgical treatment of ruptured aneurysms of the internal carotid artery at or near the point of origin of the posterior communicating artery. Lancet, *1:* 1203–1206, 1960.

20. Moniz, E. *Die Cerebrale Arteriographie und Phlebographie.* Berlin, Julius Springer, 1940.

21. Mullan, S. Experiences with surgical thrombosis of intracranial berry aneurysms and carotid-cavernous fistulas. J. Neurosurg., *41:* 657–670, 1974.

22. Mullan, S., and Dawley, J. Antifibrinolysin therapy for intracranial aneurysms. J. Neurosurg., *28:* 21–23, 1968.

23. Patterson, R. H., Jr., and Ray, B. S. Profound hypothermia for intracranial surgery. Laboratory and clinical experiences in the extra corporeal circulation by peripheral cannulation. Ann. Surg., *156:* 377–393, 1962.

24. Richardson, J. R., and Hyland, H. H. Intracranial aneurysms. Medicine, *20:* 1–83, 1941.

25. Sahs, A. L., Perret, G. E., Locksley, H. B., and Nishioka, H. *Intracranial Aneurysms and Subarachnoid Hemorrhage. A Cooperative Study.* J.B. Lippincott, Philadelphia, 1969.

26. Schorstein, J. Carotid ligation in saccular intracranial aneurysms. Br. J. Surg., *28:* 50–70, 1940.

27. Symonds, C. P. Spontaneous subarachnoid hemorrhage. Q. J. Med., *18:* 93–122, 1924.

28. Tonnis, W. Erfolgreiche behandlung eines aneurysma der art. commun. ant. cerebri. Zentralbl. Neurochir., *1:* 39–42, 1936.

29. Uihlein, A., MacCarty, C. S., Michenfelder, J. D., and Svein, H. J. Deep hypothermia and surgical treatment of intracranial aneurysms. A five year survey. J.A.M.A., *195:* 639–641, 1966.

CHAPTER

4

Use of Positron Emission Tomography Scanning in Cerebral Ischemia

DAVID G. T. THOMAS, F.R.C.S., JEREMY M. GIBBS, M.R.C.P., and
RICHARD J. S. WISE, M.R.C.P.

INTRODUCTION

Positron emission tomography (PET) uses short-lived radioisotopes of elements such as oxygen, nitrogen, and carbon as tracers *in vivo* both to image and to measure noninvasively normal physiology and pathophysiology in man. The technique has been applied to the study of cerebral ischemia both in serial observations on the pathophysiology of acute stroke and before and after neurosurgical interventions.

METHODOLOGY

Isotopes for PET

Pet involves the administration of a positron-emitting radioisotope, usually as a tracer with biological significance, and its subsequent detection with an imaging device, the positron computed tomograph (30). The positron-emitting radioisotopes of elements of basic biological importance have short half-lives (Table 4.1). The metabolism of oxygen is of great interest in cerebral ischemia, and oxygen 15 (^{15}O) is the longest-lived positron-emitting isotope of this element, with a half-life of 2.1 minutes. Hydrogen does not have a similar isotope, but fluorine-18 (^{18}F, 109-minute half-life) may be used as a substitute tracer for it in certain compounds, like the analogue of glucose, F-2-deoxy-D-glucose (^{18}F-DG). It is possible to manufacture the isotopes ^{15}O, ^{11}C, ^{13}N and ^{18}F by bombarding stable elements with high energy beams of particles from a cyclotron. Because the half-lives of such isotopes are so short, it is virtually essential to have the cyclotron on site when applying these tracers *in vivo*. However, in some cases the tracer may be made without a cyclotron by the decay of a more long-lived parent isotope, for example, rubidium-82 from strontium-82 (25 day half-life).

PET Scanners

When these radioisotopes decay, positrons (positively charged electrons) are emitted and travel only a few millimeters in tissue before being

51

annihilated on encountering one of the much more numerous negative electrons. As a result two 511-KeV photons are emitted, and these travel away from the site of the annihilation reaction at an angle of 180° to each other. The straight line path of these photons forms the essential physical basis of PET (30). The tomograph apparatus contains a series of opposing, paired detectors which record the arrival of photons at diametrically opposite sides of the patient's head. Annihilation coincidence detection of the emission of paired photons is coupled to the application of computerized axial tomography to provide sensitive and uniform spatial resolution with simultaneous collection of linear and angular data from the tracer distributed in the PET scan plane. Computer processing using a reconstruction algorithm provides a tomographic image of the distribution of radioactivity in the axial plane (Fig. 4.1). Several scanners have been developed, and the performance characteristics of some examples are summarized in Table 4.2. In order to provide quantitative data, calibration is necessary, and the recorded emission data must also be corrected for the loss of counts which results from attenuation by the tissues of the signal arising from deeper parts of the brain (4, 18). The ECAT II (EG and G Ortec) (40) scanner, in use at the MRC Cyclotron Unit in London, has a retractable ring of germanium-68. The radiation from this isotope is used to carry out a conventional

TABLE 4.1

Positron-emitting Radionuclides of Use in Cerebral Physiology

Isotope	Half-Life (min)	Tracer	Use
Oxygen-15	2.07	$C^{15}O_2$	Blood flow
		$H_2^{15}O$	Blood flow
		$C^{15}O$	Blood volume
		$^{15}O_2$	Oxygen utilization
Carbon-11	20.4	^{11}CO	Blood volume
		^{11}C-Alcohols	Cerebral blood flow
		^{11}C-2-deoxyglucose	Glucose utilization
		^{11}C-glucose	Glucose utilization
		^{11}C-methylglucose	Glucose transport
		^{11}C-aminoacids	Aminoacid uptake and protein synthesis
		$^{11}CO_2$	Cerebral pH
Nitrogen-13	10.0	$^{13}NH_3$	Blood flow
		^{13}N aminoacids	Aminoacid uptake and protein synthesis
Rubidium-82	1.25	$^{82}RbCl$	Blood brain barrier integrity
Fluorine-18	110.0	^{18}F-2-deoxy-D-glucose	Glucose utilization
Gallium-68	68.3	^{68}Ga-EDTA	Blood-brain barrier integrity

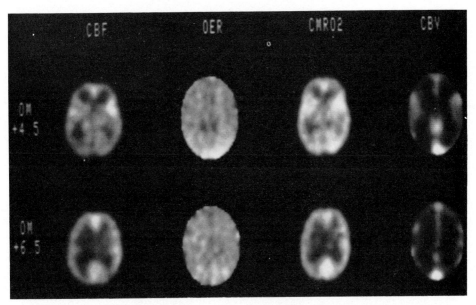

FIG. 4.1. Physiological tomographic images of CBF, OER, CMRO₂, and CBV in a normal subject, studied in two planes 4.5 and 6.5 cm above the orbitomeatal line.

transmission CT scan of the patient as well as the PET scan. The transmission scan data may then be used to make a precise regional correction for the effects of tissue attenuation.

One of the most important sources of inaccuracy in obtaining quantitative data arises from the limited spatial resolution in three dimensions (17, 26). Each PET scanner is characterized by its functional response to a point source. The full width at half the maximum height (FWHM) can be measured (Table 4.2). The counts recorded within a chosen region of interest depend on the relationship between the size of the region and the spatial resolution of the tomograph being used. Failure to record all the counts from a small region constitutes the so-called partial volume effect (17,26). It is probable that errors arise in measuring tracer concentration in brain when the object of study is smaller than twice the FWHM. This quantitative uncertainty emphasizes the need to push the spatial resolution of PET scanners to their theoretical physical limits in order to achieve the most meaningful results in quantitative clinical studies. Newer instruments exist with a spatial resolution of 6–8 mm, and others are projected with a resolution of 2 mm. Other important considerations for accuracy are the statistics of the collected data, the methods for subtraction and calculation of random coincidences, the response characteristics of the detectors, and the method of attenuation

TABLE 4.2
Performance of Typical PET Scanners

Scanner	PC384 Scanditronix	Neuroecat (Ortec)	Neuropet (NIH)	Pett VI (Nucletronix)	Therascan (Aerl)	Toppet (LET 1)
Detector	48-cm ring (×4) 96 crystals	60-cm octagon (×3) 8 crystals	38-cm ring (×4) 128 crystals	57-cm ring (×4) 72 crystals	43-cm ring (×2) 64 crystals	96-cm ring (×4) 96 crystals
Image field	26 cm	25 cm	23 cm	27 cm	30 cm	50 cm
Resolution (Full width at half the maximum height = FWHM)						
Transaxial	8 mm	8 mm	6 mm	8 mm	11.5 mm	7 mm
Axial	12 mm	15 mm	12 mm	15 mm	16 mm	
Sensitivity normalized to 1 cm of crystal height direct plane (C/sec/Ci/ml)	5500	1900	10500	2600	8300	6100

correction. Consideration of these factors is essential for critical assessment of studies performed on different scanners as well as for evaluation of serial or comparative studies on one instrument.

Tracer Procedures

In order to extract the most meaningful physiological data from PET, it is necessary to understand the fate of the labeled tracer in the body and to have a model for its behavioral distribution in the tissues. Where valid models exist, quantitation is possible. This applies now for some substances, like glucose and oxygen, which are important in cerebral ischemia. Where valid models for tracer behavior do not exist, for example, in certain labeled drugs, the studies can only be semiquantitative or qualitative. The model is used to set up mathematical equations used by the scan computer. The solution of equations requires data on the course of regional tissue concentration of isotope, provided by the tomograph, together with data on tracer input, usually provided by serial arterial blood samples.

CEREBRAL BLOOD FLOW, OXYGEN UTILIZATION, AND BLOOD VOLUME

Cerebral blood flow (CBF) may be measured by PET using steady-state or dynamic techniques. The ^{15}O steady-state inhalation method has been most widely used for the measurement of blood flow and oxygen utilization in cerebral ischemia (8, 9, 19, 21, 22, 41). Dynamic techniques (43) can be divided into washout or uptake and have been used less widely. The accuracy of the washout method for blood flow is probably similar to that of the steady-state model, while the uptake method may offer improvement. However, the error sensitivity of both of these methods for oxygen utilization is still not well defined. The blood volume-corrected, ^{15}O steady-state inhalation technique was used to produce most of the results illustrated here, and its theory and implementation will be described.

The patient lies supine on the bed of the PET scanner and inhales through a face mask first tracer amounts of cyclotron—produced $C^{15}O_2$. ^{15}O is transferred to water ($H_2^{15}O$) in the lung capillaries by the enzymatic action of carbonic anhydrase. This water circulates in the arterial blood and distributes in the brain throughout the cerebral tissue. If the patient remains at rest, the regional isotope concentration reaches equilibrium in 3–5 half-lives (6–10 minutes). At this stage, constant delivery of ^{15}O in water of circulation is matched by washout and radioactive decay. The concentration of $H_2^{15}O$ does not reach arterial levels, but the higher the flow in tissue the more closely it approaches arterial levels. At the steady state during $C^{15}O_2$ inhalation, regional tissue concentration of $H_2^{15}O$ is related to regional blood flow (rCBF) (8). The patient then inhales ^{15}O-labeled molecular oxygen ($^{15}O_2$). This becomes bound in the lungs to hemoglobin and circulates to the tissues. In the brain, it is used in aerobic respiration and is converted to $H_2^{15}O$, "water of metabolism." In the steady state during $^{15}O_2$ inhalation, regional tissue concentration of $H_2^{15}O$ is proportional to rCBF × rOER (regional oxygen extraction ratio or fraction of oxygen extracted from available arterial blood) because arterial $^{15}O_2$ concentration is constant. rOER may therefore be determined as the ratio of regional concentrations of $H_2^{15}O$ during the $^{15}O_2$ inhalation and $C^{15}O_2$ inhalation periods. Effectively, the tomograph is measuring levels of water of metabolism against water of circulation. If the regional $[H_2^{15}O]$* has been formed this way and the plasma and whole arterial blood $[H_2^{15}O]$ are measured by counting samples in a well counter, then equations may be solved to calculate rCBF and rOER in absolute units (8, 20, 41).

Using the value for water of metabolism obtained during $^{15}O_2$ inhalation and the ratio rOER, the regional cerebral metabolic rate for oxygen (rCMRO$_2$) can be derived in absolute units from the equation:

$$rCMRO_2 = rCBF \times rOER \times \text{stable oxygen content of arterial blood.}$$

Theoretical and statistical analysis shows that rOER may be overestimated unless allowance is made for the signal arising from unextracted hemoglobin-bound $^{15}O_2$ in the vascular compartment during the phase of $^{15}O_2$ inhalation, which is superimposed upon the signal arising from metabolically produced $H_2^{15}O$ within the tissues. This would lead to an overestimated value of tissue $H_2^{15}O$. A correction for this value for cerebral blood volume (rCBV) may be incorporated into the tracer equation (21, 22). In order to measure rCBV, a single bolus tracer dose of labeled carbon monoxide (^{11}CO) is given to the patient through the face mask. This isotope, with a half-life of 20.4 minutes, and the ^{11}CO bind to hemoglobin and therefore remain confined to the vascular compartment during the third phase of the PET scan. ^{11}CO is also measured in a venous blood sample, and rCBV is calculated. The fourth phase of the examination is a transmission CT scan employing the external ring source of ^{68}Ge, referred to previously. The measurement of rCBF by this method reflects capillary blood flow (tissue perfusion) since the technique is dependent on the tissue exchange of labeled water. Blood flowing through arteriovenous shunts is not measured. The measured rCBV, on the other hand, does not reflect only capillary vascularity but the volume of all blood vessels within a chosen region of interest. Images of the PET

---

* [ ] indicates "concentration of".

scan can present color-coded or grey scale quantitation of CBF, OER, CMRO$_2$, and CBV (Fig. 4.1). Further analysis may be done relating anatomical areas, like cortex *vs.* white matter, or region of interest (ROI), for example, infarct, to numerical printouts of quantitative data. The minimum size of ROI considered statistically significant was 2.6 cm^2. Results from the application of these methods in cerebral ischemia will be considered after description of a second tracer model.

METABOLISM OF GLUCOSE

The regional cerebral glucose utilization (rCMRGlu) may be measured *in vivo* in man by means of an adaptation by Phelps *et al.* (29, 34) of the model developed by Sokoloff *et al.* (39) to trace the distribution of ^{14}C-deoxyglucose (^{14}C-DG) by autoradiography in experimental animals. The labeled glucose analog competes with normal glucose for facilitated transport from the blood stream into brain cells. Once inside the cell, it competes with normal glucose for hexokinase-mediated phosphorylation. However, then the phosphorylated deoxyglucose is effectively trapped in the cell. It is an analog which cannot proceed further in the metabolic pathway of glucose. It is limited to its ability to leave the cell because of poor membrane permeability and the low levels of phosphatase in brain cells. Thus the model is free of problems associated with washout of labeled products from the tissue, and a bolus administration of the tracer can be used. Early after injection the ^{18}F-deoxyglucose (^{18}FDG) in tissue will be mainly nonphosphorylated, but by 45 minutes most of it is in the form of intracellular ^{18}F-deoxyglucose-6-phosphate (^{18}FDG-6-P). The results described below come from studies using an intravenous infusion of ^{18}FDG over a 2-minute period, with scanning of the patient 50 minutes later. Arterial blood is taken, and serial levels of ^{18}FDG were measured, initially at 20-second intervals. Mean arterial blood glucose levels were calculated from four samples at 20-minute intervals.

The analysis assumes that the distribution of ^{18}FDG follows the model and involves a lumped constant (LC) which defines the relative difference between the brain's handling of ^{18}FDG and glucose (2, 5–7, 11, 35, 37, 38, 42). LC has been measured directly in animals, but no direct regional measurements have been made in man. The value used here has been that quoted for normal cerebral tissue by Huang and colleagues (19). The equation used for calculation of CMRGlu is:

$$CMRGlu - Ci^*(T)Cp / \left(LC \int_0^T Cp^*(t) \, dt \right)$$

where Ci^* (T) is the measured tissue concentration of tracer by PET (^{18}FDG + ^{18}FDG-6-P) at a time T, p* (t) is the arterial plasma concentration of ^{18}FDG at any time between 0 and T, Cp is the measured plasma concentration of glucose, and LC is the lumped constant. Regional glucose extraction ratios (rGER) were calculated using the equation:

$$rCMRGlu = rCBF \times rGER \times Cp$$

Functional images of the PET scans for CMRGlu and rGER can be presented, as previously shown for rCBF, rCMRO, and CBV, using color or grey scale read out (Fig. 4.2). Likewise, numerical analysis is feasible for anatomical areas of interest. The equation used above is a simplified one (35), and there remains controversy about the values of the lumped constant as well as about the optimum way in which the mathematical model can be made to incorporate all of the relevant rate constants for transport, phosphorylation, and dephosphorylation. However, in spite of discussion about the accuracy of quantitative measurements of glucose utilization in cerebral ischemia by PET, several findings of interest have emerged.

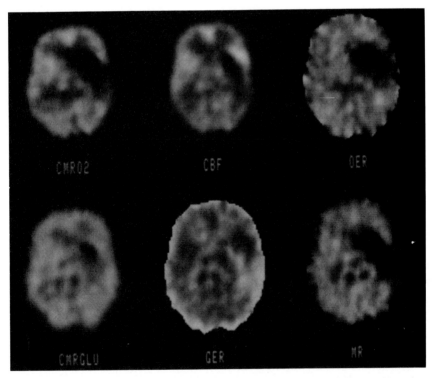

FIG. 4.2. PET images of a patient with a right hemisphere stroke studied some days after the onset. Note the low *OER*, but partial preservation of glucose metabolism (*CMRGlu*) in relation to very low *CMRO$_2$* in the infarcted area. The regional reduction of the metabolic

RESULTS OF PET STUDIES IN CEREBRAL ISCHEMIA

Acute Stroke

In cerebral ischemia, rCBF has been studied by several noninvasive methods during the past two decades (12, 24). Such studies have revealed altered regulation of blood flow in brain damaged by ischemia. However, it has become evident that rCBF alone is a poor indicator of residual tissue function. It is anticipated that oxygen utilization ($rCMRO_2$) at the onset of ischemia will be limited by oxygen delivery rather than by the brain's metabolic demand, resulting in maximal extraction of available oxygen (rOER). Later, when mitochondrial function has been impaired, the $rCMRO_2$ and rOER will fall even if rCBF is maintained, the situation of luxury perfusion related to infarction (23). A typical example is shown in Figure 4.2.

With PET scanning rCBF, $rCMRO_2$, and rCMRGlu can be measured directly simultaneously, which may be hoped to lead to more understanding than provided by rCBF measurements alone. Several studies (10, 33, 36) have shown uncoupling of rCBF and $rCMRO_2$ in ischemic or infarcted brain. Most patient studies have been done relatively late when mitochondrial function has become impaired and presumably infarction has become established with a variable degree of reflow present in the improperly autoregulated vascular bed. Consistent findings in PET studies at this stage have been depressed $rCMRO_2$, with low rOER reflecting "luxury perfusion," while rCBF has varied between high, normal, or low. A recent study (41) of 34 patients evaluated acutely as early as 3 hours after nonhemorrhagic cerebral infarction has shown, in the nine patients studied earliest after onset of the stroke, elevated rOER suggestive of ischemia rather than infarction. Serial studies were performed in these patients, and the initially raised OER fell over the next week. In some cases this was related to a fall in $rCMRO_2$ with a further fall in rCBF, while in others rCBF increased without recovery of $rCMRO_2$. Regional OER in white matter and subcortical grey matter tended to be lower than that in overlying cortex in the first few hours or days. This probably reflects an earlier transition to infarction from ischemia in the deeper parts of the hemisphere, possibly related to anatomical vascular factors.

A second study compared rCMRGlu with $rCMRO_2$ in eight patients with recent cerebral infarction, in most cases within four days of the ictus (42). Mean rCMRGlu, as well as rCBF and $rCMRO_2$, were significantly depressed within the infarcts compared to the mirror regions of the contralateral hemispheres (Table 4.3). Regional $CMRO_2$ and rCMRGlu were significantly correlated together within the infarcts, and the metabolic ratio (MR) was in the region of 0.2–0.25, compared with an MR of about 0.65 in contralateral brain (see Fig. 4.3). One may infer

TABLE 4.3

Metabolism in Infarcted and Contralateral Brain

Cortex[b]	Infarcted Brain	Contralateral
CBF (ml/100 ml/mm)	14.2 ± 7.3	32.7 ± 10.0^{c}
CMRO (ml/100 ml/mm)	0.7 ± 0.4	2.7 ± 0.7^{c}
CMRGlu (mg/100 ml/mm)	3.0 ± 1.2	4.4 ± 0.9^{d}
OER	0.3 ± 0.15	0.45 ± 0.10^{c}
GER	0.23 ± 0.09	0.13 ± 0.3^{d}
MR (ml O_2/mg glucose)	0.23 ± 0.09	0.63 ± 0.21^{d}
Lentiform nucleus		
CBF (ml/100 ml/mm)	15.9 ± 3.7	43.4 ± 6.5^{c}
CMRO (ml/10 ml/mm)	0.6 ± 0.4	3.2 ± 0.4^{c}
CMRGlu (mg/100 ml/mm)	2.7 ± 0.7	5.2 ± 0.9^{c}
OER	0.20 ± 0.14	0.40 ± 0.05^{d}
GER	0.18 ± 0.05	0.12 ± 0.02^{d}
MR (ml O_2/mg glucose)	0.19 ± 0.11	0.64 ± 0.19^{d}

[a] From R. J. S. Wise *et al.* (42).
[b] Mean values for cortex ($n = 9$) and lentiform nucleus ($N = 6$).
[c] $p < 0.001$.
[d] $p < 0.05$.

from this that in the infarct, 2 moles of oxygen were consumed per mole of glucose, that is, one-third the moles of oxygen that were consumed in the contralateral brain in the patients or in normal control brain. This suggests that the tissue in the region of a recent cerebral infarct utilizes aerobic glycolysis. It may be assumed from pathological evidence that the principal viable cell population of an early infarct consists of neutrophils and macrophages and that these cells are chiefly reliant on aerobic glycolysis for metabolism. Therefore, the low rOER and rMR found experimentally in infarcts would be compatible with the metabolism of abundant phagocytic cells clearing tissue debris. A degree of caution is necessary before accepting this conclusion on the basis of PET evidence, because of difficulties touched on in the earlier description of the methods which arise from current tracer methodology. The principal difficulty is the assumption that the lumped constant in the infarct is the same as in normal brain. Alternative PET methods (16, 32), employing labeled glucose, avoid this particular problem, and it will be important to compare the results obtained with them with the results described here.

Occlusive Carotid Artery Disease and Extracranial-Intracranial Anastomosis

The above PET studies have contributed substantially to our understanding of acute cerebral ischemia, showing in particular the important relationship between oxygen supply and cerebral metabolic demands.

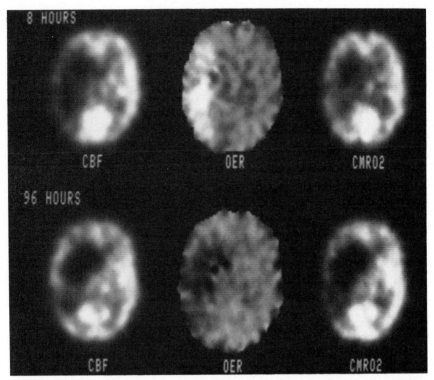

FIG. 4.3. PET images of a patient with acute cerebral infarction in left middle cerebral artery territory. Note the partial preservation of $CMRO_2$ in the acute stage (8 hours), maintained in the face of very low CBF by increased fractional oxygen extraction (OER). The later study (96 hours) shows some cortical reflow, but $CMRO_2$ has fallen further, and OER is abnormally low-relative luxury perfusion in infarcted brain.

Nevertheless, established stroke remains an irreversible and untreatable disorder in the vast majority of patients, even those admitted to hospital within hours of the onset of symptoms. One group of patients in whom medical and surgical intervention could theoretically reduce stroke risk are those with occlusive carotid artery disease. Both ulcerative and obstructive lesions of the internal carotid artery are associated with an increased risk of cerebral infarction in the ipsilateral cerebral hemisphere. Embolic events may possibly be reduced in frequency by antiplatelet medication or by surgical endarterectomy, although neither approach has yet been shown to be of definite value by adequate clinical trials. Much attention has also been focused in recent years on the technique of extracranial-intracranial (EC-IC) bypass surgery, in which the superficial temporal branch of the external carotid artery is anastomosed to the middle cerebral branch of the internal carotid system. The precise role of this procedure is still uncertain, although it should theoretically be of value when an otherwise inoperable lesion of the carotid or middle cerebral artery threatens to reduce ipsilateral cerebral blood flow to a critically low level. Although such a state of hemodynamic perfusion failure can occasionally be diagnosed on clinical grounds (3), in practice it is often difficult to establish whether continuing episodes of cerebral ischemia are due to an embolic or hemodynamic mechanism, even in the presence of complete carotid occlusion (1). It is in this situation that the combined physiological measurements possible with PET may be of practical value to the clinician.

Early studies by Grubb and colleagues, using positron-emitting isotopes with a nontomographic detector system, showed that there are patients with occlusive cerebrovascular disease in whom CBF is critically low in relation to continuing metabolic demands (15). As in acute stroke (41), this situation is characterized by increased fractional extraction of oxygen from the available blood supply, a state referred to by Baron and co-workers as "misery perfusion" (3). The finding of *inappropriately* low CBF and raised OER in a patient with carotid occlusion is therefore a conclusive indication that cerebral perfusion has fallen to a critically low level. Blood flow can no longer be matched to cerebral metabolic demands by the normal mechanism of autoregulation, and any further fall of perfusion pressure could precipitate cerebral infarction. Following the original observations of Grubb and colleagues (15), PET studies have confirmed that this mismatching of CBF and $CMRO_2$ is present in a minority of patients considered for EC-IC bypass surgery (9) and that the abnormal pattern of raised OER can be reversed by this procedure (3). Figure 4.4 shows an example of critical cerebral perfusion in a patient with bilateral occlusive carotid disease, with CBF low and OER focally raised in the territory of an occluded left internal carotid artery. In this case, endarterectomy of a severely stenosed contralateral internal carotid artery was sufficient to restore normal CBF and OER on the symptomatic side. The patient remained clinically unchanged, and there was no change of cerebral function, as judged by regional $CMRO_2$, in either hemisphere.

Earlier work in the experimental animal (13) and in patients with subarachnoid hemorrhage (14) suggested that a reduction in cerebral perfusion pressure might also be detectable as a rise in cerebral blood volume (CBV), reflecting the state of compensatory vasodilatation which maintains flow as perfusion pressure falls. This suggestion has recently been supported by studies carried out in two PET centers on patients with occlusive carotid artery disease (9, 25, 31). The findings from these studies imply that within the range of effective autoregulation, while CBF is still being maintained at an appropriate level and OER is normal, rising CBV may be the first and most sensitive index of diminishing

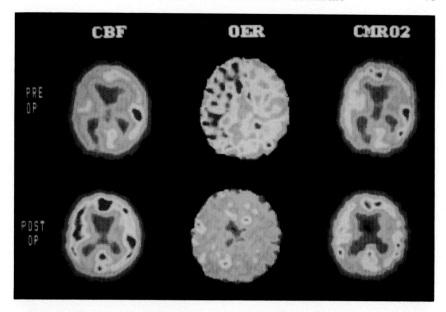

FIG. 4.4. PET images before and after surgery in a patient with bilateral carotid artery disease (complete occlusion on the left and stenosis on the right). Note the low CBF and raised OER in left carotid territory, which returned to normal after a contralateral endarterectomy.

cerebral perfusion pressure. Figure 4.5 shows a typical example of a patient with unilateral carotid artery occlusion whose cerebral blood flow was not significantly reduced but in whom cerebral blood volume was increased in the territory distal to the occluded vessel. Such a state of compensatory vasodilatation has been previously observed indirectly by other workers as impairment or loss of the capacity to increase regional CBF in response to inhaled carbon dioxide (27). The CBV changes are unlikely to be due to arteriolar dilatation alone (9) but nonetheless appear to provide useful information about cerebral perfusion pressure. It is clear that the extent of circulatory *reserve* is more important than the absolute level of cerebral blood flow when considering patients for bypass surgery. There is some evidence to suggest that even without a measurement of regional OER, which at present can be achieved only by PET, combined analysis of CBF and CBV may provide a valuable index of cerebral circulatory reserves in patients with occlusive carotid artery disease (9). Preliminary observations in our Unit (Gibbs *et al.*, unpublished data) and by Martin and colleagues (25) indicate that the predominant change after EC-IC bypass surgery may be a fall of the previously elevated CBV, often with little or no change of cerebral blood flow.

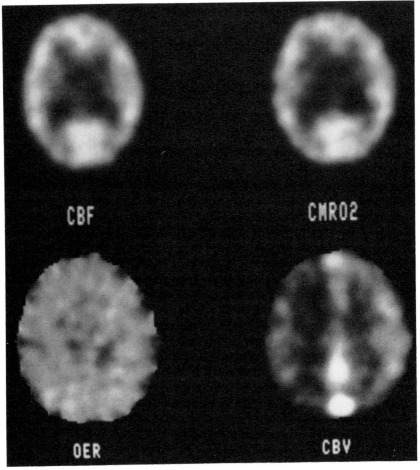

FIG. 4.5. PET images in a patient with occlusion of the right internal carotid artery. Note that there is no asymmetry of blood flow (*CBF*), but that there is a substantial increase of blood volume (*CBV*) distal to the occluded vessel.

Subarachnoid Hemorrhage

Both focal and generalized disturbances of cerebral function after subarachnoid hemorrhage (SAH) may often be attributable to secondary cerebral ischemia, rather than simply to the direct effect of hemorrhage on the brain and the presence of blood in the cerebrospinal fluid. The development of late ischemic complications does not correlate very closely with the degree of arterial spasm demonstrated angiographically and, with particular regard to the timing and risks of operative intervention, additional information obtained by other methods about the cerebral circulation may be of considerable value in the practical management of patients with SAH.

Several studies carried out with various techniques have shown that cerebral blood flow may be substantially reduced in patients with recent SAH (14, 25). However, as in the case of cerebral infarction due to occlusive vascular disease, the relationship of CBF to the prevailing metabolic demands of the tissue is more important than the absolute level of blood flow considered alone. Low CBF in a deeply comatose patient is not necessarily an indication of primary cerebral ischemia since the existing flow may be appropriately matched to the reduced metabolic requirements of a damaged brain. Again, the application of positron-emitting isotopes has allowed measurement of multiple physiological variables, rather than of CBF alone.

A major limitation of the use of PET in the study of SAH arises from the risk involved in transporting severely ill patients with aneurysms from one center to another. Unless the PET facilities are situated close to the wards of a neurosurgical referral center, such studies cannot be justified on ethical grounds. For this reason, very few patients with SAH from the National Hospitals have been studied at the MRC Cyclotron Unit in the Hammersmith Hospital.

The earliest combined measurements of cerebral blood flow and metabolism in SAH were carried out by Grubb and colleagues at the Washington School of Medicine in St. Louis, originally using ^{15}O-labeled tracers with a nontomographic detector system (14). Both CBF and $CMRO_2$ were found to be depressed after SAH, the degree of reduction correlating fairly closely with the severity of clinical grading. Among all grades of patients, those with angiographic evidence of significant vasospasm generally had lower values of CBF and $CMRO_2$ than those without spasm. Although the data for fractional oxygen extraction were not given, proportionally greater reduction of CBF than of $CMRO_2$ in all patient groups indicated that the OER was raised in these cases. Another striking observation was that CBV was increased, the extent of this increase correlating closely with the degree of clinical severity as judged by focal neurological deficit and the presence of vasospasm. Patients graded at III or IV on the Hunt and Hess scale who also had vasospasm were found to have a mean CBV 58% higher than normal controls. As in the patients with occlusive carotid artery disease discussed above, this rise of CBV may have resulted from compensatory vasodilatation in response to diminished cerebral perfusion pressure. However, the situation in acute SAH is somewhat more complicated than in patients with carotid disease studied at a time when they are asymptomatic. Although spasm of proximal arteries is likely to reduce cerebral perfusion pressure in cases of SAH, other factors such as cerebral edema and raised intracranial pressure may have profound effects on the CBV which are independent of perfusion pressure.

More recent studies from the same center using PET measurements of regional CBF, $CMRO_2$, and CBV have produced very similar results (25). Blood flow and metabolism were found to be more severely depressed in patients with marked vasospasm than in those without it. CBV was virtually normal in patients without vasospasm but was consistently increased in the vascular territory distal to arterial spasm in affected cases.

The few cases of SAH studied in our Unit have been in good clinical condition (Grade I or II), without significant spasm demonstrated angiographically. No focal abnormality of CBV, $CMRO_2$, or CBV has yet been observed in any of these patients, although values of flow and metabolism are generally lower than normal throughout the brain, as in the cases reported from St. Louis. One important technical difficulty arises in carrying out PET studies in more severely ill patients with SAH, a problem also encountered in some acute stroke cases. Strict maintenance of the patient's head position throughout all four phases of the scanning procedure ($^{15}O_2$, $C^{15}O_2$, transmission scan, and ^{11}CO scan, lasting 1½ hours in all) becomes extremely difficult. This aspect of PET procedure should always be kept in mind when evaluating quantitative results obtained from severely ill patients who may be restless and uncooperative.

CONCLUSIONS

Pet has already contributed results of interest in the study of stroke, subarachnoid hemorrhage, carotid occlusion, and in EC-IC bypass surgery, and it is probabl that it will be applied increasingly as a research method in cerebral ischemia. However, the use of PET in neurosurgery is severely limited at present, and for the forseeable future, by both theoretical and practical constraints. The problems of tracer methodology and of scanner resolution must constantly be borne in mind when interpreting the data obtained. Although less invasive than cerebral angiography, it does require cannulation of veins and often of arteries, together with the administration of radioactive isotopes. The patient's head must not move during a satisfactory scan, and this precludes the study of a restless patient. Limited studies may be made in less than an hour, but the use of multiple tracers to obtain the fullest information may take much longer. The patient, possibly gravely ill, must be brought to the scanner, which will generally be at the site of the cyclotron. The capital and running costs of the equipment are very expensive, and its use implies the collaboration of skilled scientists, both physicists and radiochemists, with clinicians. PET is likely to increase in its importance as a method of investigation for research and has a limited role in management of a small group of selected cases of cerebral ischemia.

REFERENCES

1. Barnett, H. J. M. Delayed cerebral ischaemic episodes distal to occlusion of major cerebral arteries. Neurology (Minneap.), 28: 769–774, 1978.
2. Baron, J. C. In vivo methods for measuring regional glucose metabolic rate (GLMR) (Reply). J. Nucl. Med., 24: 367, 1983.
3. Baron, J. C., Bousser, M. G., Rey, A., Guillard, A., Comar, D., and Castaigne, P. Reversal of "misery-perfusion syndrome" by extra-intracranial arterial bypass in haemodynamic cerebral ischaemia. Stroke, 12: 454–459, 1981.
4. Bergstrom, M., Litton, J., Ericsson, L., Bohm, C., and Blomgrist, G. Determination of object contour from projections for attenuation correction in cranial positron emission tomography. J. Comput. Assist. Tomogr. 6: 365–372, 1982.
5. Brooks, R. A., DiChiro, G. In vivo methods for measuring regional glucose metabolic rate (GLMR) (Reply). J. Nucl. Med., 25: 136, 1984.
6. Brooks, R. A., DiChiro, G., and Patronas, N. J. In vivo methods for measuring regional glucose metabolic rate (GLMR) (Reply). J. Nucl. Med., 24: 367, 1983.
7. DiChiro, G., Brooks, R. A., Patronas, N. J., Bairamian, D., Kornblith, P. L., Smith, B. H., Mansi, L., and Barker, J. Issues in the in vivo measurement of glucose metabolism of human central nervous system tumors. Ann. Neurol., 15 (Suppl): S138–S146, 1984.
8. Frackowiak, R. S. J., Lenzi, G. L., Jones, T., and Heather, J. L. Quantitative measurements of regional cerebral blood flow and oxygen metabolism in man using 0 and positron emission tomography: Theory, procedure and normal values. J. Comput. Assist. Tomogr., 4 (6): 727–736, 1980.
9. Gibbs, J. M., Wise, R. S. J., Leenders, K. L., and Jones, T. Evaluation of cerebral perfusion reserve in patients with carotid artery occlusion. Lancet, 1: 310–314, 1984.
10. Ginsberg, M. D., Mela, L., Wrobel-Kuhl, K., and Reivich, M. Mitochondrial metabolism following bilateral cerebral ischaemia in the gerbil. Ann. Neurol., 1: 519–527, 1977.
11. Gjedde, A. In vivo methods for measuring regional glucose metabolic rate (GLMR). J. Nucl. Med., 25: 134, 1984.
12. Glass, H. I., and Harper, A. M. Measurements of regional blood flow in cerebral cortex in man through intact skull. Br. Med. J., 1: 593, 1963.
13. Grubb, R. L., Phelps, M. E., and Raichle, M. E. The effects of arterial blood pressure on the regional cerebral blood volume by X-ray fluorescence. Stroke, 4: 390–399, 1973.
14. Grubb, R. L., Raichle, M. E., Eichling, J. D., and Gado, M. H. Effects of subarachnoid haemorrhage on cerebral blood volume, blood flow and oxygen utilisation in humans. J. Neurosurg., 46: 446–453, 1977.
15. Grubb, R. L., Ratcheson, R. A., Raichle, M. E., Kliefoth, A. B., and Gado, M. H. Regional cerebral blood flow and oxygen utilisation in superficial temporal-middle cerebral artery anastomosis patients. J. Neurosurg., 50: 733–741, 1979.
16. Hawkins, R. A., Phelps, M. E., Huang, S-C., and Kuhl, D. E. Effect of ischaemia on quantitation of local cerebral glucose metabolic rate in man. J. Cereb. Blood Flow Metab., 1: 37–51, 1981.
17. Hoffmann, E. J., Huang, S-C., and Phelps, M. E. Quantitation in positron emission computed tomography. 1. Effect of object size. J. Comput. Assist. Tomogr., 3: 299–308, 1979.
18. Huang, S-C., Hoffmann, E. J., Phelps, M. E., and Kuhl, D. E. Quantitation in positron emission computed tomography. 2. Effects of inaccurate attenuation correction. J. Comput. Assist. Tomogr., 3: 804–814, 1979.

19. Huang, S-C., Phelps, M. E., Hoffmann, E. J., Sideris, K., Selin, C. J., and Kuhl, D. E. Non invasive determination of local cerebral metabolic rate of glucose in man. Am. J. Physiol., *238*: E69–E82, 1980.

20. Ito, M., Lammertsma, A. A., Wise, R. J. S., Bernard, S., Frackowiak, R. S. J., Heather, J. D., McKenzie, C. G., Thomas, D. G. T., and Jones, T. Measurement of regional cerebral blood flow and oxygen utilisation in patients with cerebral tumours using 0 positron emission tomography: Analytical techniques and preliminary results. Neuroradiology, *23*: 63–74, 1982.

21. Lammertsma, A. A., and Jones, T. Correction for the presence of intravascular oxygen-15 in the steady state technique for measuring regional oxygen extraction ratio in the brain. 1. Description of the method. J. Cereb. Blood Flow Metab., *3*: 416–424, 1983.

22. Lammertsma, A. S., Wise, R. J. S., Heather, J. D., Gibbs, J. M., Leenders, K. L., Frackowiak, R. S. J., Rhodes, C. G., and Jones, T. Correction for the presence of intravascular oxygen-15 in the steady state technique for measuring regional oxygen extraction ratio in the brain. 2. Results in normal subjects and brain tumour and stroke patients. J. Cereb. Blood Flow Metab., *3*: 425–431, 1983.

23. Lassen, N. A. The luxury-perfusion syndrome and its possible relation to acute metabolic acidosis localised within the brain. Lancet, *2*: 1113–1115, 1966.

24. Lassen, N. A., Hoedt-Rasmussen, K., Sorensen, S. C., Skinhoj, E., Cronquist, S., Bodforss, B., and Ingvan, D. H. Regional cerebral blood flow in man determined by Krypton-85. Neurology (Minneap.), *13*: 719–727, 1963.

25. Martin, W. R. W., Baker, R. P., Grubb, R. L., and Raichle, M. E. Cerebral blood volume, blood flow and oxygen metabolism in cerebral ischaemia and subarachnoid haemorrhage: An *in vivo* study using positron emission tomography. Acta Neurochir., *70*: 3–9, 1984.

26. Mazziotta, J. C., Phelps, M. E., Plummer, D., and Kuhl, D. E. Quantitation in positron emission computed tomography. 5. Physical-anatomical effects. J. Comp. Assist. Tomogr., *5*: 734–743, 1981.

27. Norrving, B., Nilsson, B., and Risberg, J. rCBF in patients with carotid occlusion: Resting and hypercapnic flow related to collateral pattern. Stroke, *13*: 155–162, 1982.

28. Phelps, M. E., Huang, S-C., Hoffmann, E. J., and Kuhl, D. E. Validation of tomographic measurement of cerebral blood volume with C-11 labelled carboxy hemoglobin. J. Nucl. Med., *20*: 328–334, 1979.

29. Phelps, M. E., Huang, S-C., Hoffmann, E. J., Selin, C., Sokoloff, L., and Kuhl, D. E. Tomographic measurement of local cerebral glucose metabolic rate in humans with (F-18) 2-fluoro-2-deoxy-D-glucose: Validation of method. Ann. Neurol., *6*: 371–388, 1979.

30. Phelps, M. E., Hoffman, E. J., Mullani, N. A., and Ter-Pogossian, M. M. Application of annihilation coincidence detection by transaxial reconstruction tomography. J. Nucl. Med., *16*: 210–223, 1975.

31. Powers, W., Martin, W., Herscovitch, P., Raichle, M., and Grubb, R. The value of regional cerebral blood volume measurement in the diagnosis of cerebral ischemia. J. Cereb. Blood Flow Metabol., *3* (Suppl.): S-598–S599, 1983.

32. Raichle, M. E., Larson, K. B., Phelps, M. E., Grubb, R. L. J., Welch, M. J., and Ter-Pogossian, M. M. *In vivo* measurement of brain glucose transport and metabolism employing glucose ^{11}C. Am. J. Physiol., *228*: 1936–1948, 1975.

33. Rehncrona, S., Mela, L., and Siesjo, B. K. Recovery of brain mitochondrial function in the rat after complete and incomplete cerebral ischemia. Stroke, *10*: 437–446, 1979.

34. Reivich, M., Kuhl, D. E., Wolf, A., Greenberg, J., Phelps, M. E., Ido, T., Casella, V., Fowler, J., Hoffmann, E., Alavi, A., and Sokoloff, L. The ^{18}F-fluorodeoxy glucose

method for the measurement of local cerebral glucose utilisation in man. Circ. Res., *44:* 127–137, 1979.

35. Rhodes, C. G., Wise, R. J. S., Gibbs, J. M., Frackowiak, R. S. J., Hatazawa, J., Palmer, A. J., Thomas, D. G. T., and Jones, T. *In vivo* disturbance of the oxidative metabolism of glucose in human cerebral gliomas. Ann. Neurol., *14:* 614–626, 1983.

36. Schutz, H., Silverstein, P. R., Vapalathti, M., Bruce, D. A., Mela, L., and Langfitt, W. W. Brain mitochondrial function after ischemia and hypoxia. 1. Ischemia induced by increased intracranial pressure. Arch. Neurol. (Chicago), *29:* 408–416, 1973.

37. Selikson, M. H. *In vivo* methods for measuring regional glucose metabolic rate (GLMR) (Reply). J. Nucl. Med., *24:* 366–367, 1983.

38. Selikson, M. *In vivo* methods for measuring regional glucose metabolic rate (GLMR). (Reply). J. Nucl. Med., *25:* 134–136, 1984.

39. Sokoloff, L., Reivich, M., Kennedy, C., Des Rosiers, M. H., Patlak, C. S., Pettigrew, K. D., Sakurada, D., and Shinohara, M. The C deoxyglucose method for the measurement of local cerebral glucose utilisation: Theory, procedure and normal values in the conscious and anaesthetised albino rat. J. Neurochem., *28:* 897–916, 1977.

40. Williams, C. M., Crabtree, M. C., and Burgiss, S. G. Design and performance characteristics of a positron emission coupled axial tomograph ECAT-11 IEEE Trans. Nucl. Sci., *NS-26:* 619–627, 1979.

41. Wise, R. J. S., Berdardi, S., Frackowiak, R. S. J., Legg, N. J., and Jones, T. Serial observations on the pathophysiology of acute stroke. The transition from ischaemia to infarction as reflected in regional oxygen extraction. Brain, *106:* 197–222, 1983.

42. Wise, R. J. S., Rhodes, C. G., Gibbs, J. M., Hatazawa, J., Palmer, T., Frackowiak, R. S. J., and Jones, T. Disturbance of oxidative metabolism of glucose in recent human cerebral infarcts. Ann. Neurol., *14:* 627–637, 1983.

43. Yamamoto, Y. L., Diksio, M., Sako, K., Arita, N., Feindel, W., and Thompson, C. J. Pharmaco kinetic and metabolic studies in human malignant glioma. In: *Functional Radionuclide Imaging of the Brain,* edited by P. L. Magistratti, Raven Press, New York, 1983, pp. 327–335.

5

Cerebral Arterial Spasm

GEORGE S. ALLEN, M.D., PH.D.

The results of our first trial of nimodipine in patients with a subarachnoid hemorrhage provide useful data on the natural history of cerebral arterial spasm as well as the effectiveness of nimodipine (1). This data, along with other studies, will be used in this report to discuss the clinical problem of deficits from spasm; a previous hypothesis of the cause of spasm; the prevention and treatment of spasm; and the remaining clinical problem of the relationship among spasm, rebleeding, and surgery.

CLINICAL PROBLEM

An important distinction must be made between angiographic spasm and the ischemic neurological deficits due to cerebral arterial spasm as documented by angiography. The true incidence of angiographic spasm in patients following a subarachnoid hemorrhage is unknown. To arrive at this incidence, one would need to angiogram a group of patients at frequent intervals for 3 weeks following the hemorrhage, regardless of the clinical condition. This is obviously not practical, and has not been done. It is known, however, that the frequency of angiographic spasm during the first 3–4 days following the initial subarachnoid hemorrhage is extremely low (1–2%). This percentage is probably higher if patients are included who have bled a week or so prior to admission and a second bleed is the cause of their admission. In these cases, the angiographic spasm is presumably a result of the first hemorrhage.

The incidence of ischemic neurological deficits from documented angiographic spasm is better known. This incidence was 27% in our placebo group (1). The prospective tranexamic trial incidence was 28% in the group receiving tranexamic acid (28). In our nimodipine trial, over half the patients were taking aminocaproic acid; thus, the 27% in our placebo group coincides well with the 28% documented in the tranexamic acid study. About half of the patients who develop neurological deficits from spasm alone will be either dead or have permanent severe neurological deficits as a result. The remaining half will recover completely or have only minor residual deficits. In general, those patients who recover never have a severe deficit, and those who develop a severe deficit do not recover. The range of onset of neurological deficits from spasm was 4–21 days, with a peak about day 9 following the subarachnoid hemorrhage (1).

Although our study also showed a direct correlation between the amount of blood in the basal cisterns on the initial computed tomographic (CT) scan taken within 96 hours of the hemorrhage and the severity of the neurological deficit from spasm, it is not possible today to predict which patients will develop deficits from spasm. Clearly there are other factors separate from the amount of blood in the basal cisterns which also determine if a patient will develop a deficit from spasm. The lack of blood in the basal cisterns on the initial CT scan is predictive, however, especially with a high quality CT scan and careful attention to cuts through the basal cisterns. Those patients who show very little or no blood in their basal cisterns on the initial CT scan have a very reduced chance of developing deficits from spasm.

ETIOLOGY

Studies of human vessels which were in spasm from patients who sustained a subarachnoid hemorrhage have shown necrosis of smooth muscle cells several days to several weeks following the subarachnoid hemorrhage. In addition, there is some infiltration of the media and swelling of the intima, which often leads to subendothelial fibrosis (11, 18). Similar findings have been produced in animals following an experimental subarachnoid hemorrhage (27). I feel that these changes are the result of cerebral arterial spasm and are not its cause. Our working hypothesis has been that the initial event in the production of spasm is contraction of arterial smooth muscle cells. After a prolonged period of severe contraction, it is not unreasonable to suppose that morphological changes in the vessel wall then take place. The force that can be generated by contraction of these smooth muscle cells is amazing. In response to a variety of vasoactive agents, 1 mg of human basilar or anterior cerebral artery segment can generate 14,000 times its weight in tension (5).

If contraction of the smooth muscle cells is the initial event in spasm, the question then remains as to what causes the smooth muscle cells to contract. There are many different chemicals which have been shown to cause dose-dependent contractions of cerebral arterial smooth muscle. Furthermore, all have been shown to use the influx of extracellular calcium as the source of final messenger calcium for this contraction. No single chemical has been shown conclusively to be the cause of spasm. However, it is known that the occurrence and severity of the neurological deficit from spasm are directly related to the presence and amount of blood in the basal subarachnoid spaces following the hemorrhage. As mentioned previously, this is a necessary but not sufficient requirement for the production of neurological deficits from spasm. Other factors must play a role in the production of the ischemic deficit from spasm.

This critical distinction needs to be made again between spasm of the cerebral arteries and neurological deficits resulting from spasm. This distinction will be clearer if they are discussed separately.

TENTATIVE HYPOTHESIS: PRODUCTION OF CEREBRAL ARTERIAL SPASM

Serotonin (5-HT) is proposed as the vasoactive agent responsible for the contraction of cerebral arteries following a subarachnoid hemorrhage. The 5-HT$_1$ receptor (high affinity) has been shown to be the one present on large cerebral arteries and is responsible for the contractile response to serotonin (25). Half-maximal contractions are obtained with nanomolar (10^{-9} M) concentrations of *free* serotonin. However, normally in the blood there is almost no *free* serotonin (12). The platelets actively take up any free circulating serotonin and store it in their dense granules. When the aneurysm ruptures, platelets, along with the other blood elements, escape into the basal subarachnoid spaces and mix with the cerebrospinal fluid (CSF). Some of the blood clots. Two things happen to the platelets: (a) a release reaction occurs which releases serotonin and other chemicals into the CSF-blood mixture (22); and (b) the platelets become adhesive and stick to the arachnoid, the adventitia of the arterial walls, and the fibrin of the blood clots (19). The *free* serotonin which has been released and remains in basal cisterns is again actively taken up by the platelets. The platelet plasma membrane has an active uptake mechanism for serotonin and, once into the platelet, this serotonin is actively transported into dense granules, where it is stored and protected from breakdown by mitochondrial monoamine oxidase (12, 13). Thus, within a short time after the hemorrhage there is no significant *free* serotonin in contact with the 5-HT$_1$ serotonin receptors of the arterial smooth muscle cells. If any early phase of spasm occurs, it is brief and disappears as the *free* serotonin is taken up by the platelets. This accounts for the lack of spasm on the initial angiogram taken within 3 days of the hemorrhage. If angiograms were done within minutes to a few hours after the hemorrhage, spasm might be seen.

The normal concentration of serotonin in circulating blood is in the micromolar (10^{-6} M) range, and all of it is stored in the platelets. Circulating platelets have a half-life of 4–5 days (9). If this half-life is not changed by their escape into the basal cistern, then 4–5 days after the hemorrhage, half of the platelets will have disintegrated. The stored serotonin will be released by this disintegration but will be taken up and stored by the remaining half of the platelets. The storage capacity for serotonin in normal platelets far exceeds their content of serotonin (24). A second 4–5 days following the initial hemorrhage (a total of 8–10 days from the hemorrhage), half of the remaining platelets have now disintegrated. This process of gradual disintegration of the platelets continues, and at some point the reuptake capacity of the remaining platelets will be exceeded by the concentration of serotonin which is being released. At this point, for the first time (excluding the initial transient release reaction), a significant *free* level of serotonin will exist in the fluid surrounding the cerebral arteries.

There is only one other means of removing this *free* serotonin, and that is by the circulation of the CSF and drainage through the Pacchionian granulations. The formation of blood clots in the basal cisterns impedes this circulation, and antifibrinolytic agents inhibit the lysis of these clots. Finally, the degree of spasm (contraction) is directly related in a dose-dependent fashion to the amount of *free* serotonin present at the serotonin receptors on the arterial smooth muscle cell membranes (8). The degree of spasm will vary greatly from patient to patient and with time in a given patient.

In summary, according to this hypothesis, the production of spasm should be dependent on: (*a*) the amount of blood which escapes into the basal cisterns. The greater the amount of blood, the greater the incidence and severity of spasm for two reasons. First, the more blood, the more platelets and serotonin available for eventual release. Second, the more blood, the more likely CSF circulation will be impaired, which impairs the circulation of *free* serotonin out of the basal cisterns and away from the cerebral arteries. (*b*) The administration of antifibrinolytic agents should increase the incidence and severity of spasm by inhibiting the lysis of the fibrin clots. This has both the effect of keeping the fibrin clots with their adherent platelets in the vicinity of the cerebral arteries and impairing the CSF circulation of *free* serotonin out of the basal cisterns because of the continued presence of the clots. (*c*) The number of platelets per milliliter of blood and their serotonin concentration at the time of the bleed should also determine the incidence and severity of spasm.

All the evidence necessary to completely prove this theory is not available. However, it does explain the delayed time course of spasm production and accounts for the variability, the correlation with the amount of blood, and the effect of antifibrinolytic agents. The 5-HT_1 (high affinity) receptor's presence on the cerebral arteries has been demonstrated (25); serotonin has been recovered in significant concentrations from the CSF of patients several days after a subarachnoid hemorrhage (5); serotonin alone has been shown *in vitro* and *in vivo* to cause severe contraction (spasm) of the large cerebral arteries (4–7); and, finally, the platelets' release and uptake of serotonin and their adhesiveness and half-life are well documented (14–16). Zervas *et al.* (30, 31) have shown that pretreatment of blood with reserpine makes that blood incapable of causing spasm. Reserpine used as *pretreatment* eliminates serotonin from the platelets. Finally, a previous strong objection to this hypothesis was that none of the known serotonin antagonists prevent spasm. We now know that there are two serotonin receptors (26): a high affinity (5-HT_1) receptor and a low affinity (5-HT_2) receptor. We also know that the 5-HT_1 receptor is the one responsible for cerebral artery contractions (25) and that all known serotonin antagonists block only the 5-HT_2 receptor (25, 26). There are no known 5-HT_1 receptor antagonists. We are currently trying to develop a 5-HT_1 antagonist.

This hypothesis is essentially the same as the one we proposed in 1974 (4), with new supporting evidence from CT scans, knowledge of the serotonin receptor on cerebral arteries, and more knowledge of platelets.

NEUROLOGICAL DEFICITS FROM SPASM

The production of spasm is necessary but not sufficient to explain the occurrence of a neurological deficit from spasm. Many additional factors are important. The location and severity of the spasm, along with the collateral circulation to the area(s) affected by this spasm, will help determine the occurrence and severity of the deficit. For example, spasm of even a severe degree, if isolated to one A_1 segment, will usually not produce a deficit. Proximal collateral circulation via the opposite A_1 segment may be sufficient. If the recurrent artery of Heubner is involved at its origin from the A_1 segment, then the distal collateral circulation of this artery will be important.

For any given location, severity, and collateral circulation, there are still other important variables associated with the occurrence and severity of a deficit. The blood flow through the fixed lumen (resistance) of a contracted cerebral artery is dependent on the perfusion pressure, the viscosity of the blood, and the cardiac output. The perfusion pressure is the mean arterial blood pressure minus the intracranial pressure. Thus, a patient with spasm and increased intracranial pressure from any cause is more likely to develop a deficit from that spasm. A decrease in intravascular volume, which commonly occurs after a subarachnoid hemorrhage, may reduce cardiac output and increase the chances of a deficit from spasm (23).

In summary, the factors that determine the production of spasm are not the only factors which determine whether a deficit will occur from spasm and how severe that deficit will be.

THERAPEUTIC MANAGEMENT

The distinction between spasm and the deficits caused by spasm is also an important one in discussing therapy. No treatment for arterial spasm is known. Treatment has been directed toward the deficits from spasm and involves attempts at changing those additional factors involved in the occurrence of the deficits which are not involved in the production of spasm. Thus, increasing blood pressure, increasing cardiac output by increasing intravascular volume, decreasing viscosity by maintaining a hematocrit in the low 30s (21, 29) are all means of increasing flow through the decreased lumen of the arterial segment(s) in spasm (17).

For the patient who develops a deficit from spasm, the best current therapy in the author's opinion is as follows: (a) Reduce intracranial pressure to normal if it is elevated. (b) Place a Swan-Ganz catheter in the patient and increase intravascular volume with colloid and blood to achieve a hematocrit of 30–33 and an optimum cardiac output. (c) Increase blood pressure with dopamine and/or neosynephrine until the deficit disappears or a systolic pressure of 180–200 is reached. If the aneurysm has not been clipped, care must be taken not to cause it to rupture by rapidly decreasing intracranial pressure or increasing blood pressure. If the patient is developing a significant deficit from spasm, I would treat it at the risk of a rebleed.

If the spasm can be prevented, then the deficit from spasm will be prevented. If the severity of the spasm can be reduced, then the severity of the deficit should be reduced. This was the rationale behind the use of nimodipine in patients after a subarachnoid hemorrhage (1). Nimodipine prevents the influx of extracellular calcium, which is the final messenger for the contraction of the actin and myosin filaments in the arterial smooth muscle cells. Thus, *free* serotonin is still present and binds to its receptor on the smooth muscle cell. This serotonin-5-HT_1 receptor interaction does not, however, cause the influx of extracellular calcium in the presence of nimodipine. Nimodipine blocks the calcium channels and prevents the serotonin-induced influx of calcium (2, 3,10). There are many such channels in the membrane of each smooth muscle cell. From the levels of nimodipine we measured in our patients, about half of these channels were blocked by nimodipine. This should cause a reduction in the severity of the spasm but not a complete prevention of spasm. This reduction in the severity of spasm should lead to a reduction in the severity of the deficit, which is what we found (1). A second study using higher doses of nimodipine is underway. We hope that the higher doses of nimodipine will block enough calcium channels to cause a reduction in the incidence of even mild deficits.

THE RELATIONSHIP BETWEEN SPASM, REBLEEDING, AND SURGERY

In our initial nimodipine study, spasm, rebleeding, and surgery accounted together for all of the permanently severely disabled (or dead) patients. In the placebo group, approximately 50% of the patients' deficits were from spasm; 25% were from rebleeding; and 25% were a result of surgery and immediate postoperative complications of surgery. Two approaches to reduce rebleeding have been tried. Antifibrinolytic therapy is effective in reducing rebleeding but at the expense of increasing the incidence of deficits from spasm (20, 28). No overall management benefit has been shown for its use in these patients. Early surgery also reduces the incidence of rebleeding, but most surgeons would agree that, technically, early surgery is more difficult. The brain is tight, and the aneurysm is more likely to rupture at the time of surgery. It has not been proven, but it is very possible that the reduction in rebleeding gained by early surgery is counterbalanced by an increase in the severe deficits from such surgery. In addition, it is often difficult to have patients transferred to the tertiary centers, where the surgery is done with the first day or two after the hemorrhage.

In our initial nimodipine study, 55% of the placebo patients and 64% of the nimodipine patients were on Amicar. The results of our first study would suggest that nimodipine is effective in reducing the severity of the deficit from spasm even in the presence of antifibrinolytic therapy. If our second study and other studies confirm this, then the best management of these patients may be to use both nimodipine and an antifibrinolytic agent, beginning immediately after the hemorrhage, and to delay surgery for several days. To prove this, a large-scale management trial would need to be done. Both arms of the study would contain neurologically normal patients entered within 72–96 hours of their bleed and placed on nimodipine. One arm would also be given antifibrinolytic therapy, and surgery would be delayed. The other arm would have early surgery (within 72–96 hours of the bleed) and no antifibrinolytic therapy.

Regardless of the results of such a study it is clear that if nimodipine is effective in preventing spasm and its deficits, its use will alter our management strategy of these patients in many respects. Its use may allow a significant reduction in the morbidity from rebleeding and surgery, as well as from spasm.

REFERENCES

1. Allen, G. S., Ahn, H. S., Preziosi, T. J., et al. Cerebral arterial spasm: A controlled trial of nimodipine in subarachnoid hemorrhage patients. N. Engl. J. Med., 308: 619–624, 1983.
2. Allen, G. S., and Bahr, A. L. Cerebral arterial spasm. Part 10. The reversal of acute and chronic spasm in dogs with orally administered nifedipine. Neurosurgery, 4: 43–47, 1979.
3. Allen, G. S., and Banghart, S. B. Cerebral arterial spasm. Part 9. In vitro effects of nifedipine on serotonin, phenylephrine and potassium induced contractions of canine basilar and femoral arteries. Neurosurgery, 4: 37–42, 1979.

4. Allen, G. S., Gold, L. H. A., Chou, S. N., and French, L. A. Cerebral arterial spasm. Part 3. *In vivo* intracisternal production of spasm by serotonin and blood and its reversal by phenoxybenzamine. J. Neurosurg., *40:* 451–458, 1974.

5. Allen, G. S., Gross, C. J., French, L. A., and Chou, S. N. Cerebral arterial spasm. Part 5. *In vitro* contractile activity of vasoactive agents including human cerebrospinal fluid on human basilar and anterior cerebral arteries. J. Neurosurg. *44:* 594–600, 1976.

6. Allen, G. S., Gross, C. J., Henderson, L. M., and Chou, S. N. Cerebral arterial spasm. Part 4. *In vitro* effects of temperature, serotonin analogues, large nonphysiological concentrations of serotonin and extracellular calcium and magnesium on serotonin induced contractions of the canine basilar artery. J. Neurosurg., *44:* 585–593, 1976.

7. Allen, G. S., Henderson, L. M., Chou, S. N., and French, L. A. A study of cerebral arterial spasm. Part 1. *In vitro* contractile activity of various vasoactive agents on the canine basilar and middle cerebral arteries. J. Neurosurg., *40:* 433–441, 1974.

8. Allen, G. S., Henderson, L. M., Chou, S. N., and French, L. A. Cerebral arterial spasm. Part 2. *In vitro* contractile activity of serotonin in human serum and CSF on the canine basilar artery and its blockage by methysergide and phenoxybenzamine. J. Neurosurg., *40:* 442–450, 1974.

9. Chesterman, C. N., and Pennington, D. G. Platelet production and turnover: Thrombocytopenia and thrombocytosis. In: *Blood and Its Disorders*, Ed. 2, edited by R. M. Hardisty and D. J. Weatherall, Blackwell Scientific Publications, Oxford, England, 1983.

10. Cohen, R. J., and Allen, G. S. Cerebral arterial spasm—The role of calcium *in vitro* and *in vivo* analysis with nifedipine and nimodipine. In: *Cerebral Arterial Spasm: Proceedings of the Second International Workshop*, Amsterdam, The Netherlands, edited by R. H. Wilkins, pp. 527–532. Williams & Wilkins, Baltimore, 1980.

11. Conway, L. W., and McDonald, L. W. Structural changes of the intradural arteries following subarachnoid hemorrhage. J. Neurosurg., *37:* 715–723, 1972.

12. Da Prada, M., Richards, J. G., and Kettler, R. Amine storage organelles in platelets. In: *Platelets in Biology and Pathology*, Ed. 2, edited by J. L. Gordon, pp. 116–130. Elsevier/North Holland, New York, 1981.

13. Drummond, A. H. Interactions of blood platelets with biogenic amines: Uptake, stimulation and receptor binding. In: *Platelets in Biology and Pathology*, edited by J. L. Gordon, pp. 209–213. Elsevier/North Holland, New York, 1976.

14. Gordon, J. L. (ed.). *Platelets in Biology and Pathology*. Elsevier/North Holland, New York, 1976.

15. Gordon, J. L. (ed.). *Platelets in Biology and Pathology*, Ed. 2. Elsevier/North Holland, New York, 1981.

16. Hardisty, R. M., and Weatherall, D. J. (eds.). *Blood and Its Disorders*, Ed. 2. Blackwell Scientific Publications, Oxford, England, 1983.

17. Heros, R. C., Zervas, N. T., and Varsos, V. Cerebral vasospasm after subarachnoid hemorrhage: An update. Ann. Neurol., *14:* 599–608, 1983.

18. Hughes, J. T., and Schianchi, P. M. Cerebral artery spasm, a histological study at necropsy of the blood vessels in cases of subarachnoid hemorrhage. J. Neurosurg., *48:* 515–525, 1978.

19. Jaffee, R. M. Interaction of platelets with connective tissue. In: *Platelets in Biology and Pathology*, edited by J. L. Gordon, pp. 261–288. Elsevier/North Holland, New York, 1976.

20. Kassell, N. F., Torner, J. C., and Adams, H. P. Antifibrinolytic therapy in the acute period following aneurysmal subarachnoid hemorrhage. J. Neurosurg., *61:* 225–230, 1984.

21. Kee, D. B., and Wood, J. H. Rheology of the cerebral circulation. Neurosurgery, 15: 125–131, 1984.

22. MacIntyre, D. E. The platelet release reaction: Association with adhesion and aggregation, and comparison with secretory response in other cells. In: *Platelets in Biology and Pathology*, edited by J. L. Gordon, pp. 63–72. Elsevier/North Holland, New York, 1976.

23. Maroon, J. C., and Nelson, P. B. Hypovolemia in patients with subarachnoid hemorrhage: Therapeutic implications. Neurosurgery, 4: 223–226, 1979.

24. Mills, D. C. B., and MacFarlane, D. E. Platelet receptors. In: Platelets in Biology and Pathology, edited by J. L. Gordon. Elsevier/North Holland, New York, 1976.

25. Peroutka, S. J., Noguchi, M., Tolner, D. J., and Allen, G. S. Serotonin-induced contraction of canine basilar artery: Mediation by 5-HT$_1$ receptors. Brain Res., 259: 327–330, 1983.

26. Peroutka, S. J., and Snyder, S. H. Multiple serotonin receptors: Differential binding of ^{3}H-serotonin, ^{3}H-lysergic acid diethylamide and ^{3}H-spiroperidol. Mol. Pharmacol., 16: 686–699, 1979.

27. Tanabe, Y., Sakata, K., Yameda, H., et al. Cerebral vasospasm and ultrastructural changes in cerebral arterial wall: An experimental study. J. Neurosurg., 49: 229–238, 1978.

28. Vermeulen, M., Lindsay, K. W., Cheah, M. F., et al. Antifibrinolytic treatment in subarachnoid hemorrhage. N. Engl. J. Med., 311: 432–437, 1984.

29. Wood, J. H., Simeone, F. A., Kron, R. E., and Litt, M. Rheological aspects of experimental hypervolemic hemodilution with low molecular weight dextran: Relationships of cortical blood flow, cardiac output and intracranial pressure to fresh blood viscosity and plasma volume. Neurosurgery, 11: 739–753, 1982.

30. Zervas, N. T., Hori, H., and Rosoff, C. B. Experimental inhibition of serotonin by antibiotic: Prevention of cerebral vasospasm. J. Neurosurg., 41: 59–62, 1974.

31. Zervas, N. T., Kuwayama, A., Rosoff, C. B., and Salzman, E. W. Cerebral arterial spasm: Modification by inhibition of platelet function. Arch. Neurol., 28: 400–404, 1973.

6

Measurement of Regional Cerebral Blood Flow in Aneurysm Surgery

NEIL A. MARTIN, M.D., L. PHILIP CARTER, M.D., and
ROBERT F. SPETZLER, M.D.

INTRODUCTION

Despite tremendous advances in the surgical treatment of ruptured intracranial aneurysms over the past 25 years, the overall morbidity and mortality attending aneurysmal subarachnoid hemorrhage remain unacceptably high. At this point less than 35% of patients sustaining a subarachnoid hemorrhage have a full functional recovery (28). The principal causes of death and disability in patients surviving the initial hemorrhage are rebleeding and cerebral infarction (1, 49, 57). Approximately 20–30% of patients having hemorrhage will develop symptomatic cerebral ischemia, and about one-half of these patients will die or sustain a disabling neurologic deficit (22). Following surgery for ruptured aneurysm, cerebral ischemia has been considered to be the principal cause of subsequent neurologic deterioration (22).

Cerebral ischemia in patients having subarachnoid hemorrhage (SAH) results from the interaction of a number of factors: altered cerebral metabolism, increased intracranial pressure, intravascular volume depletion, loss of autoregulation and, most importantly, cerebral arterial spasm. These factors, acting separately or in concert, produce a reduction in cerebral blood flow (CBF), and it is this fall in perfusion, with its secondary reduction in oxygen and metabolite availability, that produces a failure of electrical activity, synaptic transmission, ion pumping, energy metabolism and, ultimately, irreversible cellular damage. There appears to be a distinct cerebral blood flow threshold below which neuronal electrical function fails, and a second, somewhat lower flow threshold for the disruption of structural integrity. Only when flow is persistently depressed below the lower threshold does permanent ischemic cell injury (infarction) occur. In man the normal cerebral blood flow is approximately 50–60 ml/100 gm/minute. Studies of cortical electrical activity with electroencephalography (EEG) and cerebral blood flow in man during clamping of one carotid artery for endarterectomy have established a threshold for the loss of cortical electrical activity of about 20 ml/100 g/minute, (21, 54). This threshold for failure of neuronal function

79

has been suppoted by experiments in awake primates demonstrating reversible hemiparesis when local CBF dropped below 23 ml/100 gm/ minute (during temporary middle cerebral artery occlusion) (27). The flow threshold for irreversible cellular injury is somewhat lower than that for functional impairment. Symon and Brierley (60) found that following acute vascular occlusion, infarction developed in areas where flow dropped below 10 ml/100 gm/minute. Others have demonstrated that there is a time-dependent relationship between flow and the development of infarction (4). Jones and co-workers (27) found irreversible cerebral damage in a stroke model in areas with flow temporarily (2–3 hours) below 10–12 ml/100 gm/minute, or permanently below 17–18 ml/100 gm/ minute.

It is clear that the level of cerebral blood flow has critical implications with regard to cerebral function and integrity. In recognizing the potential for CBF measurements to provide insight into the hemodynamic effects of subarachnoid hemorrhage, many investigators have carried out such studies in aneurysm patients. Most studies have employed the measurement of clearance of injected or inhaled xenon-133 by stationary detectors to determine mean hemispheric blood flow values. This chapter will describe the results of these studies as they apply to the pathophysiology of subarachnoid hemorrhage, in particular the extent and time course of the reduction in CBF caused by SAH directly, and by the subsequent complication of vasospasm. The potential for application of CBF measurements in the timing of surgery and treatment of ischemia will also be examined. Finally, the current status of techniques for clinical and intraoperative CBF measurement will be reviewed.

ACUTE EFFECTS OF SUBARACHNOID HEMORRHAGE ON CEREBRAL BLOOD FLOW AND METABOLISM

A depression in global cerebral blood flow acutely follows subarachnoid hemorrhage (Table 6.1) (11, 19, 20, 25, 26, 51, 56, 59). The diffuse fall in CBF occurs even in Grade I patients in the absence of elevated intracranial pressure or angiographically identified arterial spasm. This direct immediate effect of SAH on cerebral blood flow has been confirmed in animal models wherein, intracisternal injection of blood, under conditions in which intracranial pressure (ICP) is maintained at normal levels, caused a reduction in cerebral blood flow. Umansky and co-workers found that this decline in CBF is prompt, occurring within 5 minutes of experimental SAH in most animals, and that it can be observed in the caudate nucleus, thalamus, and internal capsule, as well as in the cortex (62).

What is the cause of this immediate fall in CBF following subarachnoid hemorrhage? Cerebral arterial spasm occurs acutely in several animal models of subarachnoid hemorrhage and possibly is implicated in the early global fall of GBF found in laboratory experiments (2, 9). Evidence for the existence of acute spasm in clinical subarachnoid hemorrhage, however, is scant. The appearance of spasm on angiograms done within 24 hours of subarachnoid hemorrhage is rare, and acute spasm has not been seen to occur immediately after hemorrhage in the reported cases of aneurysmal rupture during angiography (48, 67). Furthermore, this acute posthemorrhage reduction in CBF has been documented in patients whose angiograms were free of spasm (5, 19, 20).

At high levels, elevated ICP may cause a reduction in CBF by reducing the cerebral perfusion pressure below the lower limit of autoregulation, or by disturbing autoregulation directly. Intracranial hypertension may contribute to the fall in cerebral perfusion following SAH, but it cannot explain the frequent finding of reduced CBF in patients or in experimental SAH animal models with little or no concurrent increase in ICP (19, 51, 62).

It may be that the initial effect of subarachnoid hemorrhage on the brain is one of metabolic depression, with a decrease in CBF occurring as a secondary effect. This occurs in metabolic encephalopathies, where a primary decrease in cerebral electrical activity and energy metabolism results in reduced CBF (20). Fein (10), in primates subjected to an intracisternal injection of blood, demonstrated a disturbance of the metabolic rates of oxygen and glucose that clearly preceded any reduction in CBF. This metabolic effect has also been demonstrated in aneurysm patients. Grubb and co-workers (19), using positron emission tomography (PET), have demonstrated a fall in the cerebral metabolic rate for oxygen ($CMRO_2$) in subarachnoid hemorrhage patients that accompanies a reduction in CBF (Fig. 6.1). Other investigators (33, 63) have confirmed that $CMRO_2$, as well as CBF, is depressed after aneurysm rupture, usually in proportion to the clinical grade of the patient (Table 6.2).

THE EFFECT OF CLINICAL GRADE ON CBF

Numerous studies using xenon-133 clearance methods have shown that the degree of reduction of CBF correlated with the clinical grade of subarachnoid hemorrhage patients (Tables 6.1 and 6.2). Kelly and co-workers (30), in a study of radionuclide brain scanning in SAH patients, demonstrated an analogous tendency for patients with worse neurological grades to have abnormal perfusion (Table 6.3). Grubb and associates (19), using PET, confirmed this grade-dependent CBF reduction (Fig. 6.1). When patients are in poor neurological condition, mean hemispheric CBF may fall dangerously close to the threshold for ischemic injury. To a certain extent the reduction of CBF in Grade III and Grade IV patients is due to an increased incidence of spasm and intracranial hypertension

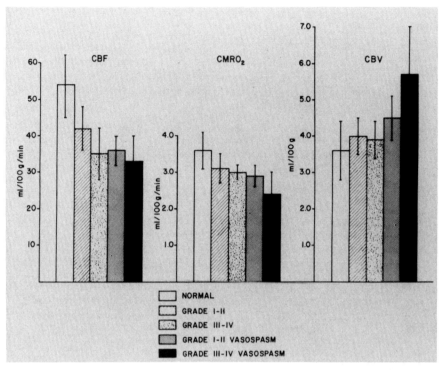

FIG. 6.1. Mean hemispheric values of cerebral blood flow (CBF), cerebral metabolic rate of oxygen (CMRO₂), and cerebral blood volume (CBV) in patients with and without cerebral vasospasm following SAH. *Vertical bars,* standard deviation of mean values. (Reproduced with permission from: R. L. Grubb *et al.* (19)).

TABLE 6.1

Cerebral Blood Flow Postsubarachnoid Hemorrhage

Author	CBF Method	CBF Normal	CBF Grades I–II	CBF Grades III–IV
James (26)	¹³³Xe (IC)ᵃ	70	65	49
Symon et al. (20)	¹³³Xe (IC)	50	39	28
Heilbrun et al. (20)	¹³³Xe (IC)		34	29
Ferguson et al. (59)	¹³³Xe (INH)		46	32
Pitts et al. (51)	¹³³Xe (IC, INH)		40	36
Grubb et al. (19)	PET	54	42	35
Weir (64)	¹³³Xe (INH)	67	60	48
Ishii (25)	¹³³Xe (IC)		42	30
Spetzler (unpublished observation)	¹³³Xe (INH)	55	45	30

ᵃ IC, intracarotid ¹³³Xe injection; INH, inhalation of ¹³³Xe ; PET, positron-emission tomography; CBF, mean hemispheric CBF.

TABLE 6.2

Relationship of CBF and CMRO₂ to Clinical Grade[a]

Clinical Grade	CBF[b]	CMRO₂
I and II	42.3	2.00
III	36.7	1.72
IV	26.9	0.93

[a] From K. Kobayashi *et al.* (33).
[b] CBF and $CMRO_2$ are mean hemispheric values.

TABLE 6.3

Relationship of Dynamic Scan Results to Clinical Grade[a]

Clinical Grade	Dynamic Scan	
	Symmetrical	Asymmetrical
I	17	4
II	4	5
III	5	6
IV	1	2

[a] Modified from P. J. Kelly *et al.* (29).

in these groups, but even in the absence of these complicating factors, CBF appears to be lower in patients with worse clinical grades (19).

IMPAIRMENT OF AUTOREGULATION AND CO₂ RESPONSE FOLLOWING SAH

Cerebrovascular autoregulation is a normal response that acts to maintain constant levels of cerebral blood flow in the face of variations in cerebral perfusion pressure. In normal humans, autoregulation is effective within a range of mean arterial pressures from approximately 60 to 160 mm Hg (41). Additionally, cerebral blood flow normally responds to changes in arterial pCO_2, with a decrease in pCO_2 inducing cerebral vasoconstriction and a fall in flow. These properties of the intracranial circulation may be impaired after cerebral injury due to trauma, compression, or hypoxia. Autoregulation and cerebrovascular reactivity to CO_2 may be abnormal following subarachnoid hemorrhage. Ishii's study (25) of 49 subarachnoid hemorrhage patients using the intraarterial xenon-133 method demonstrated a disturbed CO_2 response and impaired autoregulation in several patients (Table 6.4). Others (11, 20) have confirmed the fact that patients have a perturbation of autoregulatory function after SAH. Nornes and co-workers (46) also found a change in autoregulatory capacity in aneurysm patients. By using an electromagnetic flow probe applied to one of the main intracranial arteries, they demonstrated that the lower limit of autoregulation was

TABLE 6.4

Relationship of CO_2 Response and Autoregulation to Clinical Grade[a]

Grade	Disturbance of CO_2 Response	Disturbance of Autoregulation
I and II	5/30	2/4
III	19/25	2/2
IV	7/10	1/1

[a] From R. Ishii (25).

shifted upward in Grade III patients (mean lower limit, 76 mm Hg) when compared to that of Grades I and II patients (62 mm Hg) (46). Similar to the post-SAH reduction in CBF, the frequency of impairment of normal cerebrovascular responsiveness increases in patients in the worst clinical grades (20, 25). This vasoparalysis may be focal or global and is probably related to ischemic hypoxia, intracerebral hematoma, intracranial hypertension, or hydrocephalus.

TEMPORAL COURSE OF CBF CHANGES AFTER SAH

There are few systematic serial studies of CBF changes during the weeks after subarachnoid hemorrhage, but the extensive study of Meyer and associates (of 1265 rCBF determinations by the ^{133}Xe inhalation method in 116 SAH patients), provides valuable data on this topic (39). Their findings show a progressive fall in CBF in the first 14 days following hemorrhage, after which it stabilizes or begins to rise (Fig. 6.2). The magnitude of this fall in perfusion is related to clinical grade, but even Grade I patients showed this pattern. Interestingly, Meyer and associates found not only a decline in CBF on the side of the aneurysm but also a decline of lesser degree on the side opposite the aneurysm. The study of Weir and associates (66) also demonstrated a fall in CBF that was most pronounced between 5 and 8 days post-SAH. They found that flows increased to near normal levels by 21 days. The progressive fall in CBF could not be explained by coincident changes in blood pressure, pCO_2, or drug therapy. Changes in the cerebral microvasculature, in cerebral metabolism, or in circulating blood volume may contribute to the fall in CBF. In fact, hypovolemia, with a concomitant reduction in cardiac output, has been shown to occur after subarachnoid hemorrhage and to effect a decrease in CBF (37). Vasospasm, however, is probably the most critical factor responsible for the decline in cerebral perfusion between days 4 and 14. This is the period when the incidence of angiographic arterial spasm is greatest (34).

THE EFFECT OF CEREBRAL VASOSPASM ON CBF

Cerebral arterial spasm appears in 30–60% of angiograms done during post-SAH days 4–14 (34, 65). There have been debates in the past about

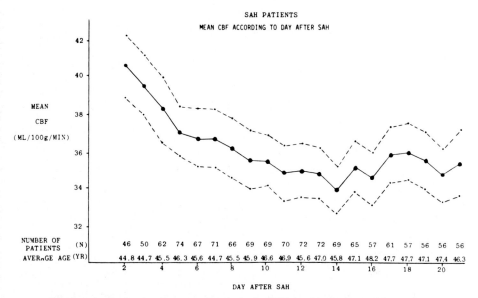

SAH PATIENTS
MEAN CBF ACCORDING TO DAY AFTER SAH

FIG. 6.2. Average value for mean hemispheric CBF (and its 95% confidence limits) on individual days after hemorrhage. (Reproduced with permission from: C. H. A. Meyer *et al.* (39).)

the clinical importance of angiographically identified arterial spasm following SAH. In contrast to the general clinical impression that vasospasm following rupture of a saccular aneurysm is a significant development that is associated with neurologic deterioration, certain studies, such as the clinicopathological study of Schneck and Kricheff (53) and the clinicoradiological study of Millikan (42) failed to find a correlation between spasm and clinical events. Fisher and his associates (13), however, in a retrospective study of SAH patients, demonstrated that delayed ischemic deficit occurred only in the presence of severe spasm (with an arterial residual lumen less than 0.5 mm), and that the deficit invariably corresponded to the site of severe spasm (Table 6.5). In a few cases severe spasm did not cause ischemic deficit, but in no case did mild or moderate spasm precipitate major neurologic symptoms. This striking correlation between the site and severity of spasm and delayed ischemic deficit has been futher established by this group and others (12, 43, 64). Overall, of the patients with angiographic spasm, approximately 50% will develop ischemic neurological deficit (7).

Examinations of regional cerebral blood flow in patients with subarachnoid hemorrhage have supported the contention that spasm diminishes perfusion (Table 6.6). The effects of spasm are manifest as a reduction in mean CBF in the hemisphere ipsilateral to the aneurysm, accompanied

TABLE 6.5

Relationship of Vasospasm to Delayed Ischemic Deficits

Degree of Vasospasm	Delayed Ischemic Deficit		
	Yes	No	Total
Severe (lumen $\leq$ 0.5 mm)	25	6	31
Absent to moderate spasm (lumen $\geq$ 1.0 mm)	0	19	19
			$\overline{50}$

[a] Modified from C. M. Fisher *et al.* (13).

TABLE 6.6

Cerebral Blood Flow in Relation to Spasm

Author	CBF Method	CBF (No Spasm)	CBF (Spasm)
James (26)	IC[a] ^{133}Xe	62	47
Ferguson *et al.* (11)	INH ^{133}Xe	45	40
Pitts *et al.* (51)	IC, INH ^{133}Xe	40	36
Grubb *et al.* (19)	PET	42 (Gr. I & II)	36 (I & II)
		35 (Gr. III & IV)	33 (III & IV)
Yamakami *et al.* (69)	INH ^{133}Xe	53 (Mild spasm)	41 (Severe spasm)

[a] IC, intracarotid ^{133}Xe injection; INH, inhalation of ^{133}Xe; CBF, mean hemispheric CBF on side of aneurysm.

in some studies by a fall in CBF of lesser degree in the contralateral hemisphere (69). Focal areas of decreased perfusion, and focal disturbances in CO_2 responsiveness and autoregulation, correlating to the distribution of severely spastic arteries, have been noted in two dimensional studies of xenon-133 clearance, but the spatial resolution of these methods is poor (20, 25). The study of SAH patients by Mickey and coworkers (40) using Xe-133 inhalation and emission computed tomography have more precisely demonstrated focal flow defects that correspond to the site of spasm, and to the patient's ischemic neurologic deficits. In our preliminary experience with xenon-enhanced CT CBF mapping, we have also seen striking focal flow abnormalities related to symptomatic cerebral vasospasm (Fig. 6.3). It has been interesting to note from these tomographic CBF studies that the somnolence that often occurs prior to or concurrent with the focal deficit due to spasm is not necessarily accompanied by a diffuse reduction in cerebral perfusion. Perhaps in these cases depression of the level of consciousness is caused by diencephalic or brainstem ischemia due to spasm of smaller perforating arteries.

As would be expected from the studies of Fisher *et al.*, severe spasm reduces CBF significantly, while mild or moderate spasm usually has little effect on perfusion. In a primate model of SAH, Simeone and coworkers (55) provided confirmatory evidence. At the minimum, a 50%

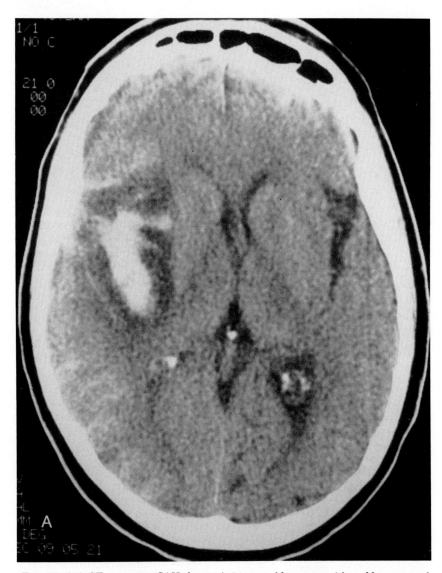

FIG. 6.3. (A) CT scan post-SAH day 1. A 54-year-old woman with sudden onset of headache, and mild hemiparesis. CT scan shows large clot in Sylvian fissure. (B) Arteriogram, post SAH-day 3. The patient is neurologically unchanged. Arteriogram shows moderate proximal middle cerebral artery (MCA) spasm and a MCA aneurysm. (C) CT scan, post-SAH day 9. The patient has become obtunded and has developed worsening of her hemiparesis. Scan demonstrates irregular decrease in density in MCA territory, with sulci not seen. (D) Arteriogram, post-SAH day 9. The study shows severe peripheral spasm with very poor filling of cortical branches of MCA. Anterior cerebral artery shows no spasm. (E) Cerebral blood flow map derived from xenon-enhanced CT scan, post-SAH day 9. Correlating with the angiogram, there is a flow defect in the MCA distribution. (Compare density of image along cortical ribbon in MCA area on *left* to that on *right*.) Although the mean flow in the MCA territory is depressed, there are certain areas of hyperperfusion (dense white areas) within the ischemic region. Note that flow is preserved in the anterior cerebral and posterior cerebral distributions. This image demonstrates the very good resolution achievable with this technique. (Note distinction between cortex and white matter, and delineation of frontal horns.)

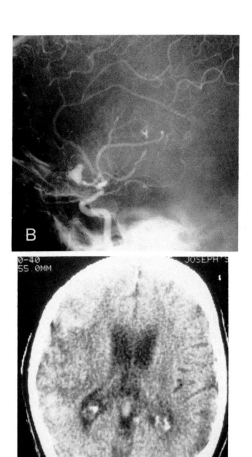

FIG. 6.3*B* and *C*

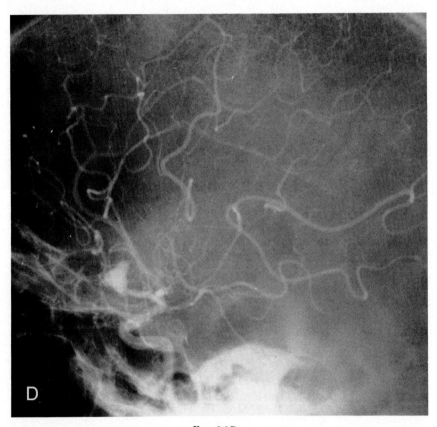

FIG. 6.3*D*

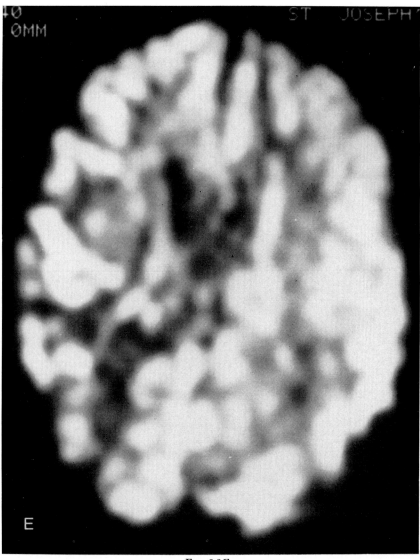

FIG. 6.3E

decrease in vessel caliber was required to effect a significant reduction in CBF (38). In addition to the severity of vessel narrowing, the location and distribution of spasm within the cerebral arterial tree also determines the magnitude of the resultant reduction of CBF. Yamakami and co-workers (69) have classified vasospasm as proximal, peripheral, or diffuse (Fig. 6.4), and correlated the type of spasm with CBF measurements and with delayed ischemic symptoms (Table 6.7). The diffuse and peripheral types of spasm are associated with low hemispheric flows and a high

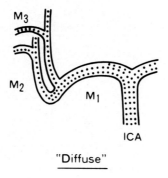

"Diffuse"

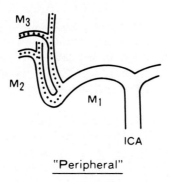

"Peripheral"

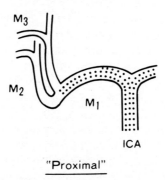

"Proximal"

FIG. 6.4. Classification of type of vasospasm by angiography. *Dots* indicate areas that showed spasm angiographically. Internal carotid artery (*ICA*) segments M_1, M_2, and M_3 of middle cerebral artery are shown. (Reproduced with permission from: I. Yamakami *et al.* (69)).

TABLE 6.7

Correlation of Ischemic Deficit and CBF to Type of Spasm

Type of Angiographic Spasm	No. of Cases	Ischemic Deficit	Mean CBF
Diffuse	4	4/4	36.5
Peripheral	3	2/3	40.7
Proximal			
Severe	6	2/6	44.8
Mild	14	1/14	52.8
No spasm	3	0/3	58.1

[a] Modified from I. Yamakami *et al.* (69).

incidence of ischemic deficit. Severe proximal spasm, involving only the internal carotid artery and vessels of the circle of Willis, causes a more modest CBF reduction and only occasional deficit. The impact of mild proximal spasm on CBF and on the clinical condition of the patients is minimal. The results of other investigators are similar. Patients with severe diffuse spasm show areas of significant hypoperfusion, while those patients with isolated focal areas of narrowing of the supraclinoid internal carotid artery or the proximal portions of the anterior and middle cerebral arteries adjacent to ruptured aneurysms often have no sign of ischemic deficit and display only mild depression of cerebral blood flow (25, 33).

While cerebral blood flow is reduced in patients with Grade III and IV subarachnoid hemorrhage with spasm, cerebral blood volume is increased in these patients (Fig. 6.1). Grubb and associates (19) postulated that this finding was attributable to a marked dilatation of intraparenchymal vessels occurring in the face of constriction of the large angiographically visualized extraparenchymal vessels. This increase in CBV is akin to that found with an acute reduction of the cerebral perfusion pressure, as seen in systemic hypotension or intracranial hypertension. The increase in CBV in the presence of vasospasm probably reflects a similar fall in the effective perfusion pressure—in this case due to the pressure drop across the spastic segments of the proximal cerebral arterial system.

Vasospasm following subarachnoid hemorrhage may have permanent neurologic effects, but it is a transient phenomenon. Serial angiography usually demonstrates the beginning of relaxation of spasm several days to a week following its onset, although it may occasionally persist for several weeks (5, 22, 65). The resolution of spasm ultimately results in the restitution of the normal caliber of the vessel. Angiographic demonstration of permanent narrowing of cerebral arteries due to spasm has not been reported (22). Corresponding sequential CBF studies have been performed, demonstrating that resolution of angiographic spasm is accompanied by an increase in CBF in the ischemic region supplied by the spastic arteries, with a restitution of normal mean hemispheric blood flow (25). The study of Mickey and co-workers (40) using a tomographic CBF method similarly showed normalization of the CBF image accompanying angiographic resolution of spasm and recovery of neurologic function. However, one patient in their study, with an infarct found on CT scanning, survived with a dense hemiplegia. As expected, a follow-up CBF study demonstrated a persistent low-flow area corresponding to the CT infarct.

THE EFFECT OF SURGERY ON CBF

The superimposition of the physiologic stress of aneurysm surgery on a cerebral circulation already compromised by the effects of SAH causes further impairment of cerebral blood flow. Ferguson and associates (11) found a decrease of CBF following surgery, from a group mean of 36 ml/100 gm/minute (preoperatively) to 31 ml/100 gm/minute (within 7 days postoperatively). While other investigators have identified a similar postoperative fall in CBF (20, 69), the study of Merory and co-workers (38) suggest that the postoperative hemodynamic changes are more variable. When taken as a whole, their group of patients had a modest increase in CBF on the first postoperative day. On closer analysis, however, the patients appeared to fall into two groups, one which had a postoperative rise in flow and one which had a postoperative fall. After 2–4 days the CBF in both groups approached the preoperative level. A significant correlation existed between the pattern of CBF change and postoperative level of consciousness. In contrast to the patients with a postoperative rise in CBF, only a minority of those with a decrease in flow were alert on the first day after surgery.

Surgery might further compromise cerebral perfusion if it caused an increase in the incidence of vasospasm. It has been suggested that the timing of surgery is important in determining the incidence of postoperative spasm. Several centers for aneurysm surgery have demonstrated that the incidence of postoperative spasm was much higher when surgery was performed during the latter half of the first week than when operation was delayed 2 weeks or more after SAH (Table 6.8) (14, 15, 18, 52, 57). As can be seen from Table 6.8, however, the incidence of preoperative spasm is significant in the patients managed with delayed surgery. It appears likely that, as Drake (8) suggests, spasm is almost entirely a consequence of the initial hemorrhage. The performance of surgery in many cases, before the time when vasospasm was predestined to occur, has led to the impression that surgery caused or aggravated spasm. Hunt's results are in accord with this suggestion. He found that the incidence and severity of vasospasm during the initial 3 weeks after hemorrhage was not related to the presence or absence of surgical intervention (24). It may be that intraoperative hypotension, dehydration and brain retraction increase the risk of postoperative infarction, partic-

TABLE 6.8

Incidence of Postoperative Spasm as Related to Timing of Surgery[a]

Author	No. of Patients	Incidence Pre-Op Spasm (%)	Timing of Surgery after SAH (Days)	Incidence of Post-Op Spasm (%)
Gianotta *et al.* (18)	86		<14	20
Saito *et al.* (52)	428	22	<4	40
			4–8	48
			9–15	7
Sundt and Whisnant (57)	310	14	<9	34
			>9	10
Fleischer *et al.* (15)	175	23	14–21	2
Flamm (14)	200	30	14–21	1.5

[a] (Modified from E. Flamm (14).)

ularly when cerebral perfusion is already marginal, but there is no convincing evidence that surgery is a significant causative factor for vasospasm.

APPLICATION OF CBF STUDIES TO THE CLINICAL MANAGEMENT OF SAH PATIENTS

As detailed in the previous sections, laboratory and clinical studies of cerebral blood flow have provided information on the effects of subarachnoid hemorrhage, vasospasm, and aneurysm surgery on cerebral perfusion. These data alone, however, are difficult to translate into practical application in the management of patients with ruptured aneurysms. On a more pragmatic level, CBF measurements may contribute to the determination of prognosis for neurologic recovery and survival. Several reports have associated the finding after SAH of low mean hemispheric blood flow with a poor outcome (Table 6.9), confirming the clinical significance of ischemia as a compliction of subarachnoid hemorrhage (30, 44, 70). Disturbed autoregulation is also associated with subsequent morbidity (20, 50). This is not surprising because, as has been discussed above, the patients with low flow and abnormal vascular reactivity are chiefly those in Grades III and IV, *i.e.*, those who are known by their poor neurological condition to have a poor prognosis.

The measurement of cerebral blood flow would most clearly be useful in the treatment of SAH patients if it identified those at particular risk for the development of critically reduced perfusion, permitting modification of management in such cases so as to avoid injurious cerebral ischemia. If CBF data defined the risks of ischemia in individual patients more reliably than other available parameters (such as clinical grade, or the degree of angiographic spasm), then its value would be obvious. Patients with significantly reduced cerebral perfusion could be treated

TABLE 6.9

Relationship of Outcome to CBF

Postop Results	No. of Cases	CBF
Excellent	26	41.8
Good	6	39.7
Fair	3	31.0
Poor	4	25.0

[a] From R. Ishii (25).
[b] CBF, mean hemispheric CBF.

in order to augment cerebral blood flow, and surgery in these patients could be delayed until their cerebral hemodynamic status was improved. Several studies have attempted to define criteria that would identify patients with borderline CBF. Kelly and associates (29) correlated the results of dynamic radionuclide brain scanning in SAH patients with their clinical outcome. Patients with normal (symmetric) scans had a better outcome, while those with abnormal (asymmetric) scans had an increased rate of cerebral infarction, particularly following aneurysm surgery. Of note in this study was the fact that the results of dynamic scanning seemed to correlate more consistently with outcome than did the presence or absence of angiographic spasm. Based on their findings, they suggested that surgery be delayed in patients with abnormal scans to reduce the risk of postoperative ischemia. In a subsequent prospective study they used the results of dynamic scanning to determine the timing of aneurysm surgery (37). Although the postoperative results were good in 29 patients undergoing operation when their perfusion scan was normal, it appears that surgery was delayed because of an initially abnormal scan in only six patients. As Peerless has pointed out in a critical review of this study, this subgroup of six patients is too small to establish the benefit of delaying surgery because of an abnormal dynamic scan.

Ferguson and associates (11) defined a group of patients in good clinical condition following SAH who had an unexpectedly low CBF ("silent spasm syndrome"). They believed that this group might be poorly tolerant of any further reduction in flow likely to follow surgery and recommended delaying operation until CBF had recovered. These investigators, however, did not report a group of patients managed according to this approach.

As noted earlier, Ishii (25) found that patients with low mean hemispheric CBF measured preoperatively had poor postoperative results. As regards timing, he simply states that surgery was delayed in his patients showing decreased CBF (or impaired cerebrovascular reactivity) and that he "obtained a good clinical response." Unfortunately, no details are provided in this report regarding this group of patients.

Nilsson (44) has used an intravenous isotope technique to obtain an estimate of cerebral perfusion. His postoperative results were correlated with measurements of perfusion. He found, as did Kelly, that patients with poor perfusion had a higher incidence of significant postoperative morbidity. Among his patients with a poor outcome, however, 33% had normal or near-normal circulatory studies. Furthermore, of 12 patients dying from rebleeding, 2 died while waiting for an improvement in their cerebral perfusion studies.

Blood flow studies, performed serially, might be of value in monitoring and titrating hemodynamic, rheologic, or pharmacologic treatment intended to increase cerebral perfusion in the face of established symptomatic ischemia. In one group of patients with spasm, CBF studies have been employed for this application (24). The use of induced hypertension was found to increase cerebral blood flow coincident with the reversal of neurologic deficit.

In summary, several reports have shown that CBF determinations can be used to predict, to a certain extent, the risk of development of delayed ischemic deficit, but the bulk of data have not established that CBF studies are better able to identify SAH patients prone to develop symptomatic ischemia than are other clinical and radiologic parameters such as the patient's neurologic grade, the degree of angiographic spasm or, more recently, the quantity of subarachnoid blood seen on the initial CT scan. While CBF measurements have been proposed as a means of determining when surgery should be performed after aneurysmal SAH, as yet the small number of studies have not firmly established a role for clinical blood flow measurement in the timing of aneurysm surgery. Finally, CBF studies may prove to be useful in monitoring therapy, involving hypervolemia, induced hypotension, calcium-channel blockers, or other drugs for symptomatic cerebral ischemia.

INTRAOPERATIVE TECHNIQUES FOR MEASUREMENT OF CEREBRAL BLOOD FLOW

In addition to the clinical CBF methods used in the studies described above, techniques are available for intraoperative monitoring of CBF. Techniques using Xe-133 have been used intraoperatively for measuring CBF, but this method does not provide continuous immediate feedback on the effects of surgical and anesthetic manipulation on flow (50). We have used a thermal diffusion flow probe calibrated against xenon-133 clearance studies to monitor cortical blood flow in more than 65 craniotomies for aneurysm (3). After opening the dura, the probe is placed on a cortical region of interest. This technique determines CBF by measuring changes in a temperature gradient established between two gold plates that are in contact with the cortex. Changes in the temperature gradient are proportional to alterations in blood flow in the underlying cortex. A continuous, quantitative recording of CBF from the underlying area is obtained during the operative procedure. Immediate changes in CBF can be detected with retraction, hypotension, vascular manipulation, and temporary vascular occlusion (Fig. 6.5). The immediate detection of significant changes in CBF provides the surgeon and anesthesiologist with an opportunity to make appropriate technical or pharmacologic adjustments so as to avoid ischemic cerebral injury. Intraoperative use of electrophysiologic methods (EEG, direct cortical response, evoked potentials) also provides a nearly continuous assessment of cerebral function. These methods, however, generally only detect changes when CBF falls to critical levels below the flow threshold for electrical dysfunction. Because this level of flow approaches the threshold for ischemic cellular death, these electrophysiologic methods provide only a "last-minute warning of impending ischemic brain damage" (671).

Intraoperative monitoring of CBF has also been done using the electromagnetic flow probe. Nornes and Wikeby (47) have measured flow during aneurysm surgery in the internal carotid artery (normally averaging 144 ml/minute), in the middle cerebral artery (97 ml/minute), and in the proximal anterior cerebral artery (65 ml/minute). Determination of flow in the middle cerebral artery after occlusion of the terminal internal carotid artery provides an indication of the adequacy of collateral through the circle of Willis, and may aid in the decision as to whether trapping procedures in this location will be tolerated. Additionally, flow may be monitored after clipping of the aneurysm to detect hemodynamically significant compromise of the parent vessel and adjacent branches.

CLINICAL CBF TECHNIQUES

The vast majority of clinical studies of CBF, including all but a few of the studies cited in this review, have utilized the technique of recording by stationary detectors, the rate of uptake, and washout of the freely diffusable radioactive tracer xenon-133. Mean hemispheric flow values or 2-dimensional flow maps are generated from these data. The xenon-133 may be delivered by intracarotid injection, which offers the advantages of achieving a high count rate and, therefore, higher resolution. Administration of xenon-133 via inhalation or intravenous injection is less invasive but, because of the lower count rates, these methods result in a loss of resolution and, because the tracer enters the external carotid system, the CBF measurements are contaminated by blood flow in scalp, bone, and meninges. Because of the 2-dimensional nature of these tech-

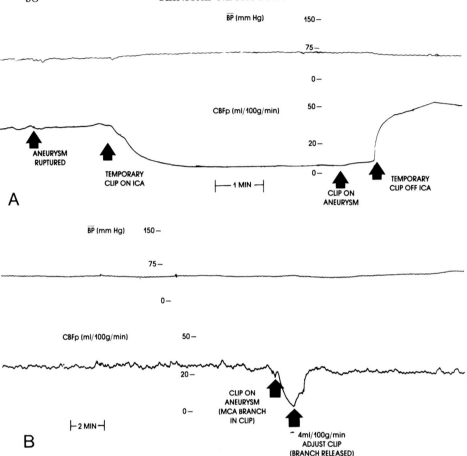

FIG. 6.5. (*A*) Graphic illustration of intraoperative mean arterial blood pressure (*top*) and cortical blood flow as determined by the thermal diffusion probe (*bottom*). In this case temporary occlusion of the internal carotid artery (*ICA*) was required when the aneurysm ruptured. Cortical flow promptly diminished. After clipping the aneurysm, the ICA was opened, and cortical flow immediately responds. (*B*) In this case a branch of the middle cerebral artery was included in a clip applied to a middle cerebral artery trifurcation aneurysm, with the result that cortical flow was reduced. With adjustment of the clip to free the branch, restoration of flow is noted. (Modified from L. P. Carter *et al.* (3).)

niques, information on CBF is primarily limited to the superficial layers of the cerebral convexities. These techniques have a serious drawback when applied to the circumstance of focal ischemia. As isotope does not enter the ischemic area, no clearance curve can be generated from it. In this case, the detector "looks through" the unlabeled region and records only activity from adjacent or deeper labeled areas (35). A tomographic method, which has the capacity to localize the tracer in three dimensions, is required to circumvent this technical problem.

Mathematical data reconstruction applied to tomographic radionuclide imaging methods can produce 3-dimensional images (emission computed tomography), and positron- or single photon-emitting radionuclides may be used as tracers (6). These techniques require specialized imaging devices and have limited spatial resolution (approximately 1–1.5 cm with current instrumentation). Positron-emitting tracers (such as oxygen-15, krypton-77, and fluorine-18) have been used with success to make functional measurements in deep cerebral structures (16, 23, 71). However, because production of the tracers is complex, costly, and requires the use of a cyclotron, and because their half-life is very brief, positron emission tomography (PET) is available at few medical centers. Xenon-133 used as a tracer with a rotating single photon emission tomograph has the capacity to demonstrate rCBF in 3 dimensions (36). The wider availability of this tracer makes this technique attractive, but it, like PET, has limited resolution. Studies of patients with stroke and subarachnoid hemorrhage have demonstrated the usefulness of this technique (36, 40). Other single photon-emitting, brain-seeking radiopharmaceuticals, such as ^{123}I-labeled amphetamine and ^{123}I-labeled HIPDM, are being investigated and may be useful (32, 68).

Rapid sequence transmission computed tomography (dynamic scanning) has the potential ability to measure the buildup and washout of tracer concentrations in the brain with excellent spacial resolution. While iodinated contrast material has been used to monitor relative changes in cerebral blood flow, it does not easily cross the blood-brain barrier and, therefore, cannot be used in the quantitative measurement of tissue perfusion (45). Because of its high atomic number, nonradioactive xenon also acts as a contrast agent and does freely diffuse across the blood-brain barrier. Sequential CT scanning during inhalation of xenon permits measurement of its time-dependent concentration in the brain, from which can be derived a measure of cerebral perfusion (72). This technique has as its primary advantages, wide availability of the requisite scanning apparatus (high resolution scanner with dynamic imaging capabilities) and of the contrast agent (stable xenon), and very good spatial resolution (to <0.5 cm). Due to the slight enhancement obtainable with xenon, the method has been felt to have the disadvantage of an unfavorable signal-to-noise ratio, but this has not prevented succesful use of the method (72).

Magnetic resonance imaging (MRI) techniques have been investigated to determine their potential for measuring flow characteristics in large vessels (17). Time-varying MR signals have been observed in the descend-

CLINICAL NEUROSURGERY

ing aorta on sequential images through the midthorax, implying that MRI can be used to determine flow velocity. Studies on *in vitro* continuous and pulsatile flow systems have confirmed that there is a defined relationship between MR signal intensity and fluid velocity (17). Further experimental and clinical studies are expected to result in the ability of MRI to describe *in vivo* velocity profiles in large vessels. Although experimental work is in progress, MRI techniques are not currently able to quantitate tissue perfusion.

It appears that the tomographic approach to CBF determination should replace the techniques using stationary scintillation probes. Even using tomographic techniques, isolated measurements of CBF may not be reliable in assessing the adequacy of cerebrovascular reserve. It may be that in order to gauge the ability of the cerebral circulation to maintain perfusion in the face of physiologic challenges, the CBF response to hemodynamic stress (such as reduction in systemic pressure) must be measured. Only the intraoperative studies of CBF during induced hypotension by Nornes *et al.* (46) and Pickard *et al.* (50) have done this in a systematic way. (30, 46). Further experience with this type of CBF study, and with the newer methods of 3-dimensional CBF mapping, will determine the optimal technique for clinical measurement of cerebral perfusion.

CONCLUSIONS

Clinical and experimental studies of cerebral blood flow have elucidated the hemodynamic consequences of aneurysmal rupture. Subarachnoid hemorrhage is accompanied by an immediate fall in CBF that is often accompanied by a disturbance of cerebrovascular reactivity and is exacerbated by the development of arterial spasm. Further clinical studies may be of value in identifying those patients at highest risk for the development of ischemic deficit, but a definite role for CBF determination in the planning of management, particularly in the timing of surgery, has yet to be established. Continuous or sequential intraoperative measurement of cerebral blood flow may be of benefit in judging the hemodynamic consequences of anesthetic or surgical manipulations. As further experience accrues with the newer tomographic methods of CBF determination, the potential benefits of CBF monitoring in aneurysm surgery will be defined and realized.

ACKNOWLEDGMENT

The authors acknowledge the invaluable editorial assistance of Georgia Frederic.

REFERENCES

1. Adams, H. P., Jr., Kassell, N. F., Torner, J. C., Nibbelink, D. W., and Sahs, A. L. Early management of aneurysmal subarachnoid hemorrhage: A report of the Cooperative

Aneurysm Study. J. Neurosurg., *54:* 141–145, 1981.

2. Brawley, B. W., Strandness, D., and Kelly, W. The biphasic response of cerebral vasospasm in experimental subarachnoid hemorrhage. J. Neurosurg., *28:* 1–8, 1968.

3. Carter, L., Erspamer, R., White, W., and Yamagata, S. Cortical blood flow during craniotomy for aneurysm. Surg. Neurol., *17:* 204–208, 1982.

4. Carter, L., Yamagata, S., and Erspamer, R. Time limits of reversible cortical ischemia. Neurosurgery, *12:* 620–623, 1983.

5. Chyatte, D., and Sundt, T. Cerebral vasospasm after subarachnoid hemorrhage. Mayo Clin. Proc., *59:* 498–505, 1984.

6. Cowan, R., and Watson, N. Special characteristics and potential of single photon-emission computed tomography in the brain. Semin. Nucl. Med., *10:* 335–344, 1980.

7. Drake, C. G. Management of cerebral aneurysm. Stroke, *12:* 273–283, 1981.

8. Drake, C. Postoperative arterial spasm. In: *Cerebral Arterial Spasm: Proceedings of the Second International Workshop,* edited by R. H. Wilkins. Williams & Wilkins, Baltimore, 1980.

9. Echlin, F. A. Spasm of basilar and vertebral arteries caused by experimental subarachnoid hemorrhage. J. Neurosurg., *23:* 1–11, 1965.

10. Fein, J. Brain energetics and circulatory control after subarachnoid hemorrhage. J. Neurosurg., *45:* 498–507, 1976.

11. Ferguson, G., Farrar, J., Meguro, K., Peerless, S., Drake, C., and Barnett, H. Serial measurements of CBF as a guide to surgery in patients with ruptured aneurysms. J. Cereb. Blood Flow Metab., *1*(Suppl. 1): S518–S519, 1981.

12. Fisher, C. M., Kistler, J. P., and Davis, J. M. Relation of cerebral vasospasm to subarachnoid hemorrhage visualized by computerized tomographic scanning. Neurosurgery, *6:* 1–9, 1980.

13. Fisher, C. M., Roberson, G. H., and Ojemann, R. G. Cerebral vasospasm with ruptured saccular aneurysms: The clinical manifestations. Neurosurgery, *1:* 245–248, 1977.

14. Flamm, E. Timing of aneurysm surgery and its relationship to cerebral vasospasm. In: *Cerebral Arterial Spasm: Proceedings of the Second International Workshop,* edited by R. H. Wilkins, pp 361–365. Williams & Wilkins, Baltimore, 1980.

15. Fleischer, A. S., and Tindall, G. T. Cerebral vasospasm following aneurysm rupture. Presented at the Annual Meeting of the American Association of Neurological Surgeons, Los Angeles, April 23, 1979.

16. Fox, P., Mintun, M., Raichle, M., and Herscovitch, P. A noninvasive approach to quantitative functional brain mapping with $H_2^{15}O$ and positron emission tomography. J. Cereb. Blood Flow Metab., *4:* 329–333, 1984.

17. George, C., Jacobs, G., MacIntyre, W., Lorig, R., Go, R., Nose, Y., and Meaney, T. Magnetic resonance signal intensity patterns obtained from continuous and pulsatile flow models. Radiology, *151:* 421–428, 1984.

18. Giannotta, S. L., McGillicuddy, J. E., and Kindt, G. W. Diagnosis and treatment of postoperative cerebral vasospasm. Surg. Neurol., *8:* 286–290, 1977.

19. Grubb, R. L., Jr., Raichle, M. E., Eichling, J. O., and Gado, M. H. Effects of subarachnoid hemorrhage on cerebral blood volume, blood flow, and oxygen utilization in humans. J. Neurosurg., *46:* 446–453, 1977.

20. Heilbrun, M. P., Olesen, J., and Lassen, N. A. Regional cerebral blood flow studies in subarachnoid haemorrhage. J. Neurosurg., *37:* 36–44, 1972.

21. Heiss, W-D. Flow thresholds of functional and morphological damage of brain tissue. Stroke, *14:* 329–331, 1983.

22. Heros, R., Zervas, N., and Varsos, V. Cerebral vasospasm after subarachnoid hemorrhage: An update. Ann. Neurol., *14:* 599–608, 1983.

23. Herscovitch, P., Markham, J., and Raichle, M. Brain blood flow measured with intravenous $H_2^{15}O$. I. Theory and error analysis. J. Nucl. Med., *24:* 782–789.

24. Hunt, W. Timing of surgery for intracranial aneurysm. In: *Cerebral Arterial Spasm: Proceedings of the Second International Workshop.* Williams & Wilkins, Baltimore, 1980.
25. Ishii, R. Regional cerebral blood flow in patients with ruptured intracranial aneurysms. J. Neurosurg., *50:* 587–594, 1979.
26. James, I. M. Changes in cerebral blood flow and in systemic arterial pressure following spontaneous subarachnoid haemorrhage. Clin. Sci., *35:* 11–22, 1968.
27. Jones, T. H., Morawetz, R. B., Crowell, R. M., Marcoux, F. W., Fitzgibbon, S. J., DeGirolami, U., and Ojemann, R. G. Thresholds of focal cerebral ischemia in awake monkeys. J. Neurosurg., *54:* 773–782, 1982.
28. Kassell, N., and Drake, C. Timing of aneurysm surgery. Neurosurgery, *10:* 514–519, 1982.
29. Kelly, P. J., Gorten, R. J., Grossman, R. G., and Eisenberg, H. M. Cerebral perfusion, vascular spasm, and outcome in patients with ruptured intracranial aneurysms. J. Neurosurg., *47:* 44–49, 1977.
30. Kelly, P. J., Gorten, R. J., Rose, J. E., and Grossman, R. G. Cerebral infarction and ruptured intracranial aneurysms. In: *Cerebral Arterial Spasm: Proceedings of the Second International Workshop,* edited by R. H. Wilkins, pp 366–371. Williams & Wilkins, Baltimore, 1980.
31. Kelly, P. J., Gorten, R. J., Rose, J. E., Grossman, R. G., and Eisenberg, H. M. Radionuclide cerebral angiography and the timing of aneurysm surgery. Neurosurgery, *5:* 202–207, 1979.
32. King, H., Tramposch, K., and Blau, M. A new brain perfusion imaging agent: [I-123] HIPDM. J. Nucl. Med., *24:* 66–72, 1983.
33. Kobayashi, K., Ishii, R., Koike, T., Ihara, I., and Kameyama, S. Cerebral blood flow and metabolism in patients with ruptured aneurysms. Acta. Neurol. Scand. Suppl. *60:* 492–493, 1979.
34. Kodama, N., Mizoi, K., Sakurai, Y., and Suzuki, J. Incidence and onset of spasm. In *Cerebral Arterial Spasm: Proceedings of the Second International Workshop,* edited by R. H. Wilkins. Williams & Wilkins, Baltimore, 1980, pp 333–337.
35. Lassen, N. Regional cerebral blood flow measurements in stroke: The necessity of a tomographic approach. J. Cerebral Blood Flow Metab., *1:* 141–142, 1981.
36. Lassen, N., Henriksen, L., and Paulson, O. Regional cerebral blood flow in stroke by xenon-133 inhalation and emission tomography. Stroke, *12:* 284–288, 1981.
37. Maroon, J. C., and Nelson, P. B. Hypovolemia in patients with subarachnoid hemorrhage: Therapeutic implications. Neurosurgery, *4:* 223–226, 1979.
38. Merory, J., Thomas, D., Humphrey, P., DuBoulay, G., Marshall, J., Ross Russell, R., Symon, L., and Zilkha, E. Cerebral blood flow after surgery for recent subarachnoid haemorrhage. J. Neurol. Neurosurg. Psychiatry, *43:* 214–221, 1980.
39. Meyer, C., Lowe, D., Meyer, M., Richardson, P., and Neil-Dwyer, G. Progressive change in cerebral blood flow during the first three weeks after subarachnoid hemorrhage. Neurosurgery, *12:* 58–76, 1983.
40. Mickey, B., Vorstrup, S., Voldby, B., Lindewald, H., Harmsen, A., and Lassen, N. Serial measurement of regional cerebral blood flow in patients with SAH using xenon-133 inhalation and emission computerized tomography. J. Neurosurg., *60:* 916–922, 1984.
41. Miller, J. D. Control of the cerebral circulation. In: *Cerebral Arterial Spasm: Proceedings of the Second International Workshop,* edited by R. H. Wilkins. Williams & Wilkins, Baltimore, 1980.
42. Millikan, C. H. Cerebral vasospasm and ruptured intracranial aneurysm. Arch. Neurol., *32:* 433–449, 1975.
43. Mizukami, M., Takeame, T., and Tazawa, T., *et al.* Value of computed tomography in

the prediction of cerebral vasospasm after aneurysm rupture. Neurosurgery, 7: 583–586, 1980.

44. Nilsson, B. W. Cerebral blood flow in patients with subarachnoid haemorrhage studied with an intravenous isotope technique: Its clinical significance in the timing of surgery of cerebral arterial aneurysm. Acta Neurochir. (Wien), 37: 33–48, 1977.

45. Norman, D., Axel, L., Berninger, W., Edwards, M., Conn, C., Redington, R., and Cox, L. Dynamic computed tomography of the brain: Techniques, data analysis, and applications. AJR, 136: 759–770, 1981.

46. Nornes, H., Knutzen, H. B., and Wikeby, P. Cerebral arterial blood flow and aneurysm surgery. II. Induced hypotension and autoregulatory capacity. J. Neurosurg., 47: 819–827, 1977.

47. Nornes, H., and Wikeby, P. Cerebral arterial blood flow and aneurysm surgery. J. Neurosurg., 47: 810–818, 1977.

48. Odom, G. L. Cerebral vasospasm. Clin. Neurosurg. 22: 29–58, 1974.

49. Pakarinen, S. Incidence, aetiology, and prognosis of primary subarachnoid hemorrhage: A study based on 589 cases diagnosed in a defined urban population during a defined period. Acta Neurol. Scand. Suppl., 43(Suppl. 29): 1–128, 1967.

50. Pickard, J. D., Matheson, M., Patterson, J., and Wyper, D. Prediction of late ischaemic complications after cerebral aneurysm surgery by the intraoperative measurement of cerebral blood flow. J. Neurosurg., 53: 305–308, 1980.

51. Pitts, L. H., Macpherson, P., Wyper, D. J., Jennett, B., Blair, I., and Cooke, M. B. D. Effects of vasospasm on cerebral blood flow after subarachnoid hemorrhage. In Cerebral Arterial Spasm: Proceedings of the Second International Workshop, edited by R. H. Wilkins, pp 333–337. Williams & Wilkins, Baltimore, 1980.

52. Saito, I., Ueda, Y., and Sano, K. Significance of vasospasm in the treatment of ruptured intracranial aneurysms. J. Neurosurg., 47: 412–429, 1977.

53. Schneck, S. A., and Kircheff, I. I. Intracranial aneurysm rupture, vasospasm and infarction. Arch. Neurol., 11: 668–680, 1964.

54. Sharbrough, F. W., Messick, J. M., and Sundt, T. M., Jr. Correlation of continuous electroencephalograms with cerebral blood flow measurements during carotid endarterectomy. Stroke, 4: 674–683, 1973.

55. Simeone, F., Trepper, P., and Brown D. Cerebral blood flow evaluation of prolonged experimental vasospasm. J. Neurosurg., 37: 302–311, 1972.

56. Spetzler, R. F. Unpublished observation.

57. Sundt, T. M., Jr., and Whisnant, J. P. Subarachnoid hemorrhage from intracranial aneurysms: Surgical management and natural history of disease. N. Engl. J. Med., 299: 116–122, 1978.

58. Symon, L. Disordered cerebrovascular physiology in aneurysmal subarachnoid hemorrhage. Acta Neurochir., 41: 7–22, 1978.

59. Symon, L., Ackerman, R., Bull, J. W. D., Du Boulay, E. P. G. H., Marshall, J., Rees, J. E., and Ross Russell, R. W. The use of the xenon clearance method in subarachnoid haemorrhage. Eur. Neurol., 8: 8–14, 1972.

60. Symon, L., and Brierley, J. B. Morphological changes in cerebral blood vessels in chronic ischemic infarction: flow correlation obtained by the hydrogen clearance method. In: The Cerebral Vessel Wall, edited by J. Cervos-Navarro et al. Raven Press, New York.

61. Teasdale G., and Mendelow D. Cortical blood flow measurements in clinical neurosurgery (editorial). J. Cereb. Blood Flow Metab., 1: 357–359, 1981.

62. Umansky, F., Kaspi, T., and Sholit, M. Regional cerebral blood flow in the acute stage of experimentally induced subarachnoid hemorrhage. J. Neurosurg., 58: 210–216, 1983.

63. Volby, B., Enevoldsen, E., and Jensen, F. Cerebral blood flow, CMRO₂, angiographic vasospasm, CSF lactate/pH and subarachnoid hemorrhage. Acta Neurol. Scand. Suppl., *60* (Suppl. 72): 482–483, 1979.

64. Weir, B. K. A. The effect of vasospasm on morbidity and mortality after subarachnoid hemorrhage from ruptured aneurysm. In: *Cerebral Arterial Spasm: Proceedings of the Second International Workshop,* edited by R. H. Wilkins, pp 333–337. Williams & Wilkins, Baltimore, 1980.

65. Weir, B., Grace, M., Hansen, J., and Rothberg, C. Time course of vasospasm in man. J. Neurosurg., *48:* 173–178, 1978.

66. Weir, B., Menon, D., and Overton, T. Regional cerebral blood flow in patients with aneurysms: Estimation by xenon-133 inhalation. Can. J. Neurol. Sci., *5:* 301–305, 1978.

67. Wilkins, R. H. Aneurysm rupture during angiography: Does acute vasospasm occur? Surg. Neurol., *5:* 299–303, 1976.

68. Winchell, H., Horst, W., Brain, L., Oldendorf, W., Hattner, R., and Parker, H. N-Isoprophyl-(¹²³I)-iodoamphetamine: Single-pass brain uptake and localization in dog and monkey brain. J. Nucl. Med., *21:* 947–952, 1980.

69. Yamakami, I., Isobe, K., Yamaura, A., Nakamura, T., and Makino, H. Vasospasm and regional cerebral blood flow (rCBF) in patients with ruptured intracranial aneurysm: Serial rCBF studies with the xenon-133 inhalation method. Neurosurgery, *13:* 394–401, 1983.

70. Yamamoto, M., Meyer, J., Naritomi, H., Sakai, F., Yamaguchi, F., and Shaw, T. Non-invasive measurement of cerebral vasospasm in patients with subarachnoid haemorrhage. J. Neurol. Sci., *43:* 301–311, 1979.

71. Yamamoto, Y., Thompson, C., Meyer, E., Nukui, H., Matsunaga, M., and Feindel, W. Three dimensional topographical regional cerebral blood flow in man, measured with high efficiency mini-B60 two ring positron device using krypton-77. Acta Neurol. Scand. Suppl. (Suppl. 72), *60:* 186–187, 1979.

72. Yonas, H., Wolfson, S., Gur, D., Latchaw, R., Good, W., Leonya, R., Jackson, D., Jannetta, P., and Reinmuth, O. Clinical experience with the use of xenon-enhanced CT blood flow mapping in cerebral vascular disease. Stroke, *15:* 443–450, 1984.

Cerebral Preservation for Intraoperative Focal Ischemia

JOHN D. MICHENFELDER, M.D.

Historically, anesthesiologists and neurosurgeons have attempted specific interventions to induce cerebral preservation since the mid-1950s. Until the mid-1970s the only intervention considered to be effective was hypothermia. However, for most practitioners the enthusiasm for hypothermia had been lost long before during the 1960s. It is perhaps instructive to briefly examine the life cycle of this interesting technique as it applied to neurosurgery and in particular to aneurysm surgery.

From the beginning it was assumed that hypothermia would preserve cerebral function as the result of a decreased oxygen demand which would permit decreased oxygen delivery. In addition, hypothermia resulted in a "relaxed" brain (presumably due to decreased cerebral blood flow) and was thought to minimize cerebral edema. It was first used in aneurysm surgery in 1955 with patient temperatures of 28–30°C (moderate hypothermia) (8). In 1960, by combining hypothermia with cardiopulmonary bypass it became possible to reduce temperatures to 12–18°C (profound hypothermia), and at these temperatures to temporarily arrest circulation (for up to 60 minutes) while the aneurysm was repaired (23). Although both the conception and application of these techniques were theoretically valid, there were problems. Whether moderate or profound, the techniques were grossly time consuming; with moderate hypothermia arrhythmias, including ventricular fibrillation, hypotension, acidosis, and so-called "rewarming shock" were all possibilities; with profound hypothermia, coagulation defects were perhaps the major problem, making hemostasis virtually impossible and resulting in a high incidence of reopenings.

By the mid 1960s, at the Mayo Clinic it became apparent that mortality from aneurysm surgery was about the same whether profound hypothermia, moderate hypothermia, or no hypothermia was used (20–25%) while the morbidity was certainly increased with the hypothermic techniques. Accordingly, hypothermia was virtually abandoned by us, and it remains in that status (we *rarely* use profound hypothermia and circulatory arrest on otherwise inoperable giant aneurysms involving the basilar system). At about the same time the entire neurosurgical approach to aneurysm surgery was changing with the introduction of the operating microscope and subspecialization by a cadre of neurovascular surgeons. This group rapidly established a new standard working through the microscope and utilizing induced hypotension without hypothermia. With these techniques our expected mortality is now approximately 5% for aneurysm surgery.

Despite such progress there continues to be an interest in developing means of improving the brain's tolerance for ischemia, both during aneurysm surgery and other neurovascular procedures (e.g., carotid endarterectomy). The cumbersome hypothermia techniques no longer seem appropriate for aneurysm surgery since they would likely introduce a higher incidence of complications. Thus the search for simple pharmacologic interventions is a logical one. The goal is not only to reduce the 5% mortality but also to reduce morbidity that results from intraoperative ischemia secondary to either temporary occlusion of a major cerebral artery or to profound degrees of hypotension that may be necessary to repair certain aneurysms. As the prototype drug, I shall consider in some detail the possible merits of thiopental therapy as a means of providing cerebral preservation in aneurysm surgery.

The thought that barbiturates might provide a degree of protection in either complete or incomplete ischemia was originally based upon a seemingly logical assumption. As already noted, it has long been assumed that the basis for the proven protection provided by hypothermia is the reduction in cerebral metabolic rate that occurs in proportion to the reduction in brain temperature. When it became recognized that deep thiopental anesthesia, such as can be achieved clinically, reduces the cerebral metabolic rate to the same degree as does a reduction in brain temperature to 30°C (18), it was rather commonly assumed that such deep levels of thiopental anesthesia should be as protective to the brain as are moderate levels of hypothermia. This was further supported by animal studies which demonstrated that the cerebral energy stores are unaffected by either deep thiopental anesthesia or hypothermia (14). Thus, with an equivalent reduction in cerebral metabolic rate and equivalent maintenance of the cerebral energy stores, it seemed appropriate to conclude that deep levels of thiopental anesthesia would provide an equivalent degree of protection.

However, subsequent animal studies demonstrated that such equivalency cannot be assumed. We showed in dogs that with induction of complete global ischemia the cerebral energy stores, as reflected by adenosine triphosphate, deplete rapidly over the initial 4 minutes of ischemia to about 20% of control at normothermia (Fig. 7.1). With hypothermia to 30°C, which reduces cerebral metabolic rate 50%, the rate of ATP depletion was reduced 50%, precisely as would be predicted. However, when deep thiopental anesthesia was examined which also

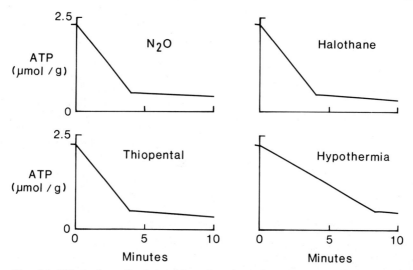

FIG. 7.1. Effect of anesthetics and hypothermia on brain energy stores during global anoxia. At normothermia with both N_2O and halothane, brain energy stores (ATP) rapidly deplete in the first 4 minutes of complete global ischemia (*upper panels*). With hypothermia (30°C), the rate of depletion is halved (*lower right*). With thiopental, despite a metabolic rate similar to that of hypothermia, energy depletion occurs at the same rate as in the other normothermic circumstances (*lower left*).

reduces the cerebral metabolic rate by 50%, it was found that the rate of ATP depletion was unaffected such that at 4 minutes the cerebral energy stores were about 20% of normal, as was seen in lightly anesthetized normothermic dogs. Thus one must conclude that despite their similarities, there is a striking difference between hypothermia and deep barbiturate therapy in terms of a potential brain protection effect.

An hypothesis which might explain these differences is based upon the interrelationship among the anesthetic state, brain function, and brain metabolism (Fig. 7.2). There is consistent evidence that anesthetics alter brain metabolic rate only to the degree that they alter brain function (9). With onset of global ischemia, brain function as reflected by the EEG is abolished within 15–30 seconds. Thereafter the energy consumed by the brain is presumably related only to that needed for maintaining the integrity of the neuron itself. Since anesthetics can only alter the metabolic rate of functioning neurons, there would be no difference between the effects of deep thiopental anesthesia and light nitrous oxide anesthesia on the metabolic demands of nonfunctioning neurons. By contrast, hypothermia presumably depresses metabolic rate by slowing the rates of all biochemical reactions, whether related to function or to the maintenance of integrity. Thus with onset of complete global ischemia during

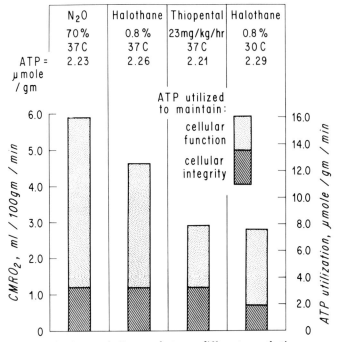

FIG. 7.2. Differences in metabolic rates between different anesthetics are accounted for only by differences in functional needs. Energy for maintenance of integrity is the same for all. By contrast, hypothermia slows the rate of all energy-consuming processes. It is coincidental that deep thiopental and moderate hypothermia (30°C) result in a similar total metabolic rate.

hypothermia, the loss of neuronal function has no impact on the effects of hypothermia on metabolic rate, and depletion of the cerebral energy stores is correspondingly slowed.

If this hypothesis is correct, thiopental could only be protective in the event of an ischemic episode wherein the function of the brain is not abolished, such as may occur in various forms of incomplete ischemia or hypoxemia. Thiopental could not be protective in the event of complete ischemia such as occurs with cardiac arrest. The latter has now been established both experimentally (5, 20) and in a randomized human trial (1). By contrast, the experimental evidence in a variety of animal models of incomplete ischemia or hypoxemia consistently demonstrates that barbiturates do provide a degree of protection consistent with their metabolic suppressive effects (10, 12). This, then, is consistent with the hypothesis.

In aneurysm surgery, should ischemia occur secondary to either transient occlusion of the parent vessel or to profound levels of hypotension, it should be comparable to that which occurs in the various animal models of incomplete ischemia. Accordingly, barbiturate therapy should prolong the brain's tolerance for such ischemia. In the event that the surgeon must temporarily occlude a major cerebral artery in order to repair an aneurysm, the logical use of barbiturate therapy should be as follows. With the surgeon ready to occlude the vessel, the anesthesiologist should administer a "sleep dose" (3–5 mg/kg) of thiopental, followed within 10–15 seconds by occlusion of the vessel. This will deliver a near maximal metabolic suppressing dose of thiopental to the area of potential ischemia. Should significant ischemia result from vessel occlusion, the delivered thiopental will not wash out, and the metabolic suppression and protection will be maintained for a prolonged period. Should the thiopental wash out, any protection will be short-lived but also will not be needed. Whether additional small doses of thiopental should be administered during the period of vessel occlusion is problematical. Presumably, if significant ischemia occurs, it will not be possible to deliver effective concentrations of thiopental to the region of ischemia. It is therefore more logical that the occluded vessel be briefly opened at arbitrary intervals (if possible and despite hemorrhage) while subsequent smaller doses of thiopental (1–2 mg/kg) are administered, followed immediately by reocclusion of the vessel.

In the event of the need for profound hypotension (mean pressure below 30–40 mm Hg) in order to repair a bleeding aneurysm, thiopental should again prolong the brain's tolerance for such incomplete global ischemia. In this circumstance a large bolus of thiopental (6–8 mg/kg) should both abruptly decrease blood pressure and produce maximum metabolic suppression. If profound hypotension must be maintained, intermittent doses of 1–2 mg/kg at 5-to-10-minute intervals would be appropriate, since although cerebral distribution of the barbiturate would be delayed by the low flow state, it should ultimately take place.

Presumably, any anesthetic drug which reduces cerebral metabolic rate would provide a degree of protection during incomplete ischemia, the magnitude of which would be directly related to the magnitude of metabolic suppression. Thiopental has always been the drug of choice because it can rapidly produce maximal metabolic suppression (isoelectric EEG with a 50–60% decrease in cerebral metabolic rate for oxygen) without totally disrupting systemic hemodynamics (although hypotension must always be anticipated). With the introduction of isoflurane, an alternative and possibly better approach appears to be available. Isoflurane is unique among volatile anesthetics in that it is possible in man and animals to produce an isoelectric EEG at concentrations that are hemodynamically tolerated (at approximately 2.0% maximum allowable concentrations (MAC) or 2.4% expired in man). We have shown in dogs that the metabolic state of the brain during isoflurane-induced EEG suppression is normal and is identical to that induced by thiopental (16). Furthermore, the magnitude of protection provided by deep isoflurane in a dog model of profound hemorrhagic hypotension (mean arterial pressure (MAP) = 20–25 mm Hg) is identical to that produced by thiopental (15). Additionally, when hypotension is induced with isoflurane to a MAP of 40 mm Hg for 1 hour in dogs, the brain is metabolically normal and is in significantly better condition than it is following 1 hour of a similar magnitude of hypotension induced by halothane, nitroprusside, or trimethaphan (13, 17).

Thus, although not nearly as extensively studied as the barbiturates, it appears that isoflurane offers the same potential for brain protection as does thiopental. If so, it offers two major advantages: first, the undesirable hemodynamic effects should be of a lesser magnitude and, second, after the period of needed protection has passed, the anesthetic concentration can be abruptly reduced. The latter is obviously not possible with barbiturates and constitutes one of the major objections to their use for brain protection. Although it would br prudent to await additional studies that confirm the above findings, isoflurane may already be the anesthetic of choice for aneurysm surgery: it is nontoxic; it has minimal effects on ICP which can be easily controlled with hyperventilation; it permits reliable control of blood pressure; and it is rapidly eliminated.

Although there has been a flurry of interest in a variety of other drugs that might provide cerebral preservation, their possible application in aneurysm surgery for that purpose is not immediately apparent. The calcium entry blocker, nimodipine, has been shown to decrease the incidence of clinically significant cerebral vasospasm in aneurysm patients (2) but has not been demonstrated to offer any other advantages. Certainly, nimodipine is a cerebral vasodilator and will increase cerebral blood flow in normal brain (6). Furthermore, it has been shown that nimodipine will significantly increase cerebral blood flow following resuscitation from complete circulatory arrest in dogs (21, 22). In primates nimodipine has been found to improve neurologic recovery following 17 minutes of complete cerebral ischemia (19), and that is presumed to be due to improved cerebral blood flow in the postresuscitation period. There is, however, no direct evidence that nimodipine will affect cerebral blood flow in areas of regional ischemia secondary to vessel occlusion or during global ischemia induced by hypotension. Neither is there evidence that following such incomplete ischemia a delayed postischemic hypoperfusion state ensues such as occurs following a period of complete cerebral ischemia. Thus, as regards cerebral blood flow (in the absence of vasospasm), further studies are needed to determine whether nimodipine offers any beneficial effects either during or following a period of incomplete ischemia.

Phenytoin has been shown in a few crude animal models to prolong the brain's tolerance for incomplete ischemia or hypoxemia (3). Phenytoin does not suppress cerebral metabolism, and therefore any protection must be by a mechanism different from the anesthetics. Phenytoin is a membrane stabilizer and has been shown to slow the release of intracellular potassium during cerebral ischemia (4). It has been postulated that high extracellular potassium contributes to ischemic brain damage and that it is the probable mechanism for the reported phenytoin protection. Although many aneurysm patients are given phenytoin, the indication is primarily (if not exclusively) for seizure control. Whether there is in addition a cerebral preservation effect needs to be determined by additional animal studies in models that are clinically relevant.

Initial animal studies with naloxone yielded remarkable results that suggested that endorphins in some way contributed to ischemic brain damage and that this could be favorably modified with naloxone (7). Subsequent studies have failed to duplicate these early findings, and it now appears that there is no place for naloxone therapy during or after a period of cerebral ischemia.

In summary, based upon a host of animal studies it does appear possible to provide a degree of cerebral protection pharmacologically during incomplete ischemia. Although it would be scientifically meritorious to determine in randomized trials whether this effect is applicable in patients undergoing aneurysm surgery, such a study seems an unlikely venture. First, it would likely be impossible to identify all of the potential causes for morbidity and mortality in these patients and then single out intraoperative ischemia as the causal event to be studied with and without pharmacologic intervention. Even if feasible to design such a study, there would be reluctance to participate. The interventions described in this chapter are relatively innocuous and short-term. Their beneficial effects are consistently demonstrable in clinically relevant animal models. That a given intervention is recognized to do little harm and perhaps much good understandably causes hesitation in embarking on a study that deliberately denies 50% of patients the possible benefits of that intervention. Given both marginal feasibility and marginal ethical considerations, any valid study in man seems unlikely.

Accordingly my current recommendation is that aneurysm patients be maintained during anesthesia on low to moderate concentrations of isoflurane with nitrous oxide while being hyperventilated ($PaCO_2 = 30$ mm Hg). If a regional ischemic event is anticipated, pretreatment with a bolus of thiopental followed by increased isoflurane concentrations (if hemodynamically tolerated) would be appropriate. If profound hypotension is required, it can be induced rapidly with a large bolus dose of thiopental or more gradually with increased concentrations of isoflurane. Either approach should provide brain protection. Possible pharmacologic "bonuses" to be found in today's aneurysm patients are maintenance levels of such drugs as nimodipine (for vasospasm) and phenytoin (for seizures). These drugs may well be providing additional cerebral effects that improve the likelihood of cerebral preservation.

REFERENCES

1. Abramson, N. S., Safar, P., Detre, K., Kelsey, S., Monroe, J., Reinmuth, O., Snyder, J., Mullie, A., Hedstrand, U., Tammisto, T., Lund, I., Breivik, H., Lind, B., and Jastremski, M. Results of a randomized clinical trial of brain resuscitation with thiopental. Abstr. Anesthesiol., 59(Suppl.): A101, 1983.
2. Alan, G. S., Ahn, H. S., Preziosi, T. J., Batty, E. R., Boone, S. C., Chou, S. N., Kelly, V. L., Weir, B. K., Crabbe, R. A., Lavik, P. J., Rosenblum, S. V., Dorsey, F. C., Ingram, C. R., Mellits, D. E., Bertsch, L. A., Boisvert, D. P. J., Hundley, M. B., Johnson, R. K., Strom, J. A., Transou, C. R. Cerebral arterial spasm—A controlled trial of nimodipine in patients with subarachnoid hemorrhage. N. Engl. J. Med., 308: 619–624, 1983.
3. Artru, A. A., and Michenfelder, J. D. Cerebral protective, metabolic and vascular effects of phenytoin. Stroke, 11: 377–382, 1980.
4. Artru, A. A., Michenfelder, J. D. Anoxic cerebral potassium accumulation reduced by phenytoin: Mechanism of cerebral protection? Anesth. Analg. (Paris), 60: 41–45, 1981.
5. Gisvold, S. E., Safar, P., Hendrickx, H. H. L., Rao, G., Moossy, J., and Alexander, H. Thiopental treatment after global brain ischemia in pigtailed monkeys. Anesthesiology, 60: 88–96, 1984.
6. Harper, A. M., Craiger, L., and Kazda, S. Effect of the calcium antagonist nimodipine on cerebral blood flow and metabolism in the primate. J. Cereb. Blood Flow Metab., 1: 349–356, 1981.
7. Hosobuchi, Y., Baskin, D. S., and Woo, S. K. Reversal of induced ischemic neurologic deficit in gerbils by the opiate antagonist naloxone. Science. 215: 69–71, 1982.
8. Lougheed, W. M., Sweet, W. H., White, J. C., Brewster, W. R. The use of hypothermia in surgical treatment of cerebral vascular lesions: A preliminary report. J. Neurosurg., 12: 240, 1955.
9. Michenfelder, J. D. The interdependency of cerebral functional and metabolic effects following massive doses of thiopental in the dog. Anesthesiology, 41: 231–236, 1974.
10. Michenfelder, J. D., Milde J. H., and Sundt, T. M., Jr. Cerebral protection by barbiturate anesthesia. Arch. Neurol. 33: 345–350, 1976.
11. Michenfelder, J. D., and Theye, R. A. The effects of anesthesia and hypothermia on canine cerebral ATP and lactate during anoxia produced by decapitation. Anesthesiology, 33: 430–439, 1970.
12. Michenfelder, J. D., and Theye, R. A. Cerebral protection by thiopental during hypoxia. Anesthesiology, 39: 510–517, 1973.
13. Michenfelder, J. D., and Theye, R. A. Canine systemic and cerebral effects of hypotension induced by hemorrhage, trimethaphan, halothane or nitroprusside. Anesthesiology, 46: 188–195, 1977.
14. Michenfelder, J. D., Van Dyke, R. A., and Theye, R. A. The effects of anesthetic agents and techniques on canine cerebral ATP and lactate levels. Anesthesiology, 33: 315–321, 1970.

15. Newberg, L. A., and Michenfelder, J. D. Cerebral protection by isoflurane during hypoxemia or ischemia. Anesthesiology, 59: 29–35, 1983.
16. Newberg, L. A., Milde, J. H., and Michenfelder, J. D. The cerebral metabolic effects of isoflurane at and above concentrations that suppress cortical electrical activity. Anesthesiology, 59: 23–28, 1983.
17. Newberg, L. A., Milde, J. H., and Michenfelder, J. D. Systemic and cerebral effects of isoflurane-induced hypotension in dogs. Anesthesiology, 60: 541–546, 1984.
18. Pierce, E. C., Jr., Lambertson, C. J., Deutsch, S., Chase, P. E., Linde, H. W., Dripps, R. D., and Price, H. L.: Cerebral circulation and metabolism during thiopental anesthesia and hyperventilation in man. J. Clin. Invest. 41: 1664, 1962.
19. Steen, P. A., Gisvold S. E., Milde, J. H., Newberg, L. A., Scheithauer, B. W., Lanier, W. L., Michenfelder, J. D.: Nimodipine improves outcome when given after complete cerebral ischemia in primates. Anesthesiology, in press, 1985.
20. Steen, P. A., Milde, J. H., Michenfelder, J. D. No barbiturate protection in a dog model of complete cerebral ischemia. Ann. Neurol., 5: 343–349, 1979.
21. Steen, P. A., Newberg, L. A., Milde, J. H., and Michenfelder, J. D. Nimodipine improves cerebral blood flow and neurologic recovery after complete cerebral ischemia in the dog. J. Cereb. Blood Flow Metabol. 3: 38–43, 1983.
22. Steen, P. A., Newberg, L. A., Milde, J. H., and Michenfelder, J. D. Cerebral blood flow and neurologic outcome when nimodipine is given after complete cerebral ischemia in the dog. J. Cereb. Blood Flow Metabol 4: 82–87, 1984.
23. Uihlein, A., Theye, R. A., Dawson, B., Terry, H. R., Jr., McGoon, D. C., Daw, E. F., and Kirlin, J. W. The use of profound hypothermia, extracorporeal circulation, and total circulatory arrest for an intracranial aneurysm: Preliminary report with reports of cases. Proceedings Staff Meeting, Mayo Clinic, 35: 567, 1960.

CHAPTER

8

Extracranial to Intracranial Bypass in the Treatment of Aneurysms

SIDNEY (SKIP) J. PEERLESS, M.D., F.R.C.S.(C), and
C. R. HAMPF, M.D.

It has long been known that ligation of the internal or common carotid artery is followed by (1) a high mortality rate and (2) a high percentage of cerebral complications... There are two causes of death and disability: (1) cerebral anemia from inadequate collateral circulation through the circle of Willis, the effects of which appear immediately and may be abrupt or progressive, and (2) cerebral thrombosis and embolism, the effects of which are late in appearing, i.e., develop twelve hours to several days later, and are usually abrupt, though at times a preceding small attack may warn of the impending event (7).

INTRODUCTION AND HISTORICAL REVIEW

With these words, Walter Dandy, M.D., began his report on the "results following ligation of the internal carotid artery" published 42 years ago in the *Archives of Surgery.* Dandy's observations were accurate and remain important today. Although the role of carotid ligation in the treatment of intracranial aneurysms has diminished with the development of modern neurosurgical techniques, there remain many giant and otherwise inaccessible aneurysms (high cervical, petrous, intracavernous) which are not amenable to direct attack; for these, other strategies are required. Hunterian ligation of the parent vessel continues to provide a reasonable alternative in the management of these lesions. Dandy stressed the importance of preoperative assessment of collateral circulation and the method of ligation (7). In the past 40 years, several techniques have been described for parent vessel occlusion. However, inherent in all of these techniques is the risk of infarction in the territory distal to the vessel occluded, secondary either to hemodynamic or embolic ischemia. Extracranial to intracranial (EC-IC) microsurgical anastomosis has been proposed as a method of decreasing the risk of these ischemic complications. A review of the literature and of the results of combined Hunterian ligation and EC-IC bypass in the treatment of aneurysms at University Hospital forms the basis of this report.

The natural history of untreated giant intracranial aneurysms is dismal. Reports on patients treated nonoperatively or with exploration only reveal that the majority of these patients were progressively disabled or died from mass effect or aneurysmal hemorrhage (2, 9, 12, 20, 23).

Direct attack on the aneurysm with clipping of the neck is the ideal treatment. This allows for the preservation of the parent artery, sparing of nearby branches or perforators, and the opportunity to immediately decompress those lesions presenting with mass effect. Direct attack is not without risk, but with improved angiographic, neuroanesthetic, and microsurgical techniques, increasing numbers of giant aneurysms can be visualized and clipped (9, 14, 23, 33). Yet, there remain many aneurysms that cannot be directly obliterated because of involvement of the parent vessel and its branches in the aneurysmal dilatation, a thick atherosclerotic or calcified neck, intraluminal thrombosis, or because the aneurysm is inaccessible.

CAROTID LIGATION

Proximal or Hunterian ligation of the parent vessel remains the mainstay of the indirect treatment of giant intracranial aneurysms. In 1785, John Hunter ligated a carotid artery of a stag belonging to King George the III. Hunter observed a few days later that the stag's antler was cold and had stopped growing. When he reexamined it a week later, he was astounded to note the antler was again warm and had resumed its growth. He ordered the stag killed and, after confirming that the carotid artery was indeed securely ligated, he noted that numerous small vessels above and below the ligature had enlarged. He reasoned that "under the stimulus of necessity" small tributary arteries will assume the functions of the larger parent artery. The principle of collateral circulation was thus established. Hunter used this principle as the basis for proximal vessel occlusion in the treatment of aneurysms when 4 months later he ligated the popliteal artery of a 45-year-old coachman with a popliteal aneurysm. This shrank the aneurysm and saved the man's leg (15, 18).

Abernethy (1) in 1798 ligated an internal carotid artery (ICA) to control the hemorrhage of a man gored in the neck by a bull. The bleeding was controlled but the patient, hypotensive from blood loss, suffered a cerebral infarction several hours later and died 30 hours after the carotid artery had been occluded (1). Ligation of the common carotid artery for an aneurysm of the ICA was first performed in 1805 by Sir Astley Cooper. The patient died 20 days later of infection (4). However, Cooper (5) repeated the procedure in 1808 with a successful result. Subsequently, carotid ligation was performed for a wide variety of neurologic disorders, including carotid cavernous fistula (29). Sir Victor Horsley (3), at the end of the 19th century, appears to have been the first to ligate the carotid artery for a saccular intracranial aneurysm, which was discovered during exploration for a presumptive middle fossa tumor. The introduction by Moniz of cerebral angiography in 1927 made the regular identification of intracranial aneurysms possible. Since then all of the extra-cranial vessels, the intracranial vessels, and their major branches have been occluded in the treatment of aneurysms (9, 26).

Carotid artery ligation was for more than half a century the primary surgical procedure to prevent enlargement and reduce the chance of rupture of aneurysms arising from the intracranial ICA, the middle cerebral artery (MCA), and in those anterior communicating aneurysms with a dominant or unilateral arterial supply (19, 21, 22). Carotid ligation for the more proximal lesions was effective in reducing the pressure and flow within the sac; its value for the anterior communicating and MCA aneurysms was less certain (11, 22).

Carotid ligation is less likely to produce cerebral ischemic complications than is more distal occlusion because of the presence of natural extra- to intracranial collaterals, the presence of the basal collateral of Willis, and the potential of cortical leptomeningeal collateral. This procedure still entails significant risk. In the pre-Listerian era, mortality rates of 38–55% and cerebral ischemic complications of 40% were reported in large series (6). Many of these complications were presumed due to sepsis. Matas (6) in 1940 reported 60 common and 6 ICA ligations with 12% mortality, and Dandy (6) in 1941 described 88 cases of extra- and intracranial ligation with 5% mortality and 7% cerebral circulatory disturbances. Nishioka's report of the Cooperative Study of 785 cases indicated a 30% cerebral ischemic complication rate, with 78% of the unruptured aneurysms and 56% of the ruptured aneurysms successfully treated (21). Because almost one-half of these ischemic events occurred within the first 6 hours, it was presumed that they were due to hemodynamic failure of the cerebral circulation. The Cooperative Study data also suggested (but because of multiple variables could not prove) that ICA ligation was slightly more effective but carried a greater risk than common carotid ligation and that gradual occlusion was safer than abrupt ligation. A more contemporary series by Jawad et al. (17) reported a 20% incidence of cerebral ischemia following carotid ligation.

Certainly, carotid ligation for aneurysms arising from the anterior cerebral complex or the MCA is less likely to be effective because the very collateral circulation that protects the brain also maintains pressure and flow to these more distal sacs. More distal occlusion of the intracranial carotid beyond the contribution of the circle of Willis or occlusion of the proximal MCA are effective in obliterating ICA bifurcation and MCA aneurysms, respectively, but at a much higher risk to the continued nutrition of the hemisphere. The collateral available to the MCA territory after proximal MCA occlusion is variable and limited almost entirely to the small connections between the central terminals of the anterior cerebral, posterior cerebral, and middle cerebral arteries. Moreover, the thalamostriate perforators coming off the terminal carotid or proximal MCA have virtually no direct or immediate collateral connections, making the central portion of the hemisphere particularly vulnerable to reduced perfusion.

EC-IC BYPASS

In an attempt to reduce the risks of ischemic complications following proximal vessel occlusion, the creation of a surgical collateral in the form of an extracranial to intracranial arterial bypass was first postulated and reported by Yasargil (35). In his 1969 monograph, he demonstrated the EC-IC bypass in the treatment of two intracranial aneurysms. Since then, several reports have described series of patients on whom the EC-IC bypass has been used in conjunction with Hunterian ligation in the treatment of aneurysms (10, 16, 26, 27, 30, 32, 36). Sindou and Keravel (31) in June 1984 summarized the reports in the literature of 113 patients treated in this fashion and noted generally good results, but with 16.8% of the patients suffering ischemic cerebral complications. Although only 5% of the surgical anastomoses were not patent, the individuals in this group had a higher risk of cerebral ischemia or infarction. However, even with a patent bypass, ischemia still occurred due to insufficient flow and embolism. Heros (13) polled 13 neurosurgeons performing EC-IC bypass for treatment of aneurysms and reported 12 cases of thromboembolic complications. From this survey and his own experience, he recommended detachable balloon occlusion of the internal carotid artery and anticoagulation.

EC-IC bypass in the treatment of giant intracranial aneurysms is today undoubtedly the best indication for the bypass and has greatly extended our ability to deal with these lesions. Even so, many questions remain unanswered. Should all patients be bypassed before proximal vessel occlusion? If not, how can patients who will benefit from preliminary bypass be identified? How does one decide whether to use the superficial temporal or the occipital artery or to interpose a high volume vein graft to irrigate the hemisphere? What is the optimum method and timing of proximal vessel occlusion? What is the role of anticoagulants and non-steroidal antiinflammatory agents to suppress platelet function in the overall management of these patients?

In addressing these questions, we will review our experience with 65 patients treated with bypass and proximal vessel occlusion. Five of these cases will be described in detail because they illustrate important considerations in the management of these lesions.

CASE REPORTS

Case 1. H.G., a 73-year-old right-handed male, was well, except for hypertension, until March 1983, when he noted diplopia. By August 1983, it had progressed to complete ophthalmoplegia and diminished acuity in the right eye. Computed tomography (CT scan) and cerebral angiography demonstrated a giant right carotid cavernous aneurysm (Fig. 8.1). On August 18, 1983, a superficial temporal to middle cerebral artery (STA-MCA) bypass was performed. Four days later, balloon occlusion of the right ICA was attempted twice within 2 hours, but with each inflation of the balloon the patient developed left-sided numbness and weakness within a few minutes. The neurologic abnormalities resolved completely with deflation of the balloon (Fig. 8.2A). Balloon occlusion of the ICA was again unsuccessful 1 week and 1 month later. In April 1984, 8 months after his STA-MCA bypass, the ICA was occluded with a detachable balloon without incident (Fig. 8.2B). Angiography demonstrated no filling of the aneurysm. During this last successful balloon occlusion, the patient was taking aspirin (ASA) and was fully heparinized. The heparin was continued for 3 days following occlusion of the internal carotid artery, and he was discharged on aspirin (325 mg twice daily). At follow-up in August 1984, his visual acuity had improved, but the ophthalmoplegia was as yet unchanged. He was otherwise neurologically well.

Comment. Despite a functioning bypass, this man could not tolerate internal carotid artery occlusion but had immediate ischemic deficit develop with the balloon inflation. He could not tolerate repeated attempts to occlude the vessel over 1 month. Eight months following the bypass, balloon occlusion was successful, suggesting that maturation of the bypass and/or other improvement of collateral flow had occurred in the interim. The importance of this case lies in its demonstration of the value of reversible occlusion of the ICA with an intravascular balloon in a fully conscious patient, permitting accurate neurological assessment with angiographic control.

Case 2. C.E., a 38-year-old right-handed male, first presented in June 1974 with a 1-year history of persistent, severe headache. Neurologic examination revealed no abnormalities. Cerebral angiography disclosed the presence of three intracranial aneurysms: a giant, partially thrombosed, right ICA bifurcation aneurysm (Fig. 8.3); a smaller left ICA bifurcation aneurysm; and a small basilar bifurcation aneurysm. At operation, the left ICA aneurysm was successfully clipped, but the right ICA aneurysm could not be secured because of a broad and calcified neck. A Selverstone clamp was applied to the right ICA. During the next year, four attempts were made to occlude the clamp, but on each occasion, the patient abruptly developed a left hemiplegia and parietal sensory deficit.

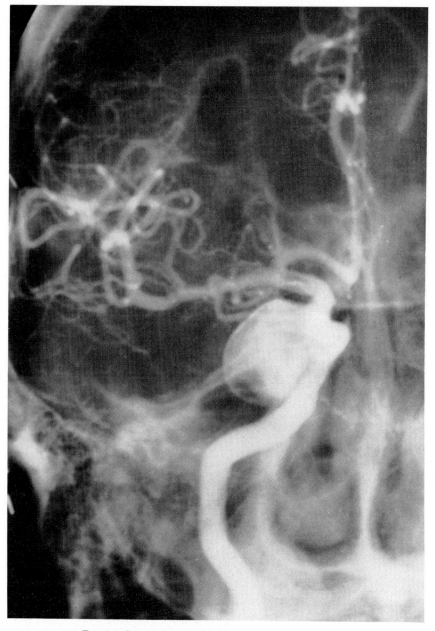

FIG. 8.1. Case 1. Giant right carotid cavernous aneurysm.

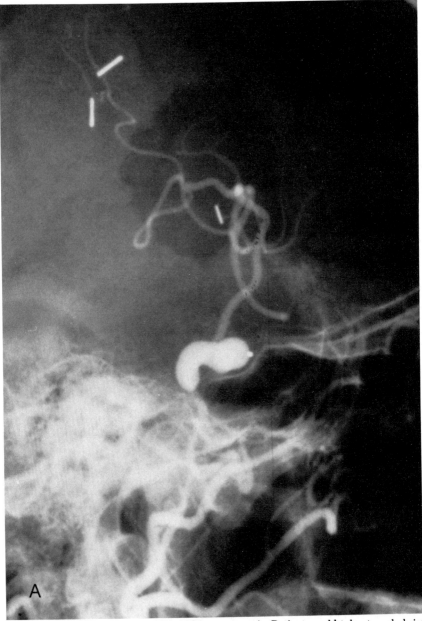

FIG. 8.2. Case 1. (A) Patent STA-MCA anastomosis. Patient would tolerate only brief periods of internal carotid artery occlusion. Note balloon inflated with contrast in cavernous portion of carotid. (B) Eight months following STA-MCA anastomosis. The bypass has enlarged with increased flow, and the internal carotid artery was successfully occluded with two detachable balloons. There was no filling of the aneurysm.

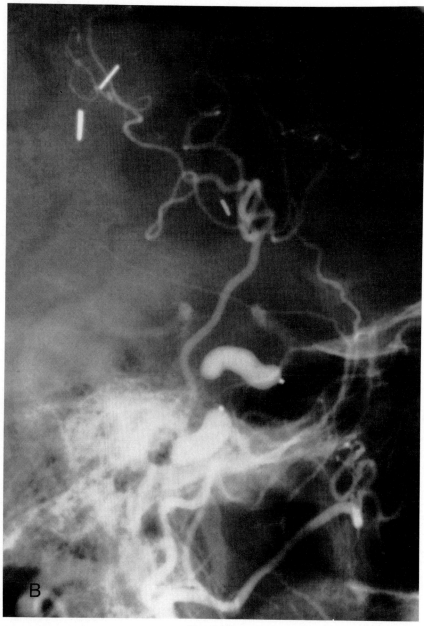

FIG. 8.2*B*

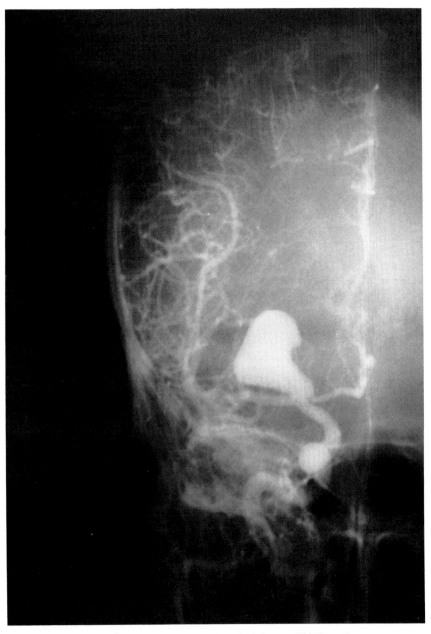

FIG. 8.3. Case 2. Giant, partially thrombosed, right carotid bifurcation aneurysm.

Repeat angiography in July 1975 demonstrated that the right ICA aneurysm had enlarged, and once again the patient did not tolerate full occlusion of the ICA but it was left with a 90% stenosis. Because of persistent headache and radiographic evidence of further enlargement of the aneurysm, an occipital artery to distal MCA bypass was performed on January 19, 1976. Following the bypass, complete ICA occlusion was tolerated without event. Angiography revealed the right ICA to be completely occluded and the bypass to be functioning well, but there was faint filling of the aneurysm via the anterior communicating artery from the left carotid injection. Because of increasing headache over the next year, the patient returned for follow-up angiography which demonstrated that the aneurysm had once again enlarged and was filling both from the left side via the anterior communicating artery (Fig. 8.4) and from the vertebral basilar system via the posterior communicating artery. He was

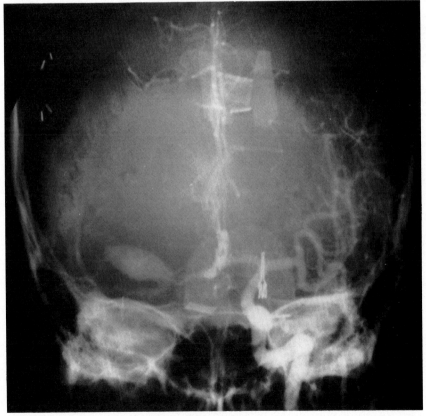

FIG. 8.4. Case 2. Persistent filling of aneurysm, following ICA occlusion, from left carotid injection via the anterior communicating artery.

taken to the operating room, and a microtourniquet was placed around the right A1, and a second tourniquet was placed around the right intracranial ICA distal to the anterior choroidal artery. These tourniquets were closed the following day under angiographic control (Fig. 8.5), thereby isolating the MCA completely from the circle of Willis. Follow-up angiography in February 1977 and July 1981 demonstrated the aneurysm to be fully thrombosed and diminished in size. The MCA was completely filled by a markedly enlarged occipital artery bypass (Fig. 8.6). The patient has remained well to date.

Comment. This case is important because it was our first experience with completely isolating the MCA from all of its proximal collateral flow, with the bypass providing perfusion to the whole central portion of the hemisphere. It also underscores the potential failure of carotid occlusion alone in preventing further enlargement of a giant aneurysm

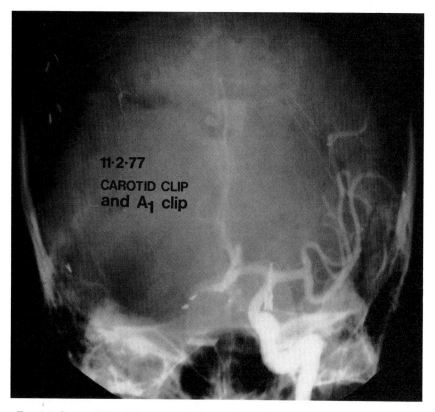

FIG. 8.5. Case 2. Right A1 and terminal carotid occluded with microtourniquets. Aneurysm no longer fills.

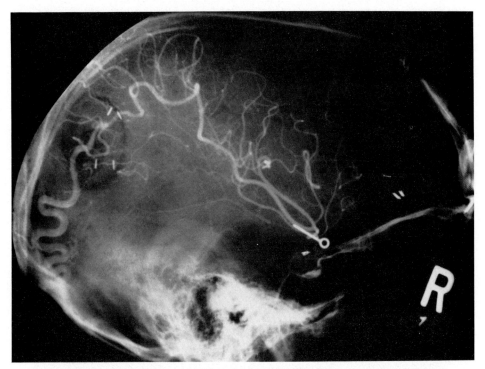

FIG. 8.6. Case 2. Excellent filling of MCA territory by occipital to MCA bypass.

of the distal ICA, and the value of the microtourniquet technique to bring
about controlled occlusion of intracranial vessels, precisely and reversibly.

Case 3. J.B., a 32-year-old male, was well until December 1, 1983,
when he suffered a coma-producing subarachnoid hemorrhage (SAH)
while on the toilet. He recovered consciousness over several hours, and
by the following day was Grade 1 (on the Hunt-Botterell scale). A CT
scan and cerebral angiography revealed the presence of a giant, left MCA
aneurysm (Fig. 8.7A). Eight days following his hemorrhage, the aneurysm
was explored, and two large branches were found to be emerging from
the dome of the sac, as well as a lenticulostriate artery arising from the
base of the lesion, preventing neck occlusion. A STA-MCA bypass was
performed. Postoperatively, he was neurologically intact. There was
marked perianeurysmal edema at surgery which prevented the placement
of a tourniquet and delayed reoperation for 3 weeks. After the swelling
had subsided, the aneurysm was reexplored, and a microtourniquet was
placed around the M1 segment and closed sufficiently to stenose but not
occlude the vessel. Following this procedure, the patient remained well

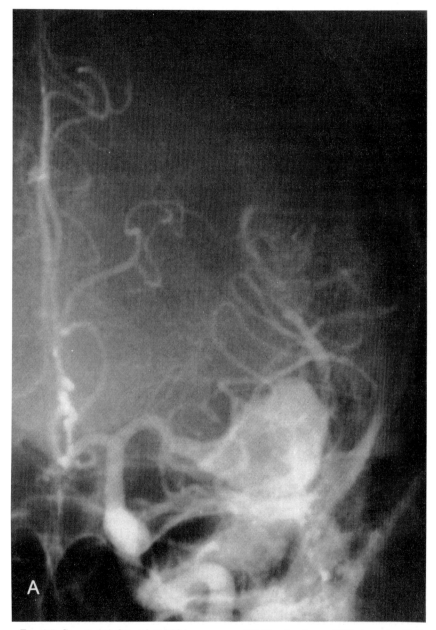

FIG. 8.7. Case 3. (*A*) Giant left MCA aneurysm. (*B*) Greater than a 90% stenosis of M1 at the site of the tourniquet (*arrow*), with massive thrombosis of the aneurysm leaving a narrow channel filling a M2 branch. (*C*) Further thrombosis of the aneurysm. A small portion of the proximal neck remains, through which a large lenticulostriate branch fills (see *arrow*).

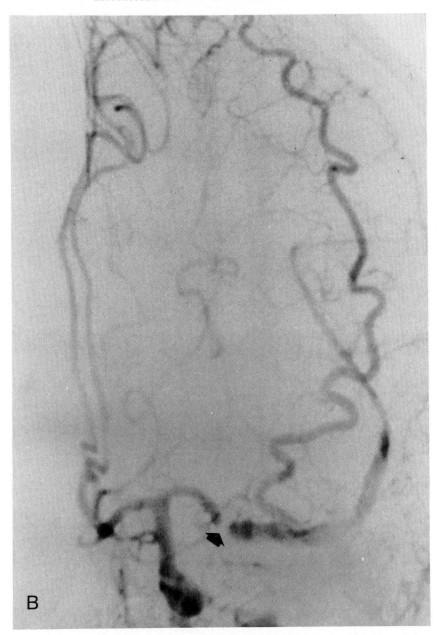

FIG. 8.7*B*

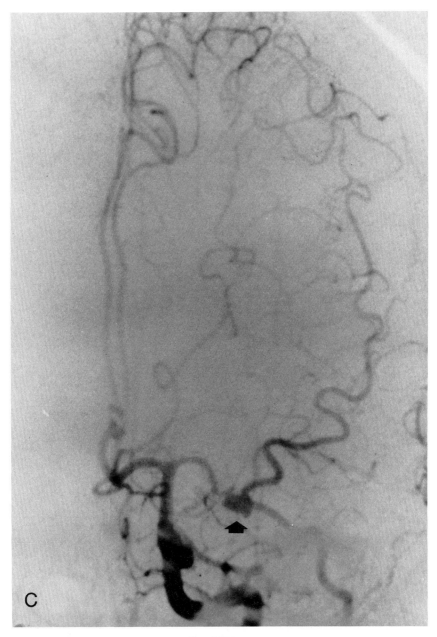

FIG. 8.7C

for 12 hours; then, he abruptly developed a severe aphasia and mild hemiparesis. With volume expansion and elevation of blood pressure, these deficits largely resolved over 24 hours. Angiography at this time revealed more than 90% stenosis of the M1 at the site of the tourniquet, with almost complete obliteration of the aneurysm except for a narrow channel filling the large M2 branch (Fig. 8.7B). The tourniquet was buried the following day, and the patient remained well, except for occasional word-finding difficulty, for 5 days, at which time he abruptly again developed increased aphasia and right upper extremity clumsiness. Repeat angiography demonstrated complete thrombosis of the aneurysm, except for a proximal funnel distal to the tourniquet through which a large lenticulostriate branch was filling (Fig. 8.7C). The patent bypass, along with leptomeningeal collateral from the anterior cerebral artery (Fig. 8.8), provided excellent collateral supply to the MCA territory. His neurologic deficits slowly improved. At discharge, he had a mild word-finding difficulty and a mild hemiparesis. At follow-up in May 1984, he had returned to work having only occasional word-finding difficulty and decreased fine finger movements of his right hand.

  Comment. In this case, we attempted to sharply reduce the flow into the aneurysm with stenosis of the MCA. This brought about partial thrombosis of the aneurysm but continued to provide flow to critical proximal lenticulostriate branches. The patient suffered two probable embolic events 12 hours and 5 days following stenosis of the vessel, despite being on ASA and dipyridamole. Heparin was not used because of the recent craniotomy and the history of massive rupture of this aneurysm in the recent past.

  Case 4. M.V., a 62-year-old right-handed female, presented with a 4-month history of bifrontal headache, a 3-month history of intermittent diplopia, and progressive loss of visual acuity in her left eye. Radiographic investigation revealed a giant left ICA aneurysm extending from the ophthalmic region to the intracranial bifurcation (Fig. 8.9). With cross-compression angiography, it was demonstrated that she had no A1 on the left and minimal posterior communicating arteries bilaterally. On May 31, 1983, she was explored at another hospital, and the aneurysm was found to involve the whole length of the intracranial carotid, ending into the left MCA. The aneurysm ruptured during attempts to clip it, and the procedure was abandoned. Six days later, we reopened her craniotomy and confirmed that the aneurysm could not be directly repaired. As the STA had been sacrificed at the initial craniotomy, a saphenous vein bypass graft was interposed between the left external carotid artery in the neck and two supra-Sylvian cortical branches and one infra-Sylvian cortical branch of the MCA. During the next 3 days, two attempts were made at balloon occlusion of the ICA, but on each

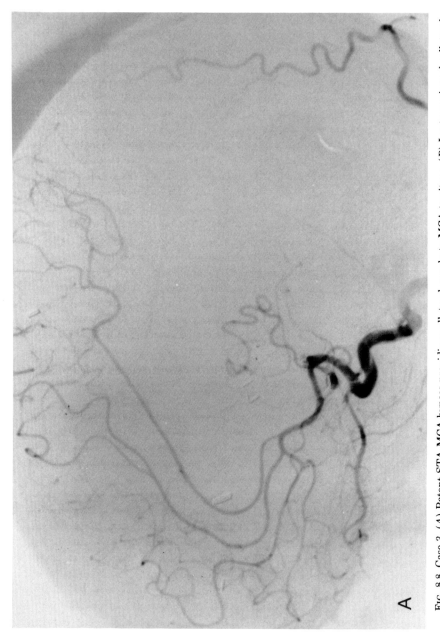

FIG. 8.8. Case 3. (A) Patent STA-MCA bypass providing collateral supply to MCA territory. (B) Leptomeningeal collateral to the supra-Sylvian branches from the anterior cerebral artery.

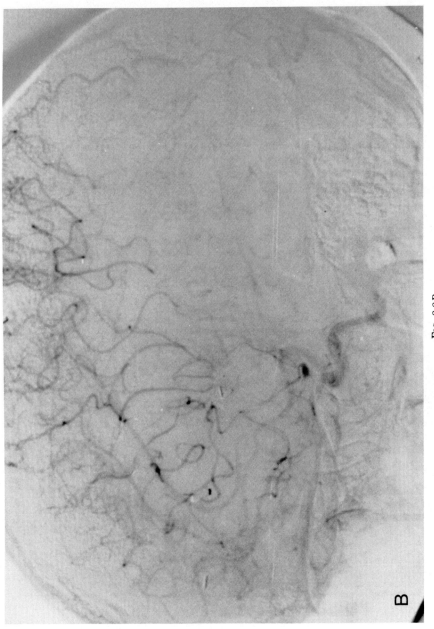

FIG. 8.8B

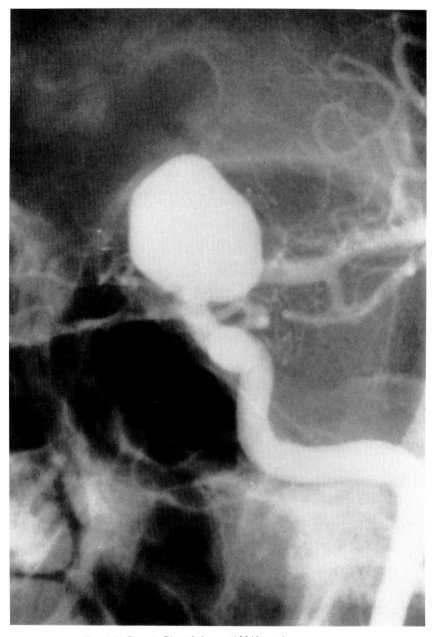

FIG. 8.9. Case 4. Giant left carotid bifurcation aneurysm.

occasion the patient developed a mild parietal dysfunction, and the balloons were deflated and removed (Fig. 8.10). Finally, on July 25, 1983, she was taken back to the angiographic suite, where repeat angiography again demonstrated excellent flow through the vein bypass and, on this occasion, the ICA was completely and uneventfully occluded with two balloons. A final angiogram on July 28, 1983, demonstrated a complete thrombosis of the aneurysm, with excellent flow to the left hemisphere via the bypass graft (Fig. 8.11). She has remained headache-free, with normal visual acuity and motor function.

Comment. It is wise to anticipate the necessity of EC-IC arterial bypass when planning the flap for exploration of a giant intracranial aneurysm. Although we have 9 years of follow-up on one patient with an interposed saphenous vein bypass, which is patent, we agree with the belief that the early and long-term patency of vein grafts is less than the patency rates of STA or occipital artery bypasses. This patient's initial failure to tolerate carotid artery occlusion, despite the presence of a high-volume bypass, may have been the result of the two previous explorations of the aneurysm, with an intraoperative rupture producing a degree of vasospasm.

Case 5. R.B., a 53-year-old architect from Tasmania, was well until March 14, 1984, when he had a sudden loss of consciousness and subsequently developed focal seizures involving his left face and extremities. A CT scan and angiography demonstrated a giant, partially thrombosed, left MCA aneurysm and a large anterior communicating artery aneurysm (Figs. 8.12 and 8.13). There was no history of SAH. The seizures were controlled with diphenylhydantoin. When the patient arrived at University Hospital, he was found to be neurologically intact. On May 25, 1984, the aneurysm was explored and could not be clipped because of massive thrombosis and multiple large perforators arising from the proximal neck of the sac. A STA-MCA bypass was performed, and a tourniquet was placed around M1. Postoperatively, he had a transient expressive aphasia, due to operative manipulation of his frontal and temporal lobes. The following day in the Angiographic Suite, the tourniquet was closed (Fig. 8.14), which the patient tolerated for 20 minutes before developing motor aphasia and right hemiparesis, which resolved slowly over 2 hours with opening of the tourniquet. The tourniquet was then retightened to produce approximately 90% stenosis, which the patient tolerated for 3 hours before again developing aphasia and right hemiparesis. The tourniquet was once more opened, and over several hours the neurologic function of his hemisphere was recovered. One month later, he was returned to the operating room, and under cardiopulmonary bypass and deep hypothermia (18°C), the aneurysm was opened and evacuated, and the MCA was reconstructed with multiple clips. The tourniquet was used

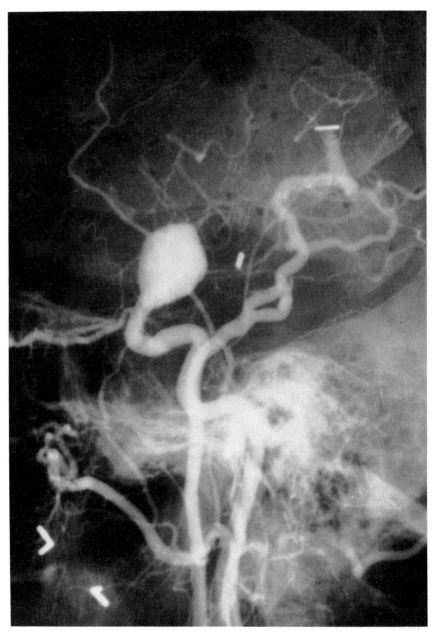

FIG. 8.10. Case 4. Postoperative angiography revealing patent vein bypass and spontaneous partial thrombosis of aneurysm. Balloon occlusion of ICA not tolerated at this time.

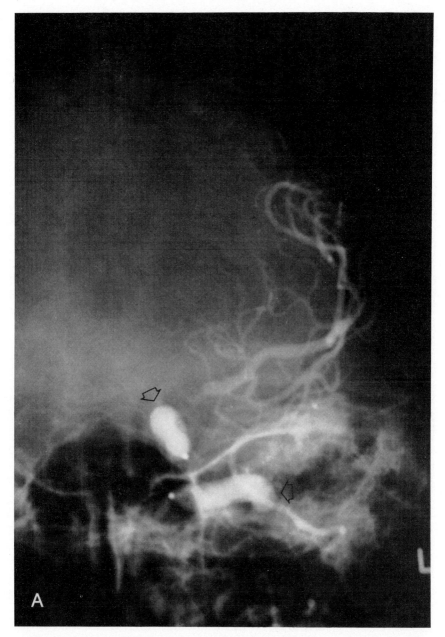

FIG. 8.11. Case 4. (*A* and *B*) Eight weeks following vein graft. Successful carotid occlusion and aneurysm thrombosis. Excellent flow to the left hemispheres. ICA balloons filled with contrast are marked with *arrows*.

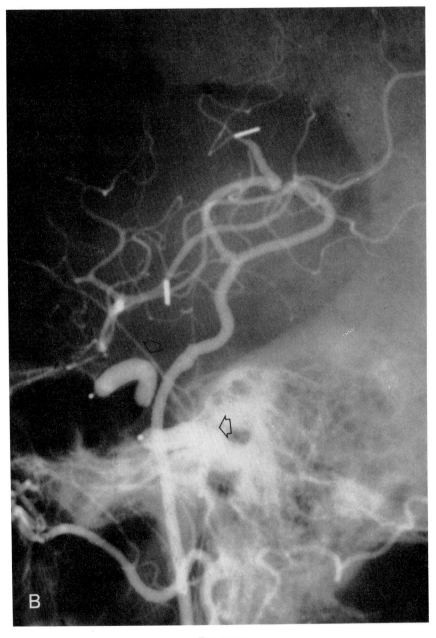

Fig. 8.11B

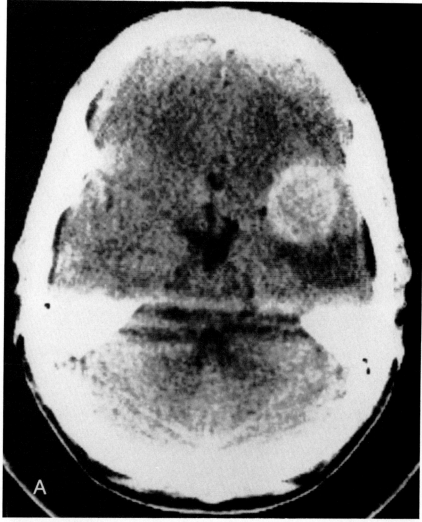

FIG. 8.12. Case 5. (*A* and *B*) Noncontrast and contrast CT scan demonstrating giant, partially thrombosed, left MCA aneurysm and large anterior communicating aneurysm. Note the edema around the aneurysm.

to occlude M1 during the dissection, evacuation, and clipping of the aneurysm but was opened at the conclusion of the procedure to provide perfusion of the proximal lenticulostriate vessels arising from the origin of the aneurysm. Postoperatively, the patient was well, with a minimal, transient expressive aphasia only. Postoperative angiograms revealed the aneurysm to be almost completely obliterated, except for a small portion

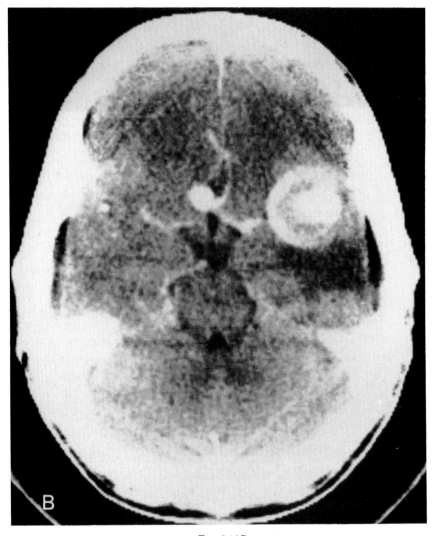

FIG. 8.12*B*

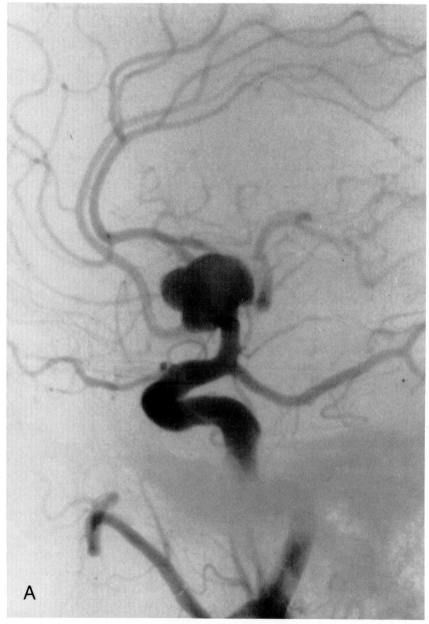

A

FIG. 8.13. Case 5. (*A* and *B*) Cerebral angiography confirming the aneurysms (*open arrows* demonstrating extent of partially thrombosed MCA aneurysm).

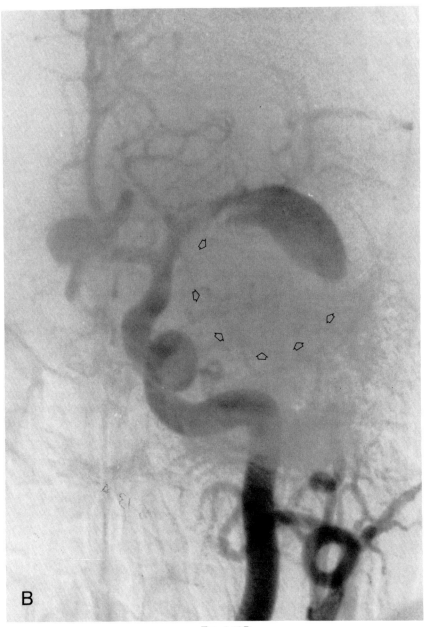

B

FIG. 8.13*B*

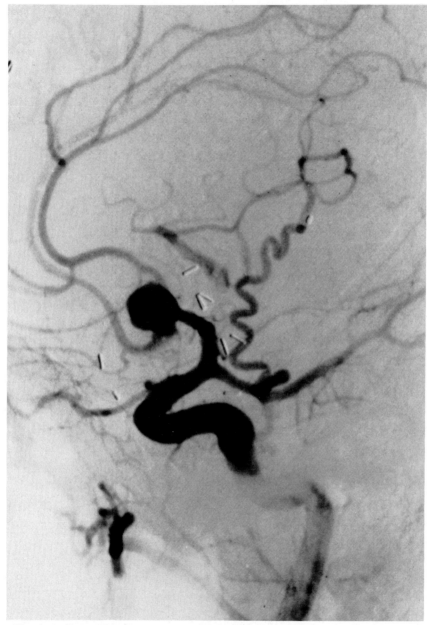

FIG. 8.14. Case 5. Tourniquet occlusion of M1 with obliteration of MCA aneurysm and patent bypass. M1 occlusion was tolerated for only 20 minutes.

remaining at the base which carried the perforating vessels (Fig. 8.15). Two months later, the anterior communicating aneurysm was successfully clipped.

Comment. In this case, the bypass was insufficient to provide perfusion of the whole MCA territory, as evidenced by the gradual emergence of neurologic dysfunction with complete occlusion and even high-grade stenosis of M1 after several hours. Because of the need to evacuate the mass of this aneurysm, as well as to protect the medial lenticulostriate perforators, an aneurysmorrhaphy was performed during low-flow, cardiopulmonary bypass, and deep hypothermia. During dissection of the aneurysm, the M1 segment was occluded with the tourniquet, but continued flow was provided to the distal territory by the bypass.

RESULTS

We have now had experience with 65 patients whose giant aneurysms we treated with EC-IC bypass and proximal vessel occlusion. In 55 of them, we used the STA or occipital artery, and in 10, a saphenous vein graft was interposed between the external carotid artery and (usually multiple) cortical middle cerebral branches to provide the surgical collateral.

Overall, the results have been encouraging. The patients were all followed up in August of 1984, and 88% were found to be in good or excellent condition, that is, neurologically normal or functioning at their normal activity but with slight neurologic deficits. Since each patient was judged to have insufficient collateral, based on the angiographic study, cerebral blood flow (CBF) study, or previous failed attempts at proximal occlusion, and since 31 of them had aneurysms that required occlusion distal to the major collateral pathway, we feel that these results represent a substantial improvement over previous methods. Certainly, proximal vessel occlusion close to the origin of the aneurysm has been very effective in preventing further enlargement or rupture of the aneurysm. In no case in which the proximal vessel occlusion has been finally accomplished has the aneurysm continued to enlarge or rupture.

Bypass Patency

All but two of the STA or occipital artery bypass grafts were patent immediately and at long-term follow-up. The interposed veins fared somewhat less well. Two of these grafts occluded within days or weeks of their anastomosis, but in both cases, the collateral perfusion provided during the critical period of proximal vessel occlusion appeared to support the hemisphere until other collateral developed. Our experience suggests that once a vein has remained patent for 1 month, the likelihood of long-term patency is high. Our first interposed vein was inserted in June 1977

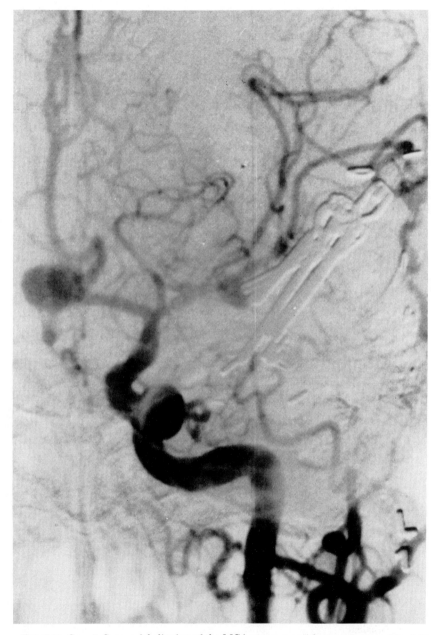

FIG. 8.15. Case 5. Successful clipping of the MCA aneurysm with preservation of the M2 branches and perforators arising from a small portion of the proximal neck.

in the treatment of a giant MCA aneurysm and remains patent today. Late neurologic complications have not been observed. No further enlargement, rupture of the aneurysm, progressive ischemic deficit, or late thromboembolic events have occurred.

Table 8.1 summarizes the results on 65 patients listed according to the site of the aneurysm. Half of the cases, that is, aneurysms arising from the cervical ICA, the petrous, the cavernous, and ophthalmic regions, should all be considered proximal to the major natural collateral flow by the ophthalmic collateral and the posterior communicating artery.

In one case an extracranial cervical carotid aneurysm presented as a painful, pulsatile mass in the neck in a 56-year-old woman. Because of an incomplete circle of Willis, an EC-IC arterial bypass was done, followed by ligation of the cervical ICA and intracranial clipping of the ICA proximal to the origin of the ophthalmic artery. The aneurysm was trapped because of its large size and the fact that it was seen, on angiography, to be partially filled with thrombus.

The single petrous carotid aneurysm presented with a history of recurrent otitis and a petrosal syndrome. Balloon occlusion of the ICA was attempted but not tolerated with the rapid development of ischemic dysfunction. A surgical collateral was, therefore, fashioned from the STA to MCA, and the ICA was closed with a Selverstone clamp. The patient tolerated this well.

There were 15 carotid cavernous aneurysms treated with EC-IC bypass and ICA occlusion. Thirteen of these patients had excellent results, but two died. Twelve of the 15 patients with carotid cavernous aneurysms presented with cavernous sinus syndromes. All of them had complete relief of their pain postoperatively and have had substantial, if not complete, reversal of their cranial nerve dysfunction. Three patients with

TABLE 8.1
Surgical Results, According to the Aneurysmal Site

| | EC/IC Bypass for Giant Aneurysms | | | | | |
| | Results | | | | | |
	No. of Patients	Excellent	Good	Fair	Poor	Dead
Carotid						
Cervical	1	1				
Petrous	1	1				
Cavernous	15	13				2
Ophthalmic	15	11	1	2	1	
Communicating	2	1	1			
Bifurcation	14	13				1
Middle cerebral	17	11	4	1	1	
Totals	65	51	6	3	2	3

carotid cavernous aneurysms presented with SAH. The fundus of the aneurysm had eroded through the temporal dura of the cavernous sinus and ruptured into the subarachnoid space. Complete obliteration of the aneurysm was effected in every instance.

Fifteen patients presented with carotid ophthalmic or para-ophthalmic aneurysms with broad or calcified necks that could not be directly clipped. Eight of these patients presented with progressive visual loss: four with subarachnoid hemorrhage (SAH), one with transient ischemic attacks (TIAs), one with embolic stroke, and one with seizures. In the last patient the aneurysm was discovered on investigation of unilateral hearing loss. Three of the 15 patients with paraophthalmic aneurysms were left with a significant neurological deficit. In one, the patient suffered an embolic cerebral complication during the preoperative angiographic study. Two suffered postoperative thromboembolic complications and, in both instances, it was clear that the embolus had arisen from the aneurysmal sac. The value of trapping the sac to prevent this disaster is evident.

There were two patients with giant aneurysms arising from the carotid communicating region. One presented with a minor embolic stroke in the MCA territory, distal to the aneurysm, and the second one with TIAs. In both instances, thromboembolic material was felt to have originated within the giant aneurysmal sac. With proximal vessel occlusion, preceded by bypass, both aneurysms thrombosed completely with no further events.

Fourteen patients presented with giant ICA bifurcation aneurysms. The clinical presentation of these patients included: three with SAH; five with headache and neurologic deficit from mass effect; five with seizures; and one with ischemic stroke. An excellent result was obtained in 13 of these patients, but one died from a fatal SAH on the day before we had planned to occlude the ICA.

Seventeen patients had giant MCA aneurysms. Six of them presented with TIA or stroke, five with SAH, three with seizures, two with intractable headache, and one with visual deficit. In nine instances, the MCA was occluded with a microtourniquet following exploration of the aneurysm and placement of the bypass. In six patients, aneurysmorraphy was carried out with reforming of the neck using clips and evacuation of a largely thrombosed mass. One patient had his MCA clipped directly distal to the lenticulostriate perforators and sparing the central sulcus branch of the MCA. The bypass was anastomosed to the angular artery, providing adequate collateral flow to the parietal and temporal distribution of the MCA. There were two embolic complications in the MCA group. One of these occurred preoperatively from a giant and largely thrombosed aneurysmal sac. This patient has been listed as fair, functioning at home independently but with a hemiparesis. The poor result occurred 24 hours after microtourniquet stenosis of the origin of the MCA. Thrombus, originating in the sac of the aneurysm, migrated to the angular artery of the dominant hemisphere, resulting in hemiparesis and severe aphasia. The value of the microtourniquet in producing reversible occlusion or controlled stenosis was dramatically underscored in this group. Six patients had transient but totally reversible neurologic signs, usually within 30 minutes of occluding the MCA but, on two occasions, within 3 hours. When the MCA is occluded at its origin, there is a very limited potential for natural collateral; therefore, the surgical collateral is called upon immediately to supply flow to a large volume of brain. With time (probably measured in days), leptomeningeal collateral and collateral provided through the choroidal and lenticulostriate arteries will augment the flow provided by the surgical anastomosis. Maintenance of critical perfusion pressure, optimum viscosity, and oxygenation and carbon dioxide levels in the blood are important until the flow has been stabilized. A particular problem unique to the giant MCA aneurysm is the mass effect produced by some of these aneurysms when they have progressed to the point of producing perianeurysmal edema, which may be dramatically worsened by an ischemic insult. As part of the treatment plan, it is frequently necessary to devise a strategy that will not only provide continued perfusion to normal brain but also will permit the surgeon to evacuate the mass. Trapping is rarely possible because of critical branches coming off the nonaneurysmal side of the neck, and aneurysmorrhaphy after opening and evacuation of the thrombus may be necessary.

Morbidity and Mortality (Table 8.2)

Five of the 65 patients were left with significant neurologic disability, and three died as the result of our attempts to deal with these aneurysms. The majority of these complications are ultimately preventable. All five of those with fair or poor results suffered embolic events. One occurred preoperatively during angiography. The ischemic deficit in the remaining four developed in the postoperative period after a delay of hours or, in one case, 2 days following proximal vessel occlusion. In each instance of the postoperative delayed ischemic event, we believe that the embolus arose from the progressing thrombosis in the aneurysmal sac and migrated into the proximal MCA, occluding the origin of the lenticulostriate vessels or critical bifurcation arteries. The two poor results came from deep hemispheric infarction causing aphasia and hemiplegia. In the patient with the carotid ophthalmic aneurysm who had a poor result, the embolus in the MCA was removed at emergency craniotomy and the aneurysm trapped with an intracranial clip. Despite the restoration of

TABLE 8.2

Results: Etiology of Morbidity and Mortality

Excellent—51 patients
  Neurologically normal
Good—6 patients
  Functioning at normal activity
  Detectable neurologic signs
  Three signs appeared after surgery
  Three preop deficits
Fair—3 patients
  Functioning at home independent
  Unable to work
  One postop embolic complication
  One preop angiographic complication
  One preop deficit
Poor—2 patients
  At home, need assistance
  Both postop embolic complications
Dead—3 patients
  One technical hemorrhage from anastomosis
  One ruptured aneurysm before occlusion
  One vasospasm + disseminated intravascular coagulation

flow in the MCA, and the excellent perfusion through a superficial temporal artery bypass, this woman has made little useful recovery.

Important lessons have been learned from all three of the fatal results, lessons that stress the risks of an inadequate bypass, of operating on patients with a high clinical grade, and of delaying proximal vessel occlusion.

One patient with a carotid cavernous aneurysm underwent a STA-MCA bypass which, because of technical problems, required revision of the microanastomosis. Postoperatively, the angiographic appearance of the bypass demonstrated slow perfusion of the middle cerebral territory. An attempt to occlude her carotid with an intravascular balloon was not tolerated, and the balloon was removed. A Selverstone clamp was then applied to the internal carotid artery and the vessel stenosed in an attempt to induce collateral flow. Over the next week, she had multiple transient ischemic attacks involving the affected hemisphere, despite vigorous attempts to maintain cerebral perfusion with blood volume expansion, heparin, and hypertensive agents. Twelve days after the placement of the EC-IC arterial bypass, she suffered an acute subdural hemorrhage from rupture of the microanastomosis. Despite the rapid removal of this clot, she died.

The second death, also with a cavernous aneurysm, occurred in a 64-

year-old woman who presented as a Grade 3 following a SAH from a 1.2-cm MCA aneurysm distal to a giant carotid cavernous aneurysm. The ruptured MCA aneurysm was repaired directly and a STA-MCA bypass fashioned in preparation for occlusion of her ICA. However, proximal vessel occlusion was never attempted because her postoperative course was complicated by severe vasospasm and then disseminated intravascular coagulation. She suffered multiple ischemic infarcts of both hemispheres and died 5 months later.

The single death that occurred in the carotid bifurcation group was a 66-year-old woman who presented with headache and was thought not to have suffered a SAH. The aneurysm was large and complex, involving the terminal carotid and both A1 and M1. A bypass was placed in preparation to occluding her ICA inflow. At the time (early in this series) we were under the impression that there was some advantage to delaying proximal occlusion until the graft had "matured." This unfortunate woman succumbed to a massive hemorrhage from this aneurysm, 7 days after the placement of the bypass and the day prior to our planned occlusion of the internal carotid artery.

DISCUSSION

While this series is small and each case presents with some unique problem, review of the series does suggest some general rules of how to proceed with the use of surgical collateral in the treatment of giant intracranial aneurysms. The first question is: Which patients require bypass as a preliminary step in the treatment of these aneurysms? Certainly it can be argued that to bypass all patients in whom proximal vessel occlusion is contemplated may be of value (8, 32). However, one cannot discount the small but very real morbidity and, rarely, mortality associated with the bypass itself (28). Certainly, any precise preoperative test that could identify those patients at risk from hemodynamic cerebral ischemia secondary to proximal vessel occlusion, would be of value. We believe that all unclippable aneurysms arising from the MCA probably require a bypass, since the natural collateral to the middle cerebral territory is limited to leptomeningeal vessels and the much slower development of deep striate and choroidal anastomoses. We would recommend that whenever proximal vessel occlusion is contemplated for the MCA, a preliminary bypass should be considered. Moreover, it is in this group that high volume bypass with the use of an interposed vein may have its greatest justification.

"At-Risk" Patients

Of the more proximal carotid lesion, some method of determining the patients at risk would seem to be of value. Detailed angiographic studies are essential, including carotid injections with cross-compression to demonstrate the patency of the anterior communicating artery and the presence of both A1s and vertebral injections with internal carotid artery compression to visualize the posterior communicating arteries (Allcock's test). Also required is injection of the external carotid artery to visualize the ophthalmic and meningeal collateral and the existence of any lepto-meningeal collateral in a careful, superselective, four-vessel study. It is critical to identify the site of origin of the first vessel or vessels distal to the point of proposed occlusion, and to estimate whether or not the natural or the surgical collateral will be sufficient to maintain perfusion of this arterial branch when the main vessel is occluded. For example, it is desirable that the anterior choroidal artery and the medial lenticulo-striate vessel must be included in the collateral network, with some certainty that their flow will be maintained.

Cerebral Blood Flow Studies

Cerebral blood flow (CBF) studies offer some promise in patient selection. Using modification of the technique of Jawad et al. (17), we have used inhalation of xenon(^{133}Xe), with flow studies carried out before and during digital compression of the affected ICA. If the flows during compression are 40 ml/100 gm/minute or more, regardless of the per-centage change from the control value, it is probably safe to ligate the carotid artery without EC-IC arterial bypass. If the flows during com-pression are less than 20 ml/100 gm/minute, then the creation of a surgical collateral is almost certainly necessary. If the CBF during compression lies between 20 and 40 ml/100 gm/minute, then the ligation of the carotid is safe, provided that the CBF reduction from control flow is less than 25%. Ligation of the carotid is also probably safe in the CBF range of 20–40 ml/100 gm/minute with up to 35% reduction in flow, provided that the internal carotid artery pressure is greater than 60 mm Hg (24). Such factors as the complexity of the test, the necessity of having a cooperative patient, the difficulty in the scheduling, the impos-sibility of obtaining accurate stump pressures in our method which is done on the ward, and the cost have all mitigated against using CBF as a standard and routine method of selection. Moreover, there remains some doubt about the accuracy of the measurement and its value when one considers that all of our serious and permanent neurologic ischemic complications have been the result of thromboembolic events which, of course, the CBF study will not predict.

Parent Vessel Occlusion

Hemodynamic microcirculatory failure is a dynamic process best eval-uated by observing the exquisitely sensitive function of the cerebral neuron in the awake patient. Belief in this concept has led us to rely increasingly on temporary occlusion of the parent vessel with the microtourniquet or the intravascular balloon. This maneuver is invaluable when coupled with angiography to document precisely the completeness of the occlusion and repeated neurologic examination to test the adequacy of neuronal function. Insufficient perfusion has usually resulted in a rapid loss of neurologic function, which is equally rapidly reversed upon opening the tourniquet or deflating the balloon. If a patient tolerates complete occlusion for 30 minutes, the likelihood is high that permanent carotid occlusion will be tolerated. Although we have not used the intravascular balloon to produce a partially occluding lesion, varying degrees of stenosis are readily accomplished with the tourniquet and, on more than one occasion, massive and indeed complete thrombosis of the aneurysm has been produced. However, we believe that the proximal vessel occlusion should be carried out as close to the neck of the aneurysm as possible to exclude the possibility of collateral crossing the neck and to avoid leaving an elongated, stagnant stump proximal or distal to the aneurysm. It is the continued low flow and a relatively stagnant column of blood that markedly increases the risk of embolic events. To this end, the intravascular balloon is placed at the base of the skull or in the intracavernous portion of the carotid; this procedure is preferable to mechanical clamping or ligation of the proximal internal carotid artery in the neck. However, an aneurysmal clip or microtourniquet is superior to the balloon when precise occlusion of the vessel is required, but meticulous care must be taken to spare any adjacent perforating branches.

Technical Aspects of the Extracranial to Intracranial Bypass

Technical aspects of the EC-IC bypass deserve evaluation (25). Considering that the STA or occipital artery can deliver only a limited volume of blood, we thought it reasonable to anastomose the extracranial vessel to a cortical vessel in the region of the hemisphere at greatest risk. For example, anastomosis in a dominant hemisphere to vessels in the speech and hand region is logically preferable to an anastomosis at the tip of the temporal lobe. The anastomosis itself should always be at least three times the diameter of the recipient vessel, and all adjacent cortical branches should be spared to maximize the runoff. If the scalp vessels are small or have been sacrificed in a previous operation, we have resorted to harvesting the long saphenous vein and interposing it between the external carotid artery in the neck and multiple cortical branches of the MCA. Two, three, or four distal anastomoses not only increase the collateral flow but also diminish the chance of slow flow and sludging and, ultimately, of thrombosis in the interposed vein. Also, we no longer delay the proximal vessel occlusion, waiting for the anastomosis and graft to "mature" (8, 32). As soon as the patient has recovered sufficiently from the anesthetic to be evaluated neurologically, we proceed with the proximal vessel occlusion. Substantial enlargement of the STA has been observed within hours of fashioning the anastomosis, and following Hunterian ligation. It would appear that as soon as the pressure drop across the anastomosis is maximized, the graft will respond to the demand by increasing flow.

The Problem of Thromboembolism

On reviewing our results, we found that the embolic complications following EC-IC arterial bypass and proximal vessel occlusion have been the most common and devastating cause of ischemic damage to these patients. In contrast to the hemodynamic failure that, although common, is usually easily reversed, an embolus lodging in the M1 segment and occluding striate vessels will almost always produce ischemic infarction. Our studies have demonstrated active platelet-fibrin deposition and turnover in the sacs of giant aneurysms, and the potential for this material to embolize into the cerebral vascular tree (34). This process is enhanced by low flows, by manipulation of the aneurysmal sac, or by a lengthy stump of vessel proximal or distal to the aneurysm itself. For these reasons, our practice has been to trap these aneurysms whenever possible, or occlude the parent artery as close to or, preferably, at the neck of the aneurysm with a detachable balloon to prevent egress of the embolic material and to minimize the dead space in the stump of the remaining parent vessel. One should attempt to produce the smallest volume of stagnant blood before the first collaterals. As well, we think it is eminently reasonable to pretreat these patients with platelet antiaggregant drugs and to carry out the occlusion of the vessel with the patient anticoagulated with heparin as soon as the general condition of the wounds permit. Finally, we have not considered it important to gradually occlude the carotid or MCA, or to wait for some hypothetical maturation of the bypass with time. Instead, the proximal vessels are occluded as soon as the graft is shown by angiography to be patent, and that is usually within 24 hours of the microvascular anastomosis. If the occlusion is tolerated, full heparinization is continued for 3 days, along with volume expansion with crystalloid and colloid. The heparin is then reduced to low dose levels for another 4 days before being discontinued. Platelet antiaggregant drugs in the form of ASA and dipyridamole are continued for another month. Because slow flow and turbulence are among the most potent factors that produce platelet aggregation and thrombosis, it seems preferable to avoid gradually stenosing a proximal vessel whenever possible. Certainly, the reduction in pressure and flow is imperceptible up to an 80 or 90% stenosis of an ICA produced by a Selverstone clamp, but the increase in turbulence and the potential for thrombus building up on the proximal side of the clamp or in the aneurysm are increased greatly. Nevertheless, there are some patients in whom a high-grade stenosis is all that can be tolerated, which would be preferable to leaving the aneurysm without protection. In this situation every effort must be made to keep the blood fluid while anticipating further maturation of the distal collateral.

Cerebral anemia from inadequate collateral circulation through the circle of Willis, as described by Dandy, can largely be prevented by microvascular anastomosis using a scalp artery or an interposed vein graft. It is now possible to isolate completely the whole of the MCA supply from the carotid and basilar circulation while still supporting normal function of the hemisphere. It is unreasonable, however, to expect even the most technically perfect bypass to prevent or even modify thromboembolism. With removal of the source of embolism and attention to those measures that will prevent unnecessary coagulation, the high mortality rate and the high percentage of cerebral complications that troubled Dandy's pioneering efforts can often be avoided.

ACKNOWLEDGMENTS

We wish to thank Drs. C. G. Drake and G. G. Ferguson for the inclusion of their cases in this report. We are grateful to Heather Carter for preparing the manuscript and to Eleanore Singer for her editorial assistance.

REFERENCES

1. Abernethy, J. *The Surgical and Physiological Works of John Abernethy, F.R.S.: Embracing Reflections on Gall and Spurzheim's System of Physiognomy and Phrenology.* Vol. 1. Longman, Hurst, Rees, Orme & Brown, London, 1825.
2. Barr, H. W. K., Blackwood, W., and Meadows, S. P. Intracavernous carotid aneurysms. A clinical-pathological report. Brain, *94:* 607–622, 1971.
3. Beadles, C. F. Aneurysms of the larger cerebral arteries. Brain, *30:* 285–336, 1907.
4. Cooper, A. A case of aneurysm of the carotid artery. Med.-Chir. Trans., *1:* 1–10, 1809.
5. Cooper, A. Second case of carotid aneurysm. Med.-Chir. Trans., *1:* 222–233, 1809.
6. Dandy, W. E. *Intracranial Arterial Aneurysms.* Cornell University Press, Ithaca, N.Y., 1945.
7. Dandy, W. E. Results following ligation of the internal carotid artery. Arch. Surg., *45:* 521–533, 1942.
8. Diaz, F. G., Ausman, J. I., and Pearce, J. E. Ischemic complications after combined internal carotid artery occlusion and extracranial-intracranial anastomosis. Neurosurgery, *10:* 563–570, 1982.
9. Drake, C. G. Giant intracranial aneurysms: Experience with surgical treatment in 174 patients. Clin. Neurosurg., *26:* 12–95, 1979.
10. Gelber, B. R., and Sundt, T. M., Jr. Treatment of intracavernous and giant carotid

aneurysms by combined internal carotid ligation and extra- to intracranial bypass. J. Neurosurg., *52:* 1–10, 1980.

11. Hamilton, J. G., and Falconer, M. A. Immediate and late results of surgery in cases of saccular intracranial aneurysms. J. Neurosurg., *16:* 514–541, 1959.

12. Heiskanen, O., and Nikki, P. Large intracranial aneurysms. Acta Neurol. Scand., *38:* 195–208, 1962.

13. Heros, R. C. Thromboembolic complications after combined internal carotid ligation and extra-to-intracranial bypass. Surg. Neurol., *21:* 75–79, 1984.

14. Heros, R. C., Nelson, P. B., Ojemann, R. G., *et al.* Large and giant paraclinoid aneurysms: Surgical techniques, complications, and results. Neurosurgery, *12:* 153–163, 1983.

15. Home, E. An account of Mr. Hunter's method for performing the operation for the popliteal aneurysm. *Lond. Med. J.*, *7:* 391–406, 1786.

16. Hopkins, L. N., and Grand, W. Extracranial-intracranial arterial bypass in the treatment of aneurysms of the carotid and middle cerebral arteries. Neurosurgery, *5:* 21–31, 1979.

17. Jawad, K., Miller, J. D., and Wyper, D. J., *et al.* Measurement of CBF and carotid artery pressure compared with cerebral angiography in assessing collateral blood supply after carotid ligation. J. Neurosurg., *46:* 185–196, 1977.

18. Kobler, J. *The Reluctant Surgeon. A Biography of John Hunter*, pp. 267–271. Doubleday, New York, 1960.

19. Love, J. G., and Dart, L. H. Results of carotid ligation with particular reference to intracranial aneurysms. J. Neurosurg., *27:* 89–93, 1967.

20. Morley, T. P., and Barr, H. W. K. Giant intracranial aneurysms: Diagnosis, course, and management. Clin. Neurosurg., *16:* 73–94, 1969.

21. Nishioka, H. Results of the treatment of intracranial aneurysms by occlusion of the carotid artery in the neck. J. Neurosurg., *25:* 660–682, 1966.

22. Odom, G. L., and Tindall, G. T. Carotid ligation in the treatment of certain intracranial aneurysms. Clin. Neurosurg., *15:* 101–116, 1968.

23. Onuma, T., and Suzuki, J. Surgical treatment of giant intracranial aneurysms. J. Neurosurg., *51:* 33–36, 1979.

24. Peerless, S. J. Comments on Diaz, F. G., Ausman, J. I., and Pearce, J. E. Ischemic complications after combined internal carotid artery occlusion and extracranial-intracranial anastomosis. Neurosurgery, *10:* 569–570, 1982.

25. Peerless, S. J. Techniques of cerebral revascularization. Clin. Neurosurg., *23:* 258–269, 1976.

26. Peerless, S. J., Ferguson, G. G., and Drake, C. G. Extracranial-intracranial (EC/IC) bypass in the treatment of giant intracranial aneurysms. Neurosurg. Rev., *5:* 77–81, 1982.

27. Peerless, S. J., Ferguson, G. G., and Drake, C. G. EC/IC bypass in the treatment of giant intracranial aneurysms. In: *Cerebral Ischemia—Clinical and Experimental Approach*, edited by H. Handa, H. J. M. Barnett, and Y. Yonekawa, pp. 56–60. Igaku-Shoin, Tokyo, 1982.

28. Reichman, O. H. Complications of cerebral revascularization. Clin. Neurosurg., *23:* 318–335, 1975.

29. Schorstein, J. Carotid ligation in saccular intracranial aneurysms. Br. J. Surg., *28:* 50–70, 1940.

30. Sindou, M., Grunewald, P., Guegan, Y., *et al.* Cerebral revascularization with extra-intracranial anastomoses for vascular lesions of traumatic, malformative, and tumorous origin. Acta Neurochir. Suppl., *28:* 282–286, 1979.

31. Sindou, M., and Keravel, Y. Intracranial giant aneurysms. Therapeutic approaches. Neurochirurgie, 30 (Suppl. 1): 88–94, 1984.
32. Spetzler, R. F., Schuster, H., and Roski, R. A. Elective extracranial-intracranial arterial bypass in the treatment of inoperable giant aneurysms of the internal carotid artery. J. Neurosurg., *53:* 22–27, 1980.
33. Sundt, T. M., Jr., and Piepgras, D. G. Surgical approach to giant intracranial aneurysms. J. Neurosurg., *51:* 731–742, 1979.
34. Sutherland, G. R., King, M., Vezina, W., *et al.* Platelet interaction within giant intracranial aneurysms. J. Neurosurg., *56:* 53–61, 1982.
35. Yasargil, M. G. *Microsurgery Applied to Neurosurgery.* Academic Press, New York, 1969, pp. 105–115.
36. Zumstein, B., Yasargil, M. G., Curcic, M., *et al.* Experiences with the extra- to intracranial bypass in the surgical management of cerebral aneurysms (9 cases). Neurol. Res., *2:* 327–343, 1980.

9

Emergency Embolectomy for Acute Embolic Occlusion of the Middle Cerebral Artery

FREDRIC B. MEYER, M.D., DAVID G. PIEPGRAS, M.D.,
THORALF M. SUNDT, M.D., and TAKEHIKO YANAGIHARA, M.D.

INTRODUCTION

The role of emergency embolectomy for acute occlusion of the middle cerebral artery remains controversial for several reasons. First, because of the paucity of case reports, the surgical results of embolectomy, as compared with the natural history of the disease, remain inconclusive. Second, the actual natural history of middle cerebral artery ischemia secondary to acute occlusion is not well defined. Third, there are good experimental data which support the concept of a critical period of reversible ischemia. This paper analyzes 20 cases of middle cerebral artery embolectomy performed at the Mayo Clinic with the aim of providing additional information with respect to patient selection, prognostic factors, surgical results, and complications.

Review of the literature disclosed 64 cases of middle cerebral artery embolecomy (5, 11, 15–21, 27, 29, 31, 33–34, 43–45, 49, 53, 55–56). These cases are summarized in Table 9.1. However, further inspection demonstrated that only 24 cases were performed within 24 hours of occlusion (Table 9.2). In these cases, the time for reestablishment of flow ranged from 40 minutes to 18 hours. The tabulated results in these 24 cases show that 14 (58%) improved, 1 was unchanged, and 9 (37.5%) died. Six of these deaths were related to either the surgery or the actual ischemic event. There were two hemorrhagic infarctions, one of which was related to the use of anticoagulation (44). Eighteen arteries were demonstrated to be patent either by angiography or autopsy, and one additional patient had partial restoration of flow (19). There was indication for good preoperative collateral flow in eight cases (11, 15, 19, 20, 21, 31, 33, 35), seven of which improved after surgery, supporting the concept initially proposed by Welch (53) of the protective effect of collateral flow.

NATURAL HISTORY

The natural history of acute occlusion of the middle cerebral artery, either embolic or thrombotic, is difficult to define. Review of the literature

CLINICAL NEUROSURGERY

TABLE 9.1

Total Case Reports of Embolectomy

Author	Year	No. of Patients	Neurological Outcome		
			Improved	No Change	Death
Welch (53)	1956	2	1	1	
Malmros (35)	1961	4	1		3
Jacobson (27)	1962	2	1	1	
Chou (11)	1963	1	1		
Shillito (43)	1964	3		3	
Shillito (44)	1967	3			3
Lougheed (34)	1965	1	1		
Donaghy (16)	1967	7	1	3	3
Sundt et al. (45)	1969	2	2		
Gilder (21)	1970	1	1		
Yasargil (55)	1970	11	8	1	2
Galibert et al. (19)	1971	4		1	3
Kapp (29)	1973	1	1		
Lapras et al. (33)	1973	6	2	4	
Khodadad (31)	1973	1	1		
Tew (49)	1974	5	4		1
Zlotnick (56)	1975	1	1		
Garrido and Stein (20)	1976	1	1		
Dolenc (15)	1978	1	1		
Gagliardi et al. (18)	1983	4	2		2
Ausman et al. (5)	1983	3	2	1	

gives a wide spectrum of information. Carter (10) in 1965 reviewed 34 patients, noting a 33% mortality rate. Of the surviving patients, 8 (29%) made good recoveries, 3 (8.8%) had moderate recoveries, and 13 (38.2%) were totally disabled. Burrows and Lascelles (9) reported on 59 patients. One-third succumbed to the initial stroke, and one-half of the remainder had severe deficits. Bladen (6) reviewed 20 cases of acute occlusion observing that eight had recanalization of the occluded artery, and two had distal migration of the clot on serial angiography. However, five patients (25%) died from the initial ischemic event. Irino et al. (26) reviewed seven cases, noting that five recanalized while two did not. However, four of five recanalized patients died within 2 weeks secondary to hemorrhagic infarction. Dalal (13) described nine cases, noting recanalization in eight patients, only two of which had improvement in neurological function. He also suggested that recanalization was associated with an increased mortality.

On the other hand, Allcock (1) reported on 40 patients with both stenosis and occlusion. This paper is often cited with an overall 5% mortality rate, with 72% of the patients making a good recovery. However, if one analyzes his subset of 29 patients with occlusions, the long-

TABLE 9.2
Embolectomy for Acute Ischemia

Author	Year	No. of Patients	Time (hr)	Source	Collateral	Improved	No Change	Death	Patency
Welch (53)	1956	1	8	Heart		1	1		1
Malmros (35)	1961	1	6–10		Yes	1			1
Jacobson (27)	1962	1	16						0
Chou (11)	1963	1	9	Heart	Yes	1			1
Shillito (43)	1964	3	5, 12	Heart				3	2
Lougheed (34)	1965	1	6	Heart	No	1			1
Sundt et al. (45)	1969	2	8, 12			2			2
Gilder (21)	1970	1	11	Shotgun	Yes	1			1
Yasargil (55)	1970	2	40 min, 18	Heart muscle		1		1	1
Galibert et al. (19)	1971	2	6, 8		Yes			2	1½
Lapras et al. (33)	1973	2	6, 12		Yes	1		1	2
Khodadad (31)	1973	1	10		Yes	1			1
Garrido and Stein (20)	1976	1	6	Aorta or carotid artery	Yes	1			1
Dolenc (15)	1978	1	6–11		Yes	1			1
Gagliardi et al. (18)	1983	4	5–6	Heart arteritis		2		2	2

term results revealed 8 (27%) with good recoveries, 11 (38%) with fair recoveries, 4 (13.8%) with poor results, and 6 (20.7%) who were totally dependent. Allcock also suggested that collateral flow was of benefit. Kaste and Waltimo (30) reviewed a series of 83 patients. The acute mortality rate was only 5%, all of which resulted from left hemispheric lesions. Fifty-three (72%) were fully independent, 20 (27%) required assistance, and 1 patient was totally dependent. It should be noted that in his fully independent group of 53 patients, only 7 were hemiparetic, and only 5 had a reduced level of consciousness at the onset of the stroke.

Krayenbuhl and Yasargil (32) reviewed 100 middle cerebral artery occlusions. There was a 5% initial mortality with an additional 5% dying within 1 year. Of the surviving patients, 54% made good recoveries, and only 18% had serious impairments.

There are also studies that show recanalization presumably due to lysis of the embolus over a period of time. Day (14) reviewed 13 patients with middle cerebral artery occlusion. Eleven patients had subsequent angiograms, six of which showed recanalization. As already discussed, Bladen (6) showed recanalization in 8 of 20, Irino *et al.* (26) in 5 of 7, and Dalal (13) in 8 of 9, with the last two series documenting a poor neurological outcome associated with recanalization.

Therefore, it remains difficult to determine the true natural history of acute occlusion of the middle cerebral artery. Review of the literature yields an initial mortality ranging from 5 to 35%, with 22–72% making a good recovery.

EXPERIMENTAL BACKGROUND

The functional integrity of the central nervous system depends on the adequate delivery of substrates for energy metabolism, particularly oxygen and glucose. Review of experimental animal and human models of stroke suggests that there are several thresholds of cerebral ischemia. First, as demonstrated by Sundt *et al.* (42, 46) and Trojanborg and Boysen (50), in man there is a change in EEG immediately if total cerebral blood flow falls below 0.16–0.18 ml/gm/min. Branston *et al.* (8) demonstrated that there is a change in evoked somatosensory potentials in the baboon if flow falls below 0.15 ml/gm/min. This has been termed the flow threshold of electrical failure in the cerebral cortex. This threshold appears to be relatively universal in various animal models (24). The second threshold has been termed pump failure, which experimentally is demonstrated by an increase in extracellular potassium during ischemia at a flow of about 0.10 ml/gm/minute, implying a depletion of ATP for the $Na+-K+$ pump (2, 3, 7). This onset of membrane pump failure may herald the start of other metabolic imbalances such as an increase in intracellular calcium (22) and the liberation of free fatty acids (54). The exact point of irreversible cell damage is unclear. The presumption is, however, that cell membrane dysfunction approximates closely the time of cell death. The reduced flow between neuronal electrical dysfunction and cell membrane pump failure has led to the concept of the "ischemic penumbra," a region of viable but nonfunctioning cerebral tissue surrounding a zone of infarction. This concept implies that there is a range of reversible ischemia between the functional threshold and cell death in which jeopardized neurons may be salvaged (4, 23).

From a second perspective, there is the element of time in the evolution of infarction. Studies by Sundt *et al.* (45, 47, 48), Crowell *et al.* (12), Watanabe *et al.* (51, 52), Dujovny *et al.* (17), and Morawetz *et al.* (38), using various animal models, have demonstrated a critical period of middle cerebral artery occlusion ranging from 2 to 7 hours which may be tolerated without infarction. Additionally, most of these studies suggest that restoration of flow after the tolerated time of occlusion increases the likelihood of hemorrhagic infarction, presumably due to increased vascular permeability secondary to ischemic damage to the endothelium. Clinically, 6 hours of no flow has been proposed as the time of permissible occlusion in humans, after which infarction is likely to occur.

Third, there is the concept of tissue vulnerability to ischemia. This can be applied both to the morphological (25, 36, 41) and physiological function of neurons (25, 28). It appears that more complex neuronal function is altered at an earlier time of reduced flow.

Fourth, the influence of collateral flow emerges as an important factor. Collateral flow may improve perfusion, perhaps critically elevating the tissue into the "ischemic penumbra," as opposed to cell death. The importance of collateral flow is supported experimentally. The variations in tolerance to middle cerebral artery occlusion in different animal models may be explained in part by differences in anatomic collateral flow. Furthermore, Michenfelder and Sundt (37) demonstrated in the squirrel monkey a slow decrease in ATP after middle cerebral artery occlusion in the first 3 hours, suggesting that there was some low level of collateral flow permitting oxidative phosphorylation. Morawetz *et al.* (38) concluded that there was good correlation between the decrease in cerebral blood flow and infarct size.

The final result when flow is restored to ischemic tissue will reflect the interaction of the various parameters discussed above: time of occlusion, collateral flow, and tissue vulnerability. The concept of the "ischemic penumbra" is critical in analyzing the goals of an emergency embolectomy. If after acute occlusion there exists a region of reversibly ischemic tissue, then the operation has a salvaging potential.

Method

CASE MATERIAL

A computerized search was made in the Mayo Clinic files for those patients undergoing emergency middle cerebral artery embolectomy from 1970 to 1983 that yielded 20 cases. These cases were reviewed extensively, along with preoperative and postoperative angiograms. All patients were seen in follow-up by a member of the Neurology Department. Further information was obtained by direct contact with the patient and family when possible.

Table 9.3 gives a summary of the clinical data. There were 10 males and 10 females with an average age of 55. The source of the embolus was the heart in seven, carotid artery in seven, aorta in three, and aneurysm in one, and was indeterminate in two. Angiographic documentation of restored flow was obtained in 16 patients (75%). The left middle cerebral artery was involved in 17 patients, the right in 3.

OPERATIVE TECHNIQUE

Each operation was performed through a pterional craniotomy. After exposure of the middle cerebral artery-internal carotid artery complex, nontraumatic aneurysm clips were placed on the main divisions of the middle cerebral artery distal to the embolus. The location of the embolus was identified by the bluish discoloration of the nonpulsatile artery. Preferably the arteriotomy was made in one of the divisions, although occasionally the main trunk of the middle cerebral artery was utilized. The embolus was milked out, utilizing suction and forceps and with the sequential use of antegrade and retrograde flow through the middle cerebral artery complex (Fig. 9.1). After the embolus was removed, the arteriotomy was closed with 9-0 or 10-0 monofilament sutures. Most patients were given pentobarbital (4 mg/kg) at the onset of the operation, and the systolic blood pressure was elevated with the purpose of enhancing collateral flow.

EVALUATION OF RESULTS

In evaluating our surgical results, we used the following definitions: "excellent" meant no demonstrable neurological deficit, "good" was defined as minimal residual neurological deficit, "fair" was defined as moderate disability but still independent, and "poor" was defined as total disability with profound deficits.

Results

Each patient prior to surgery had a severe neurological deficit, including hemiplegia, a reduced level of consciousness, and aphasia when the left middle cerebral artery was obstructed.

TABLE 9.3
Clinical Data

Patient	Age	Sex	Occlusion Site	Source	Occlusion Time (hr)	Collateral On Preop Angiogram	Backflow Surgery	Postop Angiogram	Result	Carotid Occlusion	Complication
WN	69	F	L Branch	Heart	18	Fair	Yes	Patent	Good	No	No
SR	57	F	L Trunk	Heart	14	Good	Yes	Patent	Good	No	No
KA	57	M	L Trunk	Heart	8	?	Yes	Patent	Fair	No	Hemorrhage
WX	68	M	L Branch	Aorta	5	Poor	None	No	Poor	Yes	No
WS	65	F	L Trunk	Cardiac Surgery	14	Poor	Poor	ND[a]	Death	No	No
HE	55	M	R Trunk	?	7	Fair	Yes	Patent	Fair	No	No
EY	62	M	L Trunk	?	8	Good	Yes	Patent	Excellent	No	No
SR	70	M	R Branch	Carotid	5½	Fair	Yes	Patent	Fair	No	No
CN	58	M	L Trunk	Aorta	6	None	None	No	Death	No	No
AO	53	F	L Trunk	Heart	6½	Fair	Yes	Patent	Fair	No	No
GC	52	F	L Trunk	Heart	4½	Poor	Yes	Patent	Fair	No	No
BR	67	F	L Branch	Carotid	6½	Good	Yes	Patent	Good	Yes	No
WE	76	F	L Trunk	Heart	12	Good	Yes	Patent	Good	No	No
MN	56	M	L Trunk	Carotid	7	Poor	Yes	Patent	Poor	Yes	No
CR	59	F	L Trunk	Carotid	4½	Fair	Yes	Patent	Poor	Yes	Hemorrhage
KE	18	F	L Trunk	Aneurysm	3½	Good	Yes	Patent	Good	No	No
HN	31	F	L Trunk	Carotid	5	Good	Yes	Patent	Excellent	No	No
HR	59	M	L Trunk	Carotid	3	?	Yes	Patent	Fair	Yes	No
MS	57	M	L Trunk	Aorta	4–8	Good	Yes	Patent	Fair	Yes	CSF leak
KR	16	M	R Trunk	Carotid	48	None	None	No	Poor	Yes	No

[a] ND, postoperative angiogram was not performed.

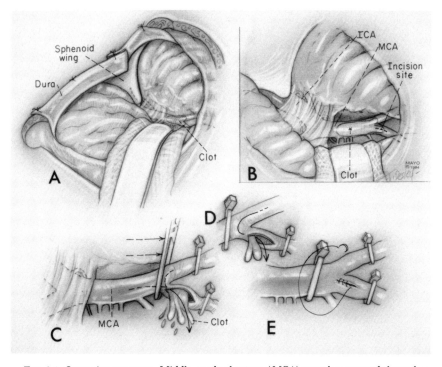

FIG. 9.1. Operative sequence. Middle cerebral artery (*MCA*) complex exposed through a pterional craniotomy (*A*). In this sequence the clot has involved the main trunk and extends proximally to the lenticulostriates. Arteriotomy is preferably made in a branch (*B*). Temporary clips are placed on branches distal to the embolus, and the clot is milked out with the aid of antegrade flow (*C*). With sequential removal of the clips, retrograde flow is used to remove the distal aspect of the embolus (*D*). Arteriotomy is closed with a running or interrupted 9-0 or 10-0 suture (*E*). ICA, internal carotid artery.

Overall, two patients (10%) had an excellent outcome, 5 patients (25%) made a good recovery, 7 patients (35%) had a fair outcome, 4 patients (20%) had a poor result, and 2 patients (10%) died. Complications included two with hemorrhagic infarction, the time for flow restoration in these cases being 4 hours 20 minutes and 8 hours. There was also one cerebrospinal fluid leak.

An aortic embolus was the source in two of the three patients in whom restoration of flow was not possible. As originally suggested (39, 40), friable atheromatous emboli are not technically suited to embolectomy, as compared with organized fibrin-platelet clots, because they tend to fragment and migrate distally (Figs. 9.2 and 9.3). The prognosis was poor in patients whose flow could not be restored (Fig. 9.4).

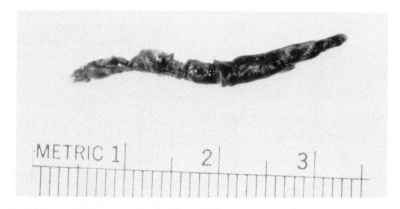

FIG. 9.2. A 3-cm fibrin-platelet embolus from the carotid artery. The organization of this clot permits total removal, as opposed to the effect of atheromatous material.

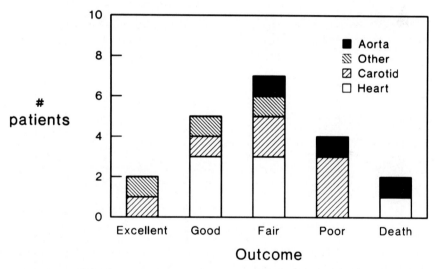

FIG. 9.3. Correlation of outcome with embolic source. Atheromatous emboli were technically more difficult to remove and also tended to migrate distally.

Although this is a small number of patients, the results can be analyzed for several variables. Figure 9.5 shows the correlation between duration of occlusion and outcome. Figure 9.6 demonstrates that there was no correlation between outcome and site of middle cerebral artery occlusion.

Patients with middle cerebral artery occlusion associated with a carotid occlusion, either intracranially or extracranially, did poorly, as depicted in Figure 9.7. This may be the sum of a profound loss of flow to the

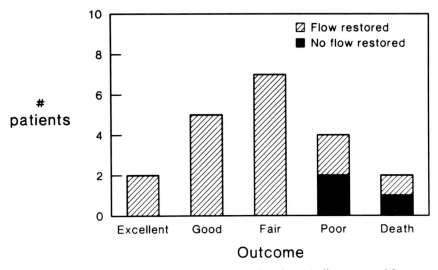

FIG. 9.4. Correlation of outcome with flow restoration. A surgically unsuccessful operation was associated with a poor prognosis.

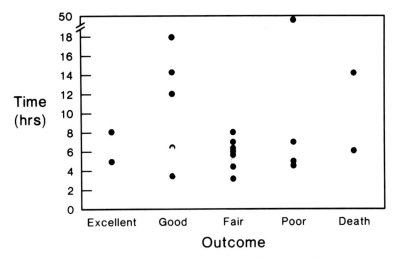

FIG. 9.5. Correlation of outcome with occlusion time. Time of no flow was not a good predictor of outcome.

lenticulostriates, which are functional end arteries, and a reflection of diminished opportunity for ipsilateral leptomeningeal collateral flow. Figure 9.11 attempts to correlate the outcome with collateral flow. The degree of collateral flow was assessed by two criteria: the leptomeningeal

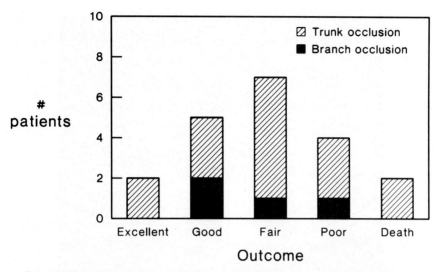

FIG. 9.6. Correlation of outcome with site of middle cerebral artery occlusion. There was no relationship between occlusion site and outcome.

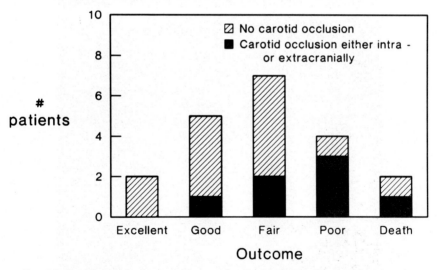

FIG. 9.7. Correlation of outcome with carotid occlusion. Ipsilateral carotid occlusion was associated with a poorer prognosis.

collateral flow on the preoperative angiogram (Figs. 9.8–9.10) and the actual backflow from the middle cerebral artery branches at the time of surgery. The results demonstrated in Figure 9.11 suggest that good collateral flow to ischemic tissue provided a better prognosis.

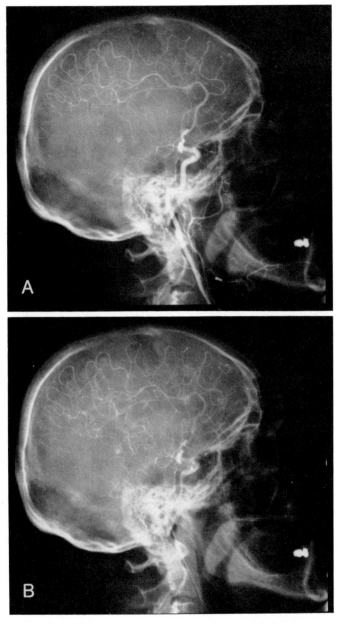

FIG. 9.8. Preoperative angiogram of a middle cerebral artery embolus (A). Good collateral flow through leptomeningeal collaterals from the ipsilateral anterior cerebral artery is seen in the arterial phase of the angiogram (B). Postoperative angiogram is shown for comparison (C).

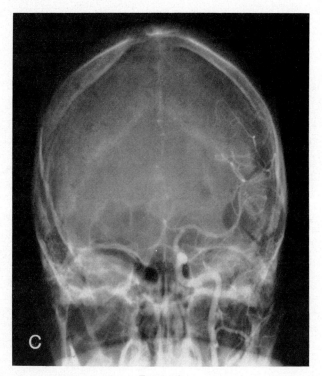

FIG. 9.8C

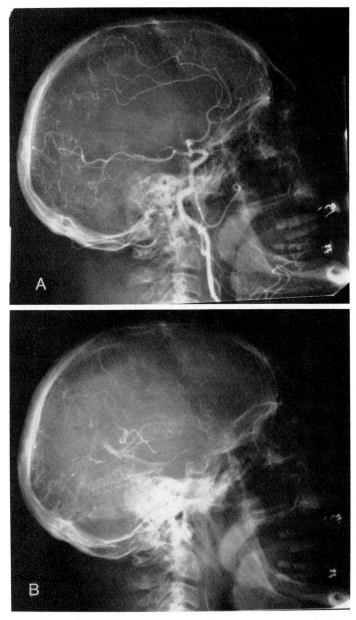

FIG. 9.9. Preoperative angiogram of a middle cerebral artery embolus (A) with fair collateral flow. In the venous phase of the angiogram there is late filling of the MCA complex through leptomeningeal collaterals (B). Postoperative angiogram is shown for comparison (C).

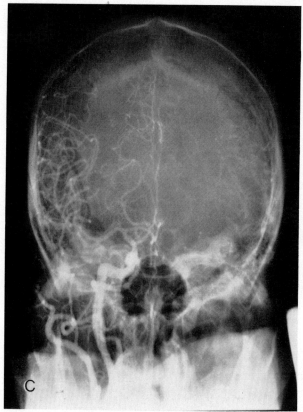

FIG. 9.9C

Analysis of Results

There are several prognostic factors that should be examined as each patient is considered for an emergency middle cerebral artery embolectomy. First, if the embolus is atheromatous debris from the aorta, the capacity to completely remove the embolic fragments and fully restore flow is poor. Second, although we could not demonstrate a good correlation between early restoration of flow and outcome, it would appear that embolectomy after a prolonged delay is unwarranted. Third, if the embolus is associated with an ipsilateral carotid occlusion, the prognosis is poor. Fourth, good collateral flow to the middle cerebral artery complex on the preoperative angiogram is a favorable prognostic indicator. Since all of our patients had acute severe neurological deficits after the occlusion, the cerebral blood flow was presumably below the threshold for electrical failure. However, seven of these patients made a remarkable

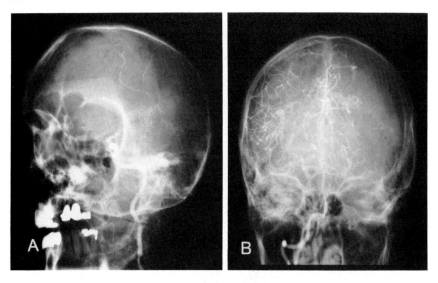

FIG. 9.10. Preoperative angiogram of a middle cerebral artery embolus with no collateral flow (A). On the contralateral carotid angiogram there is filling of the ipsilateral anterior cerebral artery; however, there is no collateral flow to the MCA complex (B). There also appears to be embolus in the carotid siphon.

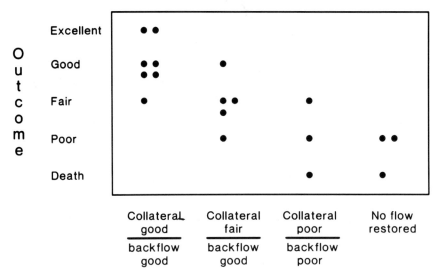

FIG. 9.11. Correlation of outcome with collateral flow. Good collateral flow, as judged by the preoperative angiogram and backflow at the time of surgery, was a good prognostic factor.

recovery, especially those judged to have had good preoperative collateral flow. Therefore, this collateral flow must have been sufficient to prevent irreversible cell damage in the majority of compromised neurons, maintaining them within this "ischemic penumbra" and, thereby, enhancing the salvaging effect of an emergency embolectomy.

The final outcome of each patient reflects the interaction of various parameters, including time of occlusion, collateral flow, and tissue vulnerability. The patients who would be expected to benefit the most by an embolectomy would be those who had good collateral flow and a short time of middle cerebral artery occlusion. However, the fact that collateral flow was the premier prognostic factor demonstrates the exquisite susceptibility of neurons to oligemia.

REFERENCES

1. Allcock, J. M. Occlusion of the middle cerebral artery. Serial angiography as a guide to conservative therapy. J. Neurosurg., 27: 353–363, 1967.
2. Astrup, J., Blennow, G., and Nilsson, B. Effects of reduced cerebral blood flow on EEG pattern, cerebral extracellular potassium, and energy metabolism in the rat cortex during bicuculline-induced seizures. Brain Res., 177: 115–126, 1979.
3. Astrup, J., Symon, L., Branston, N. M., et al. Cortical-evoked potential and extracellular K+ and H+ at critical levels of brain ischemia. Stroke, 8: 51–57, 1977.
4. Astrup, J., Symon, L., and Siesjo, B. K. Thresholds in cerebral ischemia: The ischemic penumbra. Stroke, 12: 723–725, 1981.
5. Ausman, J., Dujovny, M., and Diaz, F. Letter to the editor. Neurosurgery, 12: 639, 1983.
6. Bladen, P. A radiologic and pathologic study of embolism of the internal carotid middle cerebral arterial axis. Radiology, 82: 615–624, 1964.
7. Branston, N. M., Strong, A. J., and Symon, L. Extracellular potassium activity, evoked potential, and tissue blood flow. Relationship during progressive ischemia in baboon cerebral cortex. J. Neurol. Sci., 32: 305–321, 1977.
8. Branston, N. M., Symon, L., Crockard, H. A., and Pasztor, E. Relationship between the cortical-evoked potential and local cortical blood flow following acute middle cerebral artery occlusion in the baboon. Exp. Neurol., 45: 195–208, 1974.
9. Burrows, E. H., and Lascelles, R. G. The contribution of radiology to the diagnosis and prognosis of occlusion of the middle cerebral artery and its branches. Br. J. Radiol., 38: 481–493, 1965.
10. Carter, A. B. Prognosis of cerebral embolism. Lancet, 2: 514–519, 1965.
11. Chou, S. W. Embolectomy of the middle cerebral artery: Report of a case. J. Neurosurg., 20: 161–163, 1963.
12. Crowell R. M., Olsson Y., Klatzo, I., and Ommaya, A. Temporary occlusion of the middle cerebral artery in the monkey. Clinical and pathological observations. Stroke, 1: 439–448, 1970.
13. Dalal, P. M. Cerebral embolism. Angiographic observations on spontaneous clot lysis. Lancet, 1: 61–64, 1965.
14. Day, A. Indications for surgical intervention in middle cerebral artery obstruction. J. Neurosurg., 60: 296–304, 1984.
15. Dolenc, V. Middle cerebral artery embolectomy. Acta Neurochir., 44: 131–135, 1978.
16. Donaghy, R. M. P. Patch and bypass in microangional surgery. In: *Microvascular*

Surgery, edited by R. M. P. Donaghy and M. G. Yasargil, pp. 75–86. Stuttgart, Georg Thieme (U.S. distributor: C.V. Mosby), 1967.

17. Dujovny, M., Osgood, C. P., Barrionuevo, P. J., Hellstrom, R., and Laha, R. K. Middle cerebral artery microneurosurgical embolectomy. Surgery, *80:* 336–339, 1976.

18. Gagliardi, R., Benvenuti, L., and Guizzardi, G. Acute operation in cases of middle cerebral artery occlusion. Neurosurgery, *12:* 636–639, 1983.

19. Galibert, P., Delcour, J., Grunewald, P., Petit, P., and Rosat, P. Les obliterans de l'atere sylvienne. Neuro-Chirurgie, *17:* 165–176, 1971.

20. Garrido, E., and Stein, B. Middle cerebral artery embolectomy. J. Neurosurg., *44:* 517–521, 1976.

21. Gilder, J. V. Shotgun pellet embolus of the middle cerebral artery. J. Neurosurg., *32:* 711–714, 1970.

22. Harris, R. J., Symon, L., Branston, N. M., and Bayham, M. Changes in extracellular calcium activity in cerebral ischemia. J. Cereb. Blood Flow Metab., *2:* 203–209, 1981.

23. Heiss, W. D. Flow thresholds of functional and morphological damage of brain tissue. Stroke, *14:* 329–331, 1983.

24. Heiss, W. D., Hayaki, T., and Waltz, A. G. Cortico-neuronal function during ischemia. Arch. Neurol., *33:* 813–820, 1976.

25. Heiss, W. D., and Rosner, G. Duration verses severity of ischemia as critical factors of cortical cell damage. In: *Cerebral Vascular Disease*, edited by M. Reivich, pp. 225–236. Raven Press, New York, 1983.

26. Irino, T., Taneda, M., and Minami, T. Sanguinous cerebrospinal fluid in recanalized cerebral infarction. Stroke, *8:* 22–24, 1977.

27. Jacobson, J. H., II, Wallman, L. J., Schumaker, G. A., Flanagan, M., Suarez, E. L., and Donaghy R. M. P. Microsurgery as an aid to middle cerebral artery endarterectomy. J. Neurosurg., *19:* 108–115, 1962.

28. Jones, T. H., Morawetz, R. B., Crowell, R. M., Marcoux, F. W., Fitzgibbon, S. T., DeGirolami, V., and Ojemann, R. G. Thresholds of cerebral ischemia in awake monkeys. J. Neurosurg., *54:* 773–782, 1982.

29. Kapp, J. P., Gielchinsky, I., and Jelsma, R. Metallic fragment embolization to the cerebral circulation. J. Neurosurg., *13:* 256–261, 1973.

30. Kaste, M., and Waltimo, O. Prognosis of patients with middle cerebral artery occlusion. Stroke, *7:* 482–485, 1976.

31. Khodadad, G. Middle cerebral artery embolectomy and prolonged widespread vasospasm. Stroke, *4:* 446–450, 1973.

32. Krayenbuhl, H. A., and Yasargil, M. G. Occlusion of the middle cerebral artery. Schweiz. Arch. Neurol. Psychiatry, *94:* 287–304, 1964.

33. Lapras, J. L., Dechaume, J. P., Deruty, R., and Yasui, H. L-embolectomie arterielle intra-cranienne donnees experimentales et cliniques. Lyon Chir., *69:* 3–8, 1973.

34. Lougheed, W. M., Gunton, R. W., and Barnett, H. J. M. Embolectomy of internal carotid, middle, and anterior cerebral arteries. J. Neurosurg., *22:* 607–609, 1965.

35. Malmros, A. Cerebral embolectomy (abstr.). J. Neurol. Neurosurg. Psychiatry, *24:* 294–295, 1961.

36. Marcoux, F. W., Morawetz, R. B., Crowell, R. M., DeGirolami, and Halsey, J. H. Differential regional vulnerability in transient focal cerebral ischemia. Stroke, *13:* 339–346, 1982.

37. Michenfelder, T. D., and Sundt, T. M. Cerebral ATP and lactate levels in the squirrel monkey following occlusion of the middle cerebral artery. Stroke, *2:* 319–326, 1971.

38. Morawetz, R. B., DeGirolami, V., Ojemann, R. G., Marcouz, F. W., and Crowell, R. M. Cerebral blood flow determined by hydrogen clearance during middle cerebral artery occlusion in unaesthetized monkeys. Stroke, *9:* 143–149, 1978.

39. Piepgras, D. G., and Sundt, T. M. Operative management of intracranial arterial occlusions and acute ischemic stroke. In: *Neurological Surgery*, Ed. 6. W.B. Saunders, Philadelphia, *3:* 1619–1626, 1982.
40. Piepgras, D. G., Sundt, T. M., and Yanagihara, T. Embolectomy for acute middle cerebral artery occlusion, pp. 25 and 26. Presented at the Second Joint Meeting on Stroke and Cerebral Circulation, Miami, February 1977.
41. Scholz, W. Selective neuronal necrosis and its topistic patterns in hypoxemia and oligemia. J. Neuropathol. Exp. Neurol., *12:* 249–261, 1953.
42. Sharbrough, F. W., Messick, J. M., and Sundt, T. M. Correlation of continuous electroencephalograms with cerebral blood flow measurements during carotid endarterectomy. Stroke, *4:* 674–683, 1973.
43. Shillito, J. Carotid arteritis. A cause of hemiplegia in childhood. J. Neurosurg., *21:* 540–551, 1964.
44. Shillito, J. Intracranial arteriotomy in three children and three adults. In: *Microvascular Surgery*, edited by R. M. P. Donaghy and M. G. Yasargil, pp 138–147. Stuttgart, Georg Thieme (U.S. distributor: C.V. Mosby), 1967.
45. Sundt, T. M., Grant, W. C., and Garcia, H. J. Restoration of middle cerebral artery flow in experimental infarction. J. Neurosurg., *31:* 311–322, 1969.
46. Sundt, T. M., Sharbrough, F. W., Anderson, R. E., and Michenfelder, J. D. Cerebral blood flow measurements and electroencephalograms during carotid endarterectomy. J. Neurosurg., *41:* 310–320, 1974.
47. Sundt, T. M., and Waltz, A. G. Experimental cerebral infarction. Retro-orbital extradural approach for occluding the middle cerebral artery. Mayo Clin. Proc., *41:* 159–168, 1966.
48. Sundt, T. M., and Waltz, A. G. Cerebral ischemia and reactive hyperemia. Studies of cortical blood flow and microcirculation before, during, and after temporary occlusion of the middle cerebral artery of the squirrel monkey. Circ. Res., *28:* 426–433, 1971.
49. Tew, J. H. Reconstructive intracranial vascular surgery. MCVQ *Med. Coll. VA Q., 10:* 139–145, 1971.
50. Trojanborg, W., and Boysen, G. Relation between EEG, regional cerebral blood flow, and internal carotid artery pressure during carotid endarterectomy. EEG Clin. Neurophysiol., *34:* 61–69, 1973.
51. Watanabe, O., Brener, A. M., and West, L. R. Experimental regional cerebral ischemia in the middle cerebral artery territory in primates. Part 1. Angioanatomy and description of an experimental model with selective embolization of the internal carotid artery bifurcation. Stroke, *8:* 61–70, 1977.
52. Watanabe, O., West, L. R., and Brener, A. Experimental regional cerebral ischemia in the middle cerebral artery territory in primates. Part 2. Effects on brain water and electrolytes in the early phase of middle cerebral artery stroke. Stroke, *8:* 71–76, 1977.
53. Welch, K. Excision of occlusive lesions of the middle cerebral artery. J. Neurosurg., *13:* 73–80, 1956.
54. Wieloch, T., and Siesjo, B. K. Ischemic brain injury: The importance of calcium, lipolytic activities, and free fatty acids. *Pathol. Biol., 30:* 269–277, 1982.
55. Yasargil, M. G., Krayenbuhl, H. A., and Jacobson, J. H. Microneurosurgical arterial reconstruction. Surgery, *67:* 221–223, 1970.
56. Zlotnick, E. I. Thrombectomy of the middle cerebral artery. J. Neurosurg., *42:* 723–725, 1975.

III

Cerebellopontine Angle Tumors

10

Diagnosis of Cerebellopontine Angle Tumors*

ROBERT L. MARTUZA, M.D., STEPHEN W. PARKER, M.D.,
JOSEPH B. NADOL, JR., M.D., KENNETH R. DAVIS, M.D., and
ROBERT G. OJEMANN, M.D.

"Precise methods of examination are today in the hands of all," wrote Harvey Cushing (6) on the first page of his 1917 book *Tumors of the Nervus Acusticus and the Syndrome of the Cerebello-pontile Angle.* The precise diagnostic methods of which he wrote were the "electric ophthalmoscope, more refined perimetry, the routine use of x-ray, the revolving chair and the caloric tests of Barany." We, too, are in an age of increasing diagnostic precision. Evoked response testing allows the detection of physiologically subtle lesions, and computed tomography (CT) and magnetic resonance (MR) imaging reveal anatomic details never before seen premortem. Yet, in acquiring our new techniques, we also tend to retain many of the old, and, being in an era of great concern about medical economics, it seems timely to critically assess our techniques for the diagnosis of lesions in the cerebellopontine angle (CPA). In addition, more lesions are incidentally discovered when a diagnostic study is done for another reason, presenting the physician with a new aspect of decision making.

ACOUSTIC NEUROMA

The acoustic neuroma is the most common of all CPA lesions, and the ratio of acoustic neuromas to other angle tumors appears to have changed little with time. Cushing's series documented 42 verified angle tumors. Of these, 30 were acoustic neuromas (6). More recently, Robinson and Rudge (36) evaluated the usefulness of various diagnostic tests in patients suspected of having a CPA tumor. Of 64 patients with proven tumor, 40 had acoustic neuroma. Thus, at least two-thirds of all CPA tumors are acoustic neuroma, and it is this tumor which is usually given first consideration when a CPA lesion is suspected.

The acoustic neuroma is a benign tumor primarily formed of Schwann

* This work was supported in part by a Teacher-Investigator Development Award (NS00654) to Dr. Martuza by the National Institute of Neurological and Communicative Disorders and Stroke and by a grant from the National Institutes of Health (NS20025).

cells investing the vestibular nerve. Thus, this tumor is more appropriately termed a "vestibular schwannoma." Yet, the term acoustic neuroma is so deeply imbedded in our literature that it would do little good to change the nomenclature at this point in time. However, we should not let this naming error lead to imprecise thinking about the origins of this tumor, because it is the fact that this tumor arises on the vestibular nerve and not the auditory nerve that allows us to diagnose and to treat this tumor early enough to preserve hearing in some cases.

Most acoustic neuromas occur unilaterally in a nonhereditary fashion. In contrast, bilateral acoustic neuromas are a distinct heritable entity representing less than 5% of all acoustic neuromas (36). In this article, the term acoustic neuroma refers to the unilateral type unless otherwise stated.

Although an acoustic neuroma arises from the vestibular nerve, more than 70% of patients with an acoustic neuroma note hearing loss as the first symptom (1, 10, 27). Tinnitus, unsteadiness, vertigo, retroauricular fullness, or headache are less commonly the initial symptom. These may develop later, or they may be transient and are more easily forgotten than a hearing deficit. Facial pain or numbness, facial weakness, and hoarseness or difficulty swallowing reflect dysfunction in cranial nerves V, VII, IX, and X and are rarely seen as initial symptoms. Their presence generally suggests a large acoustic neuroma pressing on these nerves, although rare instances of sudden facial palsy from an intracanalicular tumor have been noted and have been thought to be caused by a sudden vascular compromise of the facial nerve (32).

By the time appropriate medical attention is sought, hearing loss is present in over 95% of patients (1, 10, 27). In most cases, this has been a gradually developing hearing loss, although a sudden event with loss of hearing has been described (32), and we have had several patients in whom the hearing level has fluctuated. With pure tone audiometry, the most common pattern produced by an acoustic neuroma is one of a high frequency hearing loss. However, because other patterns of hearing loss may be seen, it is not possible to determine if the hearing loss is cochlear or retrocochlear from the pure tone audiogram alone. Therefore, one should evaluate any asymmetric loss of hearing in order to reach a definitive diagnosis.

Speech discrimination should be tested in all audiograms. In general, discrimination is reduced by most acoustic neuromas greater than 1 cm in size. However, when all lesions are considered, a speech discrimination score of less than 30% is found in only 45% of the cases, and a false-positive rate of 18% is noted (43). Although speech discrimination is not accurate enough to conclusively diagnose a lesion as retrocochlear, it should be an essential part of all audiograms in order to help to decide the ultimate treatment and to help plan the route of surgery. If speech discrimination is absent or very low (<35%), translabyrinthine removal of a small tumor may be considered. In contrast, if significant speech discrimination is present, surgery to preserve hearing should be a consideration (26).

Multiple special auditory tests have been developed to improve diagnostic accuracy. Tone decay measures the ability to hear a stimulus slightly above threshold for a continuous period of time. People with normal hearing or a cochlear loss can usually hear a signal 5-dB above threshold for 1 minute. In contrast, a patient with an acoustic neuroma may require an increase in intensity to greater than 30 dB. When positive, this test is useful, but it is only positive in 70% of patients, and false-positives are noted in about 13% (43). Bekesy audiometry has also been utilized in the past, but less than half of patients with acoustic neuromas are found to have typical Type III or IV patterns (1, 43). Recruitment may be demonstrated using the alternate binaural loudness balance test. In general, cochlear disease demonstrates recruitment, and an acoustic neuroma does not. However, the rate of error approaches 50% (36, 43). Short increment sensitivity testing and acoustic reflex testing have also been utilized, but the rates of error are approximately 30 and 20%, respectively (36, 43). These more specialized audiologic tests are now primarily of historical importance in the workup of an acoustic neuroma and have been replaced by the more sensitive technique of brain stem auditory evoked response measurement.

When a sense organ or peripheral nerve is stimulated, small potentials can be recorded over the skin of the cranium using standard EEG electrodes. These tiny evoked potentials can not be easily discerned from the much larger background of EEG activity. However, the use of multiple repetitive stimuli and computerized averaging methods allow these evoked potentials to be studied. When a series of clicks is delivered to either ear, five waves can usually be detected from scalp electrodes, and these are termed the brain stem auditory evoked response (BAER). The generator of each of the waves has generally been determined from studies in the cat and then applied to analogous waves seen in the human. Wave I is thought to be generated by the portion of the auditory nerve adjacent to the cochlea and wave II by the cochlear nucleus in the pons. Recent evidence suggests the possibility that wave II is generated by the auditory nerve near the brain stem (22). Waves III and IV are from the superior olive and lateral lemniscus in the pons. Wave V is thought to originate from the rostral pons or the inferior colliculus in the midbrain. However, it must be remembered that these waves represent the summation of many potentials along the route of stimulation and may not be generated by a discrete locus.

An acoustic neuroma may leave a well-preserved wave I but will virtually always cause a delay in the appearance (increased latency) or disappearance of the remaining waves. However, since cochlear hearing loss may also prolong the absolute latency of all waves but not the interwave latencies, it is important to visualize wave I to permit determination of interwave latency. The most sensitive indicators of compression of the auditory nerve are prolongation of the I–III or I–V interwave latencies. If wave I can not be visualized, then the interear difference and the absolute latency of wave V are useful indications of eighth nerve dysfunction (3, 5, 30, 31). In the normal subject, this interval difference is usually less than 0.2 millisecond (Figs. 10.1 and 10.2).

In the first few years of its use, the reliability of BAER in predicting acoustic neuromas was uncertain, and it served as a supplement to the more traditional audiologic and vestibular tests (38). However, virtually all centers now report the superiority of this technique. In 52 cases of surgically proven acoustic neuromas, Josey et al. (13) found that the tone decay test predicted a retrocochlear lesion 63.5% of the time; the short increment sensitivity index and audiometric reflex testing were better with 69.2% and 80.8% accuracies, while the BAER was correct in 98.1% (13). The incidence of false-positives is relatively low with brain stem auditory evoked response (BAER). When the hearing loss at 4000 Hz was less than 65 dB, only 5% of nontumor patients had an abnormal BAER. However, the importance of interpreting the BAER in association with the audiogram is emphasized by the fact that when the hearing loss exceeds 65 dB, a 22% false-positive rate has been noted (4). Nonetheless, because the BAER will miss only 2–6% of all acoustic neuromas, it is currently the most accurate noninvasive screening test, and a normal BAER is good evidence against the possibility of a sizeable acoustic neuroma being present. Therefore, we now limit our audiologic testing in most cases of suspected acoustic neuroma to a pure tone audiogram measuring both air and bone conduction, speech discrimination testing, and BAER.

Caloric stimulation with electronystagmography has been useful in evaluating vestibular dysfunction in various disorders. A reduced vestibular response has been noted in a large percentage of acoustic neuroma patients; however, the usefulness of this test is severely limited by the presence of a false-positive result in one third of patients tested (1, 27, 36, 43). Therefore, while caloric testing remains valuable in the assessment of various vestibular problems, the lack of specificity in differentiating an inner ear from an eighth nerve source of dizziness limits its

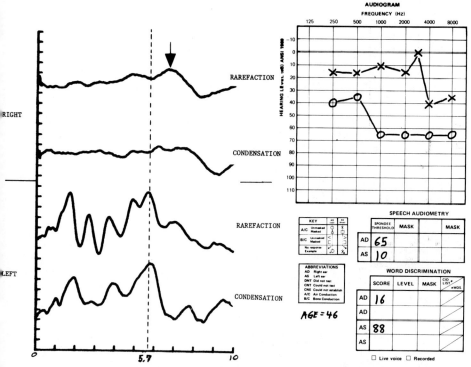

FIG. 10.1. This 46-year-old man presented with a fluctuating right-sided hearing loss. The audiogram (*top right*) demonstrated a right-sided hearing loss at all frequencies, but it was worse at the higher frequencies (0–0). A mild high frequency loss was also noted in the left ear (X–X). Speech discrimination was 16% in the right ear and 88% in the left ear (*lower right*). The BAER shows five normal waves upon left ear stimulation (*bottom left*). Rarefaction and condensation refer to the direction of the click stimulus in relation to the tympanic membrane. The normal wave V on the *left* is marked by the *ash line* at 5.7 milliseconds. The evoked response from the right ear (*top left*) shows a virtual absence of all waves. In particular, wave I is not seen, and a poorly formed wave V (*arrow*) is suggested by the rarefaction tracing and is delayed. Despite a normal contrast-enhanced CT scan, further radiologic studies are indicated in this patient. (Courtesy of Dr. A. Thornton, Massachusetts Eye and Ear Infirmary).

usefulness in identifying an acoustic neuroma. Vestibular testing may be useful when auditory testing is equivocal.

When the presenting symptoms or the neurologic findings or the audiologic results suggest the possibility of an acoustic neuroma, radiographic studies are indicated. In the recent past, these have routinely included plain x-rays of the skull and polytomes of the internal auditory meatus, followed by positive contrast myelography. However, skull x-rays and polytomes may miss 20% of small tumors and can be false-

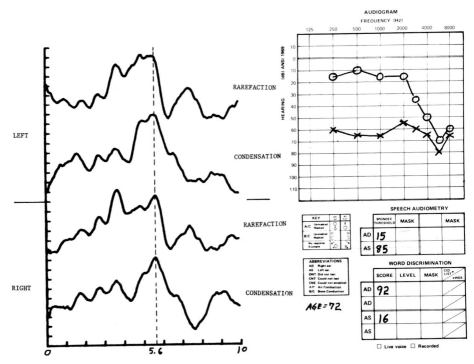

FIG. 10.2. This 72-year-old man had left-sided hearing loss due to cochlear disease. He has a 60-dB loss (*upper right*) in the left ear (X–X) at all frequencies and a moderate high frequency loss in the right ear (0–0). Speech discrimination was 16% in the left ear and 92% in the right ear (*lower right*). These results are not significantly different from those of the patient in Figure 10.1. However, the BAER is strikingly different. In this case, all wave forms are preserved with normal amplitude and latency. Wave V is 5.6 milliseconds in each ear, and the I–III and I–V interwave latencies are similar for each ear. This study suggests against retrocochlear problem, and a sizeable CPA tumor would be extremely unusual but, false-negatives do occur at approximately a 2–6% rate, particularly with small tumors. However, in a 72-year-old man, invasive studies would not be routinely indicated. (Courtesy of Dr. A. Thornton, Massachusetts Eye and Ear Infirmary).

positive in 16% (1, 43). Moreover, within the past decade, CT scan techniques have advanced to a point where a plain and intravenous contrast enhanced CT scan are all that are needed to confirm the diagnosis in most cases. The combination of a plain and a contrast-enhanced scan will show almost all acoustic neuromas greater than 1.5 cm and, using overlapping thin sections, the newer generation scanners can routinely detect smaller lesions. The CT scan also provides bone detail, obviating the need for routine plain skull x-rays and polytomes. Additionally, the CT scan can provide information not available by these other means, including tumor size and geometry, the presence of a cystic area within the tumor, relation to blood vessels, the presence of trapped arachnoid cisterns, brain stem distortion, ventricular size, and extension of tumor through the tentorium or into the cochlea. The typical CT scan of an acoustic neuroma shows a tumor which is centered at the internal auditory meatus (IAM). The IAM is usually, although not always, widened. The unenhanced scan may show an area of lower density than the cerebellum but also can appear nearly normal. The tumor enhances with intravenous contrast and is usually round with a base of attachment to the petrous bone that is less than the diameter of the tumor. Calcifications are rare, but areas of low density or relative nonenhancement are common within the tumor (Fig. 10.3).

If the clinical presentation, the audiogram, and the CT scan all are consistent with the diagnosis of an acoustic neuroma, no further tests are generally necessary. Angiography is only done if a vascular lesion, or a vascular tumor (glomus, some meningiomas) is suspected. If the CT scan with intravenous contrast is negative but the BAER and the clinical setting are highly suggestive of an acoustic neuroma, then we proceed to a subarachnoid contrast CT scan. Both gas and metrizamide have been used with great success in delineating small acoustic neuromas. However, because of its low morbidity and the better contrast resolution between tumor and subarachnoid space, we have preferred using gas. For this, the patient is placed in a lateral position, and approximately 6–10 ml of sterile carbon dioxide is introduced via a lumbar puncture. After appropriate positioning to move the gas to the CPA, a CT scan is done (Fig. 10.4). In the rare instance where gas does not adequately fill the IAM, metrizamide is instilled through the same needle, and the CT scan is repeated. Using this technique, anatomic verification can be accomplished in virtually all acoustic neuromas (10, 12, 42).

At the present time, MR imaging of CPA lesions is being studied in several centers (16, 45). The lack of x-ray exposure and the noninvasive nature of this technique are particularly appealing. McGinnis *et al.* (1, 16) reported that MR imaging could detect an acoustic neuroma in 75% of cases. The one exception was an intracanalicular tumor which was not detected by MR imaging but which was detected by a gas CT scan. Therefore, at the present time, MR must still be considered at the investigational stage, but its usefulness is increasing (Figs. 10.5 and 10.6) and we look toward it making a significant impact in the near future and perhaps replacing gas or metrizamide CT scanning in some cases.

BILATERAL ACOUSTIC NEUROMA

Bilateral acoustic neuromas are associated with a form of neurofibromatosis known as central neurofibromatosis or bilateral acoustic neurofibromatosis. This is an autosomal dominant disorder which is distinct

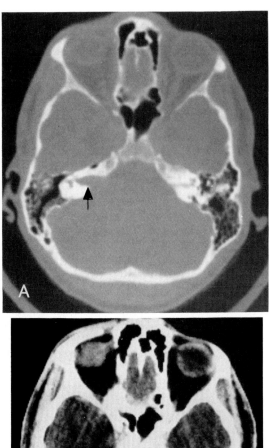

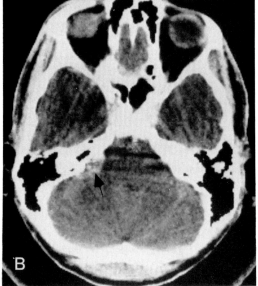

FIG. 10.3. This 36-year-old male presented with 6 months of right-sided hearing loss and 3 weeks of tinnitus. Audiologic studies revealed a high frequency hearing loss on the right with 93% speech discrimination. (*A*) CT scan on bone settings and shows a widened, flared IAM (*arrow*). (*B*) Soft tissue settings of the contrast-enhanced CT scan reveal a hetero-genenously enhancing lesion centered at the IAM (*arrow*). An acoustic neuroma was found at surgery.

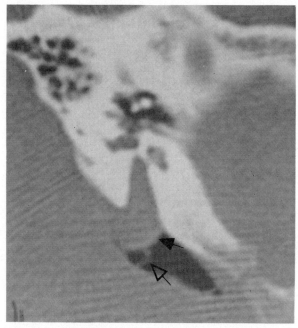

FIG. 10.4. This CO_2 CT cisternogram was performed on the patient described in Figure 10.1. The gas fails to fill the IAM and outlines the bulbous end of a small acoustic neuroma projecting from the IAM (*closed arrow*). The ends of normal sized nerves are seen medial to the tumor (*open arrow*).

from the more typical peripheral type of neurofibromatosis described by von Recklinghausen (14, 18). Currently, it is believed that these two forms of neurofibromatosis are caused either by separate genes or by separate alleles of the same gene; however, proof of this concept awaits isolation of these genes. Patients with bilateral acoustic neurofibromatosis usually become symptomatic several decades sooner than those with unilateral acoustic neuromas, and clinical presentation in the teenage years is common (19). While patients with bilateral acoustic neuromas may have café-au-lait spots or cutaneous neurofibromata, they are usually few in number and may be clinically subtle. Some patients may have no skin stigmata. The iris hamartomas (Lisch nodules) found in most patients with von Recklinghausen's neurofibromatosis are uniformly absent in patients with bilateral acoustic neurofibromatosis, although some have congenital cataracts. Therefore, since the skin and eye stigmata may be subtle or nonexistent in patients with bilateral acoustic neurofibromatosis, any patient presenting with an acoustic neuroma at an early age or with bilateral hearing loss should suggest the possibility that this gene is present. The absence of a family history of neurofibro-

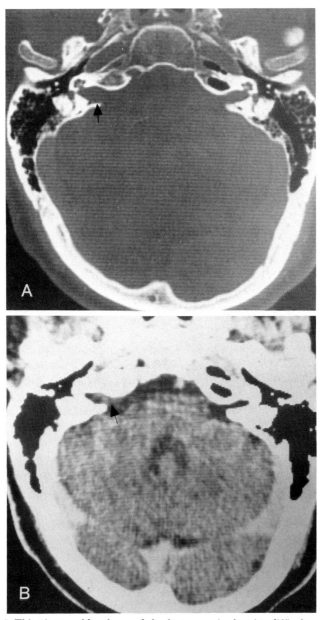

FIG. 10.5. This 49-year-old male noted slowly progressive hearing difficulty over 4 years. The audiogram showed a bilateral sensorineural hearing loss which was worse on the right. Speech discrimination was normal on the left but only 52% on the right. The BAER demonstrated a prolongation of the I–V interwave latency on the right. (A) CT scan demonstrated an enlarged right IAM (*arrow*). An initial intravenous contrast CT did not reveal a tumor. (B) GE 9800 scan with 1.5-mm cuts suggests a possible soft tissue mass in the right IAM (*arrow*). (C) CO_2 CT cisternogram confirmed a small intracanalicular tumor (*arrows*). (D) MR scan shows a right acoustic neuroma (*closed arrow*) and a normal-sized seventh and eighth nerve bundle (*open arrow*) on the left side. At surgery, an acoustic neuroma was removed, sparing hearing. With time and further experience, the MR scan may replace other studies in some cases.

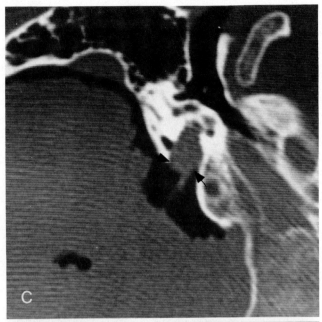

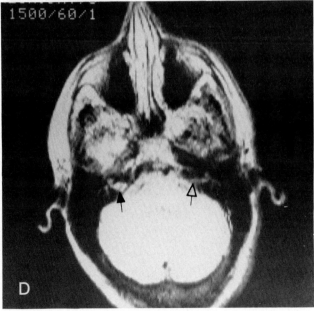

FIG. 10.5*C* and *D*

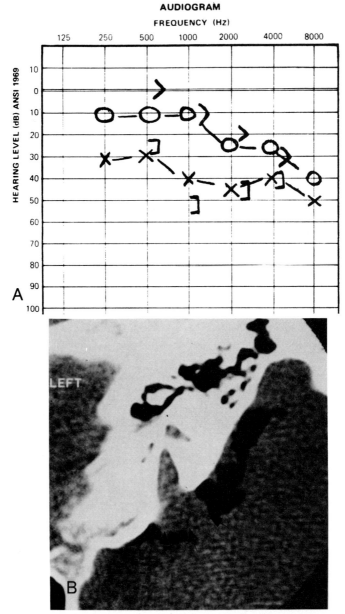

FIG. 10.6. This 36-year-old lady is in a family with hereditary bilateral acoustic neuro-fibromatosis. She presented at age 36 with decreased left-sided hearing. (A) Audiogram demonstrated bilateral hearing loss (right 0-0, left, X–X) with 96% speech discrimination. The BAER was abnormal bilaterally. The contrast enhanced CT scan was normal (not shown). (B and C) CO_2 cisternogram demonstrated bilateral small tumors projecting from the IAM (arrows). (D) MR scan revealed bilateral acoustic neuromas (arrows).

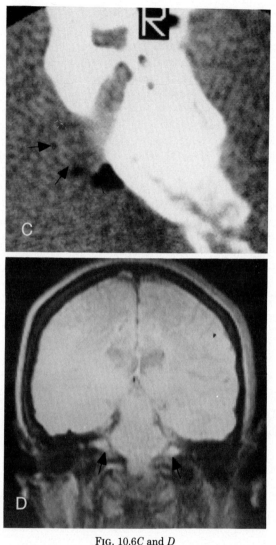

FIG. 10.6C and D

matosis does not exclude the diagnosis since more than half of the patients we have seen represent spontaneous mutations. A brain stem auditory evoked response should be done in all patients suspected of having this disorder.

Different priorities must be assigned to the patient with bilateral acoustic neuromas than are assigned to the patient with a unilateral acoustic neuroma. Patients with a unilateral acoustic neuroma are unlikely to have other associated tumors. In contrast, multiple central and peripheral nervous system tumors are common in bilateral acoustic neurofibromatosis (19). In dealing with a unilateral acoustic neuroma, an attempt to save facial nerve function is always made. Its loss may cause a significant cosmetic problem, discomfort in the face and eye, and exposure of the cornea. However, bilateral facial paralysis can also interfere with speech and mastication. Additionally, the loss of hearing for a unilateral acoustic neuroma patient, even when the surgeon has made a diligent attempt to spare it, is not a disaster since contralateral hearing remains unaffected. However, the bilateral acoustic neuroma patient faces the spectre of total deafness, and surgical planning must take this into consideration.

The tests used to diagnose an acoustic neuroma are the same whether the lesion is unilateral or bilateral (Figs. 10.6 and 10.7). The presence of bilateral lesions necessitates that a complete contrast-enhanced cranial CT scan be performed. Possible coexistence of acoustic neuromas and meningiomas or astrocytomas within the posterior fossa must be recog-

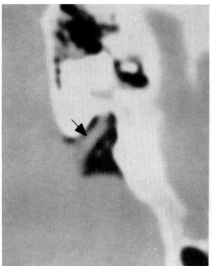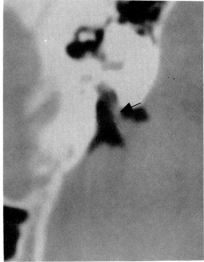

FIG. 10.7. This 30-year-old male had multiple café-au-lait marks, freckles in the inguinal creases, and small biopsy-proven neurofibromas on several scalp nerves. No iris Lisch nodules were noted. A skull x-ray demonstrated bilateral enlarged and flared internal auditory canals. The audiogram and BAER were normal. The contrast-enhanced CT scan did not demonstrate CPA tumors (not shown). A CO_2 CT cisternogram demonstrated the seventh and eighth nerve bundles (*arrows*) entering the widened IAM and confirmed the absence of acoustic neuromas. Widened IAMs without tumors can occur in von Recklinghausen's neurofibromatosis and should not be mistaken for bilateral acoustic neurofibromatosis.

nized (18, 19). If any symptoms suggest a possible spinal lesion, myelography usually is required. However, if the posterior fossa mass is large, it is often necessary to do the myelogram after the posterior fossa has been decompressed by tumor removal.

Whenever a diagnosis of bilateral acoustic neuroma is made, a thorough family history must be obtained. All susceptible family members should be examined and should have an audiogram and BAER. If any of these studies suggest the disorder, a CT scan is performed. Genetic counseling is provided to all family members.

SCHWANNOMAS OF OTHER CRANIAL NERVES

Schwannomas may arise from any nerve in the CPA, and multiple case reports appear in the literature. As an indication of their lesser incidence, one series of CPA tumors noted 177 acoustic neuromas *vs.* 5 schwannomas arising from the other nerves in the CPA and, in another report of 205 CPA tumors, there were 154 acoustic neuromas but only 6 schwannomas of other cranial nerves (29, 33). Trigeminal and facial schwannomas are the most common of these infrequent tumors and are presented to differentiate them from the acoustic neuroma. Glossopharyngeal schwannomas are discussed since they may present with signs similar to a glomus tumor.

In general, the earliest symptoms of these tumors reflect the nerve from which each arises. With trigeminal tumors, facial pain is a common symptom and usually indicates that the tumor originated in the ganglion (39). The pain is usually constant and burning, separating this problem from typical trigeminal neuralgia. Facial hypalgesia and diminished corneal sensation are also early features. Motor involvement usually occurs later. Disturbances of eye movements have been present in up to half the reported cases of trigeminal schwannoma. Tumors arising from the trigeminal root are often painless and commonly may cause hearing loss, facial palsy, and nystagmus (39).

Although trigeminal schwannomas may arise from the root or from the ganglion, they commonly involve both, and radiography demonstrates destruction of the medial portion of the petrous apex.

CT scan appearance of all schwannomas is independent of their nerve of origin. They are generally hypodense or isodense on the plain scan and enhance with contrast administration. However, because the trigeminal nerve traverses the medial petrous ridge, the anatomic location of this schwannoma is often diagnostic (Fig. 10.8).

Facial nerve schwannomas may arise from any portion of the nerve. Of 70 reviewed in the literature, 52 arose from the osseous portion of the nerve or extracranially, and 18 arose in relation to the geniculate ganglion

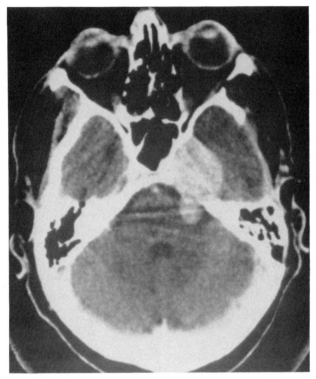

FIG. 10.8. This 59-year-old man had increasing left facial numbness for 2 years and more recent dizziness and decreased hearing on the left. His exam showed trigeminal motor and sensory dysfunction. The audiogram revealed hearing loss on the left. The enhanced CT scan shows a bilobed tumor extending from the Gasserian ganglion over the medial petrous ridge into the CPA. Surgery had proved this to be a trigeminal schwannoma.

(11). The earliest symptoms are rather uniform and consist of facial nerve dysfunction (weakness or hemispasm) and hearing loss. Tumors arising at the geniculate ganglion or proximally may also affect tear secretion, and those found proximal to the chorda tympani may also impair taste and salivation. Because the symptoms of a facial schwannoma are evident to the patient or his family at an early stage, these tumors generally present while still small in size and before causing dysfunction of other cranial nerves. The facial weakness produced distinguishes them from the acoustic neuroma.

Radiographs of the skull will reflect the location of the facial nerve tumor. Polytomes are useful for locating the tumor in relation to the geniculate ganglion, internal auditory canal, semicircular canals, and cochlea. Newer generation CT scanning can also be useful in tumor localization in lieu of polytomes. One should be aware that an epidermoid tumor in this location can also cause bone destruction and either facial weakness or spasm.

Glossopharyngeal schwannomas are rare lesions that usually present with hearing loss associated with hoarseness (8). Examination demonstrates palatal weakness, a decreased gag reflex, and decreased sensation of the oropharynx. Tomograms reveal a normal internal auditory canal with a widened jugular foramen and erosion of the jugular tubercle. The CT scan reveals a tumor similar in appearance to the acoustic neuroma but centered at the jugular foramen. An angiogram will reveal an avascular mass and will exclude a glomus tumor from the differential diagnosis.

MENINGIOMA

Meningiomas are at least three times more common in women than in men (20, 36). Twenty percent of all meningiomas occur in the posterior fossa, and half of these are located in the CPA (17, 25). Meningiomas comprise 3–13% of all CPA tumors and are second only to acoustic neuromas in this location (2, 21, 36). The presenting symptoms of a CPA meningioma are only slightly different than those of the acoustic neuroma. In a series of 32 patients with verified CPA meningiomas at the Massachusetts General Hospital and the Massachusetts Eye and Ear Infirmary (MGH-MEEI), we have noted that hearing loss (24/32), vertigo or imbalance (19/32), and tinnitus (11/32) were the most common symptoms at the time of initial evaluation (9). Fifth nerve symptoms were common; an alteration in facial sensation occurred in 9 of 32, and facial pain occurred in 5 of 32. Lower cranial nerve abnormalities occurred in 4 of 32. Headaches (7/32), visual changes (6/32), limb weakness (3/32), ear pain (2/32), and facial weakness (1/32) were less common symptoms. In contrast Sekhar and Janetta (41) noted a higher incidence of fifth nerve problems (16/22) and less hearing loss (3/28). The discrepancies between these series likely represent differences in referral patterns, such as our association with an otologic center and Janetta's interest in trigeminal neuralgia. A series of 39 acoustic neuromas and 8 CPA meningiomas from England highlights two clinical differences that are worthy of note (36). Complete unilateral hearing loss was common with acoustic neuroma (15/39) but uncommon with meningioma (1/8); milder forms of hearing loss were less predictive. In contrast, ninth nerve signs occurred in 22% of meningiomas but in no acoustic neuromas. This latter finding of an increased incidence of lower cranial nerve abnormalities with meningiomas *vs.* acoustic neuromas is also emphasized by Martinez *et al.* (17). However, these distinctions in clinical presentation are slight, and their usefulness often deteriorates in the evaluation of the individual patient.

In the MGH-MEEI series, the time of onset of symptoms until the time the patient first consulted a physician was from 1 month to 34 years, with a mean of 6 years. The delay between the first physician contact and the diagnosis of a CPA meningioma was as long as 18 years, with a mean of 4 years. These delays were due to misdiagnosis in 55%.

Meningiomas are generally larger than acoustic neuromas in most studies (9). For example, Moller et al. (21) noted that meningiomas are seldom less than 13 cm^3 at the time of diagnosis and are greater than 35 cm^3 in many instances. In contrast, acoustic neuromas only rarely reach 35 cm^3 (21).

Otologic and vestibular examination and tests were often performed in patients with CPA meningiomas who presented with hearing loss, tinnitus, or imbalance. In the MGH-MEEI series, 16 of 32 had nystagmus, 13 of 32 had ataxia, and 19 of 20 tested had reduced or absent ipsilateral caloric responses. Audiograms documented a hearing loss in 17 of 23 with a >50 dB loss in 15 (9). BAERs have been abnormal and diagnostic of a retrocochlear problem in 6 of 6 cases in the MGH-MEEI series and in all but one case in the series by Robinson and Rudge (36). However, the lack of specificity of these tests for CPA meningiomas does not allow them to be used to distinguish this lesion from the acoustic neuroma.

Radiography of the petrous bone was reported by Numaguchi et al. (24) to show IAM enlargement in 40 of 42 acoustic neuromas and 0 of 7 meningiomas. Hyperostosis of the petrous bone was uncommon and was found in only 1 of 7 meningiomas. In the MGH-MEEI series, temporal bone polytomography was done in 21 cases of CPA meningioma. Ten were abnormal showing either petrous apex erosion or bone destruction at the internal auditory meatus or both. Only one case showed hyperostosis of the petrous bone (9).

The single most useful diagnostic test is the CT scan. While a definitive diagnosis cannot be made in all cases, the CT scan provides the most information for distinguishing a CPA meningioma from an acoustic neuroma or other lesions (Figs. 10.9 and 10.10). Features which suggest a CPA meningioma on the noncontrast CT scan include: (a) a lesion which is hyperdense relative to cerebellum; (b) the presence of calcifications within the tumor or as a shell on the edge of the tumor; (c) the absence of internal auditory meatus widening. With contrast, CT scan features favoring the diagnosis of meningioma include: (a) a large tumor (greater than 35 cm^3) often extending anterior to the dorsum or extensively involving the tentorium; (b) substantial enhancement, usually in a homogenous fashion, although heterogeneity does not exclude the diagnosis; (c) a broad base of attachment to the petrous bone (9, 21). The presence of edema is of uncertain significance. Moller et al. (21) found that peritumoral edema occurred with acoustic neuromas but not

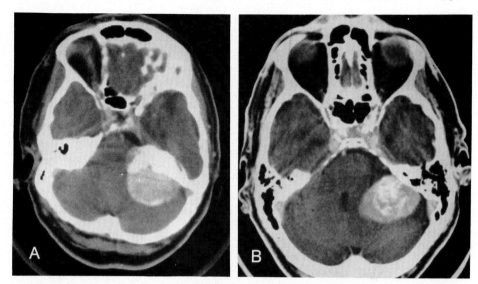

FIG. 10.9. (*A* and *B*) These scans demonstrate two types of calcification patterns noted in meningiomas. (*A*) Patient was a 56-year-old female with tinnitus. The audiogram and neurologic exam were normal. This enhanced CT scan demonstrates a hyperdense mass, with a broad base adjacent to the petrous bone and a rim of calcification at the periphery. (*B*) Patient was a 68-year-old man who presented following an episode of micturition syncope. His examination was normal. This meningioma demonstrated internal calcification. CPA meningiomas may attain large size with little or no symptoms.

with meningiomas, but Naidich *et al.* (23) found peritumoral edema in 5 of 5 of their CPA meningiomas.

The CT scan also provides other information which is critical to surgical planning. Hydrocephalus was noted in 33% of our cases (9). Additionally, the surgeon will find it useful to know if the tumor arises from or is centered anterior or posterior to the IAM. In those tumors arising anterior to the IAM, the seventh and eighth nerve will be on the posterior capsule and can be injured by the surgeon during the initial approach to the tumor. In contrast, tumors arising posterior to the IAM will usually displace the seventh and eighth nerves anteriorly (25). Other data can also be obtained from the CT scan, including petrous invasion, entrance of tumor into the jugular foramen, or the presence of major vessels within the lesion or attached to its capsule.

In the past, we employed angiography in all suspected cases of CPA meningiomas. However, since the advent of CT scanning, angiography has become somewhat less frequent. A tumor blush or an enlarged feeding vessel are more typical of a meningioma than an acoustic neuroma (21) but are not sufficiently worthwhile to outweigh the potential risk of angiography for smaller lesions. Arterial and venous displacements are

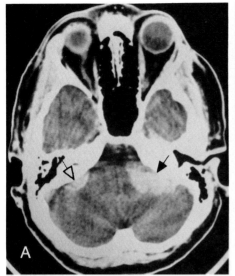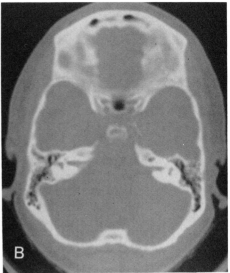

FIG. 10.10. This 45-year-old female had 3 years of progressive left hearing loss. There were no family history or clinical stigmata to suggest neurofibromatosis. The audiogram showed a severe high frequency loss on the left with 0% speech discrimination. CT scan demonstrates bilateral CPA lesions with the largest lesion on the left (*closed arrow*). Both lesions were of higher density than cerebellum on the plain scan, and both lesions enhanced with contrast administration. A large base of attachment to the petrous bone is noted (Fig. 10.10*A*). The IAMs are of normal size (Fig. 10.10*B*). An external carotid arteriogram demonstrated a homogeneous blush (not shown). Surgery on the larger left-sided lesion revealed a meningioma; the right lesion (*open arrow*) is located posterior to the IAM and is presumed to be the same. Bilateral meningiomas are very uncommon, and one might initially mistake these for bilateral acoustic neuromas.

of even less diagnostic import (24). For large lesions, arteriography is helpful in determining if vascular encasement is present and in evaluating whether or not preoperative embolization would be helpful to reduce the blood supply. Arteriography should include, in addition to a posterior circulation study, selective internal and external carotid injections since enlarged feeding arteries can come from either vessel. Additionally, in any lesion where the CT scan demonstrates profound enhancement or where significant diagnostic uncertainty exists, arteriography is essential to exclude an aneurysm, arteriovenous malformation, or glomus tumor.

EPIDERMOID TUMOR

Epidermoid tumors account for only 2–6% of all CPA lesions (2, 43). These tumors are benign and slow growing, and rather than displace major structures they often insinuate themselves around and between multiple cranial nerves and blood vessels. The clinical presentation is usually one of the abnormalities of multiple cranial nerves or of cerebellar dysfunction which develops over a period of years. By the time a diagnosis is made, the lesion may be very large and may extend extensively through the tentorial meatus or into various cranial nerve foraminae. The audiogram and BAER usually reveal a retrocochlear auditory abnormality. Skull films and polytomes may be normal. The unenhanced CT scan typically shows a lesion which is of lower density than surrounding brain and which has irregular borders. Intravenous contrast will usually not enhance the tumor mass, although enhancement of the capsule or of adjacent compressed neural tissue may be seen. The most definitive study is a metrizamide CT cisternogram (7) which demonstrates the irregular border of the lesion and which may show metrizamide "percolating" into some of the grape-like clusters of this tumor (Fig. 10.11).

Because this tumor can surround major vascular structures, angiography is often more useful for surgical planning than for diagnosis. The angiogram will show an avascular mass with some vessels traversing the lesion and other vessels displaced by the mass. At surgery, the capsule of the tumor may be densely adherent to these vessels and adjacent neural structures.

ARACHNOID CYST

Arachnoid cysts are rare and account for only 1% of all CPA lesions (2, 37). Hearing loss, headache, and imbalance are the most common complaints, although facial pain or numbness and hemifacial spasm or weakness have also been noted. In most cases, no prior history of trauma or infection can be related to cyst development.

Plain radiographs or tomograms show widening of the IAM in more than one third of the cases (2, 37), and the longstanding pressure from the cyst may also cause distortion and thinning of the suboccipital squama.

The CT scan is usually diagnostic and demonstrates a low density lesion with smooth edges. The density of the lesion is usually similar to that of CSF, although some cysts may have a slightly higher density due to their increased protein content. Enhancement does not occur with intravenous contrast. The CT scan differs from that of the epidermoid in that the edges of the arachnoid cyst are smoother and displacement of adjacent structures is more prominent. The contrast CT scan should encompass the entire limits of the lesion in order to exclude the possibility of an astrocytoma nodule within a tumor cyst. Arteriography is rarely necessary unless diagnostic uncertainty is present.

In the planning of surgery for this lesion, the operator should be aware of other possible causes of the patient's symptoms. We have had one woman who presented with hemifacial spasm and periodic retroauricular

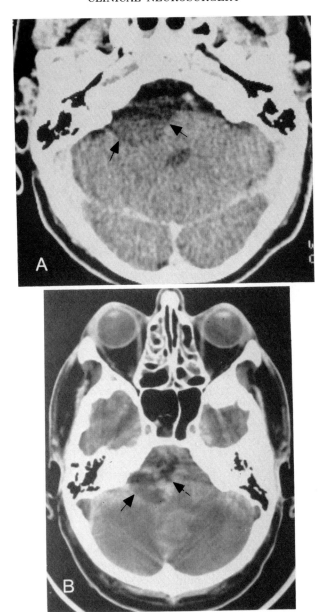

Fig. 10.11. This 39-year-old male presented with 2 months of imbalance, headache, and right-sided tinnitus. The audiogram was normal. (A) Both the noncontrast CT scan (not shown) and the contrast CT scan show a low density CPA mass with a slightly irregular border (*arrows*) and a density similar to CSF. (B) A metrizamide CT cisternogram demonstrates contrast medium around and within the lesion in an irregular fashion typical of an epidermoid tumor (*arrows*).

pain which progressed over more than a decade. The CT scan showed a large CPA arachnoid cyst which was easily fenestrated into the basal cisterns and the cervical subarachnoid space. However, microsurgical exploration also revealed significant arterial compression of her seventh nerve which was likely the cause of her hemifacial spasm, and a vascular repositioning was performed at the same operation. Her symptoms were relieved (Fig. 10.12).

LIPOMA

Lipomas are common lesions elsewhere in the body but are rare in the CPA, with only 11 of them reported in the literature. Yet, they are worthy of note because their symptoms and signs are similar to those of the acoustic neuroma while the CT scan shows a low density lesion which

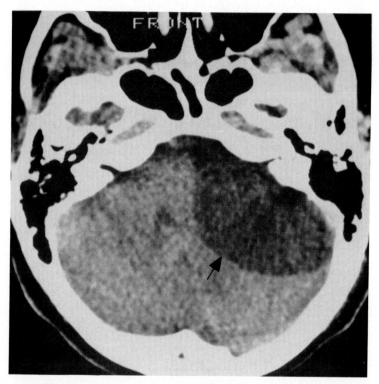

FIG. 10.12. This 50-year-old female noted progressive hemifacial spasm for 16 years and now presented because of left-sided tinnitus and decreased hearing. Examination revealed hemifacial weakness and spasm. A BAER demonstrated an increased latency of wave V and a prolonged I–V interwave latency. The CT scan with contrast reveals a low density, extraaxial, nonenhancing lesion with a smooth round margin typical of an arachnoid cyst (*arrow*).

might be initially confused with other low density lesions such as an epidermoid or an arachnoid cyst. However, careful study of the CT scan will reveal fat density of −40 to −100 Hounsfield units (Fig. 10.13) (15). The absence of calcification or other soft tissue component will exclude a teratoma.

The recognition that a CPA lesion is a lipoma is important to surgical management. Surgery should be done only if the mass is causing symptoms of compression or if the diagnosis is uncertain and a biopsy is necessary. Rapid growth or malignant change have not been reported, suggesting that the surgery should be conservative in order to accomplish decompression without harming surrounding neural structures (15). If the lipoma is an incidental finding or if symptoms are mild, sequential clinical, audiologic, and CT examinations may be preferable to surgery.

GLOMUS TUMOR

Tumors of the glomus jugulare are one of a group of vascular lesions which include carotid body tumors and other paragangliomas. When a glomus tumor presents in the CP angle, the earliest and most common symptoms are from the ninth, tenth, and eleventh cranial nerves. Plain

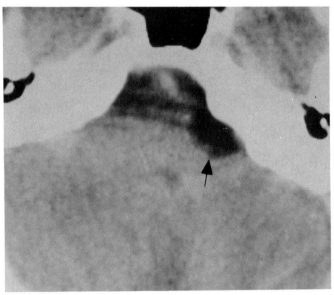

FIG. 10.13. This 41-year-old man presented with a 20-year history of facial pain. Examination revealed trigeminal hypalgesia. The audiogram demonstrated a high frequency hearing loss. This contrast-enhanced CT scan demonstrates a nonenhancing lesion with an irregular margin (*arrow*). The absorption of the tumor was measured to be −85 Hounsfield units. These features and the absence of calcification are typical of a lipoma.

skull films generally demonstrate erosion of the spur of bone between the carotid canal and the jugular fossa. The hallmark of these lesions is their extreme vascularity. The plain CT scan generally demonstrates a high density lesion centered at the jugular foramen. Intravenous contrast shows marked enhancement and variable extension into the CPA.

Arteriography is essential in evaluating a patient with any hypervascular lesion and, in the case of a glomus tumor, usually demonstrates feeding vessels from the occipital and ascending pharyngeal branches of the external carotid artery.

HEMANGIOMA, ARTERIOVENOUS MALFORMATION, AND ANEURYSM

These lesions are grouped together because of their vascular nature and because of their low incidence. Together, they account for less than 1% of all CPA abnormalities (2, 36, 44). Brackmann and Bartels have described a series of four patients with hemangiomas within the internal auditory canal. All four had dysequilibrium; 3 of 4 had a retrocochlear hearing loss; and 3 of 4 had other neurologic signs, including facial weakness and a decreased corneal reflex. One diagnostic feature which the authors felt was important was that the symptoms developed rapidly and appeared out of proportion to the relatively small size of some of these lesions. All lesions expanded the internal auditory canal, and two small lesions were not detected by routine CT scanning but required a posterior fossa contrast study.

Arteriovenous malformations or angiomas of the CPA usually present with a hemorrhage of varying neurologic severity (44). Less commonly, patients may present with trigeminal pain or fluctuating signs, suggesting a demyelinating disorder. If the ictus has been recent, the plain CT scan may show subarachnoid or intraparenchymal hemorrhage and possibly hydrocephalus. Later studies, or those done in patients who have not bled, may be unremarkable or may show areas of microcalcification. A contrast enhanced CT scan demonstrates an irregular highly enhancing mass which usually extends toward the ventricle. Serpiginous veins are often seen in the adjacent cisterns and are a tell tale sign of this lesion. Angiography is essential to define the arterial feeders and the draining veins and to help decide between several therapeutic options, including embolization, surgery, and focused radiation therapy (Fig. 10.14).

Aneurysms of the vertebral-basilar system may project into the CPA but are usually not detected unless a hemorrhage has occurred. However, even in the absence of hemorrhage, a large aneurysm may, rarely, present as a mass compressing adjacent neural structures.

INTRINSIC TUMORS

Intrinsic tumors arise within neural tissue but may present with symptoms mimicking a CPA lesion or may have an exophytic mass

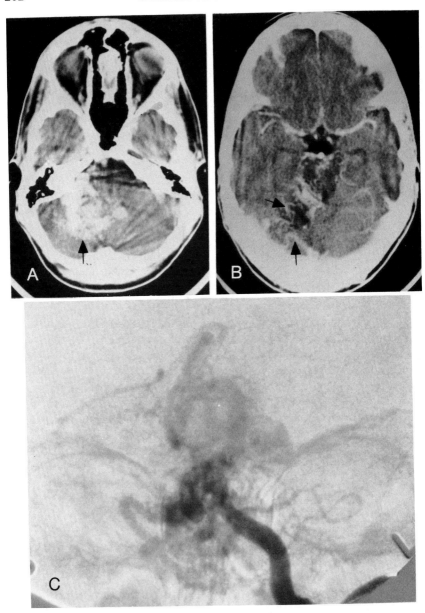

FIG. 10.14. This 12-year-old boy had the sudden onset of a headache 6 months prior to these studies. (*A*) Enhanced CT scan demonstrates an irregular lesion extending from the CPA to the fourth ventricle (*arrow*). (*B*) Higher sections demonstrate multiple serpiginous veins typical of an arteriovenous malformation (*arrows*). (*C*) Angiogram is conclusive.

projecting into the CPA. These most commonly include astrocytoma of any histologic grade, medulloblastomas, ependymomas, and choroid plexus papillomas. In one series, intrinsic lesions accounted for 9 of 92 patients presenting with CPA symptoms and represented 9 of 64 verified tumors of the CPA (36). Auditory symptoms were present in 66%, but the audiogram and other routine audiologic tests were not specific. BAER was useful in demonstrating bilateral symmetric abnormalities in 5 of 7 patients with intrinsic tumors.

The presence of rapidly developing symptoms or of any bilateral symptoms or of signs referable to the nuclei or brain stem in excess of those directly related to cranial nerves should raise the suspicion of an intrinsic lesion and should lead to a plain and contrast enhanced CT scan. Most intrinsic tumors do not widen the IAM, nor do they alter the petrous bone (2). They are generally less round and less well-defined than the acoustic neuroma and often infiltrate the cerebellum or the brain stem in a more irregular fashion than meningiomas or other extraaxial lesions (Figs. 10.15–10.17). In many cases, the diagnosis remains uncertain even after CT scanning and arteriography, and it is only discovered at the time of surgery.

It is in the area of intrinsic lesions where MR imaging may provide the greatest benefit over existing radiologic techniques. MR imaging can demonstrate the infiltrating nature of intrinsic lesions and can help differentiate them from extraaxial tumors (Fig. 10.17).

METASTATIC TUMORS

The CPA is an uncommon location for metastatic tumors. In one series of 1354 cerebellopontine angle tumors, there were only three metastatic tumors (2). While this may be an underestimate reflecting the otologic practice of the authors, metastatic tumors probably represent 1% or less of all CPA lesions in most series. Malignancies in this location can produce rapid impairment of several cranial nerves and are often associated with brain stem dysfunction (2). The plain radiographs and the CT scan may show destruction of adjacent bone or invasion of the surrounding soft tissues of the skull base; however, absence of these features does not exclude the diagnosis of a metastasis. A double dose of intravenous contrast and a delayed CT scan may be useful in searching for other lesions. If the remaining evaluation does not show a malignancy, exploration and biopsy are necessary, and the surgeon should remember to send enough tissue so that estrogen and progesterone receptors can be measured since this may alter the treatment if the lesion proves to be a metastatic breast carcinoma.

Because metastatic lesions are so uncommon in the CPA, the mere presence of a CPA mass in a patient with a known malignancy but

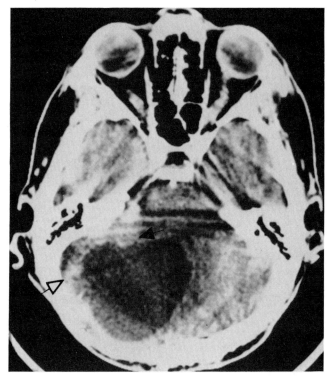

FIG. 10.15. This 43-year-old female presented with hiccoughs and vomiting. Examination showed nystagmus, bilateral dysmetria, and decreased hearing on the right. The contrast-enhanced CT scan demonstrates a prominent low density cyst. Lateral to the cyst is an enhancing rim of compressed normal cerebellum (*open arrow*). Anterolateral is a small enhancing nodule (*closed arrow*) which distinguishes this lesion from the arachnoid cyst in Figure 10.12. This nodule proved to be a low grade astrocytoma.

without other demonstrable metastases does not necessarily indicate that the lesion is a metastatic deposit. Meningiomas are three times more common in women with breast cancer than in other women (40), and we have seen three such patients with CPA meningiomas and breast cancer in the last 3 years. An additional patient with breast cancer had an acoustic neuroma and a small frontal parasagittal lesion presumed to be a meningioma (Fig. 10.18).

NONNEOPLASTIC CPA LESIONS

As surgeons, we tend to focus on the tumors or the vascular lesions which account for the vast majority of CPA lesions, but we must always remember that patients who present with auditory, vestibular, or other CPA symptoms may have disorders which are not amenable to surgery.

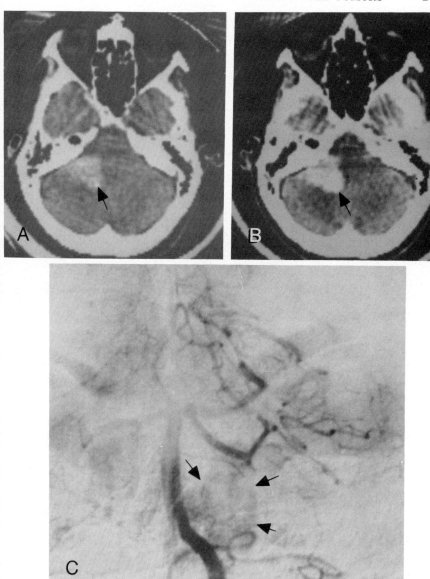

FIG. 10.16. This 61-year-old man noted bilateral hearing loss and unsteady gait for several months. The examination showed mild ataxia and absent left-sided hearing. (*A*) Unenhanced CT scan shows a left-sided lesion (*arrow*) which is denser than cerebellum and extends from the CPA to the fourth ventricle. (*B*) Contrast enhances the lesion (*arrow*). (*C*) Angiogram demonstrates a vascular blush (*arrows*) typical of a tumor. Surgery revealed a choroid plexus papilloma.

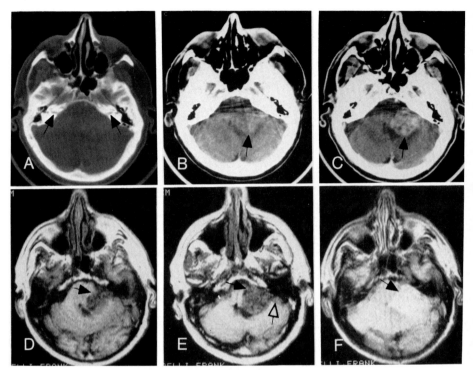

FIG. 10.17. This 60-year-old man presented with a year of progressive imbalance and hearing loss. (*A*) Plain CT scan on bone settings reveals normal sized IAMs (*arrows*). (*B*) Noncontrast CT scan shows an irregular hyperdense mass (*arrow*). (*C*) Intravenous contrast enhances the lesion in a heterogeneous fashion (*arrow*). (*D–F*) MR scans reveal a mass which appears to arise intrinsically (*closed arrow*), then extend into the CPA in an exophytic fashion (*open arrow*). The arteriogram showed only an avascular mass (not shown). A low grade partially encapsulated astrocytoma was found at surgery.

In a series of 92 patients who presented with CPA symptoms, 64 had tumors; 7 had ischemic vascular disease; 17 had other causes; and 4 remained undiagnosed (36). Among the 17 patients with other causes, migraine (5 patients), multiple sclerosis (3 patients), and sarcoidosis (2 patients) were the most common diagnoses. The hallmark of ischemic lesions is their sudden onset and their involvement of adjacent anatomic loci. All five patients with migraine had normal BAER and normal CT scans on prolonged follow-up. Both patients with sarcoidosis had normal BAER, but the three patients with multiple sclerosis had bilateral BAER abnormalities, which is common in this disorder.

DIAGNOSTIC PROBLEMS AND CONCLUSIONS

The multiplicity of cranial nerves and brain stem tracts within a small anatomic area makes the CPA one of the more challenging diagnostic

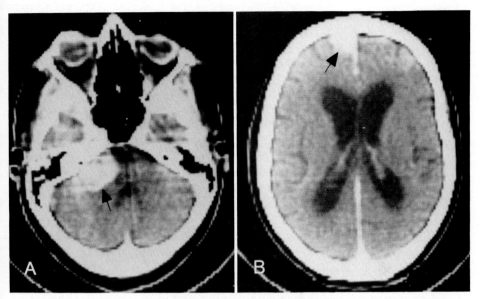

FIG. 10.18. This 70-year-old female had a mastectomy for breast cancer 5 years previously with involvement of axillary nodes. She now presented with a 6-month history of falling toward the left and recently began using a cane. This CT scan raised the suspicion of a metastasis. The remainder of her metastatic evaluation was negative. (*A*) Surgery demonstrated the posterior fossa lesion to be an acoustic neuroma (*arrow*). (*B*) Frontal lesion (*arrow*) has not been operated but is presumed to be a meningioma and remains unchanged on CT scan 3 years later.

areas for the clinician (28, 34, 35). In this report, we have drawn attention to the clinical and radiologic details which distinguish the lesions that one is likely to encounter in this area. It is now worthwhile to make a few generalizations. Clinically, hearing is most commonly impaired with acoustic neuromas, but the auditory nerve is so sensitive that an abnormal audiogram or BAER may be found with any of the other CPA lesions. Therefore, a good history will often elicit early symptoms which may direct the diagnosis toward a tumor arising in or near the trigeminal, facial, glossopharyngeal, or other nerve rather than the auditory or vestibular nerves. When auditory or vestibular sypmtoms are the only ones present, an audiogram and BAER are usually the first tests of choice. If the BAER is abnormal, a plain and contrast CT scan is done which encompasses the entire cranium and which utilizes 1.5-mm sections through the IAM. If this is negative, but the audiogram and BAER suggest a tumor, a CO_2 CT cisternogram is done. When symptoms or signs of other cranial nerves or of the cerebellum or brain stem occur with or without eighth nerve symptoms, we usually defer the BAER and perform a plain and contrast enhanced CT scan. If a lesion is seen, the

BAER will usually prove unnecessary. More refined tests are used when indicated by the prior studies. MR imaging is useful in delineating intrinsic lesions from extraaxial lesions. However, MR scan units are not readily available, and tumor can sometimes be difficult to differentiate from edema. MR must still be considered at the investigational stage. In lieu of an MR scan, metrizamide CT cisternography can be useful to differentiate intraaxial from extraaxial lesions and is particularly useful in the diagnosis of epidermoid tumors. In general, we now reserve angiography for vascular lesions, for diagnostic uncertainties, or for lesions where the angiogram is essential to treatment planning.

Toward the end of his book, Cushing noted "I have possibly spoken too lightly of the ease of diagnosis of these lesions . . . mistakes may of course be made" (6). Despite the remarkable diagnostic advances we enjoy, this statement still remains true today. To preoperatively mistake a symptomatic 2-cm acoustic neuroma for a meningioma is no great tragedy since surgery will in all likelihood be needed, and the correct diagnosis will be made at that time. However, other errors are of larger import, and a few of ours are worthy of mention.

One woman who presented with tinnitus and mild hearing loss had a contrast-enhanced CT scan which was thought to show a small intracanalicular acoustic neuroma (Fig. 10.19). A suboccipital craniectomy revealed only an abnormally formed internal auditory canal. Partial aver-

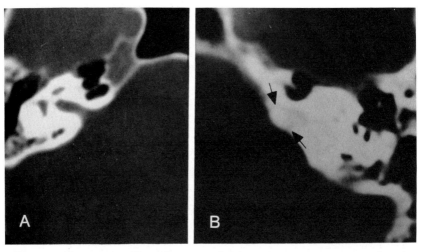

FIG. 10.19. This 56-year-old female presented with a recent onset of tinnitus and vertigo. The audiogram revealed a mild hearing loss. (A) IAM on the nonsymptomatic side was normal. (B) Contrast-enhanced CT scan was misinterpreted as showing an intracanalicular tumor within a flared IAM (arrow) on the symptomatic side. At surgery no tumor was present. A protuberance of bone was found and was decompressed. This could have been diagnosed preoperatively with tomograms or with a plain CT scan with 1.5-mm sections.

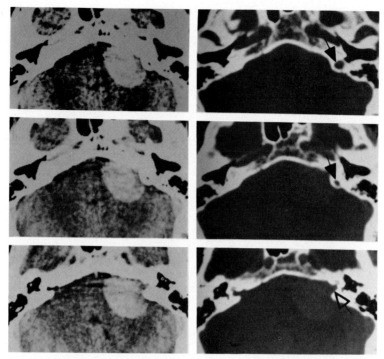

FIG. 10.20. This 39-year-old male noted 2 years of left-sided hearing loss, 1 year of left cheek numbness, and 1 month of headache. An acoustic neuroma was suggested by the three CT images on the left and was confirmed at surgery. The three images on the right are bone settings at the same levels and reveal the uppermost portion of an unusually high jugular bulb (*closed arrows*) which is adjacent to the internal auditory canal (*open arrow*). This was not noticed preoperatively, and drilling of the IAM caused profuse bleeding.

aging of a spur of bone at the IAM caused the appearance of tumor. This could have been avoided with an MR scan, a gas CT cisternogram, or simply with a noncontrast CT scan or polytomes of the canals.

A second patient did have a typical acoustic neuroma and a suboccipital removal was performed. At surgery, profuse venous bleeding ensued when the posterior lip of the internal auditory canal was drilled. In retrospect, bone settings of the CT scan revealed an aberrant jugular bulb which was immediately adjacent to the IAM (Fig. 10.20). The lesion on the CT scan should always be reviewed in relation to surrounding vascular and osseous structures.

A third case was that of an elderly lady with a large CPA mass showing enhancement at its outer rim (Fig. 10.21). The arteriogram revealed only mass effect. At surgery, a thrombosed aneurysm was found. In retrospect, the CT picture is typical of thrombosed aneurysms noted in other locations.

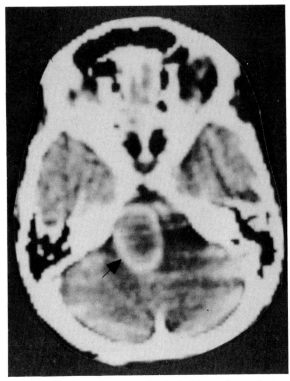

FIG. 10.21. This 70-year-old female noted left facial numbness for several years and intermittent headaches, dizziness, and unsteadiness for several months. Examination revealed papilledema, left-sided dysmetria, and facial hypalgesia and weakness. An enhanced CT scan demonstrated a CPA mass with a high density rim. The arteriogram demonstrated only mass effect (not shown). At surgery, a thrombosed aneurysm was identified.

Fortunately, for those of us who deal with CPA lesions, serious misdiagnoses are rare, and exploratory surgery in this area has been made a relic of the past. When the surgeon performs the operation, the location of the lesion in relation to the adjacent vessels, osseous structures, and nervous elements should be known, and the diagnostic possibilities should be narrowed significantly. For those who miss the intraoperative surprises of yesteryear, we offer the improvement in postoperative results of today. The treatment of CPA lesions has become one of the most challenging areas of neurosurgery. No longer shall we call it, as Cushing had, "the bloody angle . . . the gloomy corner of neurological surgery" (6).

ACKNOWLEDGMENTS

The authors thank Dr. N. Zervas and Dr. R. Kjellberg for providing clinical information on the patients discussed in Figures 10.11 and 10.14, and Dr. A. Thornton for providing the audiologic data in Figures 10.1 and 10.2. Particular appreciation is extended to Dr. T. Brady, Dr. P. F. J. New, and the MR imaging unit at the Massachusetts General Hospital for performing the MR studies and to Ms. Cynthia Campbell for assistance with the manuscript preparation.

REFERENCES

1. Brackmann, D. E. Acoustic neuroma surgery: Otologic Medical Group results. In: *Neurological Surgery of the Ear*, Chap. 35, edited by H. Silverstein and H. Norrell, pp. 248–259. Aesculapius Publishing Co., Birmingham, Ala., 1979.
2. Brackmann, D. E., and Bartels, L. J. Rare tumors of the cerebellopontine angle. Otolaryngol. Head Neck Surg., *88:* 555–559, 1980.
3. Brackmann, D. E., and Selters, W. Brain stem electric response audiometry: Acoustic tumor detection. In: *Neurologic Surgery of the Ear*, Chap. 34, edited by H. Silverstein and H. Norrell, pp. 241–246. Aesculapius Publishing Co., Birmingham, Ala., 1979.
4. Cashman, M. Z., Rossman, R. N., and Nedzelski, J. M. Cerebello-pontine angle lesions: An audiological test protocol. J. Otolaryngol., *12:* 180–186, 1983.
5. Chiappa, K. H. *Evoked Potentials in Clinical Medicine*, Chap. 5, pp. 144–202. Raven Press, New York, 1983.
6. Cushing, H. *Tumors of the Nervous Acousticus and the Syndrome of the Cerebellopontine Angle*. W.B. Saunders, Philadelphia, 1917.
7. Fein, J. M., Lipow, K., Taati, F., and Lansem, T. Epidermoid tumor of the cerebellopontine angle: Diagnostic value of computed tomographic metrizamide cisternography. Neurosurgery, *9:* 179–182, 1981.
8. Fink, L. H., Early, C. B., and Bryan, R. N. Glossopharyngeal schwannomas. Surg. Neurol., *9:* 239–245, 1978.
9. Granick, M. S., Martuza, R. L., Parker, S. W., Ojemann, R. G., and Montgomery, W. W. Clinical manifestations and diagnosis of cerebellopontine angle meningiomas. Ann. Otol. Rhinol. Laryngol., in press, 1985.
10. Hart, R. G., Gardner, D. P., and Howieson, J. Acoustic tumors: Atypical features and recent diagnostic tests. Neurology, *33:* 211–221, 1983.
11. Isamat, F., Bartumeus, F., Miranda, A. M., Prat, J., and Pons, L. C. Neurinomas of the facial nerve. J. Neurosurg., *43:* 608–613, 1975.
12. Johnson, D. W. Air cisternography of the cerebellopontine angle using high resolution computed tomography. Radiology, *151:* 401–403, 1984.
13. Josey, A. F., Jackson, C. G., and Glasscock, M. E., III. Brain stem evoked response audiometry in confirmed eighth nerve tumors. Am. J. Otolaryngol., *1:* 285–290, 1980.
14. Kanter, W. R., Eldridge, R., Fabricant, R., Allen, J. C., and Koerber, T. Central neurofibromatosis with bilateral acoustic neuroma: Genetic, clinical and biochemical distinctions from peripheral neurofibromatosis. Neurology, *30:* 851–859, 1980.
15. Leibroch, L. G., Deans, W. R., Bloch, S., Shuman, R. M., and Skultety, F. M. Cerebellopontine angle lipoma: A review. Neurosurgery, *12:* 697–699, 1983.
16. McGinnis, B. F., Brady, T. J., New, P. F. J., Buonanno, F. S., Pykett, I. L., *et al.* Nuclear magnetic resonance (NMR) imaging of tumors in the posterior fossa. J. Comput. Assist. Tomogr., *7:* 575–584, 1983.
17. Martinez, R., Vaquero, E., Areitio, E., and Biavo, G. Meningiomas of the posterior fossa. Surg. Neurol., *19:* 237–243, 1983.
18. Martuza, R. L. Neurofibromatosis and other phakomatoses. In: *Neurosurgery*, edited by R. H. Wilkins and S. S. Rengachary. McGraw-Hill, New York, 1985.
19. Martuza, R. L., and Ojemann, R. G. Bilateral acoustic neuromas: Clinical aspects, pathogenesis, and treatment. Neurosurgery, *10:* 1–12, 1982.
20. Mirimanoff, R. O., Dosoretz, D. E., Linggood, R. M., Ojemann, R. G., and Martuza, R.

L. Meningioma: Analysis of recurrence and progression following neurosurgical resection. J. Neurosurg., in press, 1985.

21. Moller, A., Hatam, A., and Olivecrona, H. The differential diagnosis of pontine angle meningioma and acoustic neuroma with computed tomography. Neuroradiology, 17: 21–23, 1978.

22. Moller, A. R., and Janetta, P. J. Compound action potentials recorded intracranially from the auditory nerve in man. Exp. Neurol., 74: 862–874, 1974.

23. Naidich, T. P., Lin, J. P., Leeds, N. E., Kricheff, I. I., and George, A. E. Computed tomography in the diagnosis of extra-axial posterior fossa masses. Radiology, 120: 333–339, 1976.

24. Numaguchi, Y., Kishikawa, T., Ikeda, J., Tsukamoto, Y., Fukui, M., et al. Angiographic diagnosis of acoustic neurinomas and meningiomas in the cerebellopontine angle— a reappraisal. Neuroradiology, 19: 73–80, 1980.

25. Ojemann, R. G. Clinical features and surgical management of meningiomas. In: Neurosurgery, edited by R. H. Wilkins and S. S. Rengachary. McGraw-Hill, New York, 1985.

26. Ojemann, R. G., Levine, R. A., Montgomery, W. M., and McGaffigan, P. Use of intraoperative auditory-evoked potentials to preserve hearing in unilateral acoustic neuroma removal. J. Neurosurg., in press, 1985.

27. Ojemann, R. G., Montgomery, W. W., and Weiss, A. D. Evaluation and surgical treatment of acoustic neuroma. N. Engl. J. Med., 287: 895–899, 1972.

28. Pait, T. G., Zeal, A., Harris, F. S., et al. Microsurgical anatomy and dissection of the temporal bone. Surg. Neurol., 8: 363–391, 1977.

29. Pool, F. L., Pava, A. A., and Greenfield, E. C. Acoustic Nerve Tumors; Early Diagnosis and Treatment, Ed. 2. Springfield, Ill., Charles C Thomas, 1970.

30. Prosser, S., Arslan, E., Conti, G., and Michelini, S. Evaluation of the monaurally evoked brainstem response in diagnosis of sensorineural hearing loss. Scand. Audiol., 12: 103–106, 1983.

31. Prosser, S., Arslan, E., and Pastore, A. Auditory brain stem response and hearing threshold in cerebellopontine angle tumors. Arch. Otorhinolaryngol., 239: 183–189, 1984.

32. Pulec, J. L., House, W. F., Britton, B. H., Jr., and Hitselberger, W. E. A system of management of acoustic neuroma based on 364 cases. Trans. Am. Acad. Ophthalmol. Otolaryngol., 75: 48–55, 1971.

33. Revilla, A. G. Differential diagnosis of tumors at the cerebello-pontine recess. Bull. Johns Hopkins Hosp., 83: 187–212, 1948.

34. Rhoton, A. L., Jr. Microsurgery of the internal acoustic meatus. Surg. Neurol., 2: 311–318, 1974.

35. Rhoton, A. L., Jr. The posterior fossa approach to the internal acoustic meatus: Laboratory dissection guide. In: Neurological Surgery of the Ear, Chap. 29, edited by H. Silverstein and H. Norrell, pp. 208–217. Aesculapius Publishing Co., Birmingham, Ala., 1979.

36. Robinson, K., and Rudge, P. The differential diagnosis of cerebellopontine angle lesions. J. Neurol. Sci., 60: 1–21, 1983.

37. Rousseaux, M., Lesoin, F., Petit, H., and Jomim, M. Les Kystes arachnoidiens de l'angle ponto-cerebelleux. Neurochirurgie, 30: 119–124, 1984.

38. Saunders, A. Z., and Jackson, R. T. CPA tumors with normal routine audiometry and positive reflex and BSER tests. Am. J. Otol., 2: 318–323, 1981.

39. Schisano, G., and Olivecrona, H. Neurinomas of the Gasserian ganglion and trigeminal root. J. Neurosurg., 17: 306–322, 1960.

40. Schoenberg, B. D., Christine, B. W., and Whisnant, J. P. Nervous system neoplasm

and primary malignancies of other sites. The unique association between meningiomas and breast cancer. Neurology, *25:* 705–712, 1975.

41. Sekhar, L. N., and Janetta, P. J. Cerebellopontine angle meningiomas. Microsurgical excision and follow-up results. J. Neurosurg., *60:* 500–505, 1984.

42. Sortland, O. Computed tomography combined with gas cisternography for the diagnosis of expanding lesions in the cerebellopontine angle. Neuroradiology, *18:* 19–22, 1979.

43. Turner, R. G., Shepard, N. T., and Frazer, G. J. Clinical performance of audiological and related diagnostic tests. Ear and Hearing, *5:* 187–194, 1984.

44. Viale, G. L., Pau, A., Viale, E. S., and Turtas, S. Angiomas of the cerebellopontine angle. J. Neurol., *225:* 259–267, 1981.

45. Young, I. R., Bydder, G. M., Hall, A. S., Steiner, R. E., and Worthington, B. S., *et al.* The role of NMR imaging in the diagnosis and management of acoustic neuroma. AJNR, *4:* 223–224, 1983.

The Neuro-Otologist's View of the Surgical Management of Acoustic Neuromas

WILLIAM F. HOUSE, M.D., and WILLIAM E. HITSELBERGER, M.D.

INTRODUCTION

The purpose of this paper was to review the experience of the Otologic Medical Group in the management of 1667 patients with surgically treated acoustic neuromas seen from 1961 through March 1984. Technical aspects of the surgery that have proven helpful to us will be reviewed, and the total mortality in this group of patients will be discussed. The 216 patients operated on in 1980 and 1981 will be reviewed in depth. Presumably, the results in this latter group of patients are representative of the best that can be obtained in our hands at this time. In this group, we will review postoperative complications, facial nerve preservation, and hearing preservation.

EPIDEMIOLOGY

In 1936, Crowe and Hardy (1) reported an incidence of 1.5% asymptomatic acoustic neuromas in consecutive autopsies carried out at the Johns Hopkins Hospital in patients without symptoms of an acoustic neuroma. If this figure is extrapolated to a population base of 200,000,000 in the United States, there should be 3 million people in this country harboring acoustic neuromas. With these figures in mind, it is apparent, then, that only a small percentage of individuals with an acoustic neuroma ever become symptomatic and require surgery. The number probably does not exceed 0.1% of the total group of patients with acoustic tumors, and even this percentage is probably an overestimate.

At the time of the Crowe and Hardy paper in 1936, it was felt that acoustic tumors constituted only 5% of all brain tumors. This was a reflection of late diagnosis and treatment for patients with this tumor and the huge reservoir of patients with smaller tumors that remained unrecognized. Generally, acoustic tumor surgery was not carried out until the patient showed fifth nerve findings, cerebellar ataxia, and symptoms of increasing intracranial pressure. At the present time, a diagnosis with the above symptoms would be considered late. It is not uncommon in the present era for the diagnosis of an acoustic neuroma to be made with symptoms of only eighth nerve involvement. This, of course, is because of the vastly improved audiologic and radiologic diagnostic capability which we now have. Consequently, many more of these tumors are being diagnosed and treated. The 5% incidence of acoustic tumors, in terms of all operated brain tumors, should probably be revised upward.

Of further epidemiologic interest, is the fact that this tumor has an extremely low incidence in the black population. In our group of 1667 patients, there were only four blacks (0.2%). This number correlates with the low incidence of inner ear pathology, such as Meniere's disease and otosclerosis in the black population.

In our patient population, 51% were male and 49 were female. The tumor occurred on the left side in 48% of our cases, on the right side in 52%.

The average age in this group of patients was 47.3 years. The occurrence of the tumor at this time in life is quite significant. Generally, at this time, patients are approaching or have reached the peak of their economic productivity. They may be completely healthy except for symptoms related to eighth nerve abnormality. The presenting symptoms usually belie the potential danger of the underlying tumor if it is allowed to grow. In earlier years (and sadly, even at the present time), surgeons were reluctant to operate on patients with small tumors because of the associated surgical morbidity and even mortality. The trade-off, apparently, was between a few more years of relatively active life as opposed to the high immediate surgical risk. Obviously, if a small tumor can be removed with minimal associated risk, this is the desirable method of therapy.

OPERATIVE TECHNIQUES

We have used two basic approaches to the cerebellopontine angle for removal of these tumors. The middle fossa approach is used for small intracanalicular tumors when we are attempting to save hearing. The suboccipital translabyrinthine approach is used for the remainder.

The basic steps in the suboccipital-translabyrinthine and the middle fossa operations for acoustic tumor removal have been described elsewhere (2, 3), and it is not our intention to go over in detail these procedures since this material is readily available. Rather, we would like to stress certain aspects of the techniques, which we feel might be helpful to the neuro-otologist attempting this type of surgery.

In the suboccipital translabyrinthine operation, bone should be removed from the subocciput posteriorly to the sigmoid sinus (Fig. 11.1). The amount of suboccipital bony removal will vary, depending on the size of the tumor—a large tumor usually requires more suboccipital bony removal than a small one. The sigmoid sinus should also be decompressed

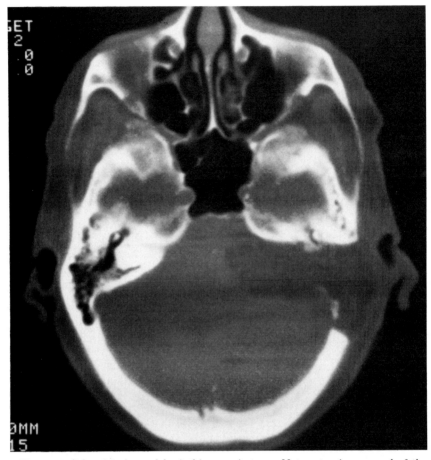

FIG. 11.1. Suboccipital-translabyrinthine craniectomy. Note extensive removal of the petrous pyramid on the left. This has the effect of exteriorizing the cerebellopontine angle tumor.

of overlying bone. This wide exposure of the subocciput, including the sigmoid sinus, in addition to the labyrinthectomy, allows extradural retraction of the underlying cerebellum if it is needed. Additionally, removal of the petrous portion of the temporal bone actually exteriorizes the underlying acoustic neuroma. In the suboccipital operation, because of the necessity for direct retraction or resection of the cerebellum before the tumor is seen, adequate visualization of the tumor can be a major problem. This is especially true when a large tumor is present. Additionally, the anterior-lying portion of the tumor next to the pons, fifth nerve, and basilar artery is not as well seen as it is using the translabyrinthine approach.

Increased intracranial pressure, especially in the case of a large tumor, is a major surgical hazard. The elevated pressure results in venous engorgement and effectively obscures the operating field until it is relieved. In the translabyrinthine approach, the underlying increased intracranial pressure tends to force the tumor outward into field of action. This by itself tends to relieve the elevated pressure. Since the acoustic tumor has been exteriorized, the underlying pressure is now a positive force in effecting its removal.

Tumor removal is always carried out anterior to the sigmoid sinus. If the sigmoid sinus is in a forward position, it is very important that the bone removal described above be complete. This means that the decompression of the sigmoid sinus must extend down inferiorly to the jugular bulb, and the labyrinthectomy must be complete.

One of the basic concepts of translabyrinthine surgery is that the removal of the neuroma centers around the facial nerve. If the facial nerve can be completely followed from the end of the internal auditory canal down to the brainstem, it is likely that the entire contour of the tumor will at various times during the operation be exposed. The labyrinthine portion of the facial nerve at the lateral end of the internal auditory canal must be seen. This can be accomplished by exposure of the vertical bony segment (Bill's bar) arising from the transverse creast at the end of the canal. The labyrinthine portion of the facial nerve is usually not involved with tumor, even in patients harboring large neuromas. Since it is generally the only point during dissection of the tumor where the exact position of the uninvolved facial nerve is known, it follows that the dissection of the facial nerve from the tumor should begin here.

It is extremely important to avoid stretching the facial nerve since this can result in postoperative weakness of the face without any obvious break in the continuity of the nerve. This can be accomplished by early identification and separation of the facial nerve from the capsule of the tumor. After this has been done, attention is turned to the tumor in the posterior fossa. If the tumor is small, continuation of the dissection in the plane between the facial nerve and the tumor will result in complete isolation of the tumor, which can then be readily removed. If the tumor is large, the anterior portion of the mass is first removed with the Urban vacuum dissector. This creates a trough which the facial nerve may fall back into. Additionally, it allows the posterior portion of the tumor to be manipulated forward without stretching the facial nerve.

When the main bulk of the tumor has been removed, the facial nerve can usually be identified as it exits the brainstem. At this point, it appears white and fasciculated. The facial nerve usually makes an intracranial bend just prior to its entrance into the brainstem. Up to the point of this bend, when the dissection has started in the internal auditory canal, the facial nerve may be very adherent to the capsule of the tumor. Once the bend has been reached, the nerve will usually change color to the normal healthy myelinated white as it disengages itself from the tumor just before it enters the brainstem. Once this point has been reached in the dissection, facial nerve preservation is almost ensured. The direction of the bend of the facial nerve corresponds to the side on which the tumor is found, *i.e.*, a right cerebellopontine angle neuroma will show the facial nerve bending towards the right, and a left angle neuroma will show the nerve bending towards the left. If the facial nerve is very adherent to the tumor capsule and appears to have been lost, another opportunity is often presented for preserving the nerve by continuing the development of the plane between the tumor and the facial nerve from the brainstem out to the internal auditory canal.

We have found the Urban dissector to be the best instrument for the rapid debulking of the tumor. In the use of this instrument, care must be exercised to keep the cutting end of the dissector under direct vision and away from important vascular and neural structures. We have used the laser in the past for removal of these tumors, but have now abandoned it. Besides the undesirable bulk and weight of the instrument on the microscope, other undesirable features of the laser have become apparent. The removal of the tumor mass is slowed down considerably when compared with the use of the Urban dissector or even removal using ordinary microinstrumentation. Additionally, and most importantly, the problem of the heat generated by the laser has not yet been solved. This has subjected a thinned facial nerve to unnecessary thermal injury. We therefore feel that the disadvantages of the laser in terms of injury to adjacent neurostructures far outweigh any claimed advantages.

Mention must be made of the anterior inferior cerebellar artery (AICA). This artery usually lies on the posterior inferior aspect of the tumor. Towards the end of the procedure, it is often seen bisecting the seventh and eighth nerves near the brainstem. It may, in fact, be used as a landmark to identify the facial nerve. Occasionally, the lateral branch of the artery, or even its main trunk, will perforate the capsule of the tumor and present in the interior of the tumor. This is obviously a very dangerous situation since the artery may be inadvertently injured. Every effort should be directed to avoid injury to the anterior inferior cerebellar artery and the lateral branch. At this time, injury to this artery constitutes the main source of morbidity and mortality in acoustic tumor surgery.

At the end of the procedure, the defect in the dura is obliterated with fat obtained from the lower abdominal wall (4). The fat is sectioned into strips, and these are individually placed in the mastoid cavity just inside the dural defect. A small piece of fat is usually placed in the aditus to the middle ear. The incus is not removed.

If the tumor is small, confined to the internal auditory canal, and hearing preservation is possible, a middle fossa approach is used. This approach to the internal auditory canal is accomplished by unroofing the internal auditory canal after elevation of the middle fossa dura. In this way, the structures of the inner ear are avoided. In our experience, the success of this procedure is not so much dependent on preservation of the cochlear nerve, which can usually be readily accomplished, as it is on preservation of the blood supply to the cochlear nerve and inner ear. This hazard is probably increased if the tumor arises from the inferior vestibular nerve because of the closer juxtaposition of the cochlear nerve to the tumor's surface, as opposed to an origin from the superior vestibular nerve.

OPERATIVE MORTALITY IN 1667 PATIENTS

In this group of patients (Fig. 11.2), we have defined operative mortality as any death resulting from changes that were initiated at the time of surgery. The length of time from surgery to death or the mode of death, in our opinion, is irrelevant if the changes resulting in a fatality were initiated by the operation.

Using this as our criteria for operative mortality in these 1667 patients, there were 30 deaths (1.8%). After case 700 (Fig. 11.3), there have been only 4 deaths in 967 patients (operative mortality, 0.4%). Between cases 807 and 1373, there were no fatalities (566 patients without a fatality).

The major cause of operative mortality in this group of patients was complications resulting from thrombosis or hemorrhage involving the anterior inferior cerebellar artery (Table 11.1).

ANALYSIS OF 216 PATIENTS OPERATED IN 1980 AND 1981

A review of patients operated on in these 2 years is important because these patients have, presumably, been the benefactors of our best surgical treatment. Additionally, an adequate time span has elapsed for adequate follow-up evaluation.

In this group of patients, we have divided the size of tumors into four groups, i.e., small, medium, large, and giant. Since the evaluation of the size of the tumor at the time of surgery is notoriously inaccurate, our measurements have been based on the size of the tumor seen on the CT scan. Small tumors were intracanalicular and measured up to 0.5 cm in diameter. Medium tumors were from 0.5 to 2.0 cm. Large tumors were

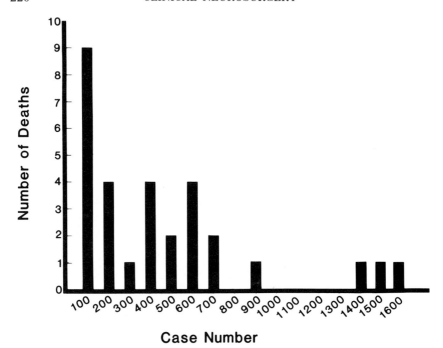

Case Number

FIG. 11.2. Number of cases of unilateral acoustic neuroma operated on each year since 1961.

from 2.0 to 4.0 cm. Giant tumors had a diameter of greater than 4.0 cm. The majority of our patients (51%) had medium-sized tumors.

Facial nerve function was judged by evaluation of function of the face at least 1 year following the surgery. Facial nerve function was normal in all of the 20 patients with small tumors. This figure decreased to 60% normal function in those patients with giant tumors. In the entire group of 216 patients, 180 patients (83%) were judged to have normal facial function 1 year postoperatively. In the group of patients not having normal facial function, 30 patients (14%) were judged to have partial paralysis not requiring further facial nerve surgery. Six patients (3%) had total paralysis. Four patients in this group had intraoperative repair of their facial nerve using a facial-facial anastomosis. Two patients required a hypoglossal facial anastomosis.

In this group of patients, we attempted to save hearing 10 times (5%) using a middle fossa approach. We were successful four times (2%). This emphasizes the futility of attempting to save hearing even when the tumor is very small. Our feeling is that the admixture of blood supply between the tumor, cochlear nerve, and inner ear is very fragile. Even with a small tumor, interference with this blood supply is quite common.

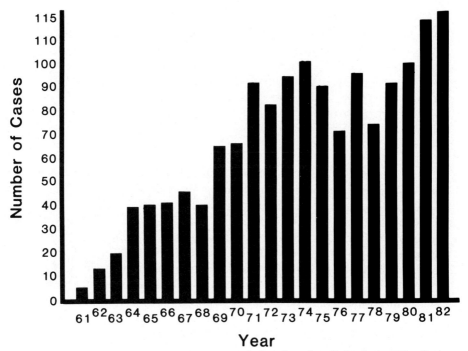

Fig. 11.3. Operative mortality. After case 700 there have been 4 deaths in 967 patients (operative mortality 0.4%). Between cases 807 and 1373 there were no fatalities (566 patients without a fatality).

TABLE 11.1

Causes of Operative Mortality in 1667 Patients

Cause of Operative Mortality	No. of Patients	%
AICA syndrome	14	(47%)
Hemorrhage	9	(30%)
Extra-axial	6	(20%)
Intracerebellar	1	(3%)
Intracerebral	1	(3%)
Extradural hem	1	(3%)
Pulmonary emboli	3	(10%)
Cardiopulmonary failure	1	(3%)
Undiagnosed arachnoid cyst	1	(3%)
G.I. hemorrhage	1	(3%)
Meningitis	1	(3%)

This factor, more than anything else, results in loss in hearing.

Total removal of the tumor was accomplished in 215 cases. In only one patient was a planned subtotal resection carried out because of overriding medical considerations.

There was no cerebellar ataxia, brainstem injury, or injury to the ninth and tenth cranial nerves in this group of patients. Seventeen patients (8%) had aseptic meningitis following removal of their tumors. There were six patients (3%) with spinal fluid rhinorrhea. Four of these sealed with the application of a pressure dressing, and two (1%) required further surgery to close the leak. There was one fatality (0.4%).

The average operating time in this group of patients was 3 hours, 12 minutes. The average stay in hospital was 10 days.

SUMMARY

The experience of our group in the management of 1667 patients with the diagnosis of an acoustic neuroma has been reviewed. Certain features of the operation have been discussed.

It is our feeling at this time that with the techniques available to the neuro-otologist for the management of patients harboring acoustic neuromas, the goals of surgery should be total removal of the tumor with preservation of the facial nerve and avoidance of injury to the adjacent important brain structures. Our patients, at this time, should reasonably expect this type of result from their surgery. Hearing preservation in the above framework continues to be frustrating and difficult to consistently attain, and obviously remains the next barrier in acoustic tumor surgery.

REFERENCES

1. Hardy, M., and Crowe, S. J. Early asymptomatic acoustic tumor. Arch. Surg., *32:* 292–301, 1936.
2. House, W. F. Transtemporal bone microsurgical removal of acoustic neuromas. Arch. Otolaryngol., *80:* 597, 1964.
3. House, W. F., and Luetje, C. M. *Acoustic Tumors*, Vols. 1 and 2. Baltimore, University Park Press, 1979.
4. House, J. L., Hitselberger, W. E., and House, W. F. Wound closure and cerebro spinal fluid leak after translabyrinthine surgery. Am. J. Otol., *4:* 126–128, 1982.

CHAPTER

12

Application of New Technology in the Treatment of Cerebellopontine Angle Tumors*

DANIEL G. NEHLS, M.D., CPT MC USA,
ROBERT F. SPETZLER, M.D., ANDREW G. SHETTER, M.D., and
VOLKER K. H. SONNTAG, M.D.

HISTORICAL PERSPECTIVE

Sir Charles Ballance is credited with the first successful removal of an acoustic neurinoma in 1894 (2, 13, 24). The tumor was approached through a suboccipital craniectomy and was removed by unsterile blunt finger dissection. According to the operative note, "... the finger had to be inserted between pons and tumour to get it away." The patient survived but was left with facial paralysis and corneal anesthesia. Since that time there has been a tremendous evolution in the treatment of cerebellopontine angle (CPA) tumors. A subtotal intracapsular resection was perfected by Cushing (10) which resulted in long-term functional survival for about 60% of patients. To Cushing goes much of the credit for defining and publicizing the progression of signs and symptoms of these tumors (24). In an effort to prevent recurrence and to avoid postoperative swelling and pontine infarction, Dandy (12) advocated complete removal of these neoplasms. Olivecrona and Givre (16) pioneered efforts to save the facial nerve and were able to achieve anatomical preservation in 30% of 300 cases. In 217 of these cases, they were able to effect a total removal of the tumor, with a mortality rate of 23.5% in this group. The work of Atkinson (1), in defining the distribution of the anterior inferior cerebellar artery (AICA) and its intimate relation to acoustic tumors, helped to reduce the incidence of brainstem infarction. The introduction of the operating microscope and the development of microsurgical technique were important advances to CPA surgery in the early 1960s (14, 23, 36, 38). The refinement of the translabyrinthine approach by House (23) and the development of the transmeatal approach by Rand and Kurze (36) provided additional routes for surgeons to use in approaching these tumors. The most recent advance in acoustic

---

* The views of the authors are their own and are not to be construed as official or reflecting the position of the Department of the Army or the Department of Defense.

tumor surgery has been the use of the laser. The ruby laser was first used in clinical neurosurgery by Rosomoff and Carroll in 1966 for irradiating tumors (15). The first use of the laser as a neurosurgical instrument was by Stellar in 1969, who used a CO_2 laser to vaporize a recurrent glioma (15).

With the advances in CPA tumor surgery, there has been a dramatic reduction in mortality and a marked improvement in preservation of facial nerve function (13, 14, 27, 39). The present techniques of microneurosurgery, with no-touch laser removal, are a far cry from the original unsterile blunt finger dissection used by Ballance. In addition, there have been improvements in electrodiagnosis, neuroradiology, and intraoperative monitoring which allow earlier detection and safer removal.

DIAGNOSIS

The size of an acoustic tumor is important in determining the nature of the signs and symptoms that it will produce (19, 20). It also has a critical influence on postoperative outcome (33). It is therefore important to detect tumors while they are still small (10). Progressive unilateral hearing loss with tinnitus is the earliest and most prominent complaint of patients with acoustic tumors (20). However, many patients ignore these symptoms, and almost one third of patients are first evaluated for nonaudiologic symptoms (21). Therefore, it is important that patients be carefully questioned about hearing loss when they present with imbalance, dysequilibrium, dizziness, or headache.

Because of the importance of early diagnosis, screening tests with a high degree of sensitivity are desirable. However, because only 5–10% of patients with unilateral hearing loss will eventually be shown to have an acoustic neurinoma (21, 45), screening tests should also have high specificity. It was estimated that in 1978, the average cost to diagnose an acoustic tumor was $15,000–$30,000 per tumor (3, 8). With the use of new techniques such as brainstem auditory evoked potentials and computed tomography, the current cost can be reduced to less than $5000 per tumor using a scheme proposed by Hart and Davenport (20). This algorithm, with minor modifications, is presented in Figure 12.1. The techniques described below have made the diagnosis of acoustic tumors specific, sensitive, and cost effective.

Brainstem Auditory Evoked Potentials

The brainstem auditory evoked potential (BAEP) is probably the most sensitive noninvasive test available for the diagnosis of acoustic tumors (6, 20, 21). It is highly sensitive for small tumors, with detection rates reported between 93 and 100% (8, 41). BAEPs may be abnormal when

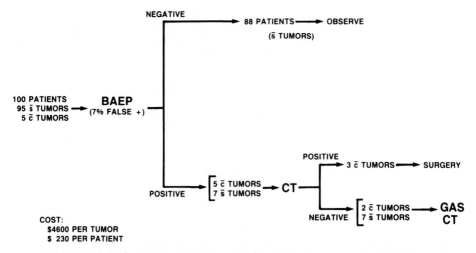

FIG. 12.1. Algorithm for the detection of acoustic tumors as proposed by Hart and Davenport (20) with minor modifications. A 7% false-positive rate is assumed for the BAEP, and five of the initial 100 patients have tumors. With these assumptions, the cost to diagnose each tumor is $4600, and the cost per patient is $230. (Modified from R. G. Hart and J. Davenport (20).)

routine audiologic tests and CT scans are normal, whereas the converse has not been seen (6). The test is especially useful in patients with nonaudiologic complaints, or mild hearing losses. The BAEP interpeak latencies (especially the Wave I–III separation) are the best indicators for acoustic tumors. The stapedius reflex is the most sensitive individual audiometric test and is abnormal in 85% of patients with tumors (20). The acoustic reflex latency has been combined with the BAEP to identify brainstem auditory evoked responses (BAER) false-positives (9).

Computed Tomography-Gas Computed Tomography

Computed tomography (CT) has been useful in detecting medium and large acoustic tumors, especially when intravenous contrast media is given. However, tumors smaller than 1.5 cm can be missed on CTs performed on third generation or older scanners (21). The sensitivity of fourth generation scanners is about 92% for tumors less than 1 cm in size (19, 44). For defining the geometry of large tumors, direct coronal CT scans and reconstructions of axial scans in various planes can be helpful.

For small tumors, and especially for intracanalicular tumors, the radiologic procedure of choice is gas CT cisternography (7, 21, 26, 34). This technique has largely replaced the metrizamide CT scan because of superior visualization of the porus acusticus and related structures. The use of filtered CO_2, instead of air, has reduced the incidence of poststudy headache (7, 21, 34), and has allowed the test to be done on an outpatient basis (34). Gas CT cisternography provides a beautiful image of the internal auditory canal and its contents (Fig. 12.2). Clark *et al.* (7) were able to visualize the neurovascular bundle in 46 of 48 examinations. However, there are pitfalls associated with this technique. These have recently been addressed by Johnson (26). He urges extreme caution in cases in which tumors are smaller than 3 mm and recommends repeat examinations at 1-year intervals. Of four patients thought to have tiny tumors, elective vestibular nerve section in two patients revealed no evidence of tumor. Three potential false-positives were avoided by persistent efforts to fill the internal auditory canals. Two patients had coexistent spinal tumors which caused difficulty in transporting the gas,

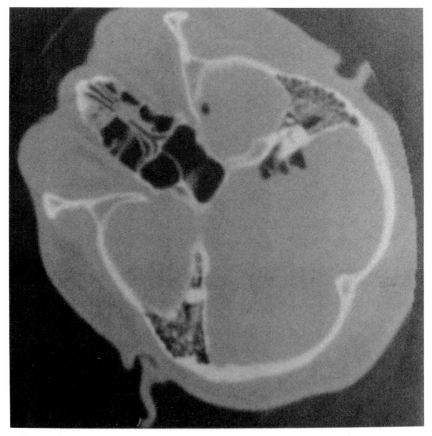

FIG. 12.2. A gas CT cisternogram demonstrates the porus acusticus and the neurovascular bundle entering it. No acoustic tumor was present.

and decompression was necessary in one case. Johnson also stresses the importance of bilateral examinations to allow comparison between the two sides.

Magnetic Resonance Imaging

Magnetic resonance imaging (MRI) uses no ionizing radiation or intravenous contrast media and is therefore a totally noninvasive technique. Because there is no signal from bone, the MRI image is unaffected by bone artifacts and is well suited to examination of the posterior fossa. On the other hand, because the bone is not imaged, sclerosis cannot be seen, and destruction of the bone can only be determined indirectly. Whether MRI is superior to CT in the diagnosis of acoustic tumors remains to be determined, although there is evidence that this may indeed be the case (30, 46).

It appears that MRI and CT may have similar sensitivities for the detection of medium and large CPA tumors, although we recently observed a large cystic acoustic tumor that was poorly visualized by contrast CT (Fig. 12.3) but was well seen by MRI (Fig. 12.4). However, small tumors may be better detected by MRI than by contrast CT. Intracanalicular tumors can be seen by MRI (Fig. 12.5). Young et al. (46) have visualized an 8-mm intracanalicular tumor; however, McGinnis et al. (30) were unable to detect any abnormalities in the inversion recovery (IR), saturation recovery (SR), or spin echo (SE) images of a purely intracanalicular tumor that was only visualized by CO_2 CT cisternography. The MRI may be the ideal screening test for patients with abnormal BAEPs or clinical features strongly suggestive of a CPA tumor. The ultimate test for ruling out small intracanalicular tumors, however, continues to be CT gas cisternography.

The specificity of the MRI may be superior to that of the CT, and MRI may be well suited to differentiating between various lesions in the cerebellopontine angle. Young et al. (46) were able to conclusively show by MRI that a lesion thought to be an acoustic tumor on CT was actually an intrinsic brainstem tumor. These authors have also reported that it may be possible to predict tumor consistency based upon the characteristics of the magnetic resonance image.

The multiplanar facility of MRI makes it useful in accurately determining the geometry of a tumor. The true dimensions of the tumor in various planes may be determined, and the position of the tumor in relation to adjacent structures may be demonstrated. This information can be helpful in preoperative planning.

Three-Dimensional CT Reconstruction

General Electric has recently developed software packages that allow construction of a three-dimensional image from CT data. This technique

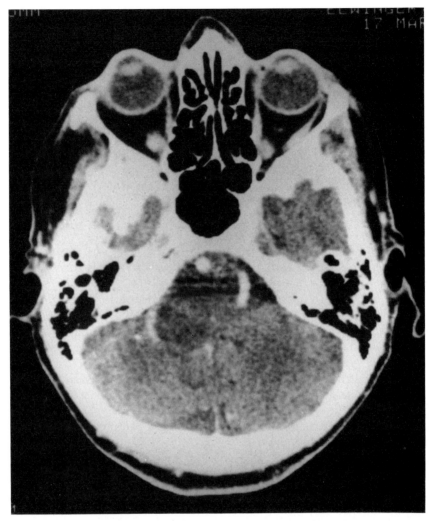

FIG. 12.3. A contrast-enhanced CT scan demonstrates a faint low density lesion with an enhancing rim in the cerebellopontine angle.

has recently been used by Hemmy *et al.* (22) to study craniofacial deformities. We have applied this technique to CPA tumors, using thin axial slices of the posterior fossa and intravenous contrast media. The images produced have demonstrated the geometry of the tumor in relation to normal boney landmarks (Fig. 12.6). Although the experience with three-dimensional CT in studying CPA tumors has been limited, this technique may be helpful to the surgeon by providing a detailed picture of the structures adjacent to the tumor, especially boney landmarks that

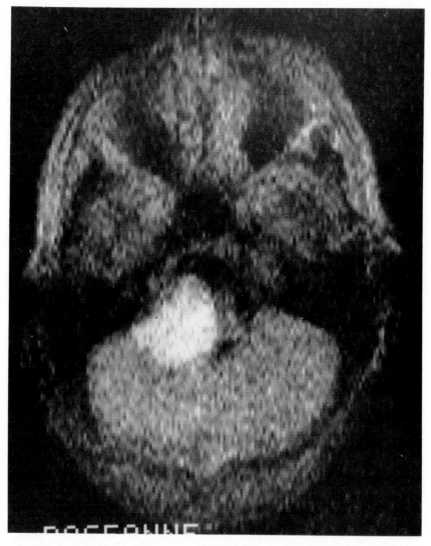

FIG. 12.4. An MRI scan of the same lesion as in Figure 12.3 does a much better job of demonstrating the large CPA tumor, which proved to be an acoustic neurinoma.

will be seen during surgery. Demonstration of inner ear structures in relation to the wall of the porus acusticus may allow the surgeon to perform a wide decompression of the porus without damaging these structures. We anticipate that three-dimensional CT studies using CO_2 cisternography may provide additional information, and we expect to perform such studies in the future.

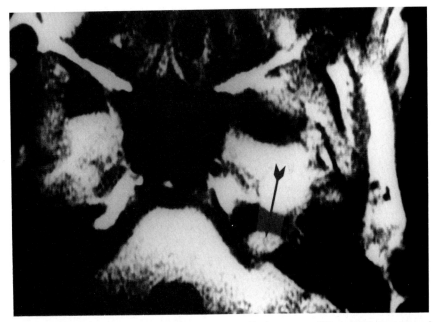

FIG. 12.5. MRI scan demonstrates an intracanalicular tumor. (Photograph courtesy of General Electric.)

INTRAOPERATIVE MONITORING

Recent advances in intraoperative monitoring have occurred which allow safer removal of CPA tumors by providing feedback on the function of the brainstem and cranial nerves. These techniques can reassure the surgeon that all is proceeding smoothly, or can signal that a problem may be developing. When dysfunction is detected by one of the following techniques, the anesthesiologist can take corrective measures such as adjusting the CO_2 tension or blood pressure, and the surgeon can remove or reposition a retractor, or change his surgical technique.

Brainstem Auditory Evoked Potentials (BAEPs)

Raudzens and Shetter (37) and Grundy et al. (18) have demonstrated the usefulness of BAEPs for intraoperative monitoring. They have shown that BAEPs can be routinely and reliably recorded in the operating room, that they do not cause intraoperative delays, and that they can provide a good prediction of postoperative auditory function. BAEPs remain stable under anesthesia and do not fatigue with repeated measurements (37). Minor changes can occur with changes in positioning, or with hypocarbia plus modest hypotension (18). Raudzens and Shetter noted

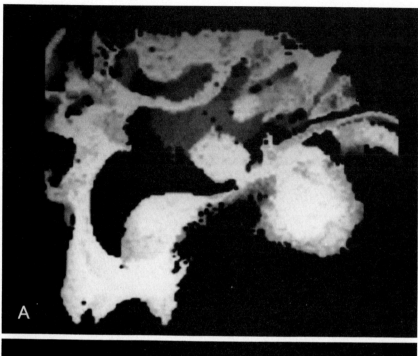

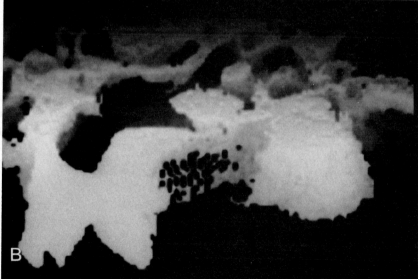

Fig. 12.6. Three-dimensional CT reconstructions of an acoustic tumor show the relationship of the tumor with adjacent structures. The images are rotated along a horizontal coronal axis, as though the observer's point of view was shifted from the vertex toward the torcular.

that the usual change in BAEPs was a failure of two consecutive averages to superimpose with progressive lengthening of wave latencies. They found that alterations of this type could first be detected within 3 minutes of the insult. Grundy *et al.* noted deterioration of the BAEP in 22 patients, typically manifesting as an increase in Wave V latency. They noted that BAEP changes returned toward normal in 19 cases after corrective measures were taken. They observed recovery of BAEP after periods of near obliteration lasting from 5 to 177 minutes. Irreversible loss of BAEPs has invariably been associated with profound postoperative hearing loss or deafness. Raudzens and Shetter observed the loss of all wave form beyond Wave I from the contralateral ear in one patient with marked cerebellar swelling. This predicted severe postoperative brainstem dysfunction.

It is probable that BAEPs have prevented permanent neurological deficits in a segment of patients monitored by this technique. If retractor placement or operative manipulation causes a change in the BAEP, the surgeon may be warned of potential danger while there is still time to take corrective actions. However, the inherent latency prevents immediate feedback and is a major drawback of the technique. At the present, however, BAEPs are the most reliable method of intraoperative monitoring. In some cases, the use of BAEPs is almost considered mandatory. Martuza and Ojemann (29) strongly suggest the use of BAEPs when operating on a patient with bilateral acoustic tumors when an attempt is being made to preserve hearing. They suggest that even minor deteriorations in the BAEP should signal the surgeon to alter his approach in these patients. They recommend settling for a partial resection, or only proceeding with a decompression of the porus.

When a very large tumor is present, it may be desirable to further monitor brainstem function. In this case, the somatosensory evoked potential (SSEP) may be helpful.

Eighth Nerve Recording

Recently, Moller and Jannetta (31) have reported the use of direct nerve recording as a means to monitor eighth nerve function during 19 craniotomies, the majority for microvascular decompression procedures. The recordings were made using Teflon-coated silver wires and provided instantaneous information about the function of the auditory nerve. They found that the direction of retraction of the cerebellum had a critical impact upon eighth nerve signals, with deterioration in nerve function with lateral-to-medial retraction. Rostral-caudal and caudal-rostral retraction were well tolerated. Such immediate feedback can be quite useful to the surgeon working in the cerebellopontine angle. It can not only warn of impending harm to the eighth nerve but may also be instructive about the relative danger of particular maneuvers and manipulations. In the series reported, no CPA tumors were included. The electrode was placed on the distal aspect of the auditory nerve as soon as it was exposed. Large tumors may obscure the distal eighth nerve, making this technique unavailable. However, for small tumors in which an effort is being made to preserve hearing, this technique may be quite useful.

Seventh Nerve Stimulation

Direct electrical stimulation of the seventh nerve can be helpful in identifying the nerve and in assessing the function of the portion of the nerve distal to the stimulus. The practice of stimulating the nerve and observing the response of the facial musculature may be refined by monitoring the facial response by EMG. This technique has several advantages. It provides an objective measure of facial nerve function and can be used even when the face is draped off and inaccessible to the observer. In addition, EMG potentials can be detected not only when the nerve is electrically stimulated (Fig. 12.7), but also when it is stimulated by touch or traction as well (Fig. 12.8). This can aid the surgeon in identifying the seventh nerve and can protect it by indicating that a particular action is mechanically stimulating the nerve. As the laser can debulk the tumor in a no-touch fashion, the EMG recording during laser debulking is unchanged from the background signal (Fig. 12.9). A direct feedback system for the surgeon can be achieved by connecting the EMG signal to a speaker. The audio signal produced gives an indication of the amount of stimulation the seventh nerve is receiving. Unfortunately, this technique only provides information on the status of the nerve distal to the stimulus, and function can be retained in the nerve distal to a transsection for some time. Therefore, a good response to stimulation does not necessarily indicate that the entire facial nerve is intact. However, this technique does seem to be helpful to the surgeon in locating the nerve and in indicating its response to various operative maneuvers.

Neurosurgical Instrumentation

Developments in instrumentation have played an important role in the evolution of CPA tumor surgery. Dramatic improvements were seen with the introduction of the microscope, microsurgical instruments, and microsurgical techniques. The most recent addition to the neurosurgeon's armamentarium is the laser.

The beam produced by the laser possesses unique qualities (15, 17, 39, 40). It has both temporal and spatial coherence. The beam is monochromatic and can be focused to varying spot diameters. The laser is able to

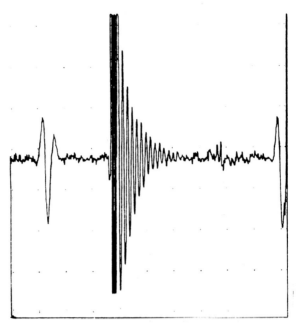

FIG. 12.7. Electrical stimulation. An EMG recording obtained from the perioral region demonstrates the effect of intracranial electrical stimulation of the seventh nerve.

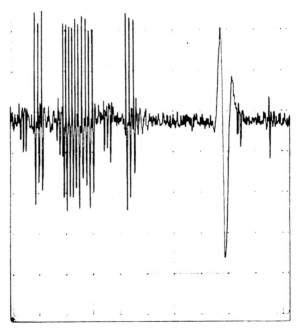

FIG. 12.8. Traction on the seventh nerve during debulking of an acoustic tumor produces EMG spikes.

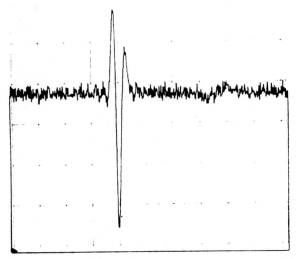

FIG. 12.9. The EMG recording during debulking with a laser shows no change from the typical background picture. An EKG artifact is present.

deliver a high concentration of energy to vaporize tissue, but it can also be used to coagulate vessels.

The carbon dioxide (CO_2) and argon lasers are the two most popular lasers for CPA tumor surgery. The CO_2 laser has the advantage of higher power, which allows rapid debulking of the tumor. Because of the high energy absorption in water, vital structures can be protected with moist patties. However, the beam presently cannot be delivered through a fiberoptic system, and this necessitates a bulky mirror apparatus. In addition, an aiming laser is necessary because the beam is not visible.

The argon laser produces a beam that can be transmitted through a fiberoptic system that can be precisely focused (15, 17). The beam is visible and is readily absorbed by hemoglobin, making the argon laser an excellent photocoagulator. However, the power is considerably less than that of the CO_2 laser, and the beam is poorly absorbed by water. Glasscock et al. (17) report that they have bounced the beam off of mirrors during middle ear surgery.

The CO_2 laser probably is the most useful laser in acoustic tumor surgery. It creates a zone of vaporization with a small zone of coagulation necrosis about 40 μm thick (15). Surrounding this zone is an area of homogeneous coagulation about 200 μm in thickness. Short high energy pulses are preferrd, as they produce less carbonization.

There are differing opinions regarding the power and spot size settings to be used in acoustic tumor surgery. Most authors, however, agree upon the general technique (15, 17, 25, 39). The laser is typically not used until the tumor has been exposed (Fig. 12.10), as conventional techniques are superior for the opening approach. Once the tumor is exposed, moist cottonoids are used to cover surrounding structures. Surface vessels smaller than 1 mm can be coagulated with the laser, but larger vessels are best coagulated with a bipolar. Coagulation of the capsule with a low power defocused beam is not only hemostatic but also shrinks the capsule and helps to free the tumor along arachnoidal planes (Fig. 12.11) (15). Gutting of the tumor is usually performed at high energy levels of 5–100-W (Fig. 12.12) (15, 39), although some authors prefer the use of lower power settings in the 5- to 10-W range (25). A wide spot diameter (defocused) beam is used in a continuous or pulsed manner. Because heat can accumulate in the bone and damage adjacent structures, the laser should never be used to remove the bone around the porus acusticus (39). Some surgeons recommend using the laser for removing small residual pieces of tumor from important structures, such as the seventh and eighth nerves or blood vessels (15, 39). For this application they use low power, small spot size, and protection of surrounding structures. Other authors strongly advise against this practice (25).

Robertson *et al.* (39) recently reported the use of a CO_2 laser for the

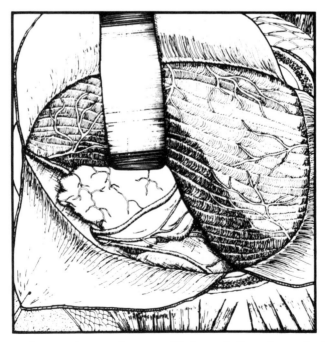

FIG. 12.10. An acoustic tumor is seen to fill the cerebellopontine angle after surgical exposure.

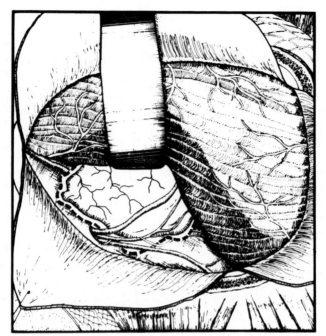

FIG. 12.11. After the capsule has been coagulated with a low power defocused beam, the capsule shrinks, which aids dissection by freeing the tumor along arachnoidal planes.

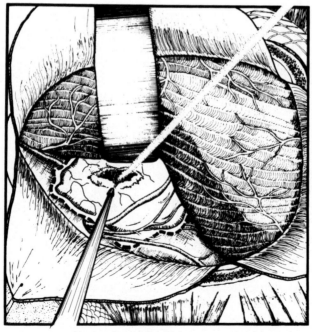

FIG. 12.12. The laser is used at high power to gut the tumor.

removal of 28 acoustic tumors. The laser was used through a variety of approaches on tumors ranging in size from 1 to 6 cm. Anatomic preservation of the facial nerve was achieved in 26 of the 28 cases. These authors found the laser to be superior to other methods for the removal of acoustic tumors. This conclusion was also reached by Cerullo (4, 5) and by Smith (42).

The advantage of the laser over conventional techniques is mostly due to its ability to remove tissue without applying traction or pressure. In this regard it is superior to the cutting loop, cavitron ultrasonic aspirator (CUSA), or rongeur (43). The laser is superior to the CUSA for the following reasons: (a) The laser achieves a no-touch removal of the tumor with minimal mechanical trauma to the adjacent seventh and eighth nerves. The CUSA must necessarily cause pressure on the tumor and adjacent structures, and the effect of vibration of the tip on the seventh and eighth nerves is unknown. (b) The laser can be used with the microscope, even in a small deep hole. The CUSA is awkward in this situation and allows poor visualization of the area undergoing debulking. (c) The laser is moderately hemostatic, whereas the CUSA is not.

A disadvantage of the laser, however, is that the surgeon must use one hand to aim the laser, and the other to manipulate a suction tip to remove the smoke. One solution is to place a side port on a suction tip. This provides a route for smoke evacuation, while the tip of the sucker can be used for dissection. The recently described microprocessor-controlled scanning manipulator may allow for more rapid and precise use of the laser (11). This device uses a microprocessor to control the path of the beam, which is directed in a scanning pattern within a previously defined area. The surgeon defines this area by tracing around the perimeter with the aiming beam. While the machine controls the beam, the surgeon's hands are freed to permit suctioning of smoke and dissection or manipulation of the tumor.

STEREOTACTIC RADIOSURGERY

Stereotactic radiosurgery has been advocated for the treatment of acoustic tumors (32, 35). Noren et al. (32) have reported the use of their Gamma II unit for the treatment of 14 acoustic tumors ranging in size from 7 to 30 mm. The Gamma II unit contains 179 ^{60}Co sources collimated to 8 or 14 mm and aimed at the center. It is possible to vary the shape and size of the area of maximal irradiation by plugging tubes or changing collimators. Each patient had a tailor-made plan calculated by computer. Eight of the 14 tumors decreased in size, from 1 to 10 mm, but three continued to increase in size. The technique was not harmless to cranial nerves in the vicinity of the tumor. Two patients developed facial numbness at 8 and 9 months. In one case this was permanent with anesthesia dolorosa. Five patients developed seventh nerve palsies 6 to 9 months after treatment, but all improved.

Convincing evidence that this technique can safely cure acoustic tumors is not available. Noren *et al.* have used this technique on two patients who had undergone surgical removal of the extracanalicular portion of the tumor, in whom the intracanalicular portion of the tumor was intentionally left for later radiosurgery. As excellent results can usually be achieved by standard microsurgical methods, this does not appear to be the optimal use of the stereotactic radiosurgery technique. Radiosurgery may be most applicable to patients who are medically unable to undergo posterior fossa surgery. It may also be found to be useful in temporizing surgery in patients with bilateral acoustic tumors.

CONCLUSIONS

Although a recent paper may have described the first case of a malignant nerve sheath tumor of the acoustic nerve (28), for the most part, acoustic nerve tumors are benign and potentially curable. Recent advances in diagnosis allow early detection of tumors, even while they remain intracanalicular. Intraoperative monitoring techniques alert the surgeon to potential dangers of operative manipulation and retractor placement. The laser is able to remove tissue in a hemostatic manner without causing pressure or traction on surrounding structures. All of these developments have helped to improve the safety and effectiveness of surgery in the cerebellopontine angle, an area once referred to by Harvey Cushing as "the gloomy corner of neurologic surgery." With advanced diagnostic tests, intraoperative monitoring techniques and modern surgical capabilities, that gloomy corner is now a region that can be approached by the neurosurgeon with confidence, surity and optimism.

ACKNOWLEDGMENTS

The authors wish to thank John A. Hodak, M.D., for providing three-dimensional CT reconstructions. They also are grateful to Alvin D. Sidell, M.D., Peter A. Raudzens, M.D., and Richard A. Flom, M.D., for reviewing the manuscript. The authors thank Georgia Frederik for editorial assistance.

REFERENCES

1. Atkinson, W. J., Jr. Anterior inferior cerebellar artery: Its variation, pontine distribution, and significance in surgery of the cerebello-pontine angle tumours. J. Neurol. Neurosurg. Psychiatry, *12:* 137–151, 1949.
2. Ballance, C. A. *Some Points in the Surgery of the Brain and Its Membranes.* Macmillan, London, 1907, p. 206.
3. Caparosa, R. J. Cost-benefit ratio in our search for cerebellopontine angle tumors. Laryngoscope, *89:* 410–420, 1979.
4. Cerullo, L. J. Acoustic nerve tumor removal with CO_2 laser: Technique and results. Presented at Congress on Laser Neurosurgery II, Chicago, Sept. 23–25, 1982.
5. Cerullo, L. J. Reviewer's comments. Neurosurgery, *12:* 290, 1983.

6. Chiappa, K. H. *Evoked Potentials in Clinical Medicine.* Raven Press, New York, pp. 159–165.

7. Clark, W. C., Acker, J. D., Robertson, J. H., Gardner, G., Dusseau, J. J., and Moretz, W. Neuroradiological detection of small and intracanalicular acoustic tumors: An emphasis on CO_2 contrast-enhanced computed tomographic cisternography. Neurosurgery, *11:* 733–738, 1982.

8. Clemis, J. D., and McGee, T. Brainstem electric response audiometry in the differential diagnosis of acoustic tumors. Laryngoscope, *89:* 31–42, 1979.

9. Clemis, J. D., and Sarno, C. N. Acoustic reflex latency test in the evaluation of nontumor patients with abnormal brainstem latencies. Ann. Otol. Rhinol. Laryngol., *89:* 296–302, 1980.

10. Cushing, H. *Tumors of the Nervus Acusticus and the Syndrome of the Cerebellopontine Angle.* W.B. Saunders, Philadelphia/London, 1917.

11. Dagan, J., Robertson, J. H., and Clark, W. C. Microprocessor-controlled scanning micromanipulator for carbon dioxide laser surgery: Technical note. J. Neurosurg., *59:* 1098–1099, 1983.

12. Dandy, W. E. An operation for the total removal of cerebellopontine (acoustic) tumors. Surg. Gynecol. Obstet., *41:* 129–148, 1925.

13. DiTullio, M. V., Jr., Malkasian, D., and Rand, R. W. A critical comparison of neurosurgical and otolaryngological approaches to acoustic neuromas. J. Neurosurg., *48:* 1–12, 1978.

14. Drake, C. G. Surgical treatment of acoustic neuroma with preservation or reconstruction of the facial nerve. J. Neurosurg., *26:* 459–464, 1967.

15. Edwards, M. S. B., Boggan, J. E., and Fuller, T. A. The laser in neurological surgery. J. Neurosurg., *59:* 555–566, 1983.

16. Givre, A., and Olivecrona, H. Surgical experience with acoustic tumors. J. Neurosurg., *6:* 396–407, 1949.

17. Glasscock, M. E., Jackson, C. G., and Whitaker, S. R. The argon laser in acoustic tumor surgery. Laryngoscope, *91:* 1405–1415, 1981.

18. Grundy, B. L., Jannetta, P. J., Procopio, P. T., Lina, A., Boston, R., and Doyle, E. Intraoperative monitoring of brain-stem auditory evoked potentials. J. Neurosurg., *57:* 674–681, 1982.

19. Harner, S. G., and Laws, E. R. Diagnosis of acoustic neurinoma. Neurosurgery, *9:* 373–379, 1981.

20. Hart, R. G., and Davenport, J. Diagnosis of acoustic neuroma. Neurosurgery, *9:* 450–463, 1981.

21. Hart, R. G., Gardner, D. P., and Howieson, J. Acoustic tumors: Atypical features and recent diagnostic tests. Neurology, *33:* 211–221, 1983.

22. Hemmy, D. C., David, D. J., and Herman, G. T. Three-dimensional reconstruction of craniofacial deformity using computed tomography. Neurosurgery, *13:* 534–541, 1983.

23. House, H. P., and House, W. F. Historical review and problem of acoustic neuroma. Arch. Otolaryngol., *80:* 601–604, 1964.

24. House, W. F. (ed.). Transtemporal bone microsurgical removal of acoustic neuromas (monograph). Arch. Otolaryngol., *80:* 597–756, 1964.

25. Hudgins, W. R. Reviewer's comments. Neurosurgery, *12:* 290, 1983.

26. Johnson, D. W. Air cisternography of the cerebellopontine angle using high-resolution computed tomography. Radiology, *151:* 401–403, 1984.

27. Koos, W. T., Spetzler, R. F., Bock, F. W., and Salah, S. Microsurgery of cerebellopontine angle tumors. In: *Clinical Microneurosurgery,* edited by W. T. Koos, F. W. Bock, and R. F. Spetzler. Georg Thieme, Stuttgart, 1976, pp. 91–112.

28. Kudo, M., Mastumoto, M., and Terao, H. Malignant nerve sheath tumor of acoustic nerve. Arch. Pathol. Lab. Med. *107:* 293–297, 1983.

29. Martuza, R. L., and Ojemann, R. G. Bilateral acoustic neuromas: Clinical aspects, pathogenesis, and treatment. Neurosurgery, *10:* 1–12, 1982.
30. McGinnis, B. D., Brady, T. J., New, P. F. J., Buonanno, F. S., Pykett, I. L., DeLaPaz, R. L., Kistler, J. P., and Taveras, J. M. Nuclear magnetic resonance (NMR) imaging of tumors in the posterior fossa. J. Comput. Assist. Tomogr., *7:* 575–584, 1983.
31. Moller, A. R., and Jannetta, P. J. Monitoring auditory function during cranial nerve microvascular decompression operations by direct recording from the eighth nerve. J. Neurosurg., *59:* 493–499, 1983.
32. Noren, G., Arndt, J., Hindmarsh, T. Stereotactic radiosurgery in cases of acoustic neurinoma: Further experiences. Neurosurgery, *13:* 12–22, 1983.
33. Olivecrona, H. Acoustic tumors. J. Neurosurg., *26:* 6–13, 1966.
34. Pinto, R. S., Kricheff, I. I., Bergeron, R. T., and Cohen, N. Small acoustic neuromas: Detection by high resolution gas CT cisternography. AJR, *139:* 129–132, 1982.
35. Rand, R. W. The stereotactic cobalt 60 gamma unit in the treatment of acoustic neuromas. In: *Neurological Surgery of the Ear and Skull Base*, edited by D. E. Brackmann. Raven Press, New York, 1982, pp. 379–389.
36. Rand, R. W., and Kurze, T. Micro-neurosurgical resection of acoustic tumors by a transmeatal posterior fossa approach. Bull. Los Angeles, Neurol. Soc., *30:* 17–20, 1965.
37. Raudzens, P. A., and Shetter, A. G. Intraoperative monitoring of brain-stem auditory evoked potentials. J. Neurosurg., *57:* 341–348, 1982.
38. Rhoton, A. L. Microsurgical removal of acoustic neuromas. Surg. Neurol., *6:* 211–219, 1976.
39. Robertson, J. H., Clark, W. C., Robertson, J. T., Gardner, L. G., and Shea, M. C. Use of the carbon dioxide laser for acoustic tumor surgery. Neurosurgery, *12:* 289–290, 1983.
40. Saunders, M. L., Young, H. F., Becker, D. P., Greenberg, R. P. Newlon, P. G., Corales, R. L., Ham, W. T., and Povlishock, J. T. The use of the laser in neurological surgery. Surg. Neurol., *14:* 1–10, 1980.
41. Selters, W. A., and Brackmann, D. E. Acoustic tumor detection with brain stem electric response audiometry. Arch. Otolaryngol., *103:* 181–187, 1977.
42. Smith, M. F. W. Hearing conservation and the CO_2 laser in acoustic neurilemmoma excision. In: *Neurological Surgery of the Ear and Skull Base*, D. E. Brackmann. Raven Press, New York, 1982, pp. 243–245.
43. Strait, T. A., Robertson, J. H., and Clark, W. C. Use of the carbon dioxide laser in the operative management and intracranial meningiomas: A report of twenty cases. Neurosurgery, *10:* 464–467.
44. Valavanis, A., Dabir, K., Hamdi, R., Oguz, M., and Wellauer, J. The current state of the radiological diagnosis of acoustic neuroma. Neuroradiology, *23:* 7–13, 1982.
45. Valvassori, G. E. The abnormal internal auditory auditory canal: The diagnosis of acoustic neuroma. Radiology, *92:* 449–459, 1969.
46. Young, I. R., Bydder, G. M., Hall, A. S., Steiner, R. E., Worthington, B. S., Hawkes, R. C., Holland, G. N., and Moore, W. S. The role of NMR imaging in the diagnosis and management of acoustic neuroma. A.J.N.R., *4:* 223–224, 1983.

CHAPTER

13

Management of Seventh and Eighth Nerve Involvement by Cerebellopontine Angle Tumors

MADJID SAMII, M.D.,
KEKI E. TUREL, M.D., M.S. (Neurosurgery), F.I.C.S., and
GOTZ PENKERT, M.D.

INTRODUCTION

Tumors in the cerebellopontine angle (CPA) have always challenged the skill of neurosurgeons. While most are benign, with total excision leading to cure, their location in the vicinity of the cranial nerves and brain stem warrants special care and expertise. Harvey Cushing (2) had to be content with partial removal of acoustic tumors in order to minimize mortality. However, in the long run, tumor recurrence led to an overall mortality rate of 56%. Dandy (3, 4) succeeded in doing 45 total acoustic tumor removals with a modest mortality rate of 11%. Although facial nerve preservation had begun to be envisioned, it was a rarity. Olivecrona (23) and Nielsen (22) reported facial nerve preservation in a high percentage of cases (65%) with an apparent gross tumor removal. However, a subsequent review of Olivecrona's cases by Horrax and Poppen (14) found half the patients either dead or with subsequent tumor recurrence (22, 23).

The otolaryngologists were the earliest to adopt the surgical microscope in routine practice and demonstrated the advantages of this device with their lower mortality rates and greater numbers of facial nerve preservations using a middle fossa approach (15, 20). However, they were unable to remove large tumors through this approach. When it was attempted, complications such as uncontrollable intraoperative bleeding occurred. The pioneering efforts of William House (16), however, paved the way for renewed optimism in the successful management of acoustic tumors with a low mortality and acceptable morbidity.

Rand and Kurze (24), Drake (11), and others showed that acoustic tumors could be removed totally, safely, and with preservation of the facial nerve. Rand and Kurze (25) discussed the possibility of anatomic preservation of the cochlear nerve, which they subsequently demon-

242

strated in 1968. Subsequent occasional reports on preservation of cochlear nerve function appeared in the literature, although these were
infrequent.

Today's neurosurgeon is able to make an earlier and more precise
diagnosis. As a result of audiometry, computed tomographic (CT) scan,
cochleomeatal scan (CMS) and magnetic resonance imaging (MRI).
When combined with modern microsurgical technique, these advances
have resulted in the preservation of an increasing number of seventh and
eighth cranial nerves.

The possibility of preservation of useful hearing in some cases of
acoustic neuroma (or neurinoma) has important implications regarding
the surgical approach. The translabyrinthine route used by the otolaryngologists to reach the acoustic tumor in the cerebellopontine angle
must destroy the cochlear organ. It is therefore limited to patients in
whom hearing ability has been lost forever. The transtemporal route has
the potential of preserving cochlear nerve function but in reality can
only be successfully employed to that end if the tumor is less than 1.5
cm in diameter. Glasscock et al. (13) have reported one case operated by
this route with useful postoperative hearing. Fisch (12) preserved cochlear
nerve function in 5 of 12 cases with acoustic tumors, but in retrospect
one-quarter of the total cases were not complete removals.

Sterkers (33) prefers the middle fossa route for intracanalicular tumors
and the retrosigmoid approach for large-size acoustic tumors. He operates
on all sizes of tumors by either of the two approaches and reported an
overall preservation of cochlear nerve function in 33% of the cases of his
94 totally removed tumors (32).

For the microsurgical removal of acoustic neuroma, we usually use the
same unilateral suboccipital approach described by Rand and Kurze (24)
in 1965. They felt that it had the following advantages over the middle
fossa and translabyrinthine routes: (a) a wide field of action; (b) direct
visualization of the anterior inferior cerebellar artery (AICA) and other
brain stem vessels; (c) dissection of all surfaces of the acoustic tumor
always under direct vision; (d) identification of the facial nerve in the
lateral angle of the internal auditory canal (IAC); and (e) ready access
to the facial nerve when either anastomosis or graft reconstruction is
necessary.

During the last 6 years, 200 CPA tumors were operated on at this
clinic by the senior author, who had already been experienced with
microneurosurgical techniques for a prior decade. The overwhelming
majority of them (167, or 83.5% of them) were acoustic neuromas. Of the
remaining 33, there were 21 meningiomas, 10 epidermoids, and 2 angioblastomas. There is an obvious and progressive tendency towards a higher
proportion of acoustic tumor referrals. Our statistics showed 78 acoustic

tumors in the first 100 CPA tumors; the second hundred CPA tumors realized 89 of them!

PREOPERATIVE WORKUP

Since this presentation deals with management of seventh and eighth nerve involvement by CPA tumors, it may suffice to say that a preoperative workup should be aimed at distinguishing the kind of tumor present. This allows the surgeon both to have a mental preparedness for the operative strategy and to preoperatively discuss the prognosis with regard to neurologic morbidity with the patient.

As for the hearing tests performed in order to detect the neural origin of the hearing disorder, it is pertinent to mention that loss of discrimination is a more sensitive index than hearing threshold. We have been doing brainstem auditory evoked potential studies (BAEPs) pre-, intra-, and postoperatively; wave V is considered significant in the diagnosis of acoustic neuromas, as its peak can be traced up to the hearing threshold. In contrast, in patients with tumors near the inner ear canal, the threshold of brain stem response is generally increased.

High-resolution cochleomeatal scanning (CMS) of the internal auditory canal (IAC) is performed by injecting intravenous ^{99m}Tc. Normally there is no radionuclear activity within the IAC, but it may be present in the presence of a tumor (Fig. 13.16A and B). The CMS may help recognize the position of the basilar vessel rostrally and the jugular vein caudally.

Computed tomographic (CT) scanning is currently the most valuable diagnostic tool. Acoustic neuromas generally appear as an irregular hyperdense mass with the porus acusticus almost at its center. Occasionally the lesion may be hypodense, but sometimes there may be no apparent tumor, or a purely intracanalicular lesion. An air CT is a necessary adjunct in such cases. The newer generation CT scanners have a higher positivity. Besides the frequent (although not mandatory) widening of the IAC, it shows the exact length of the IAC. This information is helpful when the surgeon is indecisive on how far laterally to drill. Important anatomic structures, such as the semicircular canals and jugular bulb, as well as the extent of pneumatization of the petrous and mastoid bones, are other vital pieces of information that may be useful guides for the surgeon (Fig. 13.1). Meningiomas are strongly and homogenously enhancing lesions. They may have a broad base of attachment and sometimes hyperostosis. The porus is generally eccentric and often caudal to the midpoint of the mass. Meningiomas lying in CPA may arise from the clivus, the tentorial notch, or the petrous bone. Its predominant extension may be prepontine, rostral CPA (with or without a transtentorial extension into the middle fossa), or in a caudal direction towards

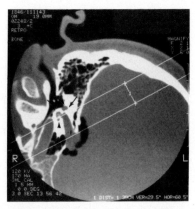

FIG. 13.1. The new generation of CT scan has the advantage of demontrating not only the characteristics of the IAC but also important anatomic features in its immediate vicinity, namely, the vestibule and semicircular canals (*arrows*), and the extent of pneumatization of the mastoid cells, as seen vividly in this picture. Such information is relevant to a safe surgical exposure of the canal.

the foramen magnum. The amount and direction of tumor extension might necessitate changing the approach from the usual retromastoid, suboccipital route to a subtemporal or combined suprainfratentorial approach. Epidermoid tumors are generally hypodense, tend to infringe into the cranial spaces, and may be seen to cross over to the opposite side in front of the pons. Epidermoids arising from within the petrous and extending into the canal are characterized by significant bone destruction.

Magnetic resonance imaging (MRI) (Fig. 13.2) shows soft tissue features of the tumor and the surrounding brain and cranial nerves while eliminating the bone.

OPERATIVE MANAGEMENT

Position

The patient is administered general anesthesia and placed in a lounging position (Fig. 13.3). A three-point fixation clamp (Mayfield) is applied to the head in the usual manner. The head is then turned to the side of the tumor so that the region of operation faces the surgeon. The neck is gripped between the surgeon's hands and stretched upwards by the length of the index fingers resting against the patient's lower jaw and the thumbs against his occiput. It is then flexed to the extent permitted without distorting the intervening hand of the surgeon. This amount of flexion will ensure that the internal jugular veins are not compressed.

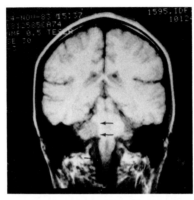

FIG. 13.2. The magnetic resonance scan shows displacement of soft tissues (cranial nerves, pons) by tumor (*arrows*) more elaborately.

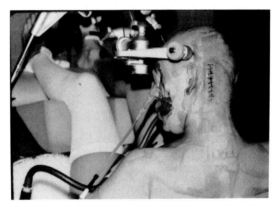

FIG. 13.3. The lounging position of the patient with head in Mayfield's fixation clamp, as described in the text, employed for exposure of all CPA tumors. Note the incision.

The patient's lower limbs are semiflexed at both hips and knees and above the horizontal level of the heart. This is necessary in order to raise the central venous pressure (CVP) as a precaution against air embolism. The CVP is also increased by using plasma volume expanders. An obstetrical Doppler device is strapped over the heart where the turbulence of the blood is best heard. The sound received is amplified by the instrument. A harsh change in its sound signals the presence of air, which can be aspirated from the right atrium via an atrial catheter.

Electrodes to record BAEPs are fixed over both mastoids and over the vertex in the midline. The sound stimulators are positioned over the external auditory meatii. BAEP recording is very useful in monitoring cochlear function. Besides employing it pre- and postoperatively, it may be extremely useful in signaling eighth nerve disturbances which may occur during operative manipulation.

Exposure

The skin incision is vertical and a thumb's breadth from the mastoid (Fig. 13.4). It is about 10 cm long, its limit extending just beyond where the transverse sinus is expected to lie. Its lower limit extends as low as is necessary to be able to gain the lower limit of the occiput. The lower limit of the subsequent muscle layers is progressively higher to make the plane of the wound somewhat oblique downwards. A small strip of uncoagulated muscle is excised for later use to cover the IAC.

The nearly circular craniectomy is 2.5–3 cm in diameter. It is directed laterally to the border of the sigmoid sinus. Superiorly, it extends to the transverse sinus. This bone opening is irrespective of the size of acoustic tumor and, in fact, for a very small tumor a slight medical extension of this craniectomy may be even more convenient. The secret of a good exposure is in being as lateral as possible in order to have the shortest and most direct access to the IAC. The dural incision is C-shaped, running only a couple of millimeters from the edges of the dural sinuses.

The surgical microscope is draped in a sterile transparent cover and brought into the operating field. We use a Zeiss Contravis model OPMI 6, which is ceiling-mounted. A 250-mm objective is used. The microscope is equipped with cameras (still, video, and 16-mm film) and an observer tube. In addition to the microscope, other microsurgical aids are: (a) an armrest to support the surgeon's arms and prevent fatigue; (b) long

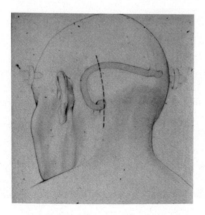

FIG. 13.4. Skin incision for CPA tumor exposure (shown by *dashed line*). The circular lateral suboccipital craniectomy abuts on the course described by the transverse and sigmoid sinuses.

microinstruments (sharp angulated dissectors of varying breadth, bayonet tumor-holding forceps, plain microdissectors, bayonet scissor, dura
knife); (c) a suction-irrigator; (d) bipolar cautery with long forceps; (e)
nerve stimulator; (f) air drill with diamond burrs ranging from 1 to 5
mm; and (g) self-retaining Leyla retractors. Finally, the operating table
should be capable of being remotely controlled in all positions to enable
the surgeon to view the tumor and surrounding structures from a variety
of positions. This is an added advantage of this approach.

The cerebellum is retracted by a single, broad-bladed, self-retaining
retractor. The CSF from the basal cisterns is allowed to flow out. This
facilitates relaxation of the brain and lessens the force of retraction. The
extracanalicular tumor is visualized. Since the vast majority of our CPA
tumors are acoustic neuromas, we shall first consider operative strategy
and then comment on other tumors of the CPA.

Opening of the IAC

It is mandatory to open the IAC. The dura over the petrous bone is
incised in a semicircular flap, with the center of its base over the porus
acusticus (Fig. 13.5). The dural flap is stripped off the bone. The dura
continues into the canal, and the raised semicircular dural flap is snipped
at the porus. The roof of IAC is now drilled. A high-speed diamond drill
placed on a light, angulated handset is used. Some surgeons place cotton
patties under the spatula and over the lower cranial nerves as an added
protection against any accident, such as injury inflicted by a slippage of
the drill. We begin with a 4- to 5-mm burr as it is both quicker and safer.

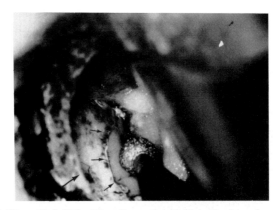

FIG. 13.5. Drilling of left IAC with a diamond drill. Note the free edge of the dura (*large
arrow*) incised along and 2–3 mm away from the dural venous sinuses. The dura over the
IAC is slit in the shape of a semicircle (*small arrows*), based on the porus, and excised.

A large size of burr is used at the beginning and, as one approaches the contents of the IAC, the burr size is reduced. While the drill works, the suction-irrigator is kept close to it to cool the bone. Heating of the bone damages the nerves within and should never be permitted. The drilling is oriented in the direction of the roof of the canal rather than its floor. With the thickness of the bone being drilled away, the last thin shell of bone is cracked out in bits with a sharp and finely angulated dissector. While drilling, it is most important to know the superolateral disposition of the semicircular canals and the inferoposterior relationship of the jubular bulb (Figs. 13.6 and 13.7). A high resolution CT scan provides the location of these structures with respect to the IAC. The exact length

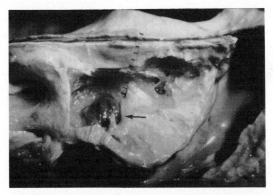

FIG. 13.6. Anatomic specimen of jugular bulb demonstrates its relationship to the floor of the IAC. The surgeon should be aware of its location to avoid inadvertently entering it during drilling of IAC.

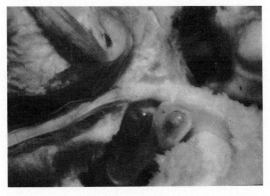

FIG. 13.7. This anatomic specimen presents the opened IAC with its contents, the facial nerve (turned upwards) and the vestibulocochlearis. Note the position of the vestibule adjacent to the fundus, and the semicircular canals just superolaterally. (Anatomic specimens were prepared by and by Prof. J. Lang, Würzburg.)

and widening of the IAC are also obtained by such a scan so that the surgeon knows how far laterally he can drill (Fig. 13.1). The lateral extent of opening of the canal is guided during operation by the bulging presence of the tumor within the dura inside the IAC. The tumor extends to a variable degree within the canal. However, it rarely reaches right up to the fundus. Hence, a full lateral opening is not routinely or randomly made (Fig. 13.8A). If the tumor bulge seems to persist far laterally, it may be advisable to stop somewhat short of the fundus and to resume drilling only after exposing and evacuating the tumor from the canal. Further drilling may then be performed with a very fine 1-mm burr from within the IAC (Fig. 13.8B and C). Finally, drilling along the floor of the canal must be performed cautiously and with the recognition of the possibility that the jugular bulb may be placed quite high.

Surgical Anatomy of CPA

Before continuing with further operative strategy it would not be out of place to recall a few points on the surgical anatomy of the region. The seventh and eighth cranial nerves arise from the pons proximal to the olive. The seventh nerve arises about one-half centimeter caudal to the emergence of the trigeminal nerve and slightly rostral and anterior to the eighth. It slopes gently downwards and dorsally to lie in front of the eighth nerve in the porus acusticus. Its course in the CPA spans 12–14 mm and in the IAC 8–10 mm. If the cross-section of the IAC is to be divided into four quadrants, the facial nerve lies in the superior and anterior quadrant. The cochlear nerve lies below the facial nerve, while the superior and inferior vestibular divisions lie in the appropriate posterior (dorsal) quadrants. The central part of the facial nerve, for about 2–3 mm, has no Schwann sheath, but acquires it, thereafter, during its course through the CPA, appearing to make it look more white and strong. The eighth nerve assumes the Schwann cell covering not in the CPA but only after entering the canal. Anatomic damage discontinuity occurs easily, and the nerves must be handled extremely gently. Both nerves have a covering of arachnoid within which arterioles follow the nerve. The AICA has enormous variations, but in at least two-thirds of normal CPAs its loop lies just in front of the porus or well within the canal.

Most acoustic neuromas arise from the Schwann cell sheath of one or more of the vestibular nerve fascicles. In only 5–7% of them it arises from the cochlear (in very rare instances a neurinoma in the CPA could arise from the seventh or fifth cranial nerves). The facts that emerge with acoustic neuroma now are:

1. The neoplasm always originates in the IAC.
2. Its growth may cause widening of the canal if the bone is relatively

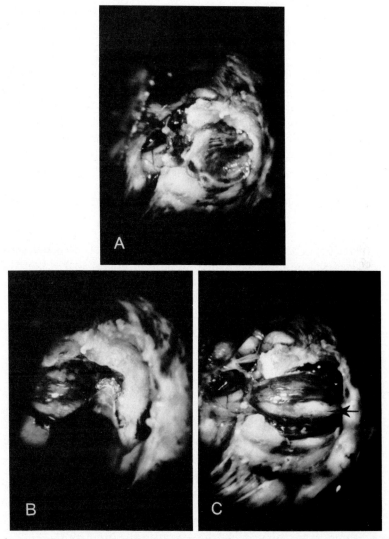

FIG. 13.8. (A) The IAC is opened to an extent just beyond the bulge produced by the tumor within the dura inside the canal. Tumor bulge in the opened canal to the right is shown. The seventh and eighth cranial nerves are seen just outside the porus acusticus. (B) If on opening the dura the tumor is found to extend beyond the extent to which the canal has already been opened, a further lateral deroofing of the IAC is done by "excavating" the canal from within outwards, using a tiny 1-mm burr, and following the tumor very carefully until its end. (C) The final appearance of the IAC and its contents. From above downwards, the vestibular fascicle, facial nerve (arrow), and cochlear nerve, after removal of an intracanalicular acoustic neuroma. Note the healthy-looking seventh and eighth cranial nerves proximal to the internal auditory meatus (IAM).

less dense. Unyielding bone may cause the tumor to compress the sensitive cochlear nerve and its vascularity more easily and to such an extent as to cause profound, rapid, or even sudden hearing loss. Such tumors carry poor prognosis with regard to recovery of hearing and at operation are also more difficult to dissect from the cochlear nerve.

3. Since most tumors arise from vestibular nerves, the seventh nerve is pushed from an anterosuperior to an anteroinferior position. The cochlear nerve is displaced from that position to a more caudal or caudodorsal location.
4. As the tumor grows out of the canal it pushes the anterior inferior cerebellar artery (AICA) progressively medially.
5. The tumor tends to grow symmetrically, with the porus generally remaining in the middle of the tumor with the tumor likened to a mushroom.
6. The fifth nerve lies only 5 mm away from the seventh, and despite its thickness, its disturbance, in case of an expansive growth, is next to follow.
7. The overlying petrous vein may also get stretched.
8. The caudal cranial nerves are less frequently compressed, and even when stretching occurs, their symptomatic involvement is uncommon.
9. The pons is the most medial structure and is reached when the extracanalicular tumor growth exceeds 1.5 cm.
10. A longstanding compression in such tumors may result in tiny blood vessels bridging between tumor and the brain stem. Handling of the pons during tumor separation or traction of such connecting blood vessels could rupture them farther away in the substance of the pons, and could result in brain stem damage.
11. The structures around are generally only displaced and compressed. Adhesion of the tumor to them is not the rule, except in the case of the facial and cochlear nerves with which the tumorous vestibular nerves are in very intimate and chronic contact. Rarely, though, there may also be adhesions to the brain stem.

SURGICAL REMOVAL OF ACOUSTIC TUMORS (Fig. 13.9)

The basic principles of surgical technique are common to all sizes of tumor, including: (a) opening of the IAC is mandatory; (b) enter tumor through posterior part of the capsule and systematically debulk it, thus making a large tumor small and a small tumor smaller; (c) achieve progressive shrinkage of tumor capsule from the neighboring compressed but nonadherent nerves; and (d) approach the parts of tumor capsule most densely adherent with neural tissue at the very end.

Tumor size is a decisive factor in the operative strategy of acoustic tumors.

Small tumors which remain within the IAC or just protrude out of the porus do not alter the anatomy of the medial cerebellopontine angle. The cerebellopontine cistern is opened in order to visualize and identify the structures. Having obtained this orientation, one should cover it with fibrin sponges. The nerves and the tumor in the canal are enclosed by the dura, which is slit horizontally across. The tumor bulges out, as it usually arises from the vestibular nerves, which face the surgeon. The tumor capsule is coagulated with bipolar current and is opened, and its core is debulked with microdissectors and tumor forceps. This reduces its volume and tension on the neighboring structures. Once the tumor bulk is reduced, the surrounding nerves become relaxed. The tumor capsule is grasped in forceps and dissected away from the adjacent nerves using a microdissector which is designed to present its rounded smooth surface to the nerve, using its internal surface bearing a sharp edge for tumor dissection. One therefore avoids handling the nerve as much as possible. The fascicles from which the tumor arises can be identified and transected in their healthy portion.

Slightly larger tumors, although still under 3 cm in size, occupy the CPA and cause a medial shift of the AICA. The seventh and eighth nerves are of course intimately related, but the remainder of the anatomy is unchanged. The AICA feeds the tumor with small branches which are coagulated and cut. The vessel is thus freed from its tumor attachment and moved to safety. Further operative management follows the same pattern as for smaller tumors. Tumors larger than 3 cm form 60% of our series of acoustic tumors.

The seventh nerve is usually not visible at the outset, being translocated anteriorly by the tumor, which obscures the surgeon's view. Large tumors may push all structures away beyond the view obtained through the microscope. Reduction of the size of the tumor in the CPA is therefore the immediate goal. An opening is made in the posterior part of the capsule using microscissors. Tumor substance is then evacuated.

One must constantly be aware of the possibility of encountering the vestibular, cochlear, and facial nerves. The dissector, which seems to excavate the tumor, should, in reality, be aiming to dissect the involved nerves. The tumor excision, in relative terms, should be a secondary issue. The dissector should be worked systematically and equally in all directions, from the center outwards. As the core is removed, the capsule starts to collapse towards the center. In doing so, it spontaneously falls away from the nerves it had been stretching. The capsule is also excised piecemeal. With shrinkage of the tumor, the nerves which were compressed and stretched begin to appear quite slack. They can be identified separate from the tumor more easily at the two extremes. Rather than discuss whether to remove tumor from lateral to medial, or *vice versa*, we would emphasize a symmetric internal decompression which "deflates" the tumor. Once it is sufficiently small, the space created in the CPA permits the tumor to be moved in all directions. The tumor capsule is therefore constantly manipulated with an attempt at freeing it from the nerves on all sides. In doing so, the operator gradually converges to the most densely adherent point. Generally such adherence of the tumor with the facial nerve is most prominent at a couple of millimeters proximal to the porus. This point is never approached at an early stage of the operation.

Occasionally, during the process of separation of the seventh nerve from the tumor, fine fascicles of the nerve may be entangled within the capsule and may resist dissection. They are best transected to avoid further traction and damage to the rest of the facial nerve.

The tumor may also be adherent to the brain stem. Until the CPA is almost completely evacuated of the space-occupying tumor, there is not enough freedom of movement nor the ability to appreciate the location of the most densely adherent points. An ideal operation would focus its activity on these points only at the very end.

During tumor dissection vestibular fascicles may be seen entering the tumor. These fascicles are transected in their nontumorous segment. The cochlear nerve, which is usually pushed under the tumor, may be identified there, and the tumor capsule may be separated away from it. It is best to dissect the tumor away from the nerve, and not vice versa, as handling the nerve could disturb its function. The strategy of removal of the intracanalicular portion has already been discussed. The point to be stressed, however, is that small and soft though the tumor may be, it should always be dissected and cut, and not "rolled over." There may be times when the intracanalicular portion extends right up to the fundus. If the canal opening has not been sufficiently lateral, it can now be done from within outwards, using a 1-mm burr (Fig. 13.8A–C). It is a good practice to remove all the tumor under direct vision. At the same time, lateral drilling must be performed very carefully so as not to damage the vestibule.

Blood vessels supplying the tumor are usually branches of the AICA. They are coagulated very close to the tumor surface, using the bipolar cautery, and are then transected. When the tumor lies close to or is attached to the brain stem, blood vessels may directly bridge between the two. Traction on these vessels may sometimes lead to intrapontine hemorrhages which can have grave consequences. As a result, the above

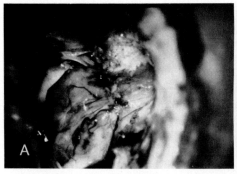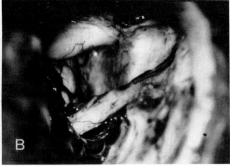

FIG. 13.9. (A) A 2.5-cm right-sided tumor almost reaching the pons. IAC opened. Tumor arising from the vestibular fascicles. Cochlear nerve pushed downwards. Vena petrosa seen superiorly. The facial nerve is pushed to the front of the tumor and is not visible. (B) Tumor excised totally. View of the facial nerve obscured by the fully preserved cochlear nerve. AICA now visible under it.

strategy should be rigidly followed in this area. Occasionally the connection of the tumor with the eighth nerve is dense and difficult to dissect. In such a situation it is preferable to transect the nerve in its healthy portion, rather than cause the nerve to pull on and possibly damage the brain stem. Nuclear lesions by such traction mechanisms may explain nerve palsies despite their apparent anatomic continuity after total tumor removal. BAEPs signal eighth nerve disturbance and are a useful tool at surgery.

Large tumors often stretch and flatten the facial nerve. As a rule, its physiologic status must be checked after the tumor is removed. The nerve is stimulated at the medial end near the brainstem, and facial contraction is observed by the anesthetist under the covering drapes. A positive contraction is a sure sign of intact facial function.

If the facial nerve does not respond to electric stimulation but is still in anatomic continuity, further management becomes a matter of judgment. One may perhaps wait for a few months postoperatively and see the result. We had one such case with a longstanding paresis and a large tumor. The tumor was excised, and the facial nerve was preserved anatomically. It had no physiologic function at operation, and we opted to wait for its late improvement. Despite a long follow-up there was no recovery, and another procedure had to be undertaken in order to restore facial nerve function. If, as a result of a large tumor, the nerve is elongated and stretched or lacks its normal luster and consistency, it is best to transect the damaged portion and do either a direct anastomosis or a nerve graft. If the facial nerve is damaged at operation, there are three possible situations: (a) the proximal and distal stumps are both available

(Figs. 13.10 and 13.11); (*b*) only the proximal stump is available; or (*c*) the proximal stump is not available.

When proximal and distal stumps are both available and there is no gap between the nerve ends, a direct end-to-end anastomosis is performed (Fig. 13.10*A* and *B*). A nerve gap within the CPA can be bridged by a graft obtained from the sural nerve (Fig. 13.11*A* –*C*).

If only the proximal stump is available and it is at least 3- to 5-mm long, the procedure of choice is an intracranial-intratemporal facial nerve grafting. If the proximal stump is not available, we must resort to peripheral anastomotic procedures (hypoglosso- or faciofacial) or plastic surgical operations.

Intracranial-Intratemporal Nerve Grafting

Ballance and Duel (1), based on their very long experience with facial nerve surgery, wrote in their authoritative paper of 1932 that autogenous grafts could be used for bridging nerve gaps with excellent results in the facial nerve. Norman Dott (6, 7) in 1958 reported his two-stage technique of intratemporal-extratemporal facial nerve graftings (Fig. 13.12). In the first stage, performed after removal of the acoustic tumor, he sutured one end of a 15- to 20-cm long sural nerve to the stump of the facial nerve at

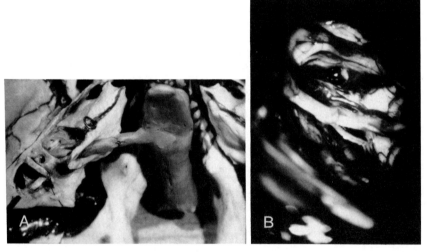

FIG. 13.10. (*A*) A model demonstrates types of facial nerve lesions during acoustic tumor surgery. Pons in the center, and left facial nerve emerging out of it, coursing towards the IAC. The "nerve" has been interrupted a couple of millimeters proximal to the porus (the site of its maximum adhesion with tumor and where it is most vulnerable to damage) and "sutured" directly in this instance to the available distal stump. (*B*) Example of the same phenomenon as above, this time at operation.

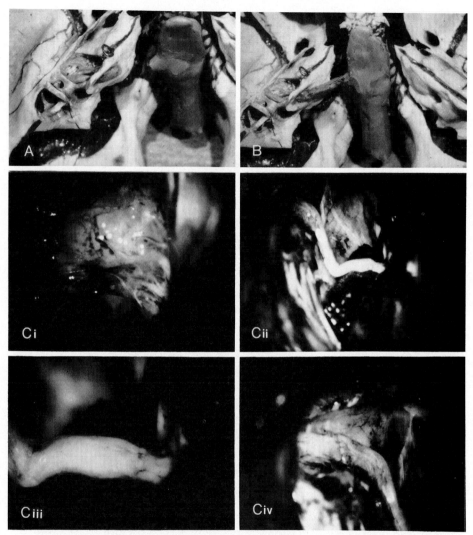

FIG. 13.11. (A) The next variety of facial nerve damage involves segmental loss but, nevertheless, availability of proximal and distal stumps; they are connected together, in picture by an appropriate length of sural nerve graft. (B). (C) Operative photographs of a right-sided tumor densely adherent to the facial nerve which necessitated its sacrifice over a small segment in favor of total tumor removal (Ci). (Cii) Proximal stump of the facial nerve sutured to a freshly obtained autologous sural nerve graft. (Ciii) The suture line is seen on this highly magnified picture. (Civ) The distal end of the graft is sutured to the distal stump of the facial nerve as it enters the now laid-open IAC.

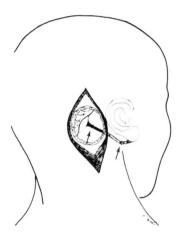

FIG. 13.12. The two-stage operation of intracranial-extracranial facial nerve anastomosis as described by Dott.

the proximal (brain stem) end. He led this graft out of the craniectomy by a subcutaneous tunnel into the retromandibular fossa. He then retrieved this end at a second operation some weeks later and sutured it to the distal stump of the facial nerve. Drake (9, 10) later reported on this method of repair of the facial nerve with encouraging results.

The technique of intracranial-intratemporal facial nerve grafting emerged as an alternative to Dott's method. It was developed by the senior author in 1975 in cooperation with his Otolaryngology colleagues Wingand, Draf and, later, Osterwald (8, 30). During the process of the removal of an acoustic tumor, if the facial nerve cannot be saved, its careful preservation at the medial end is still sought. In most instances a stump length of 1–1.5 cm is obtained, though as little as 3–5 mm would suffice. A 5–7 cm long sural nerve graft is obtained from the patient's leg. One end of this graft is prepared, carefully coapted, and anastomosed to the proximal stump of the facial nerve. Epiperineural suturing is performed with 10-0 nylon. A mastoidectomy is then performed from the outside to expose the facial nerve in its mastoidal and tympanic course. Thereafter the dura is nicked just rostral to the sigmoid sinus, and the distal end of the graft is passed out of the skull through it. This end is then prepared and anastomosed to the facial nerve, whose stump is obtained by sectioning it distal to the geniculate ganglion in its vertical course proximal to the stylomastoid foramen (Figs. 13.13 and 13.14).

Bilateral Acoustic Neuromas

Bilateral acoustic neurinomas comprise about 2.5% of all cases of acoustic neuroma (although in this series we have had 12 cases, a

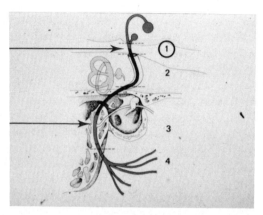

FIG. 13.13. Scheme of intracranial-intratemporal facial nerve grafting as described in the text. *Arrows* indicate sites of anastomosis of proximal stump in the CPA and distal stump in the vertical mastoidal course distal to the geniculate ganglion. The digits indicate the intracranial (*1*), intracanalicular (*2*), intratemporal (*3*), and postmastoidal (*4*) courses of the facial nerve.

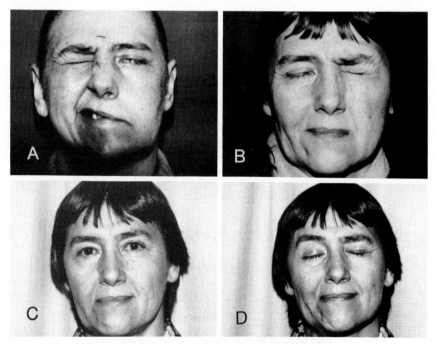

FIG. 13.14. The four photographs depict the appearance of a patient who has undergone an intracranial-intratemporal facial nerve grafting following removal of left acoustic tumor and an unavoidable section of the facial nerve. The nerve grafting was done at the same sitting. (*A*) Appearance immediately. (*B*) After 9 months. (*C* and *D*) 15 months after intracranial-intratemporal facial nerve grafting.

threefold higher figure). They differ from the conventional unilateral tumors in several ways. These tumors may represent a part of generalized von Recklinghausen's disease (VRD). Interestingly enough, most patients are detected rather late in their course. Preservation of the seventh and eighth cranial nerves in this situation is of even greater importance due to bilateral involvement, and to make matters worse, these tumors are even more difficult to operate. Unlike unilateral neuromas which arise from one side of a nerve sheath, displacing other nerves around it, the neurofibromas of VRD is a result of an unencapsulated proliferation of Schwann cells, fibrous connective tissue, and neural tissue (axons). They are lobulated and tend to grow between and around nerve fascicles. Moreover, their multifocal origin over the length of the same nerve or nerves makes their total removal even more difficult. The consequent morbidity tends to be higher than that which accompanies unilateral neurinomas. Most of our patients came with large tumors, and only two patients had tumors measuring less than 3 cm in diameter (Figs. 13.15 and 13.16).

Of 12 patients with bilateral tumors, three had already been operated on one side at another clinic and had lost their hearing on that side. The tumor on their remaining unoperated side, as well as bilateral tumors of the remaining nine patients, were all totally excised. Hearing was preserved bilaterally in two of these patients and unilaterally in one patient.

The strategy of operation does not differ significantly. However, the question that often confronts us in patients with bilateral acoustic neurinomas is which side should be operated first. Two factors come into consideration: (a) hearing ability and (b) tumor size. They may be interrelated or independent. One may have a smaller tumor with profound hearing loss, or the reverse, a larger tumor with relatively better hearing.

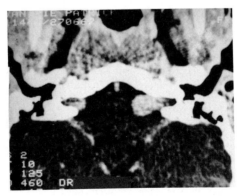

FIG. 13.15. Bilateral acoustic neuromas in an adolescent male. Note the larger 2-cm tumor on the *left* and a smaller intracanalicular growth on the other side. Both tumors were totally excised, and hearing was preserved bilaterally.

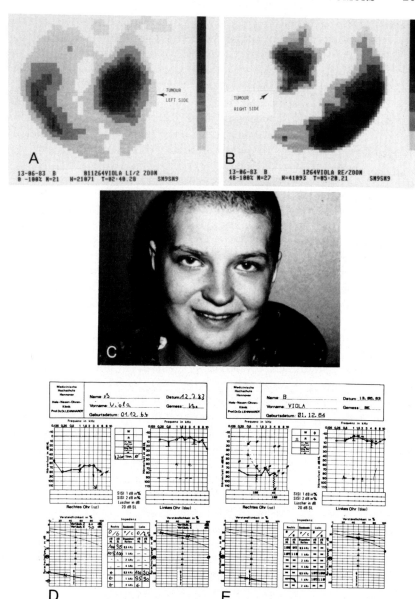

FIG. 13.16. Another case of VRD with bilateral acoustic tumors in an 18-year-old girl. (*A* and *B*) Cochleomeatal scintigraphy on left and right sides. (*C*) After total and bilateral tumor removal, her satisfaction writ on her symmetric smiling face. (*D* and *E*) Her happiness is further justified on account of her preserved bilateral hearing, as shown on audiograms done before and after surgery.

Patients with functional hearing still have a chance of its preservation, and since that is the goal of surgery, one should prefer to operate on that tumor first. On the other hand, the operative morbidity of larger tumors is decidedly higher than that of smaller ones. The process of decision-making necessarily must consider both of these factors.

Finally, a word on cystic acoustic tumors. They form only a small percentage of cases. Cystic degeneration may be of varying proportions. A largely cystic tumor is more adherent to the seventh and eighth nerves, and therefore predisposes to higher morbidity of these nerves.

OPERATIVE MANAGEMENT OF MENINGIOMAS

Meningiomas in the CPA may arise at the level of the porus acusticus, or either anterosuperior or posteroinferior to it. Meningiomas higher up in the CPA arise from the clivus, the tentorial margin and, rarely, Meckel's cave. Tumors below the porus may arise from either the jugular foramen or foramen magnum and may likewise extend downwards. Growth directions of CPA meningiomas are variable, and accordingly would involve other cranial nerves, blood vessels, and the brain stem. They would also determine the surgical approach suited for their removal, whether supratentorial, infratentorial, or combined suprainfratentorial.

From a morphological and surgical viewpoint, meningiomas are of two kinds. The more frequent variety is the rounded, expansive growth which stretches and compresses the adjacent structures. The other one is a diffuse, en plaque growth which carpets along the floor and engulfs the various structures. Fortunately, the latter is relatively uncommon.

Characteristically, meningiomas cause compression and stretching of cranial nerves without adhering to them. This is in sharp contrast to the effect an acoustic tumor tends to have on the seventh and eighth cranial nerves. In fact, the kind of compression an acoustic tumor exerts on the lower cranial nerves would be similar to the pure compressive effect meningiomas have on the cranial nerves at the base. The seventh nerve is virtually always ill-treated by the acoustic tumor. The tumor not only compresses the nerve but also elongates it in a manner so as to convert its width into its added length. With a meningioma, the nerve is clearly and separately visible, and its morphology remains unchanged. The eighth nerve in acoustic tumors undergoes considerable morphological change.

With large tumors there is often no hope of salvaging the eighth nerve. In the case of meningiomas it still retains its color and appearance, just like the facial nerve. The deficit caused is predominantly a functional one, with no degeneration and a good eventual outcome, as will be shown later. Thus, preservation of seventh and eight cranial nerves with meningiomas hardly provokes any debate.

At surgery, CPA meningiomas generally displace the trigeminal nerve rostrally and the seventh and eighth nerves downwards and backwards. A suboccipital approach would therefore have a direct view of the CPA meningioma, and unless there is a significant middle fossa extension there is no reason to consider any other route. The safety of the operation depends upon staying within the tumor substance, removing it piecemeal. The nerves need not be handled at all, as tumor debulking will in itself serve to separate the tumor from the nerves. When the tumor has a significant middle fossa extension, it is approached by a subtemporal transtentorial route. The petrous apex is also removed. Early coagulation of the basal attachment of the tumor will serve to reduce operative bleeding.

OPERATIVE MANAGEMENT OF EPIDERMOID TUMORS

These tumors fill the crevices and spaces at the skull base and may occasionally extend across the prepontine region to the opposite side. Displacement of neural and vascular structures is mild, but they are characteristically engulfed by the tumors. The more sensitive eighth nerve does occasionally manifest symptoms of involvement.

While the substance of an epidermoid tumor seems relatively easy to remove, the crucial part of the operation is removal of the tumor capsule. It is usually adherent to the arachnoid, which also usually needs to be excised. Greatest care must be taken in order to preserve the cranial nerves, blood vessels, and the brain stem enclosed within the arachnoid. However, there are no specific problems peculiar to the management of the seventh and eighth cranial nerves.

RESULTS

Of 200 CPA tumors seen during the last 6 years, 167 (83.5%) were acoustic neuromas. Of the remaining 33, there were 21 meningiomas, 10 epidermoids, and 2 angioblastomas.

Facial Nerve Function (Tables 13.1 and 13.3). Of 167 acoustic neuromas, three had a preoperative facial palsy and have been excluded from the evaluation of our operative results. Of the remaining 164, 62 had tumors smaller than 3 cm, while 102 growths measured more than 3 cm. The ratio of large to small tumors was 5:3. All patients with small tumors had their facial nerve function preserved after surgery. Of the large tumors 82 of 102, or 80.4%, had preservation of function; collectively, 144 of 164, or 87.8%, of patients operated on for an acoustic tumor, had facial nerve function after surgery.

Of 142 patients with normal preoperative facial functions, 38 (27%) showed slight immediate postoperative paresis. Two additional patients had paralysis, both of whom had cystic tumor. However, of the 22 patients

TABLE 13.1

Overall Results of Facial Nerve Function in 167 Operated Cases of Acoustic Neuroma

Preoperative Function	No. of Patients	Size	Postoperative Results
Normal (or nearly so)	142	(<3 cm)	56, 1, 44, 1, 5, 102
	61, 81		
Definite paresis	22	(<3 cm)	35, 2, 2, 18, 42
	1, 21	(>3 cm)	3, 23
Paralysis	$\dfrac{3}{167}$		$\dfrac{}{167}$

TABLE 13.2
Operative Results of the Cochlear Nerve Function in Acoustic Neuroma

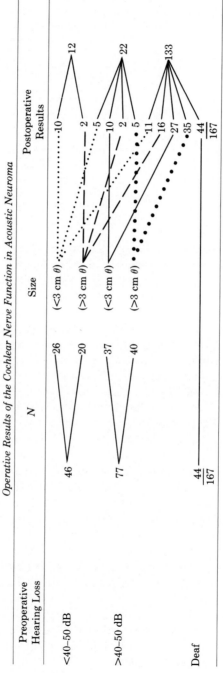

TABLE 13.3

Size-related Results of Facial Nerve Function in 164 Acoustic Neuromas Which Had Preoperative Facial Function

Size	Facial Nerve Function	
	Preop	Postop(%)
<3 cm	62	62 (100)
>3 cm	102	82 (80.4)

TABLE 13.4

Size-related Results of Cochlear Nerve Function in 123 Acoustic Neuromas in Patients Who Had Preoperative Hearing

Size	Hearing Ability	
	Preop	Postop(%)
<3 cm	63	25 (39.7)
>3 cm	60	9 (15)

with distinct preoperative weakness, 18 (81.8%) developed paralysis. There have also been two instances of patients with preoperative weakness who assumed a totally normal facial function after tumor excision. Eleven patients in this series were subjected to intracranial intratemporal nerve grafting. Ten of these have shown a good result. Two additional patients had sural nerve transplants to bridge small defects in the facial nerve when both proximal and distal stumps were available in the CPA. These cases have been done recently, and follow-up evaluation is pending. Two patients had Dott's operation, and one of them showed recovery. Of the remaining seven, five had received a hypoglossofacial anastomosis, and two have had the cross-facial operation. Adequate long-term follow-up is only available on four patients, and they have shown good function. One patient with facial palsy as a result of acoustic tumor surgery died.

Of 23 patients whose facial nerves were reconstructed, 17 have been evaluated, 16 of which have been successfully treated, giving a result of 94%. When the results of all 161 evaluated patients are combined, facial nerve function has been achieved in 160, or 99% of patients. The facial nerve was preserved in all 33 cases of meningiomas, epidermoids, and angioblastomas.

Cochlear Nerve Preservation (Tables 13.2 and 13.4). Of 167 acoustic neuromas, 44 had caused complete deafness. The remaining 123 patients with retained hearing were nearly equally divided in two groups: (a) 63 patients with tumor <3 cm in diameter and (b) 60 patients with tumor >3 cm in diameter. Of the first group, 25 (39.7%) had preservation of hearing while of the second group only 9 (15%) had hearing preserved. The overall result of 34 of 123 patients puts retained postoperative cochlear nerve function at 27.6%.

We then divided these same 123 patients into two different groups: (a) those whose preoperative hearing loss was <40 dB; and (b) those with loss >40 dB. Of 46 patients in the first group, 12 (37%) retained hearing, and of 77 patients in the second group, only 22 (28.6%) retained it. The postoperative results are better when preoperative hearing is well-preserved. It was encouraging to realize that 3 of the 34 patients had slightly improved hearing after surgery.

Hence, tumor size and preoperative hearing status are both important factors in prognosticating hearing preservation after acoustic tumor removal. The ideal situation would be when hearing is still well-preserved (loss <40 dB) and tumor size is small (<3 cm). A combination of these good prognosis factors was present in 26 of 167 patients with tumors. Postoperative hearing was retained in 10 of them (38.5%) and preserved in 15 (57.7%).

Of 21 meningiomas, 11 of 15 (73%) patients with preoperative hearing had their hearing preserved. Of 10 patients with epidermoids, eight of nine (89%) with hearing function before operation had it preserved. Of the two angioblastoma patients, one had preoperative hearing which was preserved at surgery.

Overall, of 33 patients with other CPA tumors, 20 of 25 (80%) patients with preoperative hearing ability had their hearing preserved (Table 13.5).

Complications. Considering its intricate anatomy, surgery in the CPA is certainly fraught with life-threatening consequences. Advances in microsurgical technique have made many of these procedures less risky. The complications encountered as a result of these operative procedures have been categorized as: (a) those occurring immediately and directly as the result of the operative procedure and (b) delayed complications not directly connected to the surgical technicalities.

(a) *Immediate:*

    1. Worsening of the preoperative facial and cochlear nerve function has been mentioned and discussed.

TABLE 13.5

Cochlear Nerve Preservation in CPA Tumors (200 Cases)

Tumor	Operated	Cases with Hearing Ability	
		Preop	Postop (%)
Acoustic neuroma	167	123	34[a] (27.6)
Meningioma	21	15	11[b] (73)
Epidermoid	10	9	8[b] (89)
Angioblastomas	2	2	1 (50)

[a] Includes three cases with mild improvement.
[b] Includes one case with remarkable improvement.

2. Transient trochlear nerve paresis occurred in four of our earlier cases. All of them improved spontaneously after 3–5 weeks.

3. CSF rhinorrhea was the commonest complication and occurred in seven cases. It was checked by a compression bandage in most of the cases. One patient needed continuous lumbar drainage for 2–3 days, and one patient required reopening of the wound to block the mastoidal cells.

4. Finally, some months ago we had a patient with a spinal disturbance and paraparesis which was noted immediately after surgery. This was attributed to the position during surgery. Postoperative plain x-rays, CT scan, and myelography did not demonstrate any evidence of cord compression which was likely to have occurred as the result of spinal manipulation during positioning under general anesthesia. The patient has shown gradual neurological improvement.

(b) *Delayed*

1. A *Salmonella* cerebellar abscess occurred in one patient. The origin of the bacteria seems to have been by the hematogenous route.

2. Transient facial palsy was noted in two patients after acoustic tumor removal. The patients recovered spontaneously.

3. Deaths due to medical reasons occurred. There have been four hospital deaths in this series. A 78-year-old lady who had been confined to bed for 2 months prior to surgery on account of severe brain stem compression was subjected to a total tumor excision. She had no immediate postoperative complications but died suddenly on the 4th postoperative day due to a clinically diagnosed acute myocardial infarction. The second case was of a 60-year-old man who, one year before surgery, had a severe stroke with spastic hemiparesis. He also had a lower cranial nerve palsy prior to the acoustic neuroma surgery. Postoperatively, his condition was unchanged. He suffered aspiration pneumonia postoperatively, and thereafter he gradually went downhill to die after one month. The third fatality, a 60-year-old lady, had a large tumor and suffered severe, systemic hypertension 10 years prior to surgery. As a result of her medical problems, she was operated in two stages. She did well after the first operation but did not return for the second operation until she again had developed severe increased intracranial pressure. She was readmitted in a moribund state. Placement of a ventriculo-

peritoneal shunt led to a good improvement in her general condition, and some weeks later a total excision of the tumor was performed. She recovered well and had already been transferred from the intensive care unit to the normal ward. However, 2 weeks after the operation she had a cerebral infarct in the right middle cerebral artery distribution and died in a few days. All three of these cases had large tumors, severe intracranial hypertension and, despite an uneventful postoperative course after total tumor excision, died of causes not directly related to surgery. The fourth death occurred in an elderly patient who had a small tumor but severe tinnitus. He had been subjected to coronary bypass surgery one year prior to his tumor removal. He was not a particularly good surgical candidate, but he insisted on surgery as a result of his intractable tinnitus. The operation was uneventful, but he died 48 hours later due to myocardial infarct. There were no deaths in patients with meningioma, epidermoid, and angioblastoma. The mortality rate of acoustic neuromas was 4 in 167, or 2.4%, and of all cases of CPA tumors, 2%.

SUMMARY AND CONCLUSIONS

Microsurgical techniques have made a significant contribution in the advancement of surgery. Since then, the field of neurosurgery has made great and rapid strides. Neurosurgeons now venture through the deep and delicate regions of the brain where they dared not venture only a few years ago. In particular, the morbidity and mortality of surgery in the CPA has seen a progressive decrease.

This presentation deals with 200 consecutive tumors in the CPA operated on using microsurgical techniques during the last 6 years. One hundred sixty-seven (83.5%) of them were acoustic neuromas (which included 12 patients with bilateral tumors). Of the remaining 33, there were 21 meningiomas, 10 epidermoids, and 2 angioblastomas. Preoperative investigation has been aimed at arriving at a diagnosis which is as exact as possible in order to plan the operative strategy. All patients, ranging in age from 16 to 84, have been operated upon in the lounging position (with the necessary precautions) through a unilateral suboccipital craniectomy.

The basic surgical technique, irrespective of the tumor, is to decompress it from within in order to relieve its tension and pressure on surrounding nerves, vessels, and the brain stem. The structures which are only compressed are spontaneously relieved of compression. This helps define their full anatomic course. Having been identified, they are protected from damage. The most adherent points between tumor and nerves are recognized and handled last under direct vision when there is sufficient space to allow manipulation of the tumor. In the rare event of the facial nerve being interrupted, nerve graft procedures are attempted during the same operation. Our experience with the technique of intra-cranial-intratemporal facial nerve grafting has yielded excellent results. The cochlear nerve lacks a Schwann cell cover in the CPA and is more prone to being affected, either by tumor processes or surgical manipulation.

Of our 167 acoustic nerve tumors, 60% were larger than 3 cm in diameter. The two important factors with regard to predicting the preservation of the seventh and eighth cranial nerves are tumor size (<3 cm) and preoperative hearing loss (<40 dB). The preservation of facial nerve function after tumor removal was achieved in 87.8% of patients. The facial nerve was preserved in all patients with other tumors.

With regard to hearing ability the overall result of preservation of function was achieved in 27.6%. However, when a low hearing loss (<40 dB) and small tumor size (<3 cm) are taken into account, the preservation was as high as 58%. In the other CPA tumor cases, hearing ability was preserved in 80% of patients. An important precondition while discussing results is that in every single patient the tumor removal was total.

Complications due to surgery have been mild and reversible, except with respect to seventh and eighth nerve morbidity whenever they occurred. One recent patient had paraparesis due to manipulation of his neck while being positioned under general anesthesia.

There have been four hospital deaths in acoustic tumor patients, all the result of bad medical problems. None were the direct result of the actual operative treatment.

REFERENCES

1. Ballance, C. A., and Duel, B. The operative treatment of facial palsy by the introduction of nerve grafts into the Fallopian canal and by the other intratemporal methods. Arch. Otolaryngol., 15: 1, 1932.
2. Cushing, H. Tumors of the Nervus Acusticus and the Syndrome of the Cerebellopontine Angle. W.B. Saunders, Philadelphia/London, 1917.
3. Dandy, W. E. An operation for the total removal of cerebellopontine (acoustic) tumors. Surg. Gynecol. Obstet., 41: 129–148, 1925.
4. Dandy, W. E. Results of removal of acoustic tumors by the unilateral approach. Arch. Surg., 42: 1026–1033, 1941.
5. Di Tullio, M. V., Jr., Malkasian, D., and Rand, R. W. A critical comparison of neurosurgical and otolaryngological approaches to acoustic neuromas. J. Neurosurg., 48: 1–12, 1978.
6. Dott, N. M. Facial paralysis—Restitution by extra-petrous nerve graft. Proc. Roy. Soc. Med., 51: 900–902, 1958.
7. Dott, N. M. Facial nerve reconstruction by graft bypassing the petrous bone. Arch. Otolaryngol., 78: 426–428, 1963.

8. Draf, W., and Samii, M. Intracranial-intratemporal anastomosis of the facial nerve after cerebellopontine angle tumor surgery. In: *Disorders of the Facial Nerve*, edited by M. D. Graham and W. F. House, pp. 441–449. Raven Press, New York, 1982.

9. Drake, C. G. Acoustic neuroma: Repair of facial nerve with autogenous graft. J. Neurosurg., *17:* 836–842, 1960.

10. Drake, C. G. Intracranial facial nerve reconstruction. Arch. Otolaryngol., *78:* 456–460, 1963.

11. Drake, C. G. Total removal of large acoustic neuromas. J. Neurosurg., *26:* 554–561, 1967.

12. Fisch, U. Otochirurgische Behandlung des Acusticusneurinomas. In: *Kleinhirnbrückenwinkeltumoren*, edited by D. Plester, S. Wende, and N. Nakayama, pp. 196–214. Springer Verlag, Berlin, 1978.

13. Glasscock, M. E., Hays, J. W., and Murphy, J. P. Complications in acoustic neuroma surgery. Ann. Otol., *84:* 530–540, 1975.

14. Horrax, G., and Poppen, J. L. The end results of complete *versus* intracapsular removal of acoustic tumors. Ann. Surg., *130:* 567–575, 1949.

15. House, W. F. Middle cranial fossa approach to the petrous pyramid. Arch. Otolaryngol., *78:* 460–469, 1963.

16. House, W. F. Monograph I. Transtemporal bone microsurgical removal of acoustic neurinomas. Arch. Otolaryngol., *80:* 597–756, 1964.

17. House, W. F. Monograph II. Acoustic neurinoma. Arch. Otolaryngol., *88:* 575–715, 1968.

18. House, W. F., and Hitselberger, W. W. Preservation of the facial nerve in acoustic tumor surgery. Arch. Otolaryngol., *88:* 655–658, 1968.

19. Jacobson, J. H. Microsurgical technique in the repair of the traumatized extremity. Clin. Orthop., *29:* 132, 1963.

20. Kurze, T., and Doyle, J. B. Extradural intracranial (middle fossa) approach to the internal auditory canal. J. Neurosurg., *19:* 1033–1077, 1962.

21. McCarty, C. S. Acoustic neuroma and the suboccipital approach. Mayo Clin. Proc., *50:* 15–16, 1975.

22. Nielsen, A. Acoustic tumors. Ann. Surg., *115:* 849–863, 1942.

23. Olivecrona, H. Acoustic tumors. J. Neurol. Neurosurg. Psychiatry, *3:* 141–146, 1940.

24. Rand, R., and Kurze, T. Microneurosurgical resection of acoustic tumors by a transmeatal posterior fossa approach. Bull. Los Angeles Neurol. Soc., *30:* 17–20, 1965.

25. Rand, R., and Kurze, T. Preservation of vestibular, cochlear and facial nerves during microsurgical removal of acoustic tumors: Report of two cases. J. Neurosurg., *28:* 158–161, 1968.

26. Rhoton, A. L. Microsurgical removal of acoustic neuromas. Surg. Neurol., *6:* 211–219, 1976.

27. Sachs, E. Translabyrinthine microsurgery for acoustic neuromas. J. Neurosurg., *22:* 399–401, 1965.

28. Samii, M. Neurochirurgische Gesichtspunkte bei der Behandlung der Akustikusneurinome mit besonderer Berücksichtigung des N. facialis. Laryng. Rhinol., *58:* 97–106, 1979.

29. Samii, M. Nerves of the head and neck. In: *Management of Peripheral Nerve Problems*, edited by G. E. Omer, Jr., and M. Spinner, pp. 507–547, W.B. Saunders, Philadelphia, 1980.

30. Samii, M. Facial nerve grafting in acoustic neurinoma. Clin. Plast. Surg., *11:* 221–225, 1984.

31. Smith, M. F. W., Ray, N. M., and Cox, D. J. Suboccipital microsurgical removal of acoustic neurinomas of all sizes. Ann. Otol., *82:* 407–414, 1973.

32. Sterkers, J. M. Facial nerve preservation in acoustic neuroma surgery. In: *The Cranial Nerves*, edited by M. Samii and P. J. Jannetta, pp. 451–455. Springer-Verlag, Berlin, 1981.

33. Sterkers, J. M. Retro-sigmoid approach for preservation of hearing in early acoustic neuroma surgery. In: *The Cranial Nerves*, edited by M. Samii and P. J. Jannetta, pp. 579–585. Springer-Verlag, Berlin, 1981.

34. Yasargil, M. G. Mikrochirurgie der Kleinhirnbrückenwinkel-Tumoren. In: *Kleinhirnbrückenwinkelntumoren*, edited by D. Plester, S. Wende, and N. Nakayama, pp. 215–257. Springer-Verlag, Berlin, 1978.

IV

Trigeminal Neuralgia

14

Pathophysiology of the Pain of Trigeminal Neuralgia and Atypical Facial Pain: A Neuroanatomical Perspective

JEFFREY T. KELLER, Ph.D., and HARRY VAN LOVEREN, M.D.

The history of trigeminal neuralgia is well documented in Stookey and Ransohoff's (72) monograph on this topic. However, certain historical detail is essential for a discussion of the pathophysiology of trigeminal neuralgia. Sir Charles Bell (4), in 1829, was the first to discover that the trigeminal nerve, like the spinal nerves, included a motor and sensory root. In a paper read before the Royal Society in 1821, Sir Charles Bell established "the distinct offices of the two nerves of the face" (Fig. 14.1). Bell's experiments established the fifth nerve as "the sole cause or source of the common sensibility of the head and face." It was Bell's observations which established tic douloureux as an affliction of the trigeminal, and not the facial, nerve. A full description of this disorder by a physician together, with an account of its treatment, was presented almost 150 years earlier by John Locke (71) in 1677. Locke was describing excruciating pain in the face and lower jaw in the Countess of Northumberland, whom he had been summoned to see. Locke's account of the symptoms of the Countess was an extraordinarily accurate clinical description of what we now know as trigeminal neuralgia. His observations of this disorder can stand without correction today after more than 300 years of observation. What is not clear, and still eludes neuroanatomical description, is the account that the Countess, being thoroughly purged with cathartics, was well in several weeks.

Although treatment of this disorder has progressed to more sophistocated modalities, we are still left with perplexing fundamental issues. Is Bell's thesis that the "three grand divisions of the trigeminous" are responsible for sensory supply to the face still tenable? If it is, how can one account for: (a) the persistence of pain following total section of the trigeminal sensory root (portio major); (b) the preservation of touch following complete section of the sensory root; and (c) the recurrence of pain following denervation of the face subsequent to percutaneous rhizotomy (PSR)? These clinical observations would seem to contradict

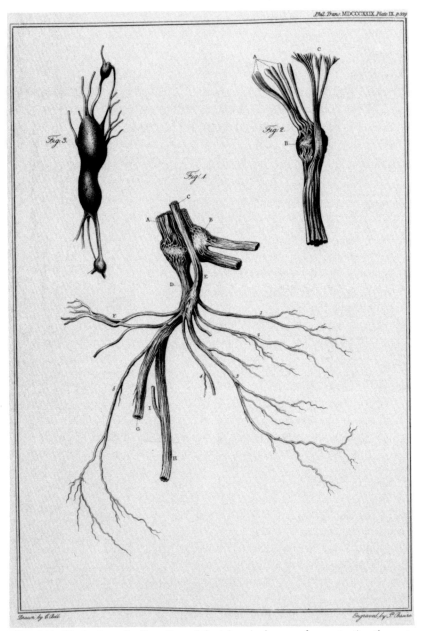

FIG. 14.1. Illustration of a dissection of the trigeminal nerve, demonstrating the motor and sensory roots. (Reproduced with permission from: C. Bell (4).)

Bell's thesis. Bell's observations were essential for an understanding of trigeminal neuralgia, and we would not detract from their importance now. However, anatomical evidence will be presented which expands his original observations and addresses inconsistencies between clinical observations and anatomical principles.

Let us proceed in addressing these issues by first discussing a common treatment modality, percutaneous stereotaxic rhizotomy (PSR), for trigeminal neuralgia. PSR is based on the theory that the neuralgia is due to demyelination of large-diameter myelinated A fibers resulting in ephaptic transmission of impulses from these fibers (A fibers) to poorly myelinated A delta and unmyelinated C fibers (6, 53, 54). The technique of PSR is similar to other classic modes of treatment such as ganglionectomy, partial or total rhizotomy, and medullary tractotomy in that it is not concerned with etiology. The mechanism of PSR is that it interrupts pain transmission (72, 73, 75, 77). Pain is eliminated but touch is preserved. Letcher and Goldring (48) and Frigyesi et al. (26) demonstrated, using radiofrequency lesions, that the compound action potential of A-delta and C fibers (nociceptive fibers) in cats is blocked at a lower current and temperature than the compound action potential of larger A-alpha and beta fibers carrying tactile sensation. These physiological studies demonstrated that temperature-dependent selective destruction of A-delta and C fibers could be achieved. Why, then, if pain conducting fibers are destroyed, does pain recur (51, 54, 55, 62, 69, 73, 76) (Table 14.1)?

As a possible explanation we propose consideration of alternate pain pathways. Victor Horsley, in a publication with May and Horsley (49), expressed the belief that the trigeminal motor root carried sensory fibers which might serve as an alternate route for pain to gain access to the CNS. The presence of sensory fibers in a motor root is not without precedent, since Sherrington (68) suggested it in the latter part of the 19th century. This observation challenged the law of Bell and Magendie,

TABLE 14.1

Results with Percutaneous Stereotaxic Rhizotomy for Typical Trigeminal Neuralgia

Author-Investigator and Yr		Cases	Initial Relief (%)	Average Follow-up	Recurrence (%)
Tew et al. (77)	1982	700	99	6 yr	19
Menzel et al. (52)	1975	315	97	12 yr	80
Sweet and Wepsic (74)	1974	274	91	4 yr	22
Siegfried (70)	1977	416	98	15 mo	4.3
Rhoton et al. (63)	1977	149	98	1–53 mo	18.7
Nugent (55)	1982	643	?	4.7 yr	23
Onofrio (57)	1975	135	98	?	12

which stated that dorsal roots of the spinal nerves are functionally sensory and ventral roots are motor. This concept has more recently been challenged by Coggeshall and colleagues (10–16), who reported a significant number of afferent fibers in the ventral roots of cats and humans. Physiological studies have yielded evidence that the afferent fibers in the ventral root are unmyelinated and that a majority of these axons with somatic receptive fields are nociceptive (10). These findings prompted Young and Stevens (81) to examine the composition of the trigeminal motor root (portio minor). Unmyelinated fibers were demonstrated in cat (9–15%) and man (12–20%). Following these initial observations, Young and Kruger (80) examined the motor root in the monkey and demonstrated afferent fibers whose cell bodies were in the semilunar ganglion, indicating the sensory nature of these fibers. Additional studies are required to determine the specific function of these fibers as well as their central termination.

Dandy (18, 19) did not believe that sensory fibers in the motor root could explain the clinical picture of preservation of touch in the ophthalmic division following trigeminal root section. It was his opinion that the motor root blends with the mandibular division, presumably carrying V3 sensory fibers and could not send fibers to the first or second divisions. Alternatively, Dandy believed that if his observations were correct "there can be but one explanation, namely, that there must be some anatomic feature of the sensory root which has not been recognized. And if this is true, that feature must be subject of considerable variation." Dandy believed that pain fibers were concentrated in a particular segment of the sensory root and were interrupted during rhizotomy while an accessory trigeminal root, independent of the portio major and minor, carried touch which accounted for the preservation of sensation following rhizotomy (Fig. 14.2). Controversy regarding these accessory fibers and their function exists. Janetta and Rand (42) and Rand (60) supported Dandy, and they termed the afferent or accessory fibers which conduct tactile information "portio intermedia." Frazier (23), in opposition to the concept of functional localization, argued that the three divisions of the trigeminal maintained their somatotopic position. Fibers subserving various sensory functions were mixed within each division. Electrophysiological studies of Pelletier et al. (58) and Poulos (59) supported Frazier's concept. Saunders and Sachs (66) concluded that the so-called "accessory rootlets" of Dandy are really components of the motor root confirming Meckel's original description of 1748. Gudmundsson et al. (30) examined 50 cadaver nerves and found accessory sensory fibers present 50% of the time. These fibers contributed primarily to the first division, and it was postulated that they were not modality specific. Finally, these investi-

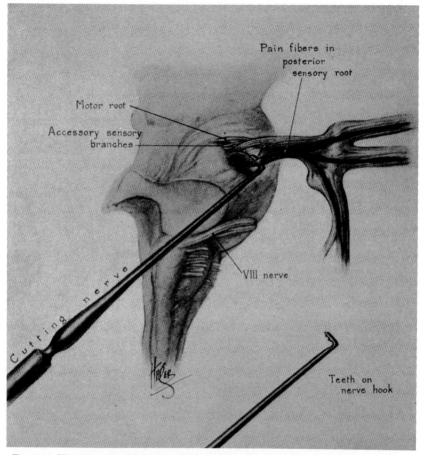

FIG. 14.2. Illustration of the trigeminal nerve, demonstrating the accessory sensory fibers presumed responsible for the preservation of touch following rhizotomy of the trigeminal (sensory) root. (Reproduced with permission from: W. E. Dandy (20).)

gators stated that "motor-to-sensory" anastomoses explained the preservation of sensation subsequent to rhizotomy of the trigeminal nerve (Fig. 14.3A and B). Therefore, there is no anatomical or physiological evidence to support Dandy's original contention that accessory branches account for preservation of touch following rhizotomy.

As demonstrated by our discussion of PSR, insight into the pathophysiology of a disorder can be gained by analysis of a specific treatment and the results obtained. Proposed modes of treatment for trigeminal neuralgia have been as diverse as proposed etiologies. A review of the literature would lead one to incriminate multiple sclerosis (46, 64), tumors

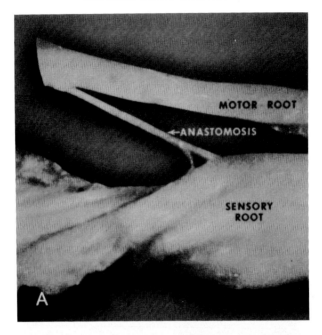

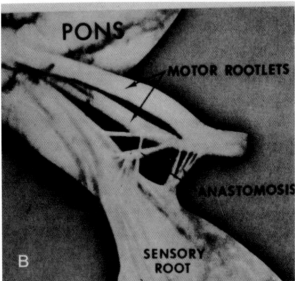

FIG. 14.3. (A) Dissection of trigeminal nerve, demonstrating numerous anastomoses between the motor and sensory roots. The proximal portion of the trigeminal root is on the right. (B) Dissection of right trigeminal nerve root, demonstrating anastomosis between the portio major and minor. (Reproduced with permission from: K. Gudmundsson *et al.* (30).)

(17, 18, 25, 26), arteriovenous malformations (21, 43), aneurysms (25), vascular compression-arterial and/or venous (1, 17, 18, 33, 40–43), petrous ridge compression (28, 56, 70), dural bands (48), congenital malformations of the base of the skull (9, 18, 27, 29), or the natural aging process (2, 3, 7, 44, 45). We will not deal with each of these entities individually but will select one, currently of major interest, and that is vascular compression.

Dandy (18) was the first to implicate compression of the trigeminal sensory root by arteries (superior cerebellar artery) (Fig. 14.4) and veins (petrosal vein) (Fig. 14.5) as a cause of trigeminal neuralgia. The first successful vascular decompression procedure was performed by Gardner and Miklos (28), who interposed Gelfoam between the offending artery and the trigeminal sensory root. Janetta and Rand (42) and Janetta (39)

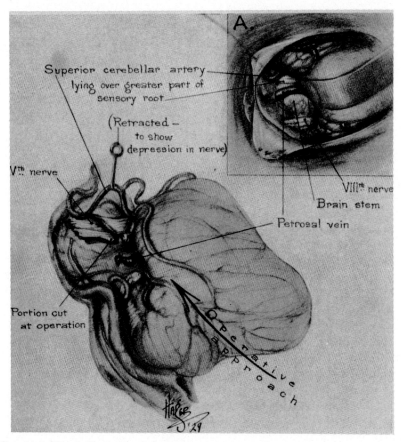

FIG. 14.4. Sketch illustrating indentation of the lateral surface of the sensory root by the superior cerebellar artery. (Reproduced with permission from: W. E. Dandy (19).)

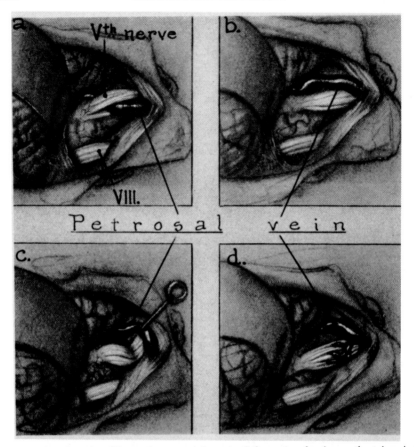

Fɪɢ. 14.5. Sketches illustrating encroachment of the petrosal vein on the trigeminal sensory root. (Reproduced with permission from: W. E. Dandy (19).)

stimulated interest in neurovascular compression as a mechanical factor in the etiology of trigeminal neuralgia and popularized the technique of microsurgical neurovascular decompression (MVD) for the treatment of this disorder. Acceptance of the theory of neurovascular compression is attributed to the work of Janetta (40, 41).

If we address neurovascular compression objectively, a number of issues are raised: (*a*) vascular compression, if present, is not always impressive; that is, the nerve is not indented (18, 77); (*b*) vascular compression is not always present in the patients with trigeminal neuralgia (1, 9, 77, 78); and (*c*) vascular compression has been demonstrated in 50% of cases examined at autopsy, even with no history of trigeminal neuralgia (32). These issues demonstrate a variability in vascular compression and its association with trigeminal neuralgia. Dandy (18) was perplexed as to why compression of the trigeminal root caused neuralgia while vascular compression of other cranial nerves did not. Although Dandy could not explain this, he stated "just as one sees many cases of gall stones without pain, so one sees lesions attacking the sensory root in the angle without the actual production of pain, but when the patient has pain and the gall stones are present, the gall stones are unquestionably the cause." We concur; Dandy was perplexed, and the question is still unanswered. Perhaps as Hardy and Rhoton (32) responded to Dandy's statement, "an equally reasonable conclusion to draw of neurovascular contact in these specimens from a "non-tic" population, may mean that the finding at operation of such neurovascular contacts is coincidental." In judging the results of any treatment for trigeminal neuralgia it must be recognized that pain may remit spontaneously for one or more years (63) or may be temporarily relieved by almost any simple manipulation of the trigeminal root (Table 14.2). We believe vascular compression is the etiology in some but not all of the cases of trigeminal neuralgia (Table 14.3).

Thus far we have considered pathophysiological mechanisms of trigeminal neuralgia with emphasis on alternate pain pathways. As intriguing as these trigeminal pathways are, they clearly do not account for all of the other facial neuralgias. The role of the facial nerve has received considerable attention with regard to this problem. Hunt (34–37), whose name is most notably associated with facial neuralgia and provides the eponym Hunt's neuralgia (geniculate neuralgia) for the condition, was first to recognize the somatic sensory component of the facial nerve (Fig. 14.6). Prior to his report the nervus intermedius (of Wrisberg) and the geniculate ganglion were only associated with secretory, vasomotor, and gustatory function.

Hunt's original description (34) discussed herpetic inflammations of the geniculate ganglion (herpetic ganglionitis) and the regions affected: internal and middle ear, tympanum, and cutaneous zone of the external ear (Fig. 14.7). He emphasized that the sensory system of the facial nerve was vestigial and regressive. There was evidence that a vestigial remnant of the facial nerve persists in a strip on the posteromedial surface of the auricle, within the buccal cavity, and in the area of distribution of the chorda tympani nerve on the palate near the anterior pillar of the fauces. Hunt viewed the sensory system of the face to be comprised of a somatic and visceral component. The cutaneous zone of innervation is well known while we believe the visceral component to be neglected, if not forgotten. The visceral component may be subdivided into an intra-oral and a "deep sensory" field supplying deep sensibility of the face. The pain involving the deeper structures of the face and posterior "orbitonasopalatal" regions was termed prosopalgia. A case of complete geniculate neuralgia accord-

TABLE 14.2
Comparative Analysis of Techniques in the Treatment of Trigeminal Neuralgia

Author and Yr		Technique	Cases	Initial Relief (%)	Average Follow-up	Recurrence (%)
Jaeger (39)	1955	Boiling water	185	96	0–5 yr	?
Sharr and Garfield (68)	1977	Alcohol injection	81	99	3.3 yr	6
Håkanson (32)	1981	Glycerol injection	75	99	17 mo	18
Dandy (17)	1929	Posterior fossa rhizotomy	88	100	2 yr	Not reported
Peet and Schneider (58)	1952	Transtemporal rhizotomy	553	95	8 yr	14
Taarnhoj (75)	1954	"Decompression"/compression	43	100	13 mo	16
Tew (77)	1982	Radiofrequency neurolysis	700	99	6 yr	19
Apfelbaum (1)	1977	Microvacular decompression	55	95	6.2 mo	24

TABLE 14.3

Comparison of Results of Posterior Fossa Exploration in Six Series of Trigeminal Neuralgia Cases

Authors and Yr		No. of Cases	Negative Results (%)	Recurrence/ Failure (%)	Average Follow-up (mo)
Apfelbaum (1)	1977	179	3	19	24
Jannetta (42)	1980	411	0.2	20	Not given
Wilson *et al.* (79)	1980	50	10	16	30
Burchiel (6)	1981	42	14	19	25
Ferguson *et al.* (24)	1981	24	2	29	28
Van Loveren *et al.* (78)	1982	50	16	16	36

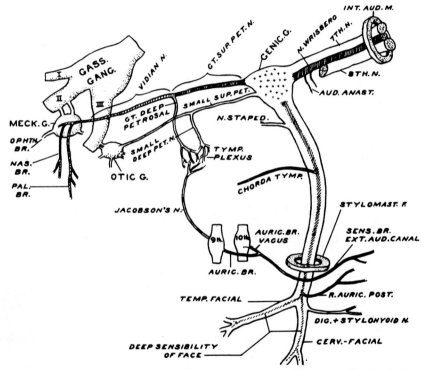

FIG. 14.6. Diagrammatic representation of the facial nerve, illustrating the distribution of the sensory components (*shaded* portions). Note branches associated with deep sensibility of the face. (Reproduced with permission from: J. M. Hunt (37).)

ing to Hunt would include otalgia and prosopalgia. Again we believe these features of Hunt's neuralgia have been forgotten. Head (33) and Davis (20) also incriminated the afferent fibers of deep sensibility to the seventh nerve. Davis (20) presented strong evidence of preservation of

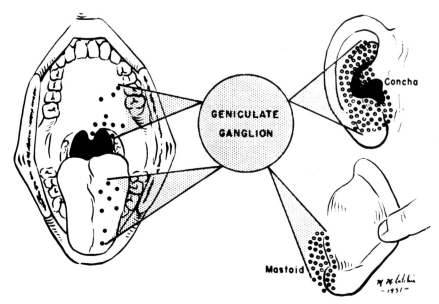

FIG. 14.7. Diagram illustrating sensory distribution of fibers passing *via* nervus intermedius through the geniculate ganglion to the periphery. Areas of herpetic vesicle eruption are indicated by *open circles*. (Reproduced with permission from: J. C. White and W. H. Sweet (79).)

deep facial sensation, including nociception, following trigeminal rhizotomy or ganglionectomy. He subsequently confirmed these clinical observations in animal studies. Deep sensation and pain could only be alleviated following section of the facial nerve.

Sachs (65), in a discussion of the role of the nervus intermedius in facial neuralgia, illustrated the historical confusion with this subject. Pain associated with the facial nerve was variously termed: atypical facial neuralgia, ciliary or periodic migrainous neuralgia, Sluder's neuralgia, sphenopalatine neuralgia, Horton's erythromelalgia of the head or histaminic cephalgia, cluster headaches, or greater superficial petrosal neuralgia. This list alone confirmed the confusion surrounding facial neuralgia. In an attempt to clarify this issue Sachs (65) reported four cases of intractable face and head pain, relieved by section of the nervus intermedius. One of those cases supported our statement that consideration should be given to alternate pain pathways in facial pain. In this case pain persisted following section of the nervus intermedius and was relieved only after the eighth nerve was sectioned. Anastomoses of fibers between the seventh and eighth nerves were noted by Bischoff (5) in 1865 (Fig. 14.8), who indicated that the vestibular portion of the eighth

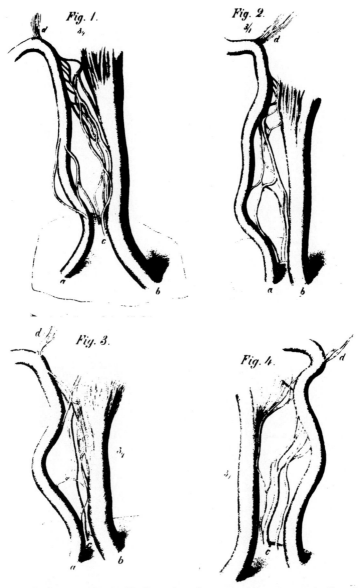

FIG. 14.8. Drawings of Bischoff's dissections demonstrating anastomotic fibers between the 7th and 8th nerves: *a*, facial nerve; *b*, auditory nerve; *c*, nervus intermedius; *d*, genu of the facial nerve with origin of the greater superficial petrosal nerve. Note labeling errors in *Figures 4* and *7*. (Reproduced with permission from: E. P. E. Bischoff (5).)

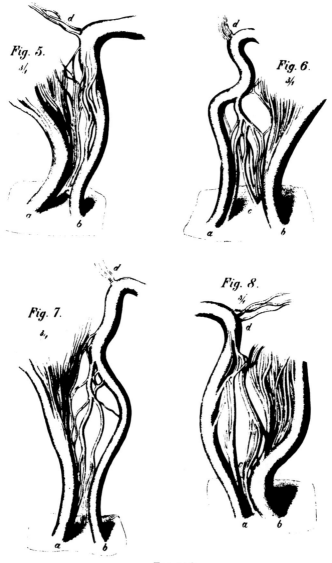

FIG. 14.8

nerve may carry fibers originating from the nervus intermedius. Such anastomoses have been subsequently confirmed by Chorobski and Penfield (8), White and Sweet (79), Rhoton *et al.* (61), and Sachs (65) (Fig. 14.9). We would not infer that the anastomoses between fibers of the seventh and eighth nerves play a significant role in all facial neuralgias.

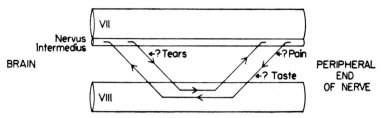

FIG. 14.9. Diagramatic representation illustrating pain fibers of the nervus intermedius anastomosing with the vestibular portion of the 8th nerve. This hypothetical scheme could account for the persistence of pain following section of the nervus intermedius, as noted by Sachs in one case. Pain was alleviated only after the 8th nerve was sectioned. (Reproduced with permission from: E. Sachs, Jr. (65).)

Rather, we would emphasize that alternate pain pathways exist and that consideration should be given to such anatomy when analyzing the so-called atypical neuralgias which are not readily classified with a specific cranial nerve. Furthermore we believe that the "deep sensory" component of the facial nerve described by Hunt (34, 37), may account for some of the neuralgias currently classified as atypical neuralgias.

This presentation began with a discussion of the studies of Sir Charles Bell establishing the fifth nerve as the "sole cause or source of a common sensibility of the head and face." This concept is no longer tenable and requires expansion if the pathophysiology of trigeminal and other facial neuralgias is to be understood. There are anastomoses between the portio major and portio minor of the trigeminal nerve, and there is strong evidence that a preponderance of sensory fibers anastomose with the motor root, rather than the converse (30). Secondly, purported sensory nociceptive fibers are present in the trigeminal motor root (80). In addition, the territory of the somatic and visceral sensory system of the seventh nerve requires reexamination. Perhaps some of the neuralgias currently categorized as atypical may be reassigned to the domain of the facial nerve rather than to the more stereotypic classification, pain of psychogenic origin.

We would encourage continued clinical observation and laboratory investigations attempting to further elucidate the pathophysiology of facial neuralgia. Currently the armamentarium for neuroanatomical and neurophysiological investigation is greater than it has ever been. Critical evaluation of the literature, particularly that of the masters of observation (Dandy, Hunt, Davis, Sweet, *etc.*), and application of modern technology should prove fruitful in unraveling some of these mysteries. Lastly, critical evaluation of treatment failures and recurrences of the neuralgia can be instructive in gaining insight into the pathophysiology of these disorders.

In closing, I have borrowed a quote from Dr. Ronald Melzack (50): "The puzzle of pain as we have seen is far from being solved and there are few problems more worthy of human endeavor than the relief of pain and suffering."

REFERENCES

1. Apfelbaum, R. I. A comparison of percutaneous radiofrequency trigeminal neurolysis and microvascular decompression of the trigeminal nerve for the treatment of tic douloureux. Neurosurgery, *1:* 16–21, 1977.
2. Beaver, D. L., Moses, H. L., and Ganote, C. E. Electron microscopy of the trigeminal ganglion. II. Autopsy study of human ganglia. Arch. Pathol., *79:* 557–570, 1965.
3. Beaver, D. L., Moses, H. L., and Ganote, C. E. Electron microscopy of the trigeminal ganglion. III. Trigeminal neuralgia. Arch. Pathol., *79:* 571–582, 1965.
4. Bell, C. On the nerves of the face, being a second paper on that subject. Philos. Trans. R. Soc. Long. *1:* 317–330, 1829. (Reprinted in Med. Classics, *1:* 123–150, 1936.)
5. Bischoff, E. P. E. *Mikroskopische Analyse der Anastomosen der Kopfnerven.* J. J. Lentner, Munchen, 1865. (Translated and edited by E. Sachs, Jr., University Press of New England, Hanover, 1977.)
6. Burchiel, K. J. Abnormal impulse generation in focally demyelinated trigeminal roots. J. Neurosurg., *53:* 674–683, 1980.
7. Burchiel, K. J., Steege, T. D., Howe, J. F., and Loeser, J. D. Comparison of percutaneous radiofrequency gangliolysis and microvascular decompression for the surgical management of tic douloureux. Neurosurgery, *9:* 111–119, 1981.
8. Chorobski, J., and Penfield, W. Cerebral vasodilator nerves and their pathway from the medulla oblongata. Arch. Neurol. Psychiatry, *28:* 1257–1289, 1932.
9. Clarke, C. R. A., and Harrison, M. J. G. Neurologic manifestations of Paget's disease. J. Neurol. Sci., *38:* 171–178, 1978.
10. Coggeshall, R. E. Afferent fibers in the ventral root. Neurosurgery, *4:* 443–448, 1979.
11. Coggeshall, R. E., Applebaum, M. L., Fazen, M., Stubbs, T. B., and Sykes, M. T. Unmyelinated axons in human ventral roots: A possible explanation for the failure of dorsal rhizotomy to relieve pain. Brain, *98:* 157–166, 1975.
12. Coggeshall, R. E., Coulter, J. D., and Willis, W. D. Unmyelinated fibers in the ventral root. J. Cell. Biol., *55:* 46A, 1972.
13. Coggeshall, R. E., Coulter, J. D., and Willis, W. D. Unmyelinated fibers in the ventral root. Brain Res., *57:* 229–233, 1973.
14. Coggeshall, R. E., Coulter, J. D., and Willis, W. D. Unmyelinated axons in the ventral roots of the cat lumbosacral enlargement. J. Comp. Neurol., *153:* 39–58, 1974.
15. Coggeshall, R. E., and Ito, H. Sensory fibers in ventral roots L7 and S1 in the cat. J. Physiol., *267:* 215–235, 1977.
16. Dandy, W. E. An operation for the cure of tic douloureux: Partial section of the sensory root at the pons. Arch. Surg., *18:* 687–734, 1929.
17. Dandy, W. E. Certain functions of the roots and ganglia of the cranial sensory nerves. Arch. Neurol. Psychiatry, *27:* 22–29, 1932.
18. Dandy, W. E. Concerning the cause of trigeminal neuralgia. Am. J. Surg., *24:* 447–455, 1934.
19. Dandy, W. E. Lesions of the cranial nerves. In: *Practice of Surgery*, Vol. 12, edited by D. Lewis and W. Walters, pp. 177–212. W.F. Prior, Hagerstown, Md., 1944.
20. Davis, L. E. The deep sensibility of the face. Arch. Neurol. Psychiatry, *9:* 283–305, 1923.

21. Eisenbrey, A. B., and Hegarty, W. M. Trigeminal neuralgia and arteriovenous aneurysm of the cerebellopontine angle. J. Neurosurg., *13:* 647–649, 1956.

22. Ferguson, G. G., Brett, D. C., Peerless, S. J., Barr, H. W. K., and Girin, J. P. Trigeminal neuralgia: A comparison of the results of percutaneous rhizotomy and microvascular decompression. Can. J. Neurol. Sci., *8:* 207–214, 1981.

23. Frazier, C. H. Subtotal resection of sensory root for relief of major trigeminal neuralgia. Arch. Neurol. Psychiatry, *13:* 378–384, 1925.

24. Frigyesi, T. L., Siegfried, J., and Groggi, G. The selective vulnerability of evoked potentials in the trigeminal sensory root to graded thermocoagulation. Exp. Neurol., *49:* 11–21, 1975.

25. Gardner, W. J. Concerning the mechanism of trigeminal neuralgia and hemifacial spasm. J. Neurosurg., *19:* 947–958, 1962.

26. Gardner, W. J. Trigeminal neuralgia. Clin. Neurosurg., *15:* 1–56, 1968.

27. Gardner, W. J. Trigeminal neuralgia. In: *Trigeminal Neuralgia: Pathogenesis and Pathophysiology,* edited by R. Hassler and A. E. Walker, pp. 153–174. W.B. Saunders, Philadelphia, 1970.

28. Gardner, W. J., and Miklos, M. V. Response of trigeminal neuralgia to "decompression" of sensory root. Discussion of cause of trigeminal neuralgia. J.A.M.A., *170:* 1773–1776, 1959.

29. Gardner, W. J., Todd, E. M., and Pinto, J. P. Roentgenographic findings in trigeminal neuralgia. A.J.R., *76:* 346–350, 1956.

30. Gudmundsson, K., Rhoton, A. L., Jr., and Rushton, J. G. Detailed anatomy of the intracranial portion of the trigeminal nerve. J. Neurosurg., *35:* 592–600, 1971.

31. Håkanson, S. Trigeminal neuralgia treated by the injection of glycerol into the trigeminal cistern. Neurosurgery, *9:* 638–646, 1981.

32. Hardy, D. G., and Rhoton, A. L., Jr. Microsurgical relationships of the superior cerebellar artery and the trigeminal nerve. J. Neurosurg., *49:* 669–678, 1978.

33. Head, H. *Studies in Neurology.* London, H. Trowde, 1920.

34. Hunt, J. M. On herpetic inflammations of the geniculate ganglion. A new syndrome and its complications. J. Nerv. Ment. Dis., *34:* 73–96, 1907.

35. Hunt, J. M. The sensory system of the facial nerve and its symptomatology. J. Nerv. Ment. Dis., *36:* 321–350, 1909.

36. Hunt, J. M. The sensory field of the facial nerve: A further contribution to the symptomatology of the geniculate ganglion. Brain, *38:* 418–446, 1915.

37. Hunt, J. M. Geniculate neuralgia (neuralgia of the nervus facialis). Arch. Neurol. Psychiatry, *37:* 253–285, 1937.

38. Jaeger, R. The relief of tic douloureux (trigeminal tic) and other pains of fifth cranial nerve by injection of hot water into Gasserian ganglion. J. Am. Geriatr. Soc., *3:* 416–423, 1955.

39. Jannetta, P. J. Arterial compression of the trigeminal nerve at the pons in patients with trigeminal neuralgia. J. Neurosurg., *26:* 159–162, 1967.

40. Jannetta, P. J. Microsurgical approach to the trigeminal nerve for tic douloureux. Prog. Neurol. Surg., *7:* 180–200, 1976.

41. Jannetta, P. J. Neurovascular compression in cranial nerve and systemic disease. Ann. Surg., *192:* 518–525, 1980.

42. Jannetta, P. J., and Rand, R. W. Transtentorial retrogasserian rhizotomy in trigeminal neuralgia by microneurosurgical technique. Bull. Los Angeles Neurol. Soc., *31:* 93–99, 1966.

43. Johnson, M. C., and Salmon, J. H. Arteriovenous malformation presenting as trigeminal neuralgia. Case report. J. Neurosurg., *29:* 287–289, 1968.

44. Kerr, F. W. L. Pathology of trigeminal neuralgia: Light and electron microscopic observations. J. Neurosurg., *26:* 151–156, 1967.
45. Kerr, F. W. L., and Miller, R. H. The pathology of trigeminal neuralgia. Electron microscopic studies. Arch. Neurol., *15:* 308–319, 1966.
46. Lazar, M. L., and Kirkpatrick, J. B. Trigeminal neuralgia and multiple sclerosis: Demonstration of the plaque in an operative case. Neurosurgery, *5:* 711–717, 1979.
47. Letcher, F. S., and Goldring, S. The effect of radiofrequency current and heat on peripheral nerve action potential in the cat. J. Neurosurg., *29:* 42–47, 1968.
48. Malis, L. I. Petrous ridge compression and its surgical correction. J. Neurosurg., *26:* 163–167, 1967.
49. May, O., and Horsley, V. The mesencephalic root of the fifth nerve. Brain, *33:* 175–203, 1910.
50. Melzack, R. *The Puzzle of Pain.* Basic Books, New York, 1973.
51. Menzel, J., Piotrowski, W., and Penzholz, H. Long-term results of gasserian ganglion electrocoagulation. J. Neurosurg., *42:* 140–143, 1975.
52. Nielsen, V. K. Pathophysiology of hemifacial spasms. I. Ephaptic transmission and ectopic excitation. Neurology, *34:* 418–426, 1984.
53. Nielsen, V. K. Pathophysiology of hemifacial spasm. II. Lateral spread of the supraorbital nerve reflux. Neurology, *34:* 427–431, 1984.
54. Nugent, G. R. Technique and results of 800 percutaneous radiofrequency thermocoagulations for trigeminal neuralgia. Appl. Neurophysiol., *45:* 504–507, 1982.
55. Onofrio, B. M. Radiofrequency percutaneous Gasserian ganglion lesions. J. Neurosurg., *42:* 132–139, 1975.
56. Orbrador, S., Queimadelos, V. G., and Soto, M. Trigeminal neuralgia secondary to asymmetry of the petrous bone: Case report. J. Neurosurg., *33:* 596–598, 1970.
57. Peet, M. M., and Schneider, R. C. Trigeminal neuralgia: Review of 689 cases with follow-up study on 65 per cent of group. J. Neurosurg., *9:* 367–377, 1952.
58. Pelletier, V. A., Poulos, D. A., and Lende, R. A. Functional localization in the trigeminal root. J. Neurosurg., *40:* 504–513, 1974.
59. Poulos, D. A. Functional and anatomical localization in the trigeminal root: In support of Frazier. In: *Current Controversies in Neurosurgery,* edited by T. P. Morley. pp. 539–545. W.B. Saunders, Philadelphia, 1976.
60. Rand, R. W. Functional and anatomical localization in the trigeminal root: In support of Dandy. In: *Current Controversies in Neurosurgery,* edited by T. P. Morley. W.B. Saunders, Philadelphia, 1976.
61. Rhoton, A. L., Kobayashi, S., and Hollinshead, W. H. Nervus intermedius. J. Neurosurg., *29:* 609–618, 1968.
62. Rhoton, A. L., Maniscalco, J., Hoagland, H. V., and Chorvat, B. D. Percutaneous stereotaxic radiofrequency lesions for trigeminal neuralgia. J. Fla. Med. Assoc., *64:* 488–493, 1977.
63. Rushton, J. G., and MacDonald, H. N. A. Trigeminal neuralgia. Special considerations of nonsurgical treatment. J.A.M.A., *165:* 437–440, 1957.
64. Rushton, J. G., and Olafson, R. A. Trigeminal neuralgia associated with multiple sclerosis. Report of 35 cases. Arch. Neurol., *13:* 383–386, 1965.
65. Sachs, E., Jr. The role of the nervus intermedius in facial neuralgia. J. Neurosurg., *28:* 54–60, 1968.
66. Saunders, R. L., and Sachs, E., Jr. Relation of the accessory rootlets of the trigeminal nerve to its motor root. A microsurgical autopsy study. J. Neurosurg., *33:* 317–324, 1970.
67. Sharr, M. M., and Garfield, J. S. The place of ganglion or root alcohol injection in

trigeminal neuralgia. J. Neurol. Neurosurg. Psychiatry, *40:* 286–290, 1977.

68. Sherrington, C. S. On the anatomical constitution of nerves of skeletal muscles: With remarks on recurrent fibers in the ventral spinal nerve root. J. Physiol., *17:* 211–258, 1894.

69. Siegfried, J. 500 percutaneous thermocoagulations of the Gasserian ganglion for trigeminal pain. Surg. Neurol., *8:* 126–131, 1977.

70. Smith, D. G., and Mumford, J. M. Petrous angle and trigeminal neuralgia. Pain, *8:* 269–277, 1980.

71. Stookey, B., and Ransohoff, J. *Trigeminal Neuralgia. Its History and Treatment.* Charles C Thomas, Springfield, Ill., 1959.

72. Sweet, W. H. Controlled thermocoagulation of trigeminal rootlets in man. In: *Current Controversies in Neurosurgery,* edited by T. P. Morley, pp. 546–549. W.B. Saunders, Philadelphia, 1976.

73. Sweet, W. H., and Wepsic, J. G. Controlled thermocoagulation of trigeminal ganglion and rootlets for differential destruction of pain fibers. Part I. Trigeminal neuralgia. J. Neurosurg., *40:* 143–156, 1974.

74. Taarnhoj, P. Decompression of the trigeminal root. J. Neurosurg., *11:* 299–305, 1954.

75. Tew, J. M., and Keller, J. T. The treatment of trigeminal neuralgia by percutaneous radiofrequency technique. Clin. Neurosurg., *24:* 557–578, 1977.

76. Tew, J. M., Tobler, W. D., and van Loveren, H. Percutaneous rhizotomy in the treatment of intractable facial pain (trigeminal glossopharyngeal, and vagal nerves). In: *Operative Neurosurgical Techniques,* edited by H. H. Schmidek and W. H. Sweet, pp. 1083–1100. Grune & Stratton, New York, 1982.

77. van Loveren, H., Tew, J. M., Jr., Keller, J. T., and Nurre, M. A. A 10-year experience in the treatment of trigeminal neuralgia. J. Neurosurg., *57:* 757–765, 1982.

78. Wilson, C. B., Yorke, C., and Prioleau, G. Microsurgical vascular decompression for trigeminal neuralgia and hemifacial spasm. West. J. Med., *132:* 481–484, 1980.

79. White, J. C., and Sweet, W. H. *Pain and the Neurosurgeon: A Forty-Year Experience.* Charles C Thomas, Springfield, Ill., 1969.

80. Young, R. F., and Kruger, L. Axonal transport studies of the trigeminal nerve roots of the cat: With special reference to afferent contributions to the portio minor. J. Neurosurg., *54:* 208–212, 1981.

81. Young, R. F., and Stevens, R. Unmyelinated axons in the trigeminal motor root of human and cat. J. Comp. Neurol., *183:* 205–214, 1979.

15

The History of the Development of Treatment for Trigeminal Neuralgia

WILLIAM H. SWEET, M.D., D.SC., D.H.C.

INTRODUCTION

There are already excellent essays on this particular facet of medical history. Rose (64), Horsley *et al.* (40), and Stookey and Ransohoff (73) have provided extensive references to the earlier literature. I have read much of this material with the specific objective of assessing why both progress and lack of progress occurred.

PERIPHERAL NEURECTOMY

The first successful surgical efforts to treat this disorder involved neurotomy of peripheral branches of the nerve. Rose (64) credits Albinus and Galen with suggesting such an operation and Schlichting and Maréchal with having first carried it out, albeit unsuccessfully. It is probably Nicholas André (2) a Parisian surgeon, who published the first detailed accounts of a small group of patients with this disorder in 1756. They were recorded in a book whose 47-word title begins *"Practical Observations on Diseases of the Urethra and on Several Convulsive Manifestations."* At no place is pain mentioned in the title. After this misleading start and 318 initial pages dealing with diseases of the urethra, largely venereal in origin, there came an excellent detailed 47-page description of five patients with paroxysms of facial pain introduced under the heading: "Remarques sur Certains Mouvements Convulsifs." His first case, seen in 1732, had had three teeth pulled from one side of the upper jaw in an effort to control repeated formation of an abscess here. The extractions dealt successfully with the infection but were followed by agonizing paroxysms, many times per day, of brief provocable pain accompanied by "hideous grimaces." His second and third patients, without predisposing infection or trauma, appeared to be completely typical for idiopathic trigeminal neuralgia. In the first patient, the distinguished surgeon to the king, Maréchal, had failed in 1730 in an effort to cut the infraorbital nerve. Two years later, after protracted reflection on what to do for the distressed woman, André decided on an innovative course of action only because of the large number of failed types of treatment for her and an analysis of what his method might offer. All of these he documented fully in an effort to meet in advance the criticisms he would encounter. His treatment was to apply a caustic stone and liquid caustic (type unspecified) "for 10 or 12 days" until the infraorbital nerve was destroyed. This achieved complete relief until a modest recurrence 18 months later. Retreatment yielded a "cure" which, persisting after 2 years, led the patient to sign a formal testimonial to this fact "after long suffering for ten full years." André followed this by a second triumph with the same method—again in a patient with third division pain on whom Maréchal had unsuccessfully operated by incision in the gums from the angle of the jaw to the incisor teeth. That operation had been followed on the 17th postoperative day by a hemorrhage which nearly killed the patient. The pains had recurred 2 months later, so André laid bare the bone and, using a trephine, exposed the canal in the bone containing nerve and vessels, destroying them with liquid caustic as far back as possible. Having encountered criticism of his handling of his first case, he asked 3 "Surgeons of the Court" and 2 "Master Surgeons of Paris" to follow the patient with him before, during, and after treatment. Finally he demonstrated the "cured" patient to the "Premier Physician to the King," who along with one of the surgeons to the King, Boisaillard, signed independent attestations as to the protracted severity of the illness and the success of the treatment at 6-month follow-up. The word of unbiased experts regarding results of treatment is as useful today as it was over 2 centuries ago. More frequent employment of such appraisals would speed medical progress.

To the disorder "with these violent agitations" André gave the name "tic douloureux." He recognized it as "exclusive and distinctive from all other diseases" and despite the explosive character of the episodes "not properly called a convulsion. . .since the movements are not involuntary." So André first recognized the disorder as a special syndrome, gave it the name "tic douloureux," which has stuck, and developed a technique for destroying the appropriate peripheral branch for a relatively long period of relief. It is fortunate that the cloak of an utterly inappropriate title did not result in complete neglect of the work. One wonders if he recognized the monumental importance of his observations or if he became discouraged by a later recurrence of the facial pain in his patients, because 2 years later in 1758 he wrote another book confined to an account of diseases of the urinary bladder and urethra.

Pujol, accepting André's name for the disorder, tic douloureux, recognized in 1787 that, although infraorbital nerve section might suffice, more than one nerve would often need to be cut "since the painful area is so richly supplied" (62). This nerve supply included of course the facial nerve, which many surgeons deliberately cut as well. Pujol also stated 2 centuries ago that dental extraction was futile and deplored the useless removal of an entire row of teeth as a diagnostic and therapeutic blunder. Such admonitions have been repeated in scores of articles; yet, most of us still see patients with this disorder who have had needless dental extractions, a sad commentary on the efficiency of our educational processes.

The writings of these early authors do not mention the pain which must have accompanied their operations, nor do they indicate what objective sensory loss may have been produced. The distinction between the main motor functions of the facial nerve and the largely sensory role of the trigeminal nerve remained to be made by Sir Charles Bell (4, 5), but surgeons, including his own brother John Bell, continued to cut the facial nerve for tic douloureux for years thereafter (11).

The tendency of the pains to undergo spontaneous remission was also not recognized for many decades. Although Fothergill (23) in 1773 gave an excellent full description of the clinical features of the disease in 14 patients, he did not realize that when his treatment of extract of hemlock in increasing doses eventually succeeded, the patient was finally benefitting from spontaneous reduction or cessation of pain. Ignorance of the mysterious factors producing remission in this disorder continues to beset our appraisal of the various treatments we try.

For a century after Pujol's paper a variety of attacks on peripheral trigeminal branches and divisions sought to preclude or delay regeneration and recurrence of pain. Von Klein's (93) 1822 tactic of crushing and cauterizing the central end of the peripheral branch was probably no improvement over André's procedure 66 years earlier. The *Boston and Medical Surgical Journal* (Volume 1, pp. 1–6, 1828) described John C. Warren's (94) experiences with six patients with "Affections of the nerves of the head, commonly called 'Tic Douloureux'." His case 3 described pains beginning near the ear and radiating forward in all directions from the scalp to the lower jaw. The patient having looked up the neuroanatomy noted that this was the course of the branches of the facial nerve and insisted it be cut despite Dr. Warren's statement that there were no recorded cases of relief of such pain after this operation. It is perhaps reassuring that also 160 years ago there were patients who were determined that they knew more than their doctors. Failure of facial neurectomy here was followed by relief from inferior alveolar neurectomy. Warren's case 6 had had brief paroxysms of supraorbital pain for 6 months with no relief from many remedies. On hearing Warren's advice that the nerve be divided "he left rather precipitately." "A considerable time after, he let me know he was entirely well, dating his recovery from the proposal of an operation."

In order to delay regeneration Malgaigne (54) in 1843 cut the second division 2 cm posterior to the lower rim of the orbit after breaking through the orbital floor and then pulled the nerve out of the canal at the infraorbital foramen. He describes the minutiae of several other procedures advised by other surgeons for denervating peripheral trigeminal branches without indicating how successful any were in terms of sensory loss, much less long-term results. Similar crucial deficiencies characterize the monograph of Vogt (92) on stretching the nerves. It remained for other surgeons to report the disappointing results of these peripheral procedures. Thus Hahn of Berlin found that of 11 cases after the Vogt nerve-stretching operation, only 1 case was really improved, and in him a portion of the nerve was also excised (64). Otto Weber (95) collected 100 cases of trigeminal neurectomy with only 18 cures, and Fowler assembled 83 such cases, but the compilation was of little value because of the short follow-up. Thus only 10 were followed for 2 or more years and only 2 for 3 or more years. Fowler (24) also collected reports on 18 cases treated by ligation of the ipsilateral common carotid artery. Relief, on the whole gratifying, was as described in Table 15.1. He adds that in one case this was the third time the patient had been reported cured. That a procedure which has utterly vanished from our armamentarium for this disorder could have been described so favorably is an eloquent admonition to us to appraise critically for many years.

As the nineteenth century wore on a huge variety of approaches and destructive gestures evolved, gradually working their way back to the base of the skull. Already by 1858 Carnochan (8) had exposed the anterior end of the foramen rotundum, emphasizing the denervation of Meckel's sphenopalatine ganglion en route. Abbë (1) added the "laceration" of Meckel's ganglion. Pancoast and Woodbury (57) in 1872 described "a new operation" for reaching the third division below the foramen ovale. Krönlein (51) in 1884 extended this to include both second and third divisions, and published one of the few postoperative sensory examinations. Rose (64) and Horsley et al. (40) described the different permuta-

TABLE 15.1

Ligation of the Ipsilateral Common Carotid Artery[a]

Relief	>3 yr in 4
	1–3 yr in 3
	<1 yr in 4
	Partial in 1
	0 in 2
	"Cure" in 2—duration unknown

[a] Data taken from 18 cases of G. R. Fowler (24).

tions of these extracranial efforts in about 30 publications as surgeons found themselves unable to overcome the psychological barrier of the skull.

NERVE AVULSION

Only one of the external procedures had much merit, *i.e.*, nerve avulsion. Blum (7) first did this in 1882 giving us a brief note. Detailed descriptions of techniques for avulsion of each peripheral trigeminal branch were given by Thiersch (83) in 1889. He reported 28 nerve avulsions in 17 patients over a 6-year period, stating that there had been but one recurrence in that time in the domain of any avulsed nerve—one of the few long term follow-ups. The distinguished Belgian neuroanatomist van Gehuchten (91) carried out a series of histologic studies on the effect in rabbits of the "abrupt tearing out of the peripheral branches of the trigeminal nerve" at their emergence from the supraorbital, infraorbital, and mental foramina. This degree of trauma injured the ganglion cells and evoked degeneration extending the length of the descending spinal trigeminal tract in the brain stem, whereas such central degeneration did not occur when he merely divided the peripheral branches. He noted that the Gasserian ganglion is so firmly attached to the dura and base of the skull in man that the direct injury stops there, so that the pontobulbar degeneration is related only to the injury to the ganglionic neurones. Moreover it is confined to those neurones from which the avulsed fibers arise. Doyen (20) carried out avulsion of the second division in front of the foramen rotundum seven times in man with relief of pain in all during "several years" of follow-up. Van Gehuchten's study (91) has been reported in detail with a 10-page translation from the original French by Spiller in the University of Pennsylvania Medical Bulletin. It led van Gehuchten to propose avulsion of the appropriate branches in man prior to consideration of an intracranial operation. From my own experience of recurrence of pain after human supraorbital and supratrochlear avulsions I suspect that the human Gasserian ganglion is less vulnerable than that of the rabbit to this type of trauma. Nevertheless I am distressed to be unable to find evidence that this rational suggestion was ever systematically pursued. Even Doyen went on to removal of the Gasserian ganglion in four patients despite early postoperative death in two of them. However, now that we can differentially destroy the pain fibers at minimal risk I do not think van Gehuchten's suggestion should be tried. I do say that our enthusiasm for demonstrating surgical prowess must not cloud our capacity to investigate the merits of lesser procedures. For example, Dandy was not willing to dignify cervical or intracranial carotid ligation for intracranial aneurysm by even classifying it as an operation. He called it a preoperative procedure (19).

APPROACHES TO THE MIDDLE CRANIAL FOSSA

Neurectomy and Ganglionectomy

Patients desperate for relief after recurrences from neurectomies at the base of the skull led four surgeons early in the final decade of the last century finally to enter the middle cranial fossa. The first to do this, William Rose of King's College Hospital, London, used an approach through the pterygoid region which involved cutting the zygomatic arch at two points, turning it and the masseter downwards and reflecting upwards the cut off coronoid process and temporal muscle (64) (Fig. 15.1). The relevant skull base was cleared, and a trephine opening was

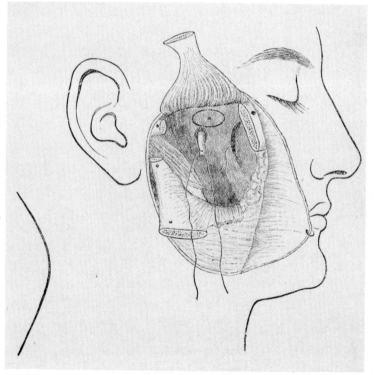

FIGS. 15.1 and 15.2   Rose's anteriolateral approach to base of middle cranial fossa via a skin flap reflected downward. (*Fig. 15.1*) The transected zygomatic arch and the masseter are turned downwards and backwards; the broken off coronoid process and temporalis muscle are reflected upwards to enter the pterygopalatine fossa, whose plexus of vessels is not shown. (*Fig. 15.2*) Diagram of bone of skull showing the track to and site of trephine opening thru skull anterolateral to foramina ovale (*F.O.*) and spinosum (*F.S.*). (Reproduced with permission from W. Rose (64).)

made in it just anterolateral to the foramen ovale. This was enlarged, and the Gasserian ganglion was dissected out (Fig. 15.2). He reported his first case in 1890 and a total of five in 1892, all free of pain. However, he saw in all "a rapid diminution of the anesthetic area," from which he cheerfully concluded, not that some of the ganglion was left behind but that "the distribution of sensation is taken up by the neighboring

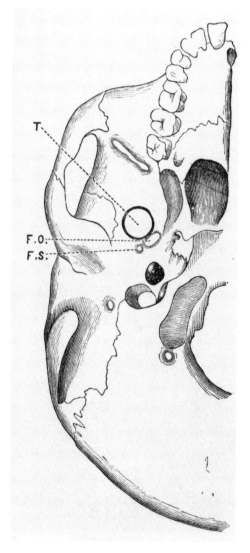

FIG. 15.2

branches much in the same way as arterial anastomosis takes place in the vascular system." In such ways are we surgeons able to keep up our spirits. I am unable to refrain from noting that Rose was a general surgeon—not a neurosurgeon. He selected this amazingly cumbersome approach after trying a variety of routes in cadavers. All the previous operations to get at the exits of foraminae rotundum and ovale had involved some sort of anterolateral attack. In 1893, both Rose (64) and the Reims surgeon, Doyen (20), were apparently unable to consider the feasibility of gentle retraction of the brain, preferring instead to achieve exposure from below and in front of the ganglion. The lesson may be that if you have decided to take a new tactic, try to avoid tethers to the old tactics.

It remained for the New Yorker, Hartley (36), in August 1891 and, independently 6 months later in February 1892, the Berliner, Krause (49), to recognize the simplicity of the straight lateral approach through the temporal squama and elevation of the temporal lobe dura. They both turned down small temporal bone flaps and tied off the middle meningeal artery. However, each used this easy exposure in his first case only to cut the peripheral second and third divisions in front of the ganglion. Krause (50) quickly followed this with a presumed removal of the Gasserian ganglion in his next case. However, like Rose, he overestimated the extent of his extirpation. His neurological colleague Dr. Nonne found, even in the 1st week after operation, a complete anesthesia to all stimuli only in the first division. The Hartley-Krause approach, as Horsley suggested it be called, quickly swept into favor, with more ganglionectomies than neurectomies being done. By 1896 Tiffany (88) had published detailed tables of round-the-world reports on 110 cases. Already there were recurrences after intracranial neurectomies, but the most disheartening feature was that 26 of the cases (24%) were postoperative fatalities. The same grim message was conveyed by the French surgeons, Marchant and Herbet (55) in 1897. Their review article records 59 cases of incomplete and 15 of complete ganglionic removal with 16 deaths (22%). Even the most experienced trio, Krause et al. (88) with 24 cases between them had had 5 deaths. Sepsis and brain trauma were thought to be the principal causes. The apprehension of surgeons about entering the intracranial cavity was born out with a vengeance. The distinguished surgeon W. W. Keen (45) concluded in 1900 that the much lower risk neurectomies were clearly preferable despite the fact that "the relief is scarcely ever permanent" Tiffany (88), under the impression that involvement of the first trigeminal division was "due entirely to reflex irritation" and recognizing the problems attendant on corneal anesthesia, urged the refinement of excision of only that part of the ganglion supplying the second and third divisions. Marchant and Herbet agreed. Tiffany also pointed out the feasibility of preservation of the motor root.

It remained for Cushing to attain a spectacular improvement over the performance of all others. He modified slightly the Hartley-Krause procedure in that he kept the middle meningeal artery intact between the foramen spinosum and its canal in the cranial vault, thereby diminishing elevation of the brain. In those days of poor control of anesthesia and intracranial pressure, the middle meningeal arterial bar to excessive retraction may have been important. He also insisted on working only in an absolutely bloodless field (11). Figure 15.3 indicates that by gentle blunt dissection he freed the stumps of peripheral divisions and ganglion and avulsed the root from the pons. His detailed 34-page report of his first 20 cases in 1905 contains photographs of many intact complete operative specimens and includes a photograph of the sensory loss in the early postoperative period for nearly every case revealing a total trigeminal anesthesia (12). There is however, a late examination in only three

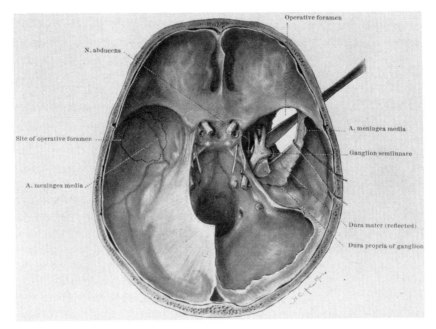

FIG. 15.3. Cushing's slight modification of Hartley-Krause approach. Cranial base after removal of brain. Note intact middle meningeal artery and separation by blunt dissection of the three peripheral trigeminal divisions, the ganglion, and rootlets from their dural envelope. (Reproduced with permission from H. Cushing (11).)

cases—two with continuing total anesthesia at 1 and 2 years, and the third (case 12) with recovery of some first division touch and pinprick pain at 18 months. By December 1919 he had done 332 Gasserian ganglion operations with 2 deaths, the 8th and 34th cases, leaving a consecutive series of 298 operations without a fatality (14).

A search for reasons for this staggeringly superior record reveals that Cushing first performed this operation on freshly autopsied patients 30 times, noting anatomical variations from person to person. During the operations, he observed that the pulse rate slowed as he elevated the temporal lobe. He monitored the vital signs and responded to changes therein, especially after the death in his case 8, with whom he persisted in surgery despite a falling blood pressure. After his extensive analysis of all the details on that patient, he concluded that he should have closed the wound promptly, despite excellent parameters on all other scores. He also said, "Injury of the cavernous sinus is by no means such a calamity as it is credited with being. The sinus is not an open canal, as usually believed, but made up of compartments in which local thromboses may occur readily and promptly, and thus hemorrhage be controlled by a few moments of (precise) pressure." Others apparently tended to pack the whole wound to control the outpouring of deep venous bleeding, close the wound, and return another day with an increased risk of sepsis.

However, Cushing's technical skill led to his persistence in using an unnecessarily extensive operation. We have no long-term follow-up of the recurrence rate, sensory loss and complications of corneal anesthesia or anesthesia dolorosa in this remarkable series. It would be of special interest to know the incidence of dysesthesias after ganglionectomy.

Open Rhizotomy

The unacceptable mortality of ganglionectomy in the hands of all but Cushing led to the next major step of substituting for it the simpler act of rhizotomy. Horsley et al. (40) reported in detail the first such operation in 1891, with the senior author having concluded that total removal of the ganglion involved too often tearing of the medially contiguous cavernous sinus, a serious matter in those days for most surgeons. His approach was intradural with elevation of temporal lobe and identification and opening of the dural roof of Meckel's cave. He described gentle avulsion of the rootlets from the pons with a dull hook, stating "this was easily accomplished." He gives a full account of the smoothness of the entire procedure, followed unfortunately by the "death from shock" of the desperately infirm patient. Horsley later credited Macewen with having done the same operation, the account of which Macewen himself never published. Their objective was to cut off all possible trigeminal connections with the pons.

Popularization of posterior rhizotomy via the extradural approach in the middle cranial fossa is largely due to the careful publications of Spiller and Frazier (69, 70), beginning in 1901. They raised the question as to whether or not the trigeminal sensory root might regenerate after it was cut but were unable to answer this question from a series of short-term experiments they did in dogs. Later, van Gehuchten (91) summarized the evidence in animals that section of the trigeminal root causes complete degeneration of all sensory bulbospinal fibers (91). The facts in man are that recurrences of pain take place after extensive partial rhizotomy in 15–20% of patients followed for long periods, whereas after total rhizotomies the rate of significant recurrence is only 2–3%. (See White and Sweet (97) for a summary of the relevant studies.)

Frazier (25) in 1915 demonstrated preservation of ophthalmic fibers and in 1918 preservation of the motor root at rhizotomy as suggested earlier by Tiffany with ganglionectomy. Frazier (25) in 1925 pointed out and Stookey (73) in 1928 confirmed that section of only the sensory rootlets from a single division may be needed if it alone is involved in the primary area of pain or trigger zone. In addition to the 24 articles of Frazier and colleagues and those of Spiller and Frazier, hundreds of other reports totalling many thousands of cases using middle fossa approaches to the trigeminal rootlets for trigeminal neuralgia were published during the subsequent 50-year period. Because of the relative ease and precision with which it could be done, it was the most widely used procedure in many services for lasting relief in the moderate and severe cases. Indeed the procedure was so successful that the neurosurgical fraternity was lulled into a state of blithe contentment with its results, and few efforts were made to improve them. Sir Geoffrey Jefferson, with much general surgical as well as neurosurgical experience, categorized it as the most successful operation in all of surgery. A few neurosurgeons preferred Horsley's original subtemporal intradural route to the extradural approach of Hartley. Henderson (39) and White and Sweet (97) have summarized the bases for this minority preference.

Although the immense gratitude of most patients is heartwarming to the surgeon there are three common problems after the operation: (a) Facial paralysis in 5–10% of patients from trauma to the greater superficial petrosal nerve transmitted to the geniculate ganglion. This results in swelling of the nerve in its tight bony case and consequent compression of the facial nerve. This is nearly always temporary and now is relatively rare with dexamethasone prophylaxis. (b) Corneal anesthesia with its attendant risk of keratitis. (c) Severe facial dysesthesias or anesthesia dolorosa. The severity of the problem of persistent constant frank pains and other disagreeable sensations came to full recognition in the latter half of this century as a consequence of late follow-ups such as those of Peet and Schneider (59), Stookey and Ransohoff (73), Grant (29), and White and Sweet (97). In an effort to minimize these complications, other intracranial tactics have been tried.

"Decompression" or "Compression" of the Trigeminal Pathways

Hypothesizing that the neuralgic pains were caused by compression of trigeminal pathways Taarnhøj (80) incised longitudinally the dural roof of the rootlets back through the superior petrosal sinus to the porus trigemini, whereas Pudenz and Shelden (62) concurrently "decompressed" the peripheral divisions at the foraminae ovale and rotundum by drilling away bone. Each method was tried in 10 patients with about equally satisfactory results in each group. Stender (71) incised the dural roof of the rootlets, stopping short of the superior petrosal sinus. Concluding that the common denominator in these operations was modest trauma to the trigeminal pathways, Shelden, Pudenz *et al.* (67) altered the "decompressive" to a "compressive" procedure in which the surgeon pushed downward vigorously on the exposed ganglion and rootlets against the floor of Meckel's cave. These operations enjoyed wide acceptance throughout the 1950s. White and Sweet (97) summarize the results given in 29 publications in that decade. For a low incidence of major dysesthesias, the price was a recurrence rate in the series with longer follow-up from 21 to over 50% (97). These results emphasize again the mysterious protracted relief from manipulations in the neighborhood of the trigeminal nerve and the need for long follow-up and caution in interpreting the results of our efforts.

APPROACHES TO THE POSTERIOR CRANIAL FOSSA

Rhizotomy

Dandy (15) was the first to advocate an intradural approach to the trigeminal rootlets in the posterior fossa. The superb description of his operative technique includes the observation of many indentations of the trigeminal rootlets by blood vessels (17). Of 215 cases in which he personally made the operative notes, he saw contact made with the rootlets by the superior cerebellar artery 66 times and by a petrosal vein 30 times, for a total of 45%. He regarded external pressure on these rootlets as a major cause of trigeminal neuralgia (18). In a 47-page comprehensive account, he reports detailed postoperative examinations on his first 23 cases (16). In 11 cases he found much residual pin and touch sensation throughout the face, although he thought he had cut the entire sensory root in all 23 of them. His attribution of this preserved sensation to intact "accessory rootlets" anterior to the main bundle of the portio major has been repeatedly confirmed. His frankly partial rhizotomies were almost always followed by preservation of touch and pin sensation throughout the face. For a time he contended that this operation gave relief because "only pain fibers are sacrificed and all forms of sensation are retained." Hence, his recommendation at this point was for a partial section of the sensory root at the pons. For this preserved sensation there proved to be the price of increased risk of recurrence. Drs. Eldridge Campbell and Frank Otenasek, later residents of Dr. Dandy, stated that he in his last years rarely did subtotal divisions of the sensory root because of this increased recurrence rate (96). This experience of Dandy appears to have been ignored by some modern neurosurgeons who do a partial rhizotomy when they see no extrinsic lesion in the cerebellopontine angle. The approach formerly entailed significant added risk over that via the middle fossa, e.g., Olivecrona's mortality was 8 times as high for rhizotomy via the posterior fossa in trigeminal neuralgia (97). Hence, few neurosurgeons had used it routinely until Jannetta perfected the technique.

Tractotomy of Bulbar Trigeminal and Other Descending Bulbar Cephalic Pain Pathways

Sjöqvist (68) noted after an extensive search of the literature that Hun (41) had described complete facial analgesia with preservation of touch on one entire side of the face associated at post-mortem with a bulbar infarct extending no higher than the middle of the inferior olive. Concluding that the pain fibers descend to this low level in man before terminating at the cells of the nucleus of the spinal or descending tract, he carried out an initial series of nine "bulbar trigeminal tractotomies" at the cross-sectional level 8–10 mm rostral to the inferior limit of the 4th ventricle, the obex. Hypalgesia or analgesia of at least some portion of the trigeminal zone ensued in seven of the nine patients, although only one had complete trigeminal analgesia (68). Nearly normal touch was preserved in all hypalgesic or analgesic zones. Grant and Weinberger (30, 31) found that clumsiness of ipsilateral hand or fingers and staggering toward the side of the lesion often occurred after these lesions apparently related to incision at the restiform body which overlies the descending trigeminal tract at this level. Accordingly they suggested making the incision 4–5 cm below the cross-sectional level of the obex, where the descending sensory tract is overlain only by external arcuate and dorsal spinocerebellar fibers. They found that in many patients transection of the tract at this lower level still produced total trigeminal analgesia. A substantial surgical experience has accumulated and was summarized by White and Sweet (97). The hope that preservation of touch on the eyeball would provide an adequate warning to the patient so that he would promptly rid the eye of foreign bodies and avoid corneal ulcers has been borne out. The preservation of nearly normal touch throughout the face has not totally precluded the development of major facial dysesthesia; 4 such cases have been reported among the 920 cases in the literature up to 1969 (97). However, many surgeons have commented on the absence of posttractotomy pains. Another feature of this descending sensory tract first noted by Sweet is that it receives the nociceptive afferents from nervus intermedius, glossopharyngeal nerve, and upper vagal fibers, as well as trigeminal fibers. He found during World War II that transverse incisions from 0 to 2 mm below the obex produced analgesia of the mucosa of oral pharynx and tonsillar fossa as well as of posterior and anterior walls of the external auditory canal in nearly all of 15 patients (97). Such a distribution had clearly been graphically depicted by Cajal in the cat and led to Sweet's check of this point in man (97).

A major problem had been the achievement of the desired trigeminal analgesia. This was solved by Sweet, who noted that the surgeon could with impunity extend the incision just ventral to the descending sensory tract into the adjoining contralateral pain pathway from the lower limb. The incision may also be extended at small cost dorsally out of the descending sensory tract into the base of the nucleus of the fasciculus cuneatus and of the nucleus magnocellularis of von Monakow. This is because the major portions of these nuclei lie caudal to the incision and have already received their afferent input from below and transmitted it to the contralateral medial lemniscus. Lateropulsion and clumsiness of the ipsilateral upper limb appearing in the early postoperative period subside quickly. The patient is tested on the operating table to ensure the presence of analgesia of V, VII, IX, X, and the contralateral distal lower limb.

These tactics to ensure extensive and persistent sensory loss led to Sweet's trial of the operation for the pain of cephalic cancer, in which patients it usually failed to give relief. Moreover, despite complete trigeminal analgesia to pinprick, a few patients with trigeminal neuralgia have continued to have typical provocable paroxysms of pain (97). The explanation for these unexpected disappointments, both in pain of cancer and much less often in trigeminal neuralgia, probably lies in the recent findings of Young and Perryman (98) that more rostral portions of the descending tract are concerned with pain. The procedure, however, does have value in the management of chronic migrainous neuralgia (78).

PERCUTANEOUS INJECTIONS TO DESTROY TRIGEMINAL PATHWAYS

Peripheral Branches

Instillation of toxic chemicals into the nerves through the intact skin or mucosa followed the demonstrations of nerve destruction by Bartholow (3) using chloroform, by Neuber (56) with osmic acid, and by Pitres and Vaillard (61) with alcohol. Schlösser was the first in 1904 to describe treatment of trigeminal neuralgia by injection of alcohol, which he did by an intraoral approach into various divisions of the nerve. Lévy and Baudouin (53) shortly described the more sterile transcutaneous approach. Long-needed follow-up reports began to appear, with Steward (72) describing relief in 80% of his patients for 12 months or more and Patrick (58) stating that the 500 injections he had done in 150 patients had brought relief from 6 months to 4 years when an effective block was achieved. *Patrick also pointed out the critical fact that the branch to inject or cut is the one supplying the area of the trigger zone, not the one to which the pain is referred, in the infrequent situation in which these are different.*

With respect to technique of these injections, Cushing (13) said, "This is more or less of a gift, and there are no rules to follow. One introduces the needle to the nerve." Others of us have, however, ventured to suggest guidelines for needle placement, the use of which has removed the mystique from the task. Grant (27) developed a special protractor, a "zygometer," to achieve more exact placement. He (27), Sweet and White (86), and Sweet (74), using radiographic control, and Stookey and Ransohoff (73) have given specific directions as to how to reach the supraorbital and infraorbital branches and the maxillary and mandibular divisions, exercises which, however, find but little use today. Combining the reports of five publications, Stookey and Ransohoff gave the average duration of relief in over 1500 patients: supraorbital nerve, 8½ months; infraorbital nerve, 12 months; second division (pterygopalatine fossa), 12 months; and third division, 16 months.

GANGLION OR ROOTLETS

Injections of Alcohol

A few critical, *patient* surgeons have developed the injection of alcohol via the foramen ovale into Meckel's cave, publishing impressive results in huge series of cases. The pioneers are Taptas (81, 82), Harris (33), and Härtel (35). Each of those last two authors produced in their earliest cases transient or lasting palsies of cranial nerves II–XII—even focal seizures or coma. Each concluded independently that once the needle was properly placed, the alcohol should be injected ½ or 1 drop at a time, with careful testing and waiting between each increment so that at the first untoward manifestation the procedure could be stopped. When they used this precaution, permanent paralysis outside the trigeminal domain virtually disappeared. Convincing testimony that Harris' method gave satisfaction was his treatment by 1940 of the enormous total of 2500 cases of idiopathic trigeminal neuralgia, and of Thurel's treatment of over 3000 cases (34, 85, 86, 87). Neither of these men was especially disturbed by the production of corneal anesthesia; indeed, Thurel sought to produce permanent anesthesia of the entire face, including the cornea, in every patient with trigeminal neuralgia who tolerated the numbness produced by alcohol injection of a peripheral branch. Härtel, however, concentrated on how to lower his disturbing incidence of 10–15% neuroparalytic keratitis. This he did by injecting no more than 0.3 ml of 70–80% alcohol at a session and stopping even sooner if the reflex from the lower half of the cornea was decreased. Härtel's caution was not emulated by many other surgeons; the numerous reports describing major percentages with loss of corneal sensation have been summarized by White and Sweet (97).

An analysis of Henderson of his 196 injections of alcohol "supposedly into the Gasserian ganglion" revealed several important new facts. He achieved acutely his objective to produce trigeminal anesthesia in 81% of the patients. He began his injections at the foramen ovale with 2–3 drops of alcohol; then, he advanced the needle by 2- to 3-mm steps, injecting 2–3 more drops at each stopping point until he had secured total sensory loss, or was about 15 mm beyond the base of the skull. The original anesthesia was maintained in only 33% of 86 patients examined 1 or more years later. An astounding pattern of recovery occurred in 37%, *i.e.*, in the third division while the first two divisions remained anesthetic. The reverse pattern of recovery only in the first two divisions was seen in only 7%; recovery occurred in all three divisions in 23%. The greater vulnerability of the first two divisions to toxic fluids injected into Meckel's cave has been confirmed by our experience with glycerol. Henderson (39) also did post-mortem dissections and injections of cresyl violet in absolute alcohol in 100 bodies. Needles passed through the skin "just lateral to the corner of the mouth," directed in the mediolateral or transverse plane toward the pupil, entered the sensory rootlets in only 12 of the 40 specimens. In the other 28, the needle emerged either from the lateral part of the ganglion or completely in front of it. He presented therewith the first critically adduced evidence that the directions given in many publications to point the needle toward the pupil are incorrect in the majority of instances. This error made by so many and the lack of patience and caution required by the later Härtel technique are perhaps the reasons why Gasserian alcohol injection never achieved popularity in the United States, despite its lower mortality than open operation.

Penman (60) in Britain and Ecker and Perl (21, 22) in this country have made several further contributions to the subject. In Ecker's latest report, 7 of 42 corneas had one or more areas of total anesthesia early after injection, but this loss decreased "in the 29 patients examined months or years later."

Injections of Phenol in Glycerine

In order to obtain better control over the injected agent after it leaves the needle, Jefferson (43) changed to 5% phenol in pure glycerine. This hyperbaric fluid remains in Meckel's cave if injected with the patient sitting and head flexed on chest. By 1966 he (44) reported on 50 patients, of whom 12 had developed corneal anesthesia following injection of an average of 0.45 ml of the agent. Chakravorty (9, 10) also has two articles reporting results with phenol and the radiopaque substance myodil in 32 patients. When he violated Jefferson's prescription of testing sensation after each 0.1-ml increment by injecting a full milliliter of 10% phenol, he produced the frightening event of temporary bilateral blindness and unilateral internal and external ophthalmoplegia.

Injections of Pure Glycerine

In August 1975 Sten Håkanson (32) of the Karolinska Institute in Stockholm, working with Lars Leksell, found to their surprise that injection of tantalum dust suspended in pure glycerol, and then injection of glycerol alone into the cerebrospinal fluid of the trigeminal cistern (Meckel's cave), stopped the paroxysmal pains of trigeminal neuralgia without producing any significant sensory loss.

Leksell (52) had published earlier a report of 2 patients relieved of their trigeminal paroxysms by single doses of 1650 or 2250 rads of photons sharply focused to the Gasserian ganglion. Relief persisted at 17 and 18 years with no trigeminal sensory loss.

I am personally indebted to Sten for instruction in his glycerol procedure, about which you will be hearing in detail from Dr. Lunsford. In my experience with the method, a major fraction of the patients do develop clinically obvious sensory loss with 0.15–0.4 ml glycerol injected into the trigeminal cisternal cerebrospinal fluid. Successful use of this method in my hands has included monitoring of that sensory loss after the injection of each 0.05 ml of the glycerol. If V1 anesthesia persists for more than 5 minutes or anesthesia in the trigger zones persists for more than 10 minutes, I empty the glycerol into the posterior fossa by extending the patient's head.

ELECTRICAL HEATING OF TRIGEMINAL GANGLION AND/OR ROOTLETS

Electrosurgical Cauterization

Kirschner (46) of Heidelberg in 1931 first proposed electrocoagulation of the Gasserian ganglion via a needle insulated except at its tip which passed current from a surgical Bovie-type unit. He (47) supplemented this in 1933 with a special frame and aiming apparatus attached to the head when a basal radiograph was taken. Using this device he (48) had been able by 1936 to pass the needle through the foramen ovale at the first thrust in 90 of his last 100 cases. By this method of electrocoagulation he relieved initially 96% of 250 patients. Although at the time of his early report there were recurrences already in 25%, he considered this no disadvantage because of the ease of repeating the procedure. Zenker (99) in Kirschner's clinic reported by 1938 on about 500 patients with 4 deaths. By 1951 Tönnis and Kreissel (89) had seen so many major sequelae of Gasserian electrocoagulation carried out in other clinics that they advised against it. The best results of the method were reported by Thiry (84) in 1962, who passed less current than Kirschner, producing only a hypesthesia or at times no sensory loss. White and Sweet have given many more details (96).

Radiofrequency Heating

An examination of the causes of death after various modifications of the Kirschner procedure and a consideration of advances in both electronics and pharmacology led Sweet in August 1965 to carry out the following procedure. He used a small, 20-gauge lumbar puncture needle insulated except at the tip and placed through the foramen ovale under radiographic control and finally in the appropriate portion of the trigeminal rootlets guided by electrophysiologic stimulation. A thermistor was then substituted for the stylet in the needle, and recordings from it measured the temperature at the tip of the needle electrode. Both the electrode placement and the episodes of heating were carried out with the patient briefly unconscious under IV methohexital. The hope was that heating of the mixed nerve by small increments would produce production of severe hypalgesia to analgesia to pin without anesthesia to touch. These hopes have been largely realized. The method has been widely utilized, with a reduced incidence of major dysesthesias and corneal anesthesia, an initial relief of pain in nearly every case, and a recurrence rate at 5–10 years of around 30% (75, 76, 97). In several series

of over a thousand cases each, there has been no mortality; Sweet and
Poletti (79) have seen no permanent neurological deficit outside the
trigeminal domain.

MEDICAL TREATMENT

The fallback position for therapy short of surgery remained morphine
for many decades. However, even this agent might be prescribed absurdly.
Thus Pancoast and Woodbury recommended "this potent amtidynous
ointment." "Morphine acetate gr 3, atropiae and aconitiae āā gr 1,
Veratriae gr 7, adipis z 3 1 misce. Rx: $\frac{1}{12}$th tsp to be rubbed over the seat
of the pain several times a day." Armand Trousseau (90) ultradistin-
guished Parisian clinician and author of many editions of a complete
text of medicine, emphasizes the disorder's intractability to all medica-
tions, with the possible exception of massive doses of opium. Although
he says "superficial electrical excitation can be of great service in the
treatment of this rebellious disorder," he then adds "unfortunately it is
usually powerless to control the neuralgia and to prevent its return." The
catalog of medicaments and maneuvers which were used month after
month until remission occurred or the patient sought surgery is a tale of
utter and poorly recognized futility, partly because of these spontaneous
remissions. Lasting 1 year or longer, these remissions occurred in 25%
of the 155 patients reported by Rushton and MacDonald (65), and one-
half of them had such a remission of 6 months or longer. Even today
there are "boobs" who recommend acupuncture for this disorder. Over
100 patients I have seen with it had had courses of acupuncture previously. In only 9 was any temporary amelioration described. A second
significant remission did not follow a second series of treatments in any
of the nine cases (77).

Beginning with and probably prior to André, the similarity between
epileptic seizures and the paroxysmal explosive character of the trigeminal pains continued to elicit comment. Indeed, Trousseau preferred the
term "Névralgie epileptiforme" to "tic douloureux." André tried the
anticonvulsant drugs then available without success (2). Rose (64), Head
(37), and Cushing (11), among many others, used "epileptiform neuralgia"
as a synonym for tic douloureux. Oddly enough, no one seems to have
thought of trying modern anticonvulsant drugs until another Frenchman,
Bergouignan (6), proposed Dilantin in 1942. Acknowledging that his
rationale for this was Trousseau's name for the disorder, he recorded
spectacular successes in three cases. Although the title of his article
described "a cure for essential facial neuralgia," this World War II report
went at first unnoticed or disbelieved. However, during the later 1940s

and up to 1958, at least eight other European publications described remissions induced by Dilantin in series of many patients. Apparently unaware of these, Iannone *et al.* (42) in this country in 1958 gave "a preliminary account" of Dilantin's efficiency in 4 patients with trigeminal and one with vagoglossopharyngeal neuralgia. Only one had not secured complete relief. This miserable failure on our part to recognize major contributions in other lands we shall need to correct. This is especially true now that the torches of progress are being snatched from our hands and left to others in consequence of fear of malpractice actions, and the restrictions of the hospital Human Studies Committees and the Federal Drug Administration.

We have in this country reported without so much delay the value of the agent Tegretol, also introduced in Europe. This has for 15 years been the initial therapy of choice for all patients in whom this disorder is suspected. Typically, relief begins in hours to a day or two after the drug is started. White and Sweet (97) gave a brief history of the medical treatments under consideration in 1969. To that list only baclofen, and perhaps Clonazepam, have been added, whereas stilbamidine, anticholinergic drugs, and mephenesin have been dropped.

Since the history of surgical treatments carries with it more valuable lessons for neurosurgeons, I have given medical management short shrift in this account. However, the availability of excellent medical management for many patients puts a greater burden on the neurosurgeon to achieve low risk operative therapies. This I think we have done, especially as I note that the toxic effects of Tegretol are far from zero. The insidious reduction of various aspects of mentation in so many patients on long-continued Tegretol is not as widely recognized as are the bone marrow, hepatic, and renal toxic effects. I personally would not take the drug over the long term, and I point out this potential impairment of drive and alertness to individuals wishing to remain in responsible roles.

ACKNOWLEDGMENTS

The author is indebted to the Neuro-Research Foundation for its support during the preparation of this chapter, and to the Wellcome Institute for the History of Medicine, London, for general provision of five of the oldest texts cited.

REFERENCES

1. Abbé, R. The surgical treatment of inveterate tic douloureux. N.Y. Med. J., *50:* 121–123, 1889.
2. André, N. A. *Observations Pratiques sur les Maladies de L'urèthre et sur Plusieurs Faits Convulsifs, et la Guérison de Plusieurs Maladies Chirurgicales avec la Décomposition d'un Remède Propre à Réprimer la Dissolution Gangréneuse et Cancéreuse, et à la Réparer: avec des Principes Qui Pourront Servir à Employer les Differens Caustiques,* Chez Delaguette. (Imprimeur de Collège et de l'Acad. Roy. de Chir., rue S. Jacq. à l'Olivier, Paris, 1756.)

3. Bartholow, R. *A Practical Treatise on Materia Medica and Therapeutics.* Appleton, New York, 1876.

4. Bell, C. On the nerves: Giving an account of some experiments on their structure and functions, which lead to a new arrangement of the system. Philos. Trans. R. Soc. Lond., *1:* 398–424, 1821.

5. Bell, C. On the nerves of the face, being a second paper on that subject. Philos. Trans. R. Soc. Lond., *1:* 317–330, 1829.

6. Bergouignan, M. Cures heureuses de névralgies faciales essentielles par le diphenylhydantoinate de soude. Rev. Laryngol., *63:* 34–41, 1942.

7. Blum, R. Arrachement du nerf sous-orbitaire. Rev. chir., *2:* 334–335, 1882.

8. Carnochan, J. M. Exsection of the trunk of the second branch of the fifth pair of nerves, beyond the ganglion of Meckel, for severe neuralgia of the face: With three cases. Am. J. Med. Sci., *35:* 134–143, 1858.

9. Chakravorty, B. G. Visual disturbance following fifth nerve ganglion injection. Report of two cases. J. Neurosurg., *23:* 354–356, 1965.

10. Chakravorty, B. G. Phenol in wax as a blocking agent in trigeminal neuralgia. Neurology (Madras), *14:* 85–88, 1966.

11. Cushing, H. A method of total extirpation of the Gasserian ganglion for trigeminal neuralgia. J.A.M.A., *34:* 1035–1041, 1900.

12. Cushing, H. The surgical aspects of major neuralgia of the trigeminal nerve. J.A.M.A., *44:* 773–779; 860–865; 920–929; 1002–1008; 1088–1093, 1905.

13. Cushing, H. The role of deep alcohol injections in the treatment of trigeminal neuralgia. J.A.M.A., *75:* 441–443, 1920a.

14. Cushing, H. The major trigeminal neuralgias and their surgical treatment based on experiences with 332 Gasserian operations. 1. The varieties of facial neuralgia. Am. J. Med. Sci., *160:* 157–184, 1920b.

15. Dandy, W. R. Section of the sensory root of the trigeminal nerve at the pons. Bull. Johns Hopkins Hosp., *36:* 105–106, 1925.

16. Dandy, W. E. An operation for the cure of tic douloureux: Partial section of the sensory root at the pons. Arch. Surg., *18:* 687–734, 1929.

17. Dandy, W. E. The treatment of trigeminal neuralgia by the cerebellar route. Ann. Surg., *96:* 787–795, 1932.

18. Dandy, W. E. Concerning the cause of trigeminal neuralgia. Am. J. Surg., *24:* 447–455, 1934.

19. Dandy, W. E. Intracranial arterial aneurysms, p. 91. Comstock, Ithaca, N.Y., 1944.

20. Doyen, E. L'extirpation du ganglion de Gasser. Arch. Prov. Chir., *4:* 429–444, 1895.

21. Ecker, A. Tic douloureux. Eight years after alcoholic Gasserian injection. N.Y. State Med. J., *74:* 1586–1592, 1974.

22. Ecker, A., and Perl, T. Selective Gasserian injection for tic douloureux. Technical advances and results. Acta Radiol. [Diagn.] (Stockh.), *9:* 38–48, 1969.

23. Fothergill, J. Observations on the use of hemlock. Medical Observations and Inquiries by a Society of Physicians, London, 1773.

24. Fowler, G. R. The operative treatment of facial neuralgia: A comparison of methods and results. Ann. Surg., *3:* 269–320, 1886.

25. Frazier, C. H. A surgeon's impression of trigeminal neuralgia based on experiences with three hundred and two cases. J.A.M.A., *70:* 1345–1350, 1918.

26. Frazier, C. H. Subtotal resection of sensory root for relief of major trigeminal neuralgia. Arch. Neurol. Psychiatry, *13:* 378–384, 1925.

27. Grant, F. C. Anatomic study of injection of second and third divisions of trigeminal nerve. J.A.M.A., *78:* 794–797, 1922.

28. Grant, F. C. Alcoholic injection of second and third divisions of trigeminal nerve. Clinical results with more exact technic. J.A.M.A., *78:* 1780–1781, 1922.

29. Grant, F. C. Discussion of R. Jaeger: The results of injecting hot water into the Gasserian ganglion for the relief of tic douloureux. J. Neurosurg., *16:* 661, 1959.

30. Grant, F. C., and Weinberger, L. M. Experiences with intramedullary tractotomy. IV. Surgery of the brain stem and its operative complications. Surg. Gynecol. Obstet., *72:* 747–754, 1941.

31. Grant, F. C., and Weinberger, L. M. Experiences with intramedullary tractotomy. I. Relief of facial pain and summary of operative results. Arch. Surg., *42,* 681–692, 1941.

32. Håkanson, S. Trigeminal neuralgia by injection of glycerol into the trigeminal cistern. Neurosurgery, *9:* 638–646, 1981.

33. Harris, W. Alcohol injection of the Gasserian ganglion for trigeminal neuralgia. Lancet, *1:* 218–221, 1912.

34. Harris, W. An analysis of 1433 cases of paroxysmal trigeminal neuralgia (trigeminal-tic) and the end-results of Gasserian alcohol injection. Brain, *63:* 209–224, 1940.

35. Härtel, F. Üeber die intracranielle Injektionsbehandlung der Trigeminusneuralgie. Med. Klin., *10:* 582–584, 1914.

36. Hartley, F. Intracranial neurectomy of the second and third divisions of the fifth nerve: A new method. N.Y. Med. J., *55:* 317–319, 1892.

37. Head, H. Trigeminal neuralgia. In: *A System of Medicine,* Vol. 6, edited by T. C. Allbutt, MacMillan, New York, 1900.

38. Henderson, W. R. The anatomy of the Gasserian ganglion and the distribution of pain in relation to injections and operations for trigeminal neuralgia. Ann. R. Coll. Surg. Engl., *37:* 346–373, 1965.

39. Henderson, W. R. Trigeminal neuralgia: The pain and its treatment. Br. Med. J., *1:* 7–15, 1967.

40. Horsley, V., Taylor, J., and Colman, W. S. Remarks on the various surgical procedures devised for the relief or cure of trigeminal neuralgia (tic douloureux). Br. Med. J., *2:* 1139–1143; 1191–1193; 1249–1252, 1891.

41. Hun, H. Analgesia, thermic anaesthesia and ataxia, resulting from foci of softening in the medulla oblongata and cerebellum, due to occlusion of the left inferior posterior cerebellar artery. A study of the course of the sensory and co-ordinating tracts in the medulla oblongata. N.Y. Med. J., *65:* 513–519; 613–620, 1897.

42. Iannone, A., Baker, A. B., and Morrell, F. Dilantin in the treatment of trigeminal neuralgia. Neurology, *8:* 126–128, 1958.

43. Jefferson, A. Trigeminal root and ganglion injections using phenol in glycerine for the relief of trigeminal neuralgia. J. Neurol. Neurosurg. Psychiatry, *26:* 345–352, 1963.

44. Jefferson, A. Trigeminal neuralgia: Trigeminal root and ganglion injections using phenol in glycerin. In: *Pain,* edited by R. S. Knighton and P. R. Dumke, pp. 365–371. Little, Brown, Boston, 1966.

45. Keen, W. W., and Spiller, W. G. Peripheral resection of fifth nerve. Three cases with microscopic examination of the portions of the nerves removed and report on the later condition of patients. J.A.M.A., *34:* 1023–1026, 1900.

46. Kirschner, M. Zur Elektrochirurgie. Arch. Klin. Chir., *167:* 761–768, 1931.

47. Kirschner, M. Die Punktionstechnik und die Elektrokoagulation des Ganglion Gasseri. Arch. Klin. Chir., *176:* 581–620, 1933.

48. Kirschner, M. Zur Behandlung der Trigeminusneuralgie: Erfahrungen an 250 Fällen. Arch. Klin. Chir., *186:* 325–334, 1936.

49. Krause, F. Resection des Trigeminus innerhalb der Schädelhohle. Arch. Klin. Chir., *44:* 821–832, 1892.

50. Krause, F. Entfernung des Ganglion Gasseri und des central davon gelegenen Trige-minusstammes. Dtsch. Med. Wochenschr., *19:* 341–344, 1893.

51. Krönlein. Ueber eine Methode der Resection des zweiten und dritten Astes des N. trigeminus unmittelbar am Foramen rotundum und ovale. Dtsch. Z. Chir., *20:* 484–492, 1884.

52. Leksell, L. Stereotaxic radiosurgery in trigeminal neuralgia. Acta Chir. Scand., *137:* 311–314, 1971.

53. Lévy, F., and Baudouin, A. Les injections profondes dans le traitement de la névralgie faciale rebelle. Presse Méd., *14:* 108–109, 1906.

54. Malgaigne, J-F. Manuel de Médecine Opératoire, Fondée sur l'anatomie normale et l'anatomie pathologique, Ed. 4, pp. 150–154. Germer-Baillière, Paris, 1843.

55. Marchant, G., and Herbet, H. De la résection du ganglion de Gasser dans les névralgies faciales rebelles. Rev. Chir. (Paris), *17:* 287–318, 1897.

56. Neuber, G. Ueber Osmiumsäure-Injectionen bei peripheren Neuralgieen. Mitt. Chir. Klin. Kiel, *1:* 19–23, 1883.

57. Pancoast, J., and Woodbury, F. New operation for the relief of persistent facial neuralgia. Philadelphia Med. Times, *2:* 285–287, 1872.

58. Patrick, H. T. The technic and results of deep injections of alcohol for trifacial neuralgia. J.A.M.A., *58:* 155–163, 1912.

59. Peet, M. M., and Schneider, R. C. Trigeminal neuralgia. A review of six hundred and eighty-nine cases with a follow-up study on sixty-five per cent of the group. J. Neurosurg., *9:* 367–377, 1952.

60. Penman, J. Some developments in the technique of trigeminal injection. Lancet, *1:* 760–764, 1953.

61. Pitres, J. A., and Vaillard, L. Des névrites provoquées par le contact de l'alcool pur ou dilué avec les nerfs vivants. C.R. Soc. Biol. (Paris), *5:* 550–553, 1888.

62. Pudenz, R. H., and Shelden, C. H. Experiences with foraminal decompression in the surgical treatment of tic douloureux. Presented at the American Academy of Neurological Surgery, New York, October 1, 1952.

63. Pujol, A. *Essai sur la Maladie de la Face Nommée le Tic Douloureux, avec quelques Réflexions sur le Raptus Caninus de Coelius Aurelianus, par M. Pujol.* Théophile Barrois, Paris, 1787.

64. Rose, W. Abstract of the Lettsomian lectures on the surgical treatment of trigeminal neuralgia. Lancet, *1:* 71–73; 182–184; 295–302, 1892.

65. Rushton, J. G., and MacDonald, H. N. A. Trigeminal neuralgia. Special considerations of nonsurgical treatment. J.A.M.A., *165:* 437–440, 1957.

66. Schlösser, K. Erfahrungen in der Neuralgiebehandlung mit Alkoholeinspritzungen. Klin Wochenschr., *44:* 533–534, 1907; Verhandel. Kongr. Inn. Med, *24:* 49–55, 1907.

67. Shelden, C. H., Pudenz, R. H., Freshwater, D. B., and Crue, B. L. Compression rather than decompression for trigeminal neuralgia. J. Neurosurg., *12:* 123–126, 1955.

68. Sjöqvist, O. Eine neue Operationsmethode bei Trigeminus-neuralgie: Durchschneidung des Tractus spinalis trigemini. Zentralbl. Neurochir., *2:* 274–281, 1937.

69. Spiller, W. G., and Frazier, C. H. The division of the sensory root of the trigeminus for relief of tic douloureux: An experimental, pathological and clinical study with a preliminary report of one surgically successful case. Philadelphia Med. J., *8:* 1039–1049, 1901.

70. Spiller, W. G., and Frazier, C. H. Tic douloureux: Anatomic and clinical basis for subtotal section of sensory root of trigeminal nerve. Arch. Neurol. Psychiatry, *29:* 50–55, 1933.

71. Stender, A. "Gangliolysis" for the surgical treatment of trigeminal neuralgia. J. Neurosurg., *11:* 333–336, 1954.

72. Stewart, P. Tic douloureux: The technique and results of Schlösser's method of treatment. Br. Med. J., *2:* 848–851, 1909.

73. Stookey, B., and Ransohoff, J. *Trigeminal Neuralgia.* Charles C Thomas, Springfield, Ill., 1959.
74. Sweet, W. H. Trigeminal injection with radiographic control: Technic and results. J.A.M.A., *142:* 392–396, 1950.
75. Sweet, W. H. Trigeminal neuralgias. In: *Facial Pain,* edited by C. C. Alling, pp. 89–106. Lea & Febiger, Philadelphia, 1968.
76. Sweet, W. H. Treatment of facial pain by percutaneous differential thermal trigeminal rhizotomy. In: *Progress in Neurological Surgery,* Vol. 7, edited by H. Krayenbühl, P. E. Maspes, and W. H. Sweet, pp. 153–179. S. Karger, Basel, Switzerland, 1976.
77. Sweet, W. H. Some current problems in pain research and therapy (including needle puncture, "acupuncture"). Pain, *10:* 297–309, 1981.
78. Sweet, W. H., Graham, J. R., and Poletti, C. E. Periodic (chronic) migrainous neuralgia. (Chronic) cluster headache. Presented at the International Association for the Study of Pain, Seattle, Washington, August and September, 1984.
79. Sweet, W. H., and Poletti, C. E. Comparison between radiofrequency heat and glycerol lesions in the treatment of trigeminal neuralgia. Presented at the American Association of Neurological Surgeons, San Francisco, April 10, 1984.
80. Taarnhøj, P. Decompression of the trigeminal root and posterior part of the ganglion as treatment in trigeminal neuralgia. Preliminary communication. J. Neurosurg., *9:* 288–290, 1952.
81. Taptas, N. Les injections d'alcool dans le ganglion de Gasser à travers le trou ovale. Presse méd., *19:* 798–799, 1911.
82. Taptas, N. Maux de Tête et Névralgies. In: *Douleurs Craniofaciales.* Masson & Cie, Paris, 1953.
83. Thiersch, C. Ueber Extraction von Nerven, mit Vorzeigung von Präparaten. Verhandl. Dtsch. Ges. Chir., *18:* 44–52, 1889.
84. Thiry, S. Expérience personnelle basée sur 225 cas de névralgie essentielle du trijumeau traités par électrocoagulation stéréotaxique du ganglion de Gasser entre 1950 et 1960. Neurochirurgie, *8:* 86–92, 1962.
85. Thurel, R. Névralgie faciale et alcoolisation du ganglion de Gasser. Semin. Ther., *37:* 608–610, 1961; also Rev. Neurol., *104:* 75–77, 1961a.
86. Thurel, R. Alcoolisation du ganglion de Gasser et diffusion de l'alcool aux formations nerveuses du voisinage. Rev. Neurol., *104:* 78–79, 1961b.
87. Thurel, R. Névralgie faciale et sclérose en plaques. Rev. Neurol., *105:* 346–347, 1961c.
88. Tiffany, L. M. Intracranial operations for the cure of facial neuralgia. Ann. Surg., *24:* 575–619; 736–748, 1896.
89. Tönnis, W., and Kreissel, H. Die Bedeutung einer sorgfältigen Differentialdiagnose für die chirurgische Behandlung der Trigeminusneuralgie. Dtsch. Med. Wochenschr., *76:* 1202–1205, 1951.
90. Trousseau, A. Névralgie éileptiforme. In: *Clinique Médicale de L'Hotel-Dieu de Paris,* Vol. 2, pp. 156–167. Librairie J.-B. Baillière et Fils, Paris, 1877.
91. van Gehuchten, A. (transl. by W. G. Spiller). Surgical treatment of trifacial neuralgia. Univ. Penn. Med. Bull., *17:* 50–59, 1904.
92. Vogt, P. Die Nerven-Dehnung als Operation in der chirurgischen Praxis. In: *Eine experimentelle und klinische Studie,* pp. 69–73. F. C. W. Vogel, Leipzig, 1877.
93. von Klein, A. Ueber die Möglichkeit der Zerstörung des Gesichtsnerven bei seinem Austritt aus dem Schädel. J. Chir. Augenlt., *3:* 46–61, 1822.
94. Warren, J. C. Cases of neuralgia, or painful affections of nerves. Boston Med. Surg. J., *1:* 1–6, 1828.
95. Weber, O. Cited by Rose, p. 72, 1631.
96. White, J. C., and Sweet, W. H. *Pain: Its Mechanisms and Neurosurgical Control,* pp.

192–193. Charles C Thomas, Springfield, Ill., 1955.

97. White, J. C., and Sweet, W. H. *Pain and the Neurosurgeon. A Forty Year Experience*, pp. 96, 157–165, 169–178, 185–187, 193–196, 197–207, 208–210, 232–251, 447–449, 463, Charles C Thomas, Springfield, Ill., 1969.

98. Young, R. F., and Perryman, K. M. Rostral trigeminal brainstem lesions abolish dental pain in Macaque. Presented at the American Association of Neurological Surgeons Meeting, San Francisco, April 1984.

99. Zenker, R. I. Behandlung der Trigeminusneuralgie unter besonder Berücksichtigung der Grundlagen, der Ausführung und der Ergebnisse der Punktion und Elektrokoagulation des Ganglion Gasseri nach Kirschner. Ergeb. Chir. Orthop., *31:* 1–82, 1938.

CHAPTER

16

Choice of Surgical Therapeutic Modalities for Treatment of Trigeminal Neuralgia: Microvascular Decompression, Percutaneous Retrogasserian Thermal, or Glycerol Rhizotomy

L. DADE LUNSFORD, M.D., and RONALD I. APFELBAUM, M.D.

Surely one of the most horrid afflictions in its full fury, trigeminal neuralgia affects an estimated 15,000 new people per year in the United States (11). This paroxysmal condition of the nervous system is generally responsive to both medical and surgical therapy. Rarely are cachectic, end-stage tic douloureux patients now seen, since effective medical therapies including carbamazepine and phenytoin, and secondary drugs such as baclofen almost always can ameliorate some of the pain or the frequency of attacks. Improved surgical techniques also have evolved over the past several decades, allowing excellent pain control with fewer risks and side effects than ever before. Surgery, therefore, should not be withheld if patients become refractory to or intolerant of medical therapy.

Few diseases of solitary nerves have been subjected to more ingenious attacks than trigeminal neuralgia. To obtain relief, the trigeminal nerve, ganglion, or tract has been frozen, boiled, pickled, massaged, resected, decompressed and, more recently, even inflated (Table 16.1) (20). Each treatment has proven beneficial to many patients, and each treatment has reflected technology available for its era. Neurosurgeons should take heart that so many effective treatments have been devised but also must recall those patients whose tic douloureux has been eliminated, only to be replaced by the fearful and virtually untreatable result of trigeminal deafferentation, anesthesia dolorosa.

Current concepts of treatment for trigeminal neuralgia reflect emerging knowledge about etiology and pathogenesis. In many patients, trigeminal neuralgia is associated with arterial or venous vascular compression, strategically located at the junction of the nerve with the pons (root entry zone), where central myelin merges into peripheral myelin (14). This leads to localized demyelination and altered physiology within the trigeminal system which has been described as neural short-circuiting or ephap-

TABLE 16.1

Surgical Options for Treating Trigeminal Neuralgia

Type of Therapy	Site	Technique
Ablative	Peripheral nerve	Local blocks
		Phenol
		Alcohol
		Avulsion (neurectomy)
	Gasserian ganglion	Subtemporal section
		Radiofrequency rhizotomy
		Balloon compression
	Retrogasserian (postganglionic) nerve	Radiofrequency rhizotomy
		Glycerol rhizotomy
	Root entry zone	Selective nerve section
	Brain stem	Tractotomy
Nonablative	Gasserian ganglion	Mechanical, rubbing
	Root entry zone	Microvascular decompression (MVD)

tic transmission (15) but in reality is probably more complex (8). Therapy directed at removal of the offending vessel (microvascular decompression (MVD)), while eliminating the etiologic factor, does not guarantee that the abnormal axonal transmission will be prevented, since this presumably requires remyelinization to occur.

Other causes of pain resembling tic douloureux also have been noted. Neoplastic lesions of the cerebellopontine angle can result in neural compression directly or can displace vessels across the nerve. Direct surgical attack, when feasible in these cases, may not only cure the trigeminal neuralgia but also prevent other symptoms due to further tumor growth and the resultant neural compromise. In 1–2% of patients with multiple sclerosis, demyelination with plaque formation at the root entry zone results in trigeminal neuralgia. This condition requires treatment other than vascular decompression.

Not all patients will be able to undergo posterior fossa exploration and MVD because of medical infirmity or advanced age. At the present time sufficient evidence has accumulated to suggest that 60–80% of patients with tic douloureux can have long-term (possibly permanent) elimination of pain, and as many as 95% can be relieved initially by surgery but may have some recurrences (4, 5, 14, 26). Pain can be eliminated without the need to totally destroy facial sensation in most patients, regardless of whether percutaneous or open neurosurgical procedures are selected.

The final decision regarding surgical modalities can only be made by the patient after he has had a full explanation of all the options, including the benefits and risks of each. The surgeon can offer a recommendation, but it is the patient who on one hand is suffering with the pain but who, on the other hand, must accept the risks and live with the sequelae of treatment.

MICROVASCULAR DECOMPRESSION OF THE TRIGEMINAL ROOT ENTRY ZONE

A vascular etiology of tic douloureux in many patients was noted originally by Dandy (9), confirmed by Gardner (10), and thoroughly verified by the work of Jannetta (12–14). Jannetta deserves the credit for extending these observations and suggesting that relief of pain was possible by moving or removing the offending vessel while sparing the nerve. Subsequently his observations and conclusions were confirmed by many others (1, 5, 26). With this approach, employing microscopic illumination, magnification, and microsurgical technique, a potential surgical cure became possible for at least the most common cause of tic douloureux: vascular compression (Fig. 16.1). Although posterior fossa exploration by retromastoid craniectomy and MVD is generally well tolerated, we now tend to restrict this approach to patients younger than 65 years and to those without significant additional medical or systemic risk factors, such as poorly controlled hypertension or coronary artery disease. Others (5) have operated on patients well into their 90s by this approach, apparently without complications, but our personal experience indicates higher risk in the older age group.

Long-term results suggest that MVD is effective, resulting in complete and longlasting relief of tic douloureux in about 70% of patients followed for up to 10 years (Table 16.2). An additional 20% of patients can expect improvement but may have recurrent, though medically controllable, pain. The vast majority of these patients have no change in facial sensation after surgery, and no cases of anesthesia dolorosa have been reported. Other cranial nerve deficits have been reduced to less than 5% and are most often transient, except for those related to hearing reduction. Mortality rates have declined from 3% to virtually zero in experienced hands. Jannetta (13) has reported no mortality in the last 200 patients in his series. One of the authors (R.I.A.) noted no deaths in his early experience (1), but recently has reported an overall 1% mortality rate (4), although none occurred in the last 110 patients (4½ years).

The operative technique has become relatively standardized at the University of Pittsburgh, where surgery is performed in the lateral decubitus position. This position has eliminated the need for central venous pressure (CVP) line placement and bladder catheterization. Jan-

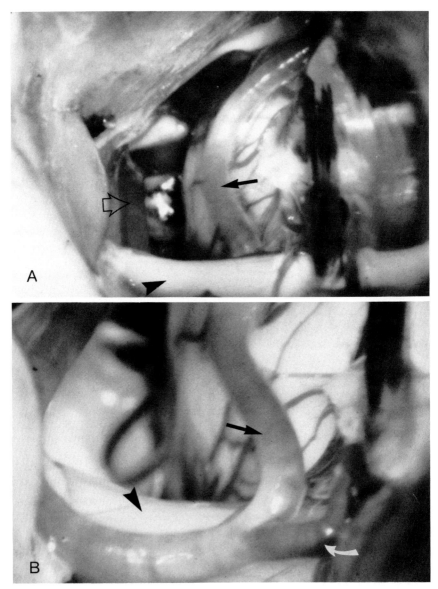

FIG. 16.1. Typical vascular cross-compression of the root entry zone of the trigeminal nerve by a loop of the superior cerebellar artery (SCA), resulting in lower division (maxillary and mandibular) tic douloureux. (*A*) Loop of SCA (*open arrow,* proximal portion; *closed arrow,* a distal branch of the artery) prior to decompressing the left trigeminal nerve (*arrowhead*). (*B*) Same vessel dissected free of the root entry zone. A second distal branch (*curved arrow*) which was embedded in the anterior surface of the nerve is now seen.

TABLE 16.2
Surgical Options for Trigeminal Neuralgia[a]

Technique	Long-term Results (Excellent Relief) (%)[a]	No. of Cases	Published Series (Date)	Average Length or Range of Follow-up (yr)
Microvascular decompression (MVD)	83.8	411	Jannetta (14) (1981)	3–16
	70.4	289	Apfelbaum (4) (1984)	5.2
	73.0	37	Barba and Alksne (5) (1984)	3.5
	84.0	50	Van Loveren, Tew et al. (26) (1982)	3
Percutaneous retrogasserian radiofrequency rhizotomy (PRRR)	72	484	Sweet (23) (1976)	4.5–9
	61	700	Van Loveren, Tew, et al. (26) (1982)	6
	75	135	Siegfried (22) (1981)	5–7
	77	643	Nugent (21) (1982)	4–7
	52	96	Latchaw et al. (16) (1983)	5
	35	78	Burchiel et al. (7) (1981)	5
Percutaneous retrogasserian glycerol rhizotomy (PRGR)	69	100	Håkanson (11) (1983)	2.5
	67	112	Lunsford (19) (1984)	1.5

[a] Pain free or rare pain not requiring medication.

netta and his associates have used shredded Teflon felt as the implant placed between the nerve, vessel, and brain stem. This agent is easy to manipulate and promotes minimal arachnoidal scarring, in contrast to muscle. One of the authors (R.I.A.), however, prefers the semisitting position but also has eliminated CVP catheters (3). Ivalon and shredded Teflon felt are both used, depending on the anatomy. We feel that absorbable material such as muscle and Gelfoam should not be used. At present, the role and dosage of perioperative corticosteroid administration is being investigated. Between 3 and 7 days after surgery, approximately 20% of patients will develop a benign aseptic meningeal reaction characterized by headache, meningismus, and culture-negative CSF pleocytosis. This condition responds promptly to spinal tap and a 2- or 3-day course of oral corticosteroids.

MVD done by surgeons experienced in posterior fossa surgery is an excellent treatment for tic douloureux; it attacks the etiology of the tic in many patients and reduces the risk of facial deafferentation. Recent evidence that prior deafferentation procedures may significantly reduce the subsequent likelihood of benefit from MVD (5) may mitigate for early or primary treatment of tic by MVD if no other contraindications exist and the patient so desires. MVD probably has a greater likelihood of longlasting pain relief than any other procedure (7). This is a real consideration in the younger patient.

PERCUTANEOUS RETROGASSERIAN RADIOFREQUENCY RHIZOTOMY (PRRR)

Selective destruction of the postganglionic retrogasserian trigeminal nerve by graded radiofrequency lesions has become a benchmark by which new therapies for tic douloureux can be compared. Originally designed by Sweet and Wepsic (25), using temperature-monitored electrodes of a rather large size, relatively large lesions were created. This procedure has also been called radiofrequency lesioning, radiofrequency trigeminal neurolysis, radiofrequency gangliolysis, or thermocoagulation stereotaxic rhizotomy. Radiofrequency rhizotomy recently has undergone several technical modifications that significantly have reduced the complications associated with earlier experiences (26). Usage of an angled smaller electrode has allowed more precise exploration and lesioning of the various divisions (Fig. 16.2). While temperature monitoring has been claimed to add more precise control of the lesion capability, Nugent (21) has reported long-term success using a 6-mm angled cordotomy electrode without using temperature monitoring (21). His experience extends to more than 700 patients with follow-up up to 10 years. We concur with

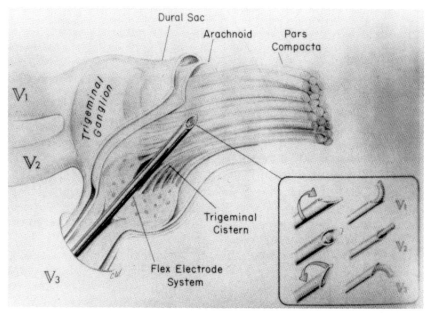

FIG. 16.2. Technical modification of the electrode system for percutaneous retrogasserian radiofrequency rhizotomy, allowing temperature monitoring during lesioning. (Reproduced with permission from: H. Van Loveren *et al.* (26).)

Nugent's observation that the smaller electrode allows more precise lesions with less postoperative sensory loss.

PRRR must be performed with a cooperative patient who can respond appropriately to physiological stimulation during the procedure. Local anesthesia, supplemented by ultrafast-acting barbiturates and narcotics such as fentanyl, are sufficient for transovale needle placement, but a delicate balance is required to provide patient comfort, reduce anxiety, and still retain cooperation. Once lost, lack of patient cooperation may lead to lesioning in unwanted locations or insufficient lesions. Long-term results are variable and may reflect the degree of facial sensory loss (both analgesia and anesthesia) since the best results reported (92% long-term relief) have occurred with creation of dense lesions but at the expense of an approximate 6% risk of anesthesia dolorosa (23). Long-term control rates as low as 35% at 5 years have been reported (7, 16). Nonetheless, it may be better to risk recurrence and yet retain a good method of treatment by repeat operation, rather than risk anesthesia dolorosa, a condition for which virtually no treatment exists.

To date, despite the large number of patients treated by this technique since 1974, virtually no experimental animal or human autopsy data exist regarding the extent and nature of radiofrequency lesions of the trigeminal nerve. We believe that the most appropriate target site for trigeminal radiofrequency lesion is the retrogasserian trigeminal nerve, not the gasserian ganglion. Destruction of the cell bodies themselves may be associated with greatly increased incidence of postoperative deafferentation pain. It remains unclear as to whether PRRR effects are primarily against the C fiber or A delta fiber population mediating the pain response, or whether fast-conducting (light touch) fiber pathways must be lesioned as well in order to reduce the trigger mechanism. It is obvious, however, that PRRR provides symptomatic relief in many patients without directly attacking the etiology of tic douloureux. This treatment has enjoyed widespread success (22) but is dependent upon sophisticated lesion generating equipment and fine cordotomy or temperature-monitored electrodes. In addition it requires, at the very least, a cooperative patient.

Finally, during our performance of trigeminal cisternography using metrizamide in more than 275 patients, we have been distressed to confirm that seemingly appropriate transovale needle placement, and egress of CSF does not ensure that a needle is successfully placed within the trigeminal cistern of Meckel's cave (17). Cisternography occasionally has shown subtemporal or subdural needle placement. In such patients subsequent stimulation with an electrode in these locations resulted in referred pain to the ophthalmic or maxillary divisions of the nerve. Thus, stimulation may be useful but is not always a sufficient indicator of proper intracisternal retrogasserian trigeminal needle placement.

Burchiel et al. (7) have summarized some advantages of radiofrequency rhizotomy: (a) avoiding the risks of craniotomy and general anesthesia; (b) virtually no risk of mortality; and (c) reduced expense. These benefits must be balanced against the discomfort of the procedure and the sensory loss produced, which often is significant, and may include the cornea and the well-documented dysesthetic sequelae.

PERCUTANEOUS RETROGASSERIAN GLYCEROL RHIZOTOMY (PRGR)

Håkanson (11) first demonstrated the benefit of glycerol injection into the postganglionic fibers of the trigeminal nerve as a treatment for tic douloureux. This procedure uses chemical rather than thermal injury to the nerve. His approach is predicted on anatomic rather than physiological confirmation of proper needle placement within the cistern of Meckel's cave after transovale needle placement (Fig. 16.3). Trigeminal cisternography performed with a water-soluble contrast agent (presently metrizamide, 300 mg iodine per ml) remains the only method to both confirm the proper target and estimate the cistern size so that the volume of glycerol needed for pain relief can be determined. Furthermore, metri-

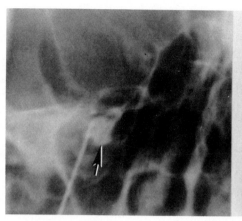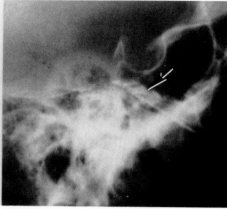

FIG. 16.3. Intraoperative trigeminal cisternogram with metrizamide (300 mg iodine per ml, total volume 0.25 ml). Proper delineation of both the size and location of the cistern is mandatory prior to glycerol injection. (Reproduced with permission from: L. D. Lunsford and M. H. Bennett (19).)

zamide can be used to spare the lower division trigeminal fibers from the glycerol effects when only upper division fibers are to be treated (11, 18). A normal constituent of human plasma, glycerol in 99% anhydrous form, is a weak neurolytic alcohol. The mechanism of action of glycerol has not been completely resolved since both large fiber and small populations can be affected by the glycerol (19, 24). Sweet and Poletti (24) noted changes in the late component evoked response measurements, presumably mediating the slower conducting C-fiber afferents (19). However, in our view the most likely explanation of relief after glycerol rhizotomy lies in selective destruction of the previously damaged large fiber population that can be implicated in the etiology of tic douloureux, and in part may be responsible for the trigger mechanism (6, 19). We have found that the trigeminal evoked response measurements that reflect fast fiber activity tend to improve after successful rhizotomy, indicating that glycerol attacks the presumably abnormal partially demyelinated fibers and perhaps leaves a pool of more normally conducting fibers in order to restore the trigeminal evoked potential towards normal (19). Recent experience with trigeminal rhizotomy using glycerol injected into the retrogasserian trigeminal nerve in cats has shown significant large and small fiber effects and can result in complete elimination of the trigeminal evoked response if efficient lesions develop in maxillary portions of the nerve (6).

The initial experience of one of the authors (L.D.L.) with PRGR has been reported (18, 19). At the University of Pittsburgh 225 patients have been treated by glycerol rhizotomy, many of whom had already relapsed after prior surgical treatments. Sixty-five percent remain pain free at follow-up, extending to 3 years, although a few patients have required a repeat procedure. The majority note no major increase in postoperative facial sensory loss. Patients with prior deafferentation procedure and those who develop postoperative eruptions of herpes simplex perioralis are most likely to develop increased sensory loss. No patient in this series has developed anesthesia dolorosa, although 6% did develop annoying paresthesias or frank dysesthesias when surgery resulted in significant facial deafferentation or severe postoperative herpes simplex perioralis eruptions occurred.

The experience of the other author (R.I.A.), although less extensive, is similar. Seventy-three patients have been treated at Montefiore Medical Center, New York City, by this modality over the last 26 months. Complete pain relief was achieved in 86% after one procedure and in 90% of patients after two procedures (usually repeated within 2–4 weeks). The average duration of follow-up of these patients was 15 months, with 16 recurrences noted (23%). No recurrences have yet occurred in patients who had two procedures. Nine of these patients could not be controlled by medication. Repeat PRGR in seven and a PRRR in another gave good relief, so that 89% of patients treated at Montefiore Medical Center (R.I.A.) remained completely pain free at follow-up.

Facial sensory loss was absent or slight in most patients but six had substantial loss, including three cases of corneal anesthesia. Dysesthesia, however, rarely occurred, and when it did it was only of major intensity in two patients. No cases of anesthesia dolorosa have yet been seen. This is in sharp contradistinction to our previous series of 130 patients with PRRR, wherein we observed 21% incidence of numbness, with an 18% incidence of decreased corneal sensation and 20% dysesthesia and a 4% incidence of anesthesia or analgesic dolorosa.

The procedure has been well described (11). We have found no reason to alter Håkanson's original procedure other than to perform it in an operating room or radiographic suite with anesthesia in attendance. High quality intraoperative imaging with hard copy films is mandatory. This can be achieved with a C-arm (as preferred by L.D.L.) or by using a standard fluoroscope and implementing the hanging head position (as preferred by R.I.A.) (2). No percutaneous procedure, especially if it is performed in elderly or medically infirm patients, is free of stress: approximately 15% of patients developed signs of increased vagal output, resulting in anything from brief bradycardia to profound slowing and hypotension after manipulation of the trigeminal nerve. We accordingly premedicate our patients with an anticholinergic (Atropine or Robinul) and an anxiolytic (Vistaril, L.D.L.) or with Droperidol (0.075 mg/kg,

R.I.A.), begin sedation with fentanyl (0.5–3 ml), and now frequently add methohexital sodium (Brevital) in 10-mg I.V. increments during needle placement. The only perioperative mortality in our combined experience occurred at the University of Pittsburgh in a 77-year-old patient who suffered a fatal myocardial infarction in the recovery room.

Whenever a new procedure is introduced for treatment of facial pain, expanded indications and technical variations are subsequently suggested. We have reviewed many of these and find them to offer no advantages. PRGR is not recommended for patients with atypical trigeminal neuralgia or atypical facial pain. It does not work in these conditions and occasionally may exacerbate such problems, especially when additional facial deafferentation is superimposed upon the original pain problem. Large volumes of glycerol injected until facial sensory loss develops represent no advantage over radiofrequency rhizotomy, and in fact, represent a less well-controlled way to make a trigeminal lesion. The amount of glycerol injected is dependent upon the cisternal volume and divisions affected (17–19). No advantage to prophylactic treatment of presently unaffected divisions has emerged in our experience, since the procedure is relatively simple to perform and can be easily repeated. Approximately 10% of patients selected for glyerol rhizotomy will be found to have a suboptimal cisternogram or improper needle placement. In such cases, glycerol should not be injected. Rather, it has been our practice to attempt glycerol rhizotomy as a second procedure using an 18-gauge needle instead of a 20-gauge spinal needle. If an abnormal cisternogram is encountered, an angled cordotomy electrode can be introduced through the needle for radiofrequency rhizotomy after physiological testing. When easy penetration of the foramen ovale is followed by free emergence of CSF and a normal cisternal appearance after metrizamide injection, we can confidently predict that patients with tic douloureux will have relief in more than 95% of cases. Complete relief will be sustained in more than 75% of cases followed for up to 3 years. Recurrence may reflect further ongoing demyelination of the trigeminal nerve, regardless of whether the demyelination is due to cross-compression or other mechanisms.

SELECTION OF A SURGICAL THERAPY FOR TRIGEMINAL NEURALGIA

Surgical therapy (Fig. 16.4) is reserved for patients refractory to or toxic from medical treatment. Several variables should be discussed with the patient and should enter the decision tree for surgical therapy (Table 16.3). We now tend to reserve MVD for those patients less than 65 years of age, although older patients who are "physiologically younger" may be candidates, as may those older than 65, when percutaneous treatment fails.

SURGICAL OPTIONS FOR TRIGEMINAL NEURALGIA

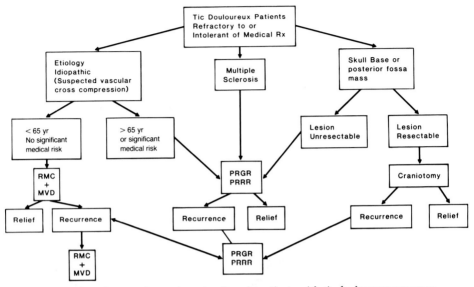

FIG. 16.4. Decision tree for treatment options in patients with tic douloureux unresponsive to or intolerant of medical therapy. *RMC + MVD*, retromastoid craniectomy and microvascular decompression.

TABLE 16.3

Variables in Surgical Choices for Trigeminal Neuralgia

Type	Variable	Surgical Choice
Age	<65	MVD
	>65	PRGR
		PRRR
Associated conditions	Multiple sclerosis	PRGR
	Intracranial mass (unresectable)	PRRR
	Medical infirmity	
Prior surgical treatment for tic	Minor sensory loss	MVD, PRRR, PRGR
	Major sensory loss	MVD
Psychological status	Major anxiety (general anesthesia recommended)	MVD
		PRGR
	Minor anxiety (I.V. sedation sufficient)	PRGR
		PRRR

Previously, one of us (R.I.A.) was offering MVD to patients up to the age of 72. An analysis of complications indicates that a disproportionate number of these occurred in those patients over age 65, including two of our three fatalities. With the introduction of PRGR, with its lowered incidence of facial numbness and dysesthesia, we have therefore lowered the "cut off" age. However, those patients with a history of prior destructive surgery for tic douloureux may also warrant MVD if major facial sensory loss is already present, since the addition of further deafferentation may greatly increase the risk of anesthesia dolorosa.

Percutaneous therapy is recommended as the procedure of choice for patients with tic associated with multiple sclerosis, significant medical infirmities, or unresectable intracranial masses. Patients with multiple sclerosis fare well after either glycerol or radiofrequency lesion, but patients with arteriovenous malformations have responded much less satisfactorily after glycerol (19).

We prefer to start with PRGR when a percutaneous approach is indicated. The procedure is much less painful for the patient, doesn't require him to make discriminatory judgments, and is usually quicker. More importantly, however, PRGR produces significantly less facial sensory loss and significantly less dysesthesia than PRRR while providing equal initial relief. If localization within the trigeminal cistern cannot be obtained on two separate occasions, then a radiofrequency lesioning is performed.

The patient's mental state and cooperation is obviously important for satisfactory performance of any procedure. Those with moderate anxiety can be sedated well for either glycerol or radiofrequency rhizotomy, but when excessive anxiety is detected, general anesthesia should be considered. Microvascular decompression and glycerol rhizotomy can be performed with the patient asleep.

CONCLUSION

There are several excellent treatments for tic douloureux. A procedure can best be recommended after considering the patient's age, associated conditions, general health, state of facial sensation, acceptance of associated risks, and response to prior surgical procedures, if any. No doubt additional surgical procedures will be added to the armamentarium in the future. Present evidence indicates that most patients with tic douloureux can be made pain free by surgery and that they may retain either normal or minimally reduced facial sensation. There seems to be little benefit to creating extensive facial deafferentation by surgery simply to relieve tic douloureux, an eminently treatable symptom complex that has fascinated the medical world for more than 300 years.

REFERENCES

1. Apfelbaum, R. I. A comparison of percutaneous radiofrequency trigeminal neurolysis and microvascular decompression of the trigeminal nerve for the treatment of tic douloureux. Neurosurgery, 1: 16–21, 1977.

2. Apfelbaum, R. I. Technical considerations for facilitation of selective percutaneous radiofrequency neurolysis of the trigeminal nerve. Neurosurgery, *3:* 396–399, 1978.

3. Apfelbaum, R. I. Surgical management of disorders of the lower cranial nerve. In: *Operative Neurosurgical Techniques.* Vol. 2, edited by H.H. Schmidek and W.H. Sweet. New York, Grune & Stratton, 1982, pp. 1063–1082.

4. Apfelbaum, R. I. Surgery for tic douloureux. Clin. Neurosurg., *31:* 667–683, 1984.

5. Barba, D., and Alksne, J. F. Success of microvascular decompression with and without prior surgical therapy for trigeminal neuralgia. J. Neurosurg., *60:* 104–107, 1984.

6. Bennett, M. H., and Lunsford, L. D. Percutaneous retrogasserian glycerol rhizotomy for tic douloureux. Part 2. Results and implications of trigeminal evoked potential studies. Neurosurgery, *14:* 431–435, 1984.

7. Burchiel, K. J., Steege, T. D., Howe, J. F., and Loeser, J. D. Comparison of percutaneous radiofrequency gangliolysis and microvascular decompression for the surgical management of tic douloureux. Neurosurgery, *9:* 111–119, 1981.

8. Calvin, W. H., Loeser, J. D. and Howe, J. F. A neurophysiological theory for the pain mechanism of tic douloureux. Pain, *3:* 147–154, 1977.

9. Dandy, W. E. Treatment of trigeminal neuralgia by the cerebellar route. Ann. Surg., *96:* 787–795, 1932.

10. Gardner, W. J. Concerning the mechanism of trigeminal neuralgia and hemifacial spasm. J. Neurosurg., *19:* 947–958, 1962.

11. Håkanson, S. Retrogasserian glycerol injection as a treatment of tic douloureux. Adv. Pain Res. Ther., *5:* 927–933, 1983.

12. Jannetta, P. J. Observation on the etiology of trigeminal neuralgia, hemifacial spasm, acoustic nerve dysfunction, and glossopharyngeal neuralgia. Definitive microsurgical treatment and results in 117 patients. Neurochirurgica, *20:* 145–154, 1977.

13. Jannetta, P. J. Microvascular decompression for trigeminal neuralgia. Surg. Rounds, *6:* 24–35, 1983.

14. Jannetta, P. J. Vascular decompression in trigeminal neuralgia. In: *The Cranial Nerves,* edited by M. Samii and P. J. Jannetta, pp. 331–340. New York, Springer-Verlag, 1981.

15. Kerr, W. L., and Miller, R. H. The pathology of trigeminal neuralgia. Arch. Neurol., *15:* 308–319, 1966.

16. Latchaw, J. P., Hardy, R. W., Forsythe, S. B., and Cook, A. F. Trigeminal neuralgia treated by radiofrequency coagulation. J. Neurosurg., *59:* 479–484, 1983.

17. Lunsford, L. D. Identification of Meckel cave during percutaneous glycerol rhizotomy for tic douloureux. A.J.N.R., *3:* 680–682, 1982.

18. Lunsford, L. D. Treatment of tic douloureux by percutaneous retrogasserian glycerol injection. J.A.M.A., *248:* 449–453, 1982.

19. Lunsford, L. D., and Bennett, M. H. Percutaneous retrogasserian glycerol rhizotomy for tic douloureux. Part 1. Technique and results in 112 patients. Neurosurgery, *14:* 424–430, 1984.

20. Mullan, S., and Lichton, T. Percutaneous microcompression of the trigeminal ganglion for trigeminal neuralgia. J. Neurosurg., *59:* 1007–1012, 1983.

21. Nugent, G. R. Technique and results of 800 percutaneous radiofrequency thermocoagulations for trigeminal neuralgia. Appl. Neurophysiol., *45:* 504–507, 1982.

22. Siegfried, J. Percutaneous controlled thermocoagulation of Gasserian ganglion in trigeminal neuralgia. Experience with 1000 cases. In: *The Cranial Nerves,* edited by M. Samii and P. J. Jannetta, pp. 322–330. Springer-Verlag, New York, 1981.

23. Sweet, W. H. Treatment of facial pain by percutaneous differential thermal trigeminal rhizotomy. Prog. Neurol. Surg., *7:* 153–179, 1976.

24. Sweet, W. H., and Poletti, C. E. Retrogasserian glycerol injection as a treatment for

trigeminal neuralgia. In: *Operative Neurosurgical Techniques,* edited by H. H. Schmidek and W. H. Sweet, pp. 1107–1112, Grune & Stratton, New York, 1982.

25. Sweet, W. H., and Wepsic, J. G. Controlled thermocoagulation of trigeminal ganglion and rootlets for differential destruction of pain fibers. Part 1. Trigeminal neuralgia. J. Neurosurg., *40:* 143–156, 1974.

26. Van Loveren, H., Tew, J. M., Keller, J. T., and Nurre, M. A. A 10 year experience in the treatment of trigeminal neuralgia. Comparison of percutaneous stereotaxic rhizotomy and posterior fossa exploration. J. Neurosurg., *57:* 757–764, 1982.

17

Management of the Failed Patient with Trigeminal Neuralgia

PETER J. JANNETTA, M.D., and DAVID J. BISSONETTE, P.A.-C.

Failure, relative or absolute, is a common end result of many human endeavors and is frequently easier to deal with than success. Such is human nature. Currently, in most areas of surgery and neurosurgery, our endeavors are successful for the great majority of patients. Failure in a life-threatening disease is more acceptable to us than in nonlethal problems. The patient with complications of a nonlethal nature, having a severe problem, and especially with the side effects of our treatment, becomes a frustrating embarrassment to us. This can occur despite the fact that we have done our well-intentioned best. Neurosurgeons would like to be perfect and, like all physicians, want our patients to do well. A "failed" patient is a signal that we are not perfect and that the forces of nature have again outwitted us. We cannot hide these failures, avoid them, or ignore them. Rather, we can learn from them and, frequently, can make the patients feel better or even cure them.

As we collect data on our patient series, we gather information potentially useful to our subsequent patients. It is unfortunate that better results are submitted for publication more frequently than series with bad results, as this sets unrealistic standards which are then compared unfavorably with one's own (unpublished) patient results. Perhaps neurosurgery, like diving competitions, should have a "degree of difficulty" in the formulae for evaluation of success or failure.

As we do and must deal with data when evaluating the results of patient care, we must ensure that these data are as complete, precise, and as accurate as possible. Errors creep into analyses of patient results, and the reader is well aware of them. A common error is the assumption that patients you have not heard from are doing well. This is not unknown in series evaluating the results of the surgical treatment of trigeminal neuralgia. All too often, the patients are somewhere else, seeing someone else for their recurrent pain or the disabling side effects of your procedure. Another, perhaps more common error, is physician bias regarding results. It has been demonstrated that the results in a series vary according to who collects, collates, and evaluates the information. This is not necessarily because the surgeon, as mentioned above, wants his patients to do well; it also may occur because many patients with whom we have good rapport also want us as surgeons to do well. This group, who are fond of their surgeon, may complain to others while telling the surgeon that all is well. Such has been, and probably always will be, functional as a source of error.

Presuming then that we are being as complete, precise, and accurate as possible, and that as much personal error and bias are obviated as possible, many questions can be asked, and some can even be answered about any operative series. Again, the reader is familiar with these questions, some of which are reiterated below.

Some questions to be asked may include: What has been the true effect of a certain form of therapy for a specific syndrome? Do subgroups exist where the rates of success or failure may vary, depending upon specific or general characteristics of the population being treated? Is one form of treatment to be preferred over another in these various subgroups? Is it ethical, indeed is it moral, to subject all or certain patients to a specific form of treatment? What is the risk of temporary or permanent morbidity or death with a given procedure? Is a procedure which offers better quality of survival and a greater chance for permanent cure but which may carry a higher risk of morbidity or mortality justified? Are the risks of a specific operative procedure higher or lower if it is a repeat operation? Under what circumstances is a surgeon justified in trying an operation he has not performed before? Finally, when an operation has failed, what are the results of the various techniques which can be utilized?

Such are some of the important questions to be asked of *any* operative treatment. Such are the questions which can be and should be asked about the experience with operations upon intractable trigeminal neuralgia, which represents in many ways the epitome of our treatment of nonlethal neurosurgical problems, the neurosurgical dilemma, as it were, in microcosm.

The present authors cannot give satisfactory answers to all of the above questions, many of which remain moot. And yet, we can study our patient population and evaluate the results in the patients who have come to us with recurrence of pain or other complications following operations for trigeminal neuralgia. In doing this analysis, we feel somewhat handicapped in attempting to generalize because of the demographic variations in the patient population we have treated.

The patients analyzed in this chapter are those who have undergone one or more prior operations for intractable trigeminal neuralgia and in whom the symptom of lancinating facial pain has recurred on the same side of the face, and who continue to have pain despite adequate medical treatment or have had complications of medical treatment (usually drug toxicity or allergic reactions). In addition, some patients who have undergone various destructive procedures on the trigeminal nerve and now have sensory aberrations (up to frank anesthesia dolorosa) are considered in this chapter, but only if they also have recurrent intractable trigeminal neuralgia. Patients with anesthesia dolorosa or severe hypesthesia dolorosa and no tic pain are excluded from this analysis. They are not relieved of their pain by procedures which we can perform. The risks and results of central ablative and stimulatory functional-stereotactic procedures in patients have been analyzed elsewhere by others and will not be discussed here.

PATIENT POPULATION AND METHODOLOGY

Fifty-one patients (23 men and 28 women, ages 28–71) with recurrent trigeminal neuralgia were treated by the authors from January 1, 1972 to December 31, 1982. Data from all our tic patients have been obtained from primary office records, correspondence, hospital records, and questionnaires. These data were computerized by one of us (D.J.B.). Initial computer programs were devised by Doctor John K. Vries of our department. The computerized data were analyzed including the latest follow-up information (1984), and the "failed" population was identified. Demographic data are summarized in Tables 17.1 and 17.2.

DECISION-MAKING REGARDING OPERATIVE PROCEDURE

A number of decisions, *ad seriatum*, can be made regarding choice of operative procedure for a particular patient (Table 17.3). These decisions are generally straightforward. First, of course, is the decision whether to do something operatively or not. Occasionally, a patient will return for operation who has not undergone adequate medical treatment. Fre-

TABLE 17.1

Patient Population: Recurrent Trigeminal Neuralgia after Microvascular Decompression

51 patients, 23 M, ages 36–71 (mean, 54.9 yr)	
28 F, ages 28–68 (mean, 52.5 yr)	
Duration of symptoms (mean)	3.3 yr
Time to recurrence	0.77 yr
Length of follow-up (mean)	52.5 mo

TABLE 17.2

Location of Recurrent Pain (51 Patients)

Distribution	V_1	V_2	V_3	$V_{1,2}$	$V_{2,3}$	$V_{1,2,3}$	All
Left ($N = 28$)	3	5	4	3	13	0	
Right ($N = 23$)	0	6	4	3	9	1	
Totals	3	11	8	6	22	1	51

TABLE 17.3

Options in Treatment of Failed Trigeminal Neuralgia

1. Medical
   a. Phenytoin, carbamazepine, baclofen
   b. Centrally acting drugs
2. Surgical
   a. Destructive
      Radiofrequency lesion, nerve section,
      Glycerol rhizolysis (?)
   b. Nondestructive
      Glycerol rhizolysis (?)
      Microvascular decompression

quently, a good reason exists for lack of completion of a medical regimen. Most commonly, we find that the patient will not take carbamazepine (Tegretol) in an adequate dose because of one or more disabling side effects (slowing of mentation, nausea, ataxia, *etc.*) which are or have been particularly troublesome to him. Many of these patients simply will not take the drug again. Some physicians, having had a prior bad experience with a drug, will not prescribe it again. Let us assume, for purposes of this discussion, that all patients to be considered have had an adequate trial of medication and have reached an unsatisfactory end point.

Patients who are elderly, frail, or ill with other chronic disease or who do not want to undergo an open operation should have a glycerol rhizolysis or radiofrequency lesion (4, 9, 13, 15–18). We presently prefer the glycerol procedure to the radiofrequency lesion because of the decreased incidence of sensory loss and sensory aberrations with the former. Healthy patients with an estimated 5-year survival are candidates for exploration of the trigeminal nerve in the cerebellopontine angle. We have not performed selective section of the portio major routinely at reoperation. Perhaps this should be done along with microvascular decompression in those patients who have had prior destructive procedures, as demonstrated by Barba and Alksne (2), or tic of long duration (over 8 or so years), as discussed by Apfelbaum (1). Selective section may be considered at the primary microvascular decompression (MVD) under these circumstances.

TECHNICAL CONSIDERATIONS IN REPEAT MVD

If repeat MVD is decided upon, the prior operative note and any photographs or videotapes should be reviewed if possible. This information is helpful both in reviewing relationships for ease and safety of operation and in trying to find the cause of the recurrence. Patient positioning (lateral), anesthetic, and monitoring methods are the same as in a primary operation and have been previously reported (3, 5–8, 10).

A new incision should be made if the old one is unsuitable. We have done this several times because the prior incision was too posterior and/or low. After draping, the incision is carried down to the dura mater and to the bony margins of the craniectomy using sharp, blunt, and Bovie dissection. If bone chips are present from the prior operation, they aid considerably in finding the dura. The craniectomy is enlarged laterally and rostrally over the lateral sinus as necessary. It is important that the lateral sinus be exposed (Fig. 17.1). The dura mater is opened away from the prior incision, and traction sutures are placed on the edges. Microdissection is begun at this point. Adhesions between the cerebellum and dura are usually present under the area of the old dural incision. A cottonoid is placed under a narrow self-retaining microsurgical retractor blade, and constant mild tension is applied with the retractor and the sutures so as to separate the cerebellum from the dura. A plane is established, using bipolar forceps and microscissors, working rostrally, laterally, or caudally until normal arachnoid is reached. Adhesions are almost always more dense in large muscular men and less so in slender women. When a normal arachnoid-dura plane is found, a long narrow cottonoid can be unfolded into the superolateral angle between cerebellum, tentorium cerebelli, and petrous bone. Adhesions decrease as dissection continues anteriorly following the junction between tentorium

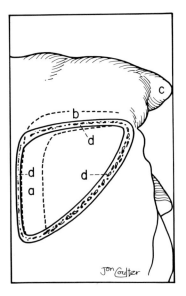

FIG. 17.1. Craniectomy for microvascular decompression of trigeminal nerve (right side). Patient in lateral position. (*a*) Lateral sinus. (*b*) Sigmoid sinus. (*c*) Mastoid eminence. (*d*) Margins of craniectomy.

and petrous bone. Finding the auditory nerve early is helpful, but the surgeon must be careful not to retract the cerebellum in a lateral-to-medial direction. The most common error in a reoperation is to dissect too rostrally to the trigeminal nerve. The nerve is best found at the brainstem under the ala of the cerebellum or, occasionally, it may be found first at Meckel's cave. If adhesions are extensive, painstaking sharp and blunt microdissection using continued countertraction techniques is necessary to find the normal subdural space.

At reoperation, it is usually more difficult to find the trigeminal nerve than to dissect it free of the surrounding tissue reaction (if any) or to establish and treat the cause of the recurrent pain. The usual causes of immediate and persistent lack of pain relief at prior operation are a missed causative blood vessel or an inadequate implant. An additional common cause of early recurrence (usually within 6 months) is recollateralization of intrinsic pontine veins. Late recurrence appears to be due most commonly to continued elongation of arteries which come into the root entry zone of the nerve or displacement of the implant off the nerve. An exception to this is the group of patients in whom we used muscle as the implant. Despite animal studies which showed that autologous muscle persists in the subarachnoid space without dissolution or atrophy, we found that muscle does shrivel up, and that it may dissolve away, and that over a period of 3–5 years an artery can pulsate right through a muscle implant, even if it is quite large and again causes pulsatile compression of the nerve.

Dissection should be performed on the nerve side of previously placed implants. This can be done without injury to neural tissue. The nerve should be inspected in its entirety, including the underside of the ala of the cerebellum (which may contain arteries or veins) and the surface of the nerve to Meckel's cave. Intrinsic pontine veins recollateralize in the same area in which they were found at the prior operation. This phenomenon is fascinating because of the multiple questions which can be asked regarding mechanisms of tissue regrowth. Because the root entry zone of the portio major extends for a considerable distance out the nerve as a cone of central myelin surrounded by the multiple entering trigeminal sensory fascicles (Fig. 17.2), distal vascular compression is not infrequently the cause of trigeminal neuralgia. In fact, the most common cause of isolated V2 tic is a so-called aberrant trigeminal vein coursing from pons to the dura somewhere adjacent to Meckel's cave and causing compression relatively distal on portio major. It is quite easy to coagulate and divide or decompress this vein. The implant material which we have used for over 4 years is shredded Teflon felt (C.R. Bard Inc. Billerica, Mass.). It has excellent handling characteristics, causes minimal tissue reaction, and is permanent.

OPERATIVE FINDINGS AND RESULTS

Operative findings at the first and second operations are collated in Table 17.4. These data include patients without relief who were reoperated on on the same admission as well as true recurrences, that is, patients who were relieved of their pain for a period of time. As collated, the data do demonstrate several significant factors in recurrence including the following. (*a*) Continuing elongation of vessels can cause new vascular compression. (*b*) Intrinsic veins recollateralize over the path of the prior vein, occurring commonly at about 4 months after the initial procedure. (*c*) Implants of muscle atrophy under arteries, allowing compression again, with this phenomenon taking 3 or 4 years or more to develop.

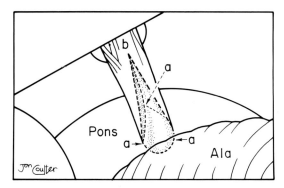

Fig. 17.2. Representation of right trigeminal nerve in cerebellopontine angle. Cone-shaped central myelin extends distally in portio major of trigeminal nerve. Root entry zone "junctional area" may extend to Meckel's cave; *a-a-a* is circumference of portio major at pons (central myelin); *ab-ab-ab* is the cone of central myelin extending peripherally.

TABLE 17.4

Operative Findings at Retromastoid Craniectomy (RMC) for Trigeminal Neuralgia: Recurrence after First Operation in 51 Patients

	First RMC	Second RMC
Arterial	19	10
Venous	10	17
Mixed A&V	20	15
Implant	0	5
Cyst + vein	0	1
Scar + vein + artery	0	1
"Negative" exploration	0	1
Tumor	1	1
Total	50[a]	51

[a] Plus one patient who had nerve section at first operation.

Case Reports

Case 1. A 73-year-old woman presented with severe recurrent trigeminal neuralgia and anesthesia dolorosa following multiple operations including total section of the nerve in the posterior fossa. At operation (Fig. 17.3), the superior cerebellar artery was found to be compressing the stump of the completely severed trigeminal nerve on the pons. Microvascular decompression completely relieved the tic. The anesthesia dolorosa was unchanged.

Case 2. A 48-year-old woman presented with right-sided V2 and 3 trigeminal neuralgia. At the first operation, a branch of superior cerebellar artery (SCA) was mobilized from the trigeminal nerve root entry zone rostrally and held away with Teflon felt implant (Fig. 17.4). There was

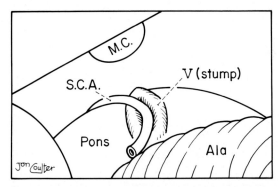

FIG. 17.3. Case 1. Right upper cerebellopontine angle in 73-year-old woman with trigeminal neuralgia and anesthesia dolorosa. *Ala*, ala of cerebellum; *M.C.*, Meckel's cave; *V (stump)*, pontine stump of transected trigeminal nerve compressed by *S.C.A.*

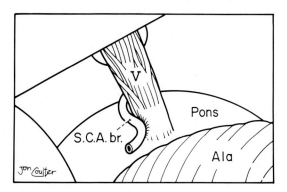

FIG. 17.4. Case 2. First operation. Right $V_{2,3}$ trigeminal neuralgia. Tortuous superior cerebellar artery branch compressing nerve rostrally mobilized and held away with shredded Teflon felt. No relief of pain.

no response to treatment. One week later at reoperation (Fig. 17.5), the more proximal segment of the same artery was noted to be compressing the anterior aspect of root entry zone of nerve. It was decompressed using Teflon felt, and provided total relief of pain. Lesson: The entire circumference of nerve was not adequately visualized or decompressed.

Case 3. A 41-year-old man presented with intractable right-sided V2 trigeminal neuralgia following multiple peripheral procedures and three posterior fossa explorations. At operation (Fig. 17.6), branches of superior cerebellar artery were found to have been nicely separated from the trigeminal nerve by a large implant. An aberrant trigeminal vein causing compression and grooving of the lateral aspect of portio major was found just proximal to Meckel's cave. The vein was coagulated and divided with total relief of pain.

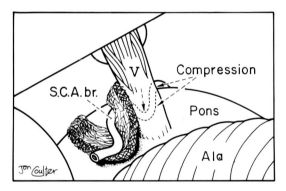

FIG. 17.5. Case 2. Second operation, 1 week later. Further compression by proximal segment of artery found and relieved, with excellent result.

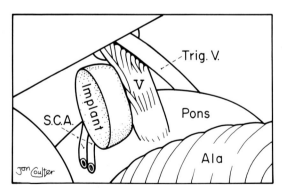

FIG. 17.6. Case 3. Right trigeminal nerve in 41-year-old man with persistent V$_2$ pain. Trigeminal vein causing persistent compression of lateral distal portio major. See text for details.

Results of repeat microvascular decompression (Table 17.5) are satisfactory but not perfect. Fortunately, reoperation appears to carry low morbidity, but not everyone is cured (Tables 17.5–17.7). Two subgroups of failed patients, those with no relief after MVD who had reoperation during the same hospitalization and those who had an implant of Ivalon sponge pulsating into the trigeminal nerve as a secondary pulsatile "missile" are considered in Tables 17.8 and 17.9. Reoperation early is easy on both patient and surgeon and should be considered if there is no relief. We stopped using Ivalon sponge because of the "secondary missile"

TABLE 17.5

Results of Repeat Microvascular Decompression in Trigeminal Neuralgia in 51 Patients

Relief	Complete	Partial	No
Immediate	31	18	2
Long-term	26	6	19

TABLE 17.6

Cranial Nerve Complications following Repeat Microvascular Decompression

Cranial Nerve	Complication	
	Temporary	Permanent
IV	0	0
V	0	0
VI	1	0
VII	2	1
VIII	0	0

TABLE 17.7

Other Complications following Repeat Microvascular Decompression

Delayed headache	15
Pulmonary embo-lism	1
Acute hydrocephalus (self-limited)	1
Infection	0
Death	0

TABLE 17.8

Lack of Relief and Immediate Reoperation

6 patients—2F, 4M
Ages 41, 47, 48, 55, 57, 60
Findings—inadequate MVD
Results—5 total relief
        1 failure

phenomenon of this fairly hard implant. Several mechanical factors may be functional in this lack of improvement. Scar formation and gliosis, although mild, may be such as to prevent reformation of normal myelin and axis cylinders; the intrinsic disease within the nerve may be too extensive for repair of the damage. Still other vascular compression may be missed. Secondary changes may have occurred more centrally in the trigeminal system. Patients who have had prior destructive procedures do not do as well after microvascular decompression as those who have not experienced them, as recently shown by Barba and Alksne (2). A high proportion of our recurrences (22 of 51 patients) had prior destructive operations (Table 17.10), in contrast to 1 of 8 of the remaining patients. Furthermore, as Apfelbaum (1) has noted, patients with many years of trigeminal neuralgia do not do as well following microvascular decompression as those whose time with it is of briefer duration.

DISCUSSION

Patients with recurrent pain, lack of relief, or unpleasant sequelae after operations for trigeminal neuralgia have been discussed in many articles over the years as part of the analysis of results of operation (1, 4, 5–7, 9, 11–18). Most operations for tic have had as their aim the interruption or modification of trigeminal nerve or ganglion tissue by various mechanical, chemotoxic, or thermal trauma. The development of recurrent pain has been followed generally by another such traumatic procedure. The "trade-off" of numbness for pain and the complications of denervation up to and including frank anesthesia dolorosa have been acceptable exchanges. As trauma-producing procedures have become perhaps more specific to the problem and caused less destruction of

TABLE 17.9

Recurrence due to Implant as "Secondary Missile" from Adjacent Artery

5 Patients
Implant type—5 Ivalon
Results—2 total relief
3 failures

TABLE 17.10

Prior Destructive Operation (before First Retromastoid Craniectomy) of 51 Patients with Recurrent Trigeminal Neuralgia

Total no. of patients	22
Peripheral nerve destruction	15
Radiofrequency lesion	5
Retrogasserian section	2

neural tissue, the recurrence rates have risen. This is not to denigrate the use of such procedures, which are often the best available procedures for a given patient by a given surgeon. As tissue destruction has decreased, quality of survival has certainly been improved. Repeat controlled destructive lesions, in a patient with moderate sensory loss, may be very effective in relieving pain. Contributions which specifically address the question of failure are rare.

A longitudinal prospective study of young patients with trigeminal neuralgia would be of interest. It would mean that two or more generations of neurosurgeons would have to be involved. The social, psychological, and economic aspects of the lives of such patients might be usefully addressed in such a study. Similarly, quality of life as affected by the primary problem, as well as the results and side effects of treatment, should be studied and may be meaningful in future decision making (1, 18). Older surgeons develop expertise in specific areas and treat large populations of patients. The patients, if young, outlive their treating surgeons. One transgenerational study on trigeminal neuralgia patients treated by Dandy was published by Revilla (12) in 1947, 1 year after Dandy's death. A few studies from "old-line" excellent institutions have included patients treated across the years. Accurate later follow-ups are hard to achieve. Such a prospective study might be useful in seeing what we are doing to and for our patients.

We would like to share a perspective regarding the operative treatment of trigeminal neuralgia, a perspective which deserves a careful look at what we do to and for patients. First, a question: Why treat a symptom primarily with a trade-off procedure? We do not burn or transect dorsal spinal roots as the primary operative treatment for a herniated disc. We remove the disc when conservative therapy has failed. Destruction of a dorsal root, even with ganglion removal, gives temporary relief and has side effects. We do such a procedure as a last resort only. With our expanded knowledge of the pathophysiology of trigeminal neuralgia, and with the knowledge that definitive treatment (*i.e.*, MVD) is less likely to be successful in a patient who has had a prior destructive operation, does it not make sense to save the destructive procedures for later (Table 17.10) (2). This is posed as a point for consideration. Quality of survival after these procedures is another point which has been discussed in recent papers and may mitigate against use of destructive operations as the first procedure of choice (1, 18). Here, as you see, we are discussing indications for operation, *when* one may be preferred over another, not whether one is "bad" and another "good."

We are certainly not totally happy with our success rates in primary and repeat MVD for trigeminal neuralgia (80+ percent good or excellent results; two operative deaths in over 800 operations). Our data include

59 patients who have occasional mild pain, 39 of whom have had or now take medicines (phenytoin, dilantin). We would like to do better.

In conclusion, our data agree with those of Barba and Alksne (2) that prior destructive operations have an adverse effect on the outcome of microvascular decompression for trigeminal neuralgia. The history of the failed patient does provide information helpful in the choice of a primary operative procedure. Furthermore, a repeat operation has a good chance of giving permanent relief of pain. At reoperation, further vascular compression of the trigeminal nerve is usually found and can be relieved, but scarring and gliosis, tic of prolonged duration, and perhaps irreversible changes centrally in the trigeminal system may prevent relief by repeat vascular decompression alone. In patients with these factors and/ or recurrent intrinsic pontine venous recollateralization, a selective section or the portio major in addition to repeat vascular decompression may be the procedure of choice. Destructive procedures therefore are well indicated as secondary or tertiary procedures.

REFERENCES

1. Apfelbaum, R. I. A comparison of percutaneous radiofrequency trigeminal neurolysis and microvascular decompression of the trigeminal nerve for the treatment of tic douloureux. Neurosurgery, 47: 16–21, 1977.
2. Barba, D., and Alksne, J. F. Success of microvascular decompression with and without prior surgical therapy for trigeminal neuralgia. J. Neurosurg., 60: 104–107, 1984.
3. Grundy, B. L., Jannetta, P. J., Procopio, P. T., Lina, A., and Doyle, E. Intraoperative monitoring of brain-stem auditory evoked potentials. J. Neurosurg., 57: 674–681, 1983.
4. Håkanson, S. Trigeminal neuralgia treated by the injection of glycerol into the trigeminal cistern. Neurosurgery, 9: 638–646, 1981.
5. Jannetta, P. J. Vascular decompression in trigeminal neuralgia. In: The Cranial Nerves, edited by M. Samii and P. J. Jannetta, pp. 312–315. Springer-Verlag, Berlin, 1981.
6. Jannetta, P. J. Microvascular decompression for trigeminal neuralgia. Surg. Rounds, 6: 24–35, 1983.
7. Jannetta, P. J. Treatment of trigeminal neuralgia by micro-operative decompression. In: Neurological Surgery, Ed. 2, Vol. 6, edited by J. Youmans, pp. 3589–3603. W.B. Saunders, Philadelphia, 1982.
8. Jannetta, P. J., Abbasy, M., Maroon, J. C., Morales-Ramos, F., and Albin, M. S. Etiology and definitive microsurgical treatment of hemifacial spasm. Operative techniques and results in forty-seven patients. J. Neurosurg., 47: 321–328, 1977.
9. Lunsford, L. D., and Bennett, M. H. Percutaneous retrogasserian glycerol rhizotomy for tic douloureux. Part 1. Technique and results in 112 patients. Neurosurgery, 14: 424–430, 1984.
10. Moller, A. R., and Jannetta, P. J. Monitoring auditory functions during cranial nerve microvascular decompression operations by direct recording from the eighth nerve. J. Neurosurg., 59: 493–499, 1983.
11. Nugent, G. R., and Berry, B. Trigeminal neuralgia treated with percutaneous radiofrequency lesions. J. Neurosurg., 40: 517–523, 1974.

12. Revilla, A. G. Tic douloureux and its relationship to tumors of the posterior fossa. J. Neurosurg., *4:* 233–239, 1947.
13. Schurmann, K., Butz, M., and Brock, M. Temporal retrogasserian resection of trigeminal root *versus* controlled elective percutaneous electrocoagulation of the ganglion of Gasser in the treatment of trigeminal neuralgia. Report on a series of 531 cases. Acta Neurochir., *26:* 33–35, 1972.
14. Stookey, B., and Ransohoff, J. *Trigeminal Neuralgia. Its History and Treatment.* Charles C Thomas, Springfield, Ill., 1959.
15. Sweet, W. H. Percutaneous differential thermal trigeminal rhizotomy for the management of facial pain. In: *Advances in Neurosurgery,* Vol. 3, *Brain Hypoxia: Pain,* edited by H. Penzholz, M. Brock, J. Hamer, M. Klinger, and O. Spoerri, pp. 274–286. Springer-Verlag, Berlin, 1975.
16. Sweet, W. H., and Wepsic, J. G. Controlled thermocoagulation of trigeminal ganglion and rootlets for differential destruction of pain fibers. Part 1. Trigeminal neuralgia. J. Neurosurg., *39:* 143–156, 1974.
17. Tew, J., and Mayfield, F. Trigeminal neuralgia. A new surgical approach. (Percutaneous electrocoagulation of the trigeminal nerve.) Laryngoscope, *83:* 1096–1101, 1973.
18. van Loveren, H., Tew, J. M., Keller, J. T., and Nurre, M. A. A 10-year experience in the treatment of trigeminal neuralgia. J. Neurosurg., *57:* 757–764, 1982.

V

Pineal Tumors

18

Neuropathology of Pineal Region Tumors

BERND W. SCHEITHAUER, M.D.

EMBRYOLOGY

As a structure, the epiphysis cerebri or pineal gland has been known for millennia, yet despite numerous embryologic, comparative anatomic, physiologic, biochemical, and morphologic studies, its function remains poorly understood. Identifiable in embryos at 6 mm crown-rump (CR) length, the gland is seen to develop as an evagination of the posterosuperior diencephalic roof (22). The pineal begins as cellular anterior and posterior anlagen surrounding a diverticular extension of the third ventricle (Fig. 18.1). With their fusion, the lumen of the pineal diverticulum is cut off, forming an intrapineal cavity, the cavum pineale, lined by ependyma and subependymal glia. With astroglial proliferation, the cavum undergoes an obliterative process which is frequently incomplete, resulting in the formation of single or multiple cavities. In fetal life, two neuroectodermal cell types are identified within the pineal: small dense and large pale parenchymal cells termed pineocytes, and astroglial cells, the latter forming a stromal matrix in the gland. The fetal pineal has a pronounced lobular architecture (Fig. 18.2). A delicate connective tissue envelope of meningeal mesenchyme surrounds the gland and forms a delicate framework about its vasculature.

HISTOLOGY

Microscopically, the adult pineal consists of sheets, lobules, and cords of monomorphous pinealocytes embedded in a glial stroma separated by scant vascular connective tissue septae. The principle functional cells of the pineal, the pineocytes, are unipolar. Their argyrophilic processes terminate in bulbous expansions, often abutting the microvasculature (Fig. 18.3*A* and *B*). Ultrastructurally, pineocytes (60) possess all the organelles necessary for hormone synthesis, a feature consistent with the concept that they are neurosecretory in nature. This conclusion is in keeping with biochemical studies which have demonstrated the production of the indole hormone melatonin (50). Blood levels of the latter

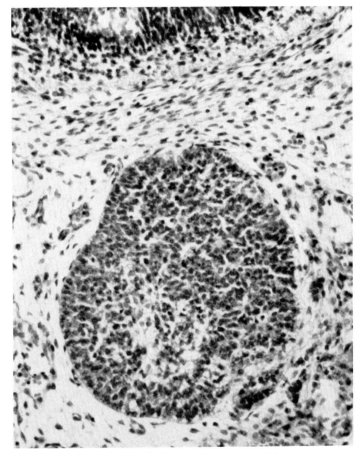

FIG. 18.1. The developing pineal gland in a 9½-week-old, 30 mm CR fetus. The gland, sectioned above the level of the cavum pineale, is composed of a uniform population of pineoblasts demonstrating ill-defined rosette formation. H&E, × 250.

undergo diurnal variation and diminish in response to light exposure, an interesting property in view of the role of the pineal gland as a photoreceptor organ in lower vertebrates (96). Interestingly, photoreceptor differentiation of pineocytes has also been documented in neonatal rats (114).

Delicately fibrillated astrocytes both form plaques within the gland and line the commonly occurring microcavities within its substance (Fig. 18.4A). Calcareous bodies, composed of carbonates and phosphates of calcium and magnesium, form in and around the gland (Fig. 18.4B), often increasing in abundance with age. The cellular origin of such bodies and their mechanism of formation are unsettled.

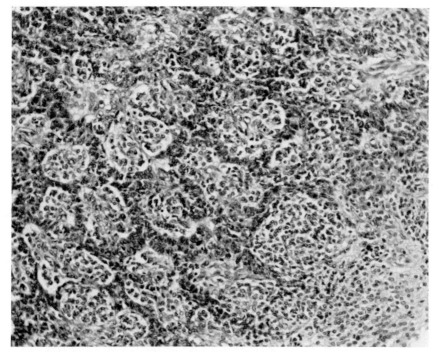

FIG. 18.2. Microsection of the late fetal pineal gland showing a prominent lobular architecture. Note the small peripherally placed pineoblasts as well as centrally situated more fully differentiated cells resembling pineocytes. H&E, × 200.

NEOPLASMS OF PINEAL REGION

The common clinical presentation and distinct morphologic features of most neoplasms occurring in relation to the pineal gland forms the basis of the regional approach to pineal area tumors.

A variety of neoplasms occur in the pineal region, the most common being derived from germ cells (Table 18.5). The remainder are a combination of pineal parenchymal tumors (Table 18.1), gliomas of the pineal or its surroundings, a variety of rare neuroectodermal or mesenchymal lesions, metastatic tumors, and malformations (Table 18.3).

Pineal Parenchymal Tumors

Pineal parenchymal neoplasms are rare. Ten examples were encountered in the Mayo Clinic experience over a 53-year period (27) representing an incidence of less than 0.1% of intracranial tumors. In view of their morphologic similarity to and presumed common derivation from pineocytes or their precursors, the tumors are designated pineoblastoma and pinealocytoma. The former is a highly malignant neoplasm, truly

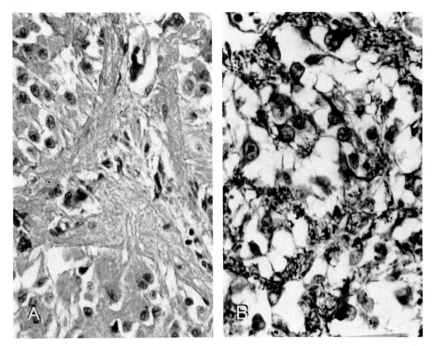

FIG. 18.3. (A) Microsection of the adult pineal gland demonstrating lobules composed of unipolar pineocytes with processes directed to the vasculature. H&E, × 400. (B) The morphology of pineocytes is highlighted by silver stains. Note the polarity of the cells as well as their knob-like terminations. DeGirolami-Zvaigne method, × 480. (Courtesy of Dr. L. J. Rubinstein, Department of Pathology, University of Virginia, Charlottesville, Va.)

one of the class of primitive neuroectodermal tumors. The pineocytoma is a less malignant, better differentiated lesion composed of cells resembling mature pineocytes. Transitional tumors sharing the features of pineoblastoma and pineocytoma are common (36). Pineocytomas not infrequently demonstrate divergent differentiation to glial cells and neurons (36). The resultant histopathologic spectrum of pineal parenchymal tumors is summarized in Table 18.1.

PINEOBLASTOMA

Several series of this rare tumor have been reported (17, 25, 36, 67). A highly malignant, poorly differentiated neuroectodermal tumor, the pineoblastoma occurs most commonly in the first 3 decades of life. The symptoms are of short duration and reflect the tumors' location but are otherwise nonspecific. Survival is short; all patients in the series of Borit *et al.* (17) died within 2 years of surgery. Pineoblastomas are unencapsulated, soft, friable, and gray; they characteristically infiltrate surround-

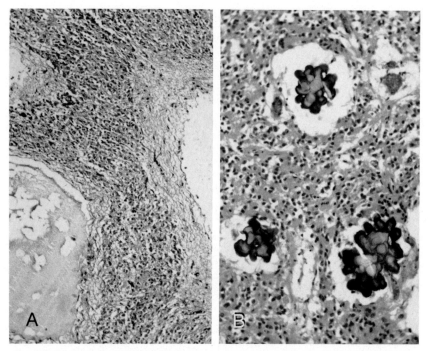

FIG. 18.4. (A) Cystic cavities within the normal pineal gland. Such spaces, representing remnants of the cavum pineale, may be single or multiple and are lined by a dense hypocellular layer of fibrillary astrocytes. H&E, × 100. (B) Calcareous bodies in the pineal gland of an adult. H&E, × 160.

ing structures, including the posterior third ventricle; and they show a marked tendency to cerebrospinal dissemination (Fig. 18.5). Systemic metastasis is a rare phenomenon (7).

The resemblance of pineoblastoma to medulloblastoma is based upon the clinical features noted above, as well as their radiosensitivity and tendency to craniospinal spread. It is further reinforced by their light and electron microscopic features (18, 36, 46, 52). They are highly cellular tumors composed of small mitotically active cells with scant cytoplasm disposed in patternless sheets (Figs. 18.6 and 18.7A and B). Occasionally, tumor giant cell formation is noted, as is arrangement of cells in a nodular mosaic pattern reminiscent of the structure of the fetal pineal gland. When early differentiation is present, it is manifested by the formation of Homer Wright rosettes similar to those of neuroblastoma, the delicate centrally directed processes being argyrophilic. Perivascular rosette formation, also a feature of pineocytic differentiation, is frequently observed. The bulbous terminal expansions characteristic of

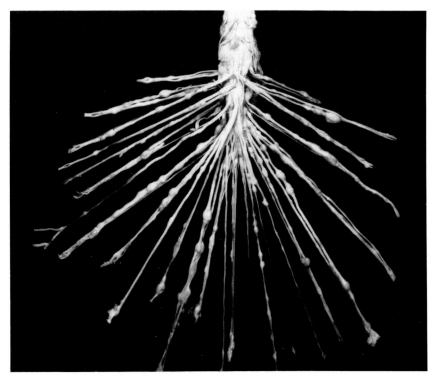

FIG. 18.5. Pineoblastoma implants on the cauda equina. Such seeding, although less frequent, is also noted in association with pineocytomas.

mature pineocytes are not evident, except in the transitional tumors with combined features of pineoblastoma and pineocytoma.

Few pineoblastomas have been studied by electron microscopy (35, 46, 52). As expected, the ultrastructural features are those of a poorly differentiated neurectodermal neoplasm with variable photoreceptor or neuroblastic differentiation.

PINEOCYTOMA

Unlike the pineoblastoma, this better differentiated variant of pineal parenchymal neoplasm occurs primarily in adult life, is somewhat slower in evolution, and is thus accompanied by a longer period of preoperative symptoms. Pineocytomas are spherical to irregular, soft, grey tumors which demonstrate a somewhat lesser tendency to local invasion and craniospinal metastasis (Fig. 18.8). Although some available data indicate a prolonged survival in patient with pure pineocytoma (17), the patients

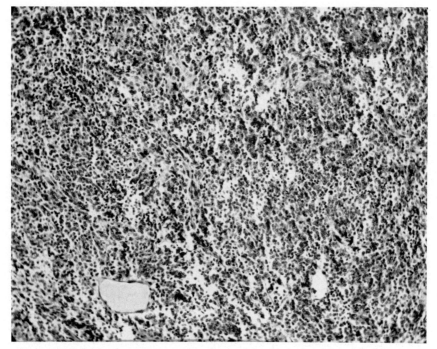

FIG. 18.6. Photomicrograph of a pineoblastoma demonstrating morphologic features similar to those of medulloblastoma. The tumors are highly cellular and poorly differentiated, and may show the formation of Homer Wright rosettes. H&E, × 160.

reported by Herrick and Rubinstein (36) experienced a similar survival to those with pineoblastoma, prolonged survival being associated primarily with pineocytomas showing extensive glial or neuronal differentiation or both (see below).

Pineocytomas are moderately cellular, variably mitotically active neoplasms composed of differentiated unipolar cells disposed in lobules or irregular clusters. The cytoplasmic processes are engaged either in the formation of perivascular pseudorosettes or exaggerated large versions of Homer Wright rosettes (Fig. 18.9). On occasion, a pseudopapillary growth pattern is observed (92, 106). The cells, which resemble mature pineocytes, are argyrophilic, and their terminations take the form of knob-like expansions (Fig. 18.10A and B). Argyrophilia of the cytoplasm and processes of the tumor cells are best visualized in paraffin sections utilizing the DeGirolami and Zvaigzne method (26). Ultrastructural studies show a resemblance between pineocytoma cells and normal adult mammalian pineocytes (35, 69).

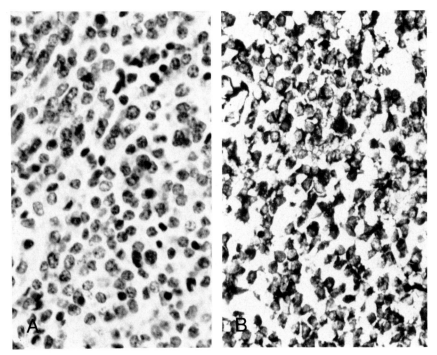

FIG. 18.7. (A) Cytology of the cells of a pineoblastoma. The cells are cytologically malignant, possess scant cytoplasm, and are highly mitotically active. H&E, × 640. (B) Silver method for pineal parenchymal cells, demonstrating staining of the cytoplasm and processes. DeGirolami-Zvaigne method, × 480. (Courtesy of Dr. L. J. Rubinstein, Department of Pathology, University of Virginia, Charlottesville, Va.)

Pineal Parenchymal Neoplasms with Divergent Differentiation

PINEOBLASTOMA

Unlike the occurrence of pineocytic differentiation in transitional tumors, *i.e.*, mixed pineoblastoma-pineocytoma, a feature unassociated with an improved prognosis, divergent differentiation to other neuroectodermal elements is a process primarily observed in pineocytomas (Table 18.1). Photoreceptor differentiation, a rare form of specialization in pineoblastomas, deserves mention. The latter is evidenced by the formation of Flexner-Wintersteiner rosettes, as well as "fleurettes," and has been reported in two cases of pineoblastoma (36, 100) (Fig. 18.11); both cases occurred in 2-year-old male patients, were accompanied by craniospinal seeding, and were associated with a short postoperative survival. Fleurette formation has also been described in ocular retinoblastomas (107). In view of the photoreceptor function of the pineal gland in both

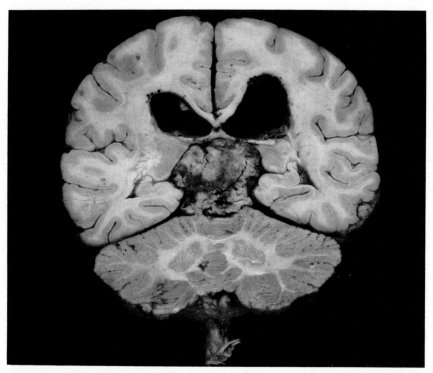

FIG. 18.8. The gross appearance of a pineocytoma demonstrating lobularity and expansive growth with displacement of surrounding structures. Note the presence of hydrocephalus resulting from aqueductal compression. (Reproduced with permission from: A. H. Baggenstoss and J. G. Love. Arch. Neurol. Psychiatry, *41:* 1187–1206, 1939.)

fish and amphibians (96), and since photoreceptor differentiation has been documented in the development of the pineal in lower mammals (114), this phenomenon is of particular interest in that it recapitulates the phylogeny of the pineal gland and suggests a homology of pineoblastomas with retinoblastoma. The rare concurrence of retinoblastoma and pineoblastoma further highlights the relationship (40).

A unique pineoblastoma with melanin formation has also been reported (8). Interestingly, melanin pigment production is transiently expressed in the fetal pineal (60).

PINEOCYTOMA

Astrocytic and neuronal differentiation in pineocytomas and rarely in pineoblastoma (98) is a process analogous to the finding of neuroglial differentiation in primitive neuroectodermal tumors at other sites. In pineocytomas, the presence of such elements may be of favorable prog-

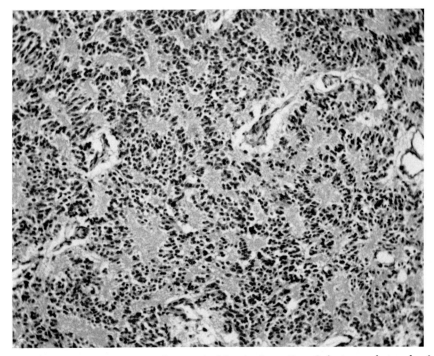

FIG. 18.9. Pineocytomas are characterized by the formation of clusters and strands of cells resembling normal pineocytes. The cells often form exaggerated Homer Wright rosettes. H&E, × 160.

nostic significance (Table 18.2). The finding of neuronal components has particularly been associated with an indolent clinical course (36) (Table 17.2). Astrocytic (18) neuronal (36) and combined ganglionic-astrocytic differentiation (so-called "ganglioglioma of the pineal") have been reported (36, 69, 86) (Fig. 18.12).

In view of the occurrence of scant nerve cell processes as well as abundant astrocytes within the normal pineal gland, the finding of such structures by electron microscopy alone should be interpreted with caution. A substantial ganglionic or glial component should be documented by light microscopy before accepting a pineocytic tumor as demonstrating clinically significant divergent differentiation.

Pineal Gliomas and Rare Tumors of the Pineal Region

Astrocytic neoplasms of the pineal gland are a rarity. Their origin from pluripotential pineal parenchymal cells is likely in view of the known occurrence of neuronal, astrocytic, and ganglioglial differentiation in

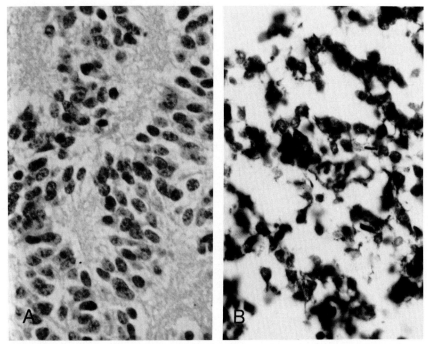

FIG. 18.10. (A) The cytology of pineocytoma cells often shows little atypia or mitotic activity and resembles that of normal pineocytes. Note the lack of atypia and paucity of mitotic activity. H&E, × 460. (B) Note argyrophilic cell processes, some with knob-like terminations. DeGirolami-Zvaigne method, × 480. (Courtesy of Dr. L. J. Rubinstein, Department of Pathology, University of Virginia, Charlottesville, Va.)

TABLE 18.1

Classification of Pineal Parenchymal Neoplasms[a]

Pineoblastoma
    with pineocytic differentiation (transitional tumors)
    with retinoblastomatous differentiation
Pineocytoma
    with neuronal differentiation
    with astrocytic differentiation
    with neuronal and astrocytic differentiation (*i.e.*, "ganglioglioma" of the pineal)

   [a] (From M. K. Herrick and L. J. Rubinstein (36).)

pineocytic neoplasms (36). An alternative source of such tumors might be from resident astrocytes within the gland. As previously noted, the latter are a component of the stroma of the pineal. Their presence has long been known and has recently been further documented by immunocytochemistry (77) and by electron microscopy (69).

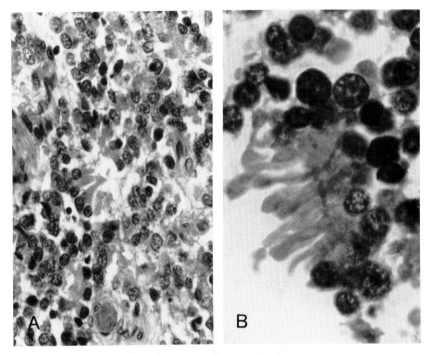

FIG. 18.11. (A and B) Pineoblastoma with photoreceptor differentiation demonstrating the formation of fleurettes. (A) H&E, × 400. (B) H&E, × 1000. (Courtesy of Dr. L. J. Rubinstein, Department of Pathology, University of Virginia, Charlottesville, Va.)

Reported examples of astrocytoma include the full spectrum of malignancy and of histologic patterns, including pilocytic, fibrillary, and astroblastic types. Extrapineal extension or partial pineal involvement in some reported examples make their site of origin conjectural (21, 25, 80, 113). Few tumors can with confidence be stated to have originated within the pineal gland (24, 25, 77, 84, 85, 88). The finding of astrocytic differentiation in a significant proportion of pineocytomas requires adequate tissue sampling to exclude the coexistence of a pineal parenchymal component before a diagnosis of astrocytoma is substantiated.

Examples of oligodendroglioma, ependymoma, and glioblastomas of the pineal region have been published, but the tumors were not specifically localized to the gland (25). A variety of rare primary neuroectodermal and nonneuroectodermal neoplasms as well as miscellaneous lesions of the pineal region have been reported (Table 18.3).

PINEAL CYST

The processes of pineal development and of aging have been carefully studied (22, 105). As previously noted, the formation of the gland involves

TABLE 18.2

Cytologic Variants of Pineal Parenchymal Tumors and Their Biologic Behavior[a]

Pineoblastomas	Malignant
With pineocytic differentiation	Malignant
With retinoblastomatous differentiation	Malignant
Pineocytomas	Malignant
With astrocytic differentiation	Malignant or benign
With neuronal differentiation	Benign
With neuronal and astrocytic differentiation	Benign
("ganglioglioma of the pineal")	

[a] (From M. K. Herrick and L. J. Rubinstein (36).)

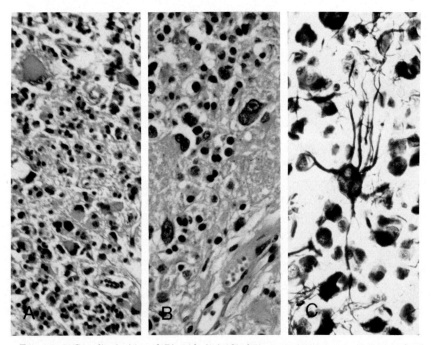

FIG. 18.12. Ganglionic (A and B) and glial (C) differentiation in a pineocytoma. Such tumors have been termed "ganglioglioma of the pineal gland" and are associated with a favorable prognosis. (A) H&E, × 400. (B) Bielschowski method, × 400. (C) H&E, × 250. Case in Reference 27. (Courtesy of Dr. H. Okazaki, Department of Pathology, Mayo Clinic, Rochester, Minn.)

fusion of the anterior and posterior pineal anlagen with entrapment of a portion of the pineal diverticulum, a continuation of the third ventricle, within the substance of the gland. The result is the formation of the cavum pineale. Although the latter undergoes partial or complete obliteration in later life, it not uncommonly enlarges to form one or several

TABLE 18.3
Rare Neoplasms and Tumor-like Lesions of the Pineal Region

Neuroectodermal tumors
  Astrocytoma variants (21, 24, 25, 77, 80, 84, 113)
  Oligodendroglioma (25)
  Ependymoma (25)
  Glioblastoma (25)
  Medulloepithelioma (30, 57)
  Paraganglioma ("chemodectoma") (97)
  Ganglioneuroma (84)
  Melanoma (28)
Nonneuroectodermal Tumors
  Hemangioma (39)
  Meningioma (89)
  Hemangiopericytoma (73)
  Craniopharyngioma (99)
Miscellaneous
  Pineal cyst (22, 93)
  Arachnoid cyst (101)
  Epidermoid cyst (55, 62, 91, 117)
  Dermoid Cyst (32, 87)
  Lipoma (37)
  Plasma cell leukemia (38)
  Metastatic carcinoma (34, 74)

macroscopic cysts within the pineal (Fig. 18.13). The inspissated fluid content of such a pineal cyst is a presumed secretory product of its lining cells, which are in large part astroglial but may focally resemble ependyma. Small cysts are common autopsy findings, but only rare examples become clinically symptomatic (22, 93).

Epidermoid (55, 62, 91, 117) and dermoid cysts (32, 87) of the pineal region are rare.

GERM CELL TUMORS

The occurrence of germ cell tumors within the central nervous system has been related to the midline migration pathway of germ cells during embryogenesis. An alternative explanation related to the midline position of most germ cell tumors is that they may result from a disturbance in primitive streak development (20). This group of neoplasms, presumably derived from developmental germ cell rests, conceptually lends itself to an orderly histogenetic classification which reflects the process of development (Table 18.4).

Intracranial germ cell tumors are rare, representing an incidence of 0.3% of intracranial neoplasms operated at Mayo Clinic (11). Marsden *et al.* (53) identified only 13 examples in the Manchester University

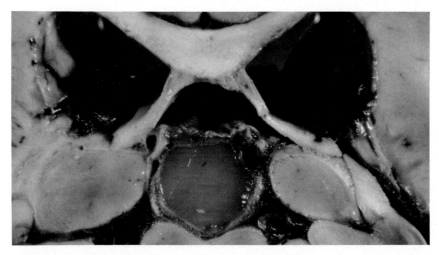

FIG. 18.13. Pineal cyst. This large cyst was an incidental autopsy finding unaccompanied by clinical symptoms. (Courtesy of Dr. Ellsworth Alvord, Department of Neuropathology, University of Washington, Seattle, Wash.)

Children's Tumor Registry over a 25-year period, representing 9.5% of all germ cell tumors in patients under 14 years of age.

The analogy between germ cell tumors of the central nervous system and those of the gonads is complete (12, 29, 87). The World Health Organization (WHO) classification of germ cell tumors of the gonads, presented in Table 18.5 (61), is not only applicable to craniospinal examples but is preferable to the simplistic, imprecise format offered by the present WHO classification of germ cell tumors of the central nervous system (116). The latter does not distinguish between mature and immature teratomas, nor does it provide a category for endodermal sinus tumors.

Bjornsson *et al.* (12) in their recent clinicopathologic and immunocytochemical review of intracranial germ cell tumors from this institution, described the features of 70 cases. Males predominated in all categories, comprising 63% of the overall patient population. Most occurred in young patients (97% in the first four decades), with the peak incidence being the second decade (46%). The tumors were characteristically midline and showed a geographic preference, in decreasing order of frequency, for the pineal region, third ventricle, and suprasellar area. Fifty percent of tumors involved the pineal gland and the posterior third ventricle. The relative proportions of histologic tumor types was as follows: germinoma (61%), immature teratoma (23%), mature teratoma (10%), embryonal carcinoma (3%), yolk sac tumor (1.5%) and choriocarcinoma (1.5%).

TABLE 18.4

Histogenesis of Germ Cell Tumors

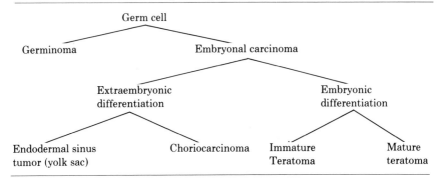

TABLE 18.5

World Health Organization Classification of Testicular Germ Cell Tumors[a]

A. Tumors of one histologic type
    1. Seminoma
    2. Spermatocytic seminoma
    3. Embryonal carcinoma
    4. Yolk sac tumor
    5. Polyembryoma
    6. Choriocarcinoma
    7. Teratomas
        Mature
        Immature
        With malignant transformation
B. Tumors of more than one histologic type
    1. Embryonal carcinoma and teratoma (teratocarcinoma)
    2. Choriocarcinoma and any other types
    3. Other combinations

[a] From F. K. Mostofi and L. H. Sobin (61).)

Specific features of these histologic variants are discussed below, and their association with tumors markers is summarized in Table 18.6.

Reports of systemic metastases of pineal germ cell tumors are infrequent (12, 90). All but rare examples (33) do so only after surgical intervention.

Germinoma

In that most germ cell tumors involve the pineal gland and since the histologic appearance of this, the most common variant, superficially resembles that of the normal fetal pineal gland, germinomas have in the past been incorrectly designated "pinealoma." When occurring in the

TABLE 18.6

Immunocytochemistry of Germ Cell Tumors

	HCG[a]	AFP[a]	a-1-AT
Germinoma	±	−	−
Embryonal carcinoma	−	−	−
Endodermal sinus tumor	−	+	+
Mature and immature teratoma	−	±	±
Choriocarcinoma	+	−	−

[a] AFP, α-fetoprotein; α-1-AT, α-1-antitrypsin.

hypothalamic region, the term "ectopic pinealoma" has been applied. The nosologic distinction between germinoma and pineal parenchymal tumors is well established (29, 87). In that germinomas are not histogenically related to pineal parenchymal neoplasms, this confusing terminology should be abandoned.

The early combined literature review and series report of Dayan (23) analyzed the clinicopathologic features of a large number of germinomas. In our institutional experience with 43 cases (12), they were noted to arise most often in males (70%) and occurred most frequently in the second and third decades of life (67%). Germinomas are unusually common in Japan (104). The ratio of pineal to hypothalamic involvement is approximately 3:1; one third of cases are said to involve both sites.

Germinomas situated in the hypothalamic region characteristically produce the triad of diabetes insipidus, visual disturbance, and hypopituitarism. Diabetes insipidus is reported in as many as 95% of patients and may precede other symptoms by years. In contrast, visual abnormalities occur in only approximately 30%, but are the most frequent presenting complaint (83). Hypogonadism and occasionally precocious puberty have also been reported in hypothalamic involvement (10). Mental disturbance has been associated with germinomas diffusely involving the ventricular system (5, 23, 31, 68).

A recently reported suprasellar germinoma in a patient with Kleinfelter's syndrome is of interest in that such patients are at increased risk for the development of extragonadal germ cell neoplasms (1).

Unlike other tumors of germ cell type, germinomas often do not form circumscribed masses but rather infiltrate locally and spread by discontinuous growth in the craniospinal subarachnoid space (Fig. 18.14). Invasion of the quadrigeminal plate may produce aqueductal destruction and resultant hydrocephalus. Parenchymal metastases as well as extradural spread are rare (81, 95). Six reported cases associated with hematogenous systemic metastases were reviewed by Borden *et al.* (15); all occurred subsequent to surgery and were primary in the pineal region. A

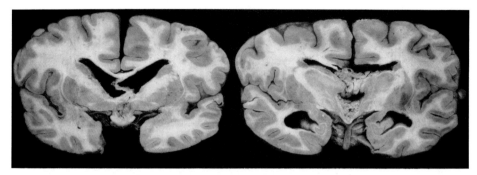

FIG. 18.14. Germinoma of the pineal gland with widespread ventricular and subarachnoid seeding. (Reproduced with permission from: J. F. Donat *et al.* (27).)

postoperative pulmonary metastasis was noted in 1 of 43 germinomas in the Mayo Clinic experience (12).

Microscopically, germinomas consist of an admixture of primitive germ cells and reactive lymphocytes. The cells grow in sheets and lobules and are characterized by large round vesicular nuclei, prominent often irregular nucleoli, and pale ill-defined cytoplasm (Fig. 18.15). The cells are rich in glycogen, a helpful diagnostic feature. Mitoses are readily identified and focal necrosis may be seen. Human chorionic gonadotropin-immunoreactive syncytiotrophoblastic giant cells were observed in one-half of cases in our institutional review (12), a much higher incidence than is observed in extragonadal germ cell tumors. Such trophoblastic cells may be responsible for elevations of HCG in cerebrospinal fluid and serum, are of no prognostic significance and, most importantly, do not indicate the coexistence of choriocarcinoma (13). Unlike gonadal and mediastinal germinomas, granulomatous reaction is uncommon in intracranial examples. Ultrastructural studies report morphologic features identical to those of testicular seminoma and ovarian disgerminoma (41, 59, 79, 103).

In view of the radiosensitivity of germinomas and their favorable prognosis in comparison to other germ cell tumors, it is of clinical importance to exclude the presence of other germ cell components. The morphologic heterogeneity of such tumors understandably requires adequate and thorough tissue sampling. Measurements of α-fetoprotein and human chorionic gonadotropin in serum and cerebrospinal fluid obtained at the time of surgery may also be of assistance in that they serve as a marker for the presence of endodermal sinus tumor and choriocarcinoma elements, respectively.

Embryonal Carcinoma

Among the least frequently reported intracranial germ cell tumors (12, 16, 42), the embryonal carcinoma is conceptually the most primitive of

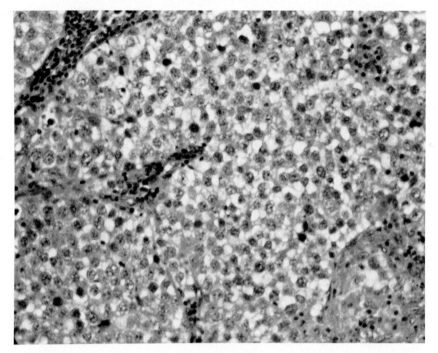

FIG. 18.15. Germinomas are composed of sheets and lobules of large cells with vesicular nuclei, prominent nucleoli, and indistinct glycogen-rich cytoplasm. An associated lymphocytic infiltrate is common, but significant granulomatous inflammation is rarely observed in germinomas of the nervous system. H&E, × 250.

neoplasms composed of pluripotential epithelial cells. This highly malignant lesion forms a mass, most often in the pineal region, and is rarely found in its pure form (Fig. 18.16). It is composed of sheets of mitotically active cuboidal to columnar cells with large vesicular nuclei and prominent nucleoli (Fig. 18.17). Embryoid body formation is rarely noted. Focal embryonic (teratoid) or extraembryonic (yolk sac, trophoblastic) differentiation is not uncommon and is the likely basis for reports of α-fetoprotein and human chorionic gonadotropin production in what are presumed to be pure embryonal carcinomas (3). The clinical behavior and prognosis of this neoplasm are similar to those of endodermal sinus tumor.

Endodermal Sinus Tumor

Initially thought to represent merely a morphologic variant of embryonal carcinoma, the endodermal sinus tumor (EST) or "yolk sac tumor" has come to be considered a specific form of germ cell tumor due primarily to its elaboration of protein markers. It morphologically reca-

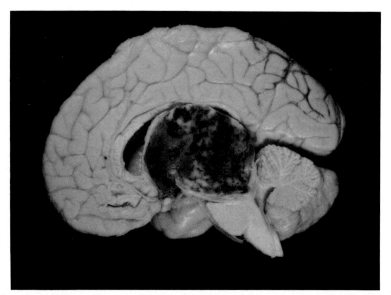

FIG. 18.16. Embryonal carcinoma forming a large, discreet, focally hemorrhagic pineal and third ventricular mass. This tumor also contained an EST component. Embryonal carcinomas express behavioral similarities to those of endodermal sinus tumor and may widely seed the neuroaxis. (Reproduced with permission from: J. F. Donat *et al.* (27).)

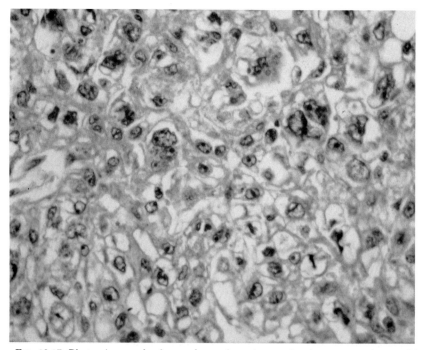

FIG. 18.17. Photomicrograph of an embryonal carcinoma showing a patternless proliferation of large discreet epithelial cells with vesicular nuclei, prominent nucleoli, and abundant mitotic figures. H&E, × 250.

pitulates the yolk sac or endodermal sinus, an extraembryonic endodermal derivative in lower mammals.

Since Bestle's first description of an intracranial endodermal sinus tumor (9), nearly 40 cases have been reported, the most recent example with accompanying literature review being that of Kleinman *et al.* (45). Nearly two-thirds were pure, being unassociated with other germ cell elements. Approximately one-half arose in the pineal region. Alternate sites of origin, in order of decreasing frequency, were the third ventricle, sellar region, and posterior fossa. The patients ranged in age from 10 months to 24 years (mean, 13 years); approximately 70% were male. The nonspecific nature of the symptoms reflected the tumors' location and as of short duration. Of interest is the reported occurrence of endodermal sinus tumor in two female siblings (65).

Craniospinal spread has been reported to occur in one-third of patients (Fig. 18.18), whereas abdominal spread via ventriculoperitoneal shunts has been noted in five instances (6, 44, 110). Systemic metastasis is an uncommon occurrence, having been reported in only two cases (64, 71). Endodermal sinus tumors are highly aggressive, with the mean survival in reported cases being less than one year. Optimal therapy appears to be a combination of surgery with adjuvant radio- and chemotherapy.

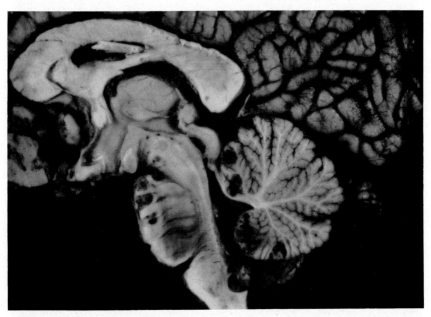

FIG. 18.18. Gross appearance of an endodermal sinus tumor of the pineal region with associated multifocal cerebrospinal metastases involving the cerebellum and brain stem. (Courtesy of Dr. Ellsworth Alvord, Department of Neuropathology, University of Washington, Seattle, Wash.)

Although several histologic patterns, including solid and microcystic forms have been described, the classic morphologic feature of endodermal sinus tumor is the formation of Schiller-Duval bodies (Fig. 18.19). The latter are structures composed of a blood vessel invaginating a space, with both being enshrouded by a layer of cuboidal tumor cells with clear cytoplasm, small dark nuclei, and distinct nucleoli. By immunocytologic methods, eosinophilic, PAS-positive, and diastase-resistant cytoplasmic globules, as well as extracellular hyaline spheres, are seen to be composed of α-fetoprotein or α-1-antitrypsin, respectively (Fig. 18.20) (45, 64, 76).

Serum and cerebrospinal fluid α-fetoprotein levels are elevated in patients with endodermal sinus tumor and have been shown to be useful in the diagnosis, monitoring of therapy, detection of recurrences, and formulation of prognosis (63, 71). In that the half-life of α-fetoprotein is 5–7 days, meaningful levels may be determined even in the postoperative period.

Teratomas: Immature and Mature

Teratomas represent the expression of embryonic differentiation in germ cell tumors. Two principle forms are encountered, mature and

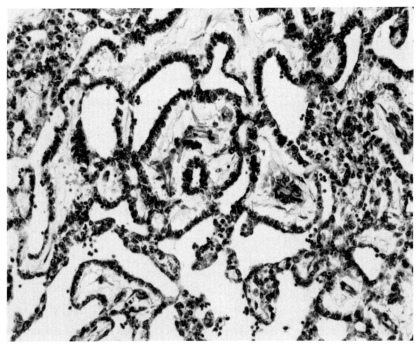

FIG. 18.19. Photomicrograph of an endodermal sinus tumor demonstrating the formation of Schiller-Duval bodies, characteristic features recapitulating the endodermal sinus, an endodermal sinus, an endodermal derivative in lower mammals. H&E, × 250.

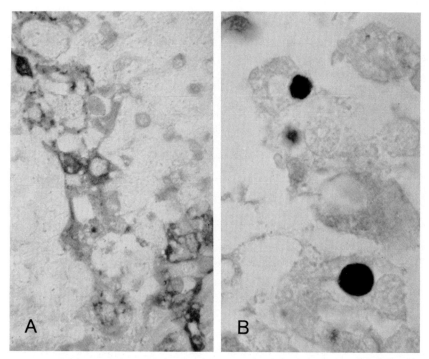

FIG. 18.20. Immunocytochemical reaction of an endodermal sinus tumor for α-fetoprotein (A) as well as α-1-antitrypsin (B). (A) Immunoperoxidase method, × 400; (B) immunoperoxidase method, × 800. (Courtesy of Dr. G. Kleinmann, Bridgeport Hospital, Bridgeport, Conn.)

immature; either may be accompanied by other germ cell elements. The designation "immature" denotes resemblance to embryonic or fetal tissues, whereas "mature" indicates full maturation to adult tissue. This distinction is of more than pathologic interest in that their prognosis differs greatly. The numerically more frequent immature tumors follow an aggressive or malignant course. The latter is also more often associated with other primitive germ cell elements such as embryonal carcinoma, a combination termed "teratocarcinoma."

Teratomas most frequently involve the pineal or suprasellar region, are lobulated and multicystic, and may be massive (Fig. 18.21). Most patients present in the first decade. In our institutional experience (12), the teratomas, both mature and immature, appeared clinicopathologically similar to those reported by others (2, 41, 43, 70, 75, 108). By definition, teratomas consist of tissues representing all three germ layers. In practice, less complete tumors, termed "imperfect," are not uncommon. Neuroectodermal components are no more frequently encountered or

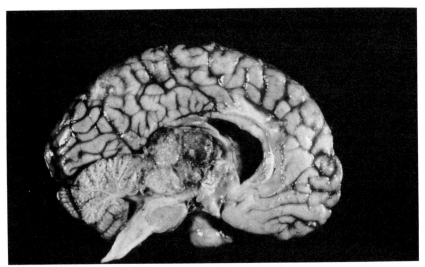

FIG. 18.21. Teratoma of the pineal region. Such tumors, both mature and immature, are characteristically globular, multicystic, and heterogeneous in texture. (Courtesy of Dr. Ellsworth Alvord, Department of Neuropathology, University of Washington, Seattle, Wash.)

extensively represented in intracranial tumors than they are in teratomas at other locations.

IMMATURE TERATOMA

The large series of germ cell tumors of Bjornsson *et al.* (12) disclosed 16 immature teratomas, 10 of which involved the posterior third ventricle or pineal region. Nine were pure teratomas consisting of fetal-appearing tissues (Fig. 18.22), whereas seven contained additional malignant germ cell elements, including either or both germinoma and embryonal carcinoma, and endodermal sinus tumor. Syncytiotrophoblastic giant cells, immunocytochemically reactive to HCG, were observed in one case. Of particular interest were two examples with extensive rhabdomyoblastic components, both of which demonstrated widespread cerebrospinal dissemination of the same (Fig. 18.23). Such tumors should be distinguished from the rare rhabdomyosarcoma of the central nervous system (48, 49, 54, 56, 66, 78, 94, 111) as well as from the medullomyoblastoma (14, 51, 58, 88); both lack other features of germ cell tumors.

Grading schemes such as those applied to gonadal germ cell tumors (72) have not been successfully applied to intracranial teratomas, due primarily to incomplete tissue sampling, high operative mortality, and the small number of tumors available for study. The poor prognosis

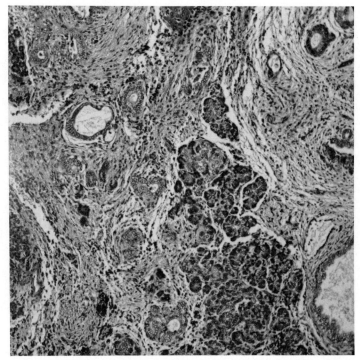

FIG. 18.22. Photomicrograph of an immature teratoma. Note the resemblance of the varied tissues to those of a fetus. H&E, × 100.

associated with immature teratomas was also apparent in our series (12). Eleven of the 16 patients with immature teratoma survived the postoperative period. Of these, seven died of their tumor. Twenty-five percent of all patients developed metastases, three in the form of craniospinal dissemination and one with peritoneal metastases via a ventriculoperitoneal shunt (12).

MATURE TERATOMA

Of the 23 teratomas included in our study (12), seven were mature teratomas. The tumors consisted entirely of fully differentiated tissue; none contained other malignant germ cell elements. All were midline, and six involved the posterior third ventricle and pineal region. Eleven patients (69%) were males.

Histologically, ecto- and endodermal epithelia were associated with well-differentiated fibrous, cartilaginous, osseous, and nervous tissues (Fig. 18.24). Again, neuroectodermal elements were no more extensively

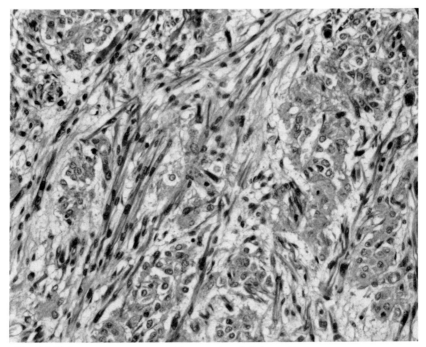

FIG. 18.23. Immature teratoma with extensive rhabdomyoblastic differentiation. Elongate myotubes are well seen and represent the component which disseminated widely in the craniospinal leptomeninges. H&E, × 160.

represented than in teratomas at other locations. Three patients who survived the postoperative period were alive at 4–13 years without evidence of recurrence; the high operative mortality in our series reflects the long period of case study (1925–1983).

CHORIOCARCINOMA

Extragenital choriocarcinomas are rare, arising in the midline in such locations as the retroperitoneum, mediastinum, gastrointestinal tract, and central nervous system. Yamagami *et al.* (12), in a recent exhaustive review of intracranial choriocarcinomas, summarized the clinicopathologic features of 24 pure examples. Among our 70 cases of primary intracranial germ cell neoplasm, only one such tumor was identified (11, 12).

Patients with choriocarcinoma of the nervous system are often in the second decade. Most present with a short duration of symptoms, including Parinaud's syndrome in posteriorly situated tumors and visual dis-

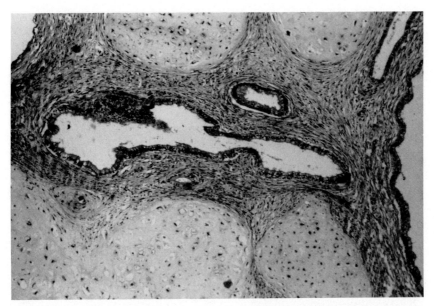

FIG. 18.24. Mature teratoma. The tumor is less cellular than the immature teratoma (Fig. 18.21) and is composed of histologically mature epithelial and mesenchymal elements. H&E, × 100.

turbances as well as diabetes insipidus in the less frequently occurring sellar and suprasellar examples. Precocious puberty is uncommon (19, 82, 115).

The diagnosis of choriocarcinoma may be presumed on the basis of highly elevated serum and cerebrospinal fluid HCG levels (3, 109, 112). It must be kept in mind that elevated levels of this product are not pathognomonic of choriocarcinoma. Syncytiotrophoblastic giant cells, present in approximately half of germinomas as well as in a small number in other germ cell tumors, may also produce elevated HCG levels (12).

Choriocarcinomas at all sites tend toward hemorrhage. Aside from its obvious catastrophic clinical consequences, such hemorrhage may thwart the pathologist's attempts to identify viable tumor tissue.

Choriocarcinomas are pathologically characterized by the presence of a bilaminar or plexiform pattern of syncytiotrophoblastic giant cells overlying cords of cytotrophoblast (Fig. 18.25A). This neoplastic recapitulation of the cell arrangement observed in chorionic villi is further mimicked by the presence of extensive blood-filled spaces. True chorionic villi are not observed. Immunocytochemical stains for HCG are strongly reactive within syncytiotrophoblastic cells (Fig. 18.25B).

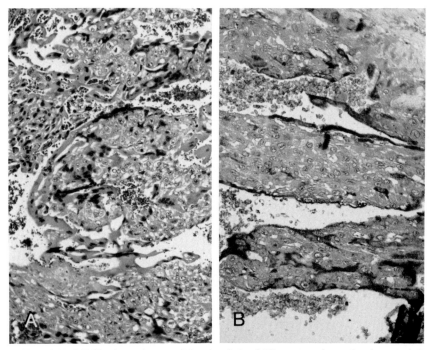

FIG. 18.25. (A) Choriocarcinoma of the pineal gland. The tumor shows the characteristic bilayer arrangement of syncytio- and cytotrophoblast associated with blood-filled spaces. H&E, × 100. (B) Immunostains for human chorionic gonadotropin are strongly reactive in syncytiotrophoblastic cells. Immunoperoxidase method (anti-HCG), × 100.

In that metastases of genital choriocarcinoma to the nervous system are without doubt more common than are primary tumors at this site (4, 47) it remains questionable as to whether any investigation, short of a detailed autopsy, can resolve the issue in a given case. Intracranial choriocarcinoma has been documented to metastasize outside the central nervous system (70, 102).

REFERENCES

1. Ahagon, A., Yoshida, Y., Kusuno, K., et al. Suprasellar germinoma in association with Klinefelter's syndrome: Case report. J. Neurosurg., 58: 136–138, 1983.
2. Albrechtsen, R., Klee, J. G., and Moller, J. E. Primary intracranial germ cell tumors including five cases of endodermal sinus tumor. Acta Pathol. Microbiol. Scand. (A) Suppl. 233: 32–38, 1972.
3. Allen, J. C., Nisselbaum, J., Epstein, F., et al. Alphafetoprotein and human chorionic gonadotropin determination in cerebrospinal fluid. J. Neurosurg., 51: 368–374, 1979.
4. Athanassiou, A., Begent, R. H. J., Newlands, E. S., et al. Central nervous system metastases of choriocarcinoma: 23 years' experience at Charing Cross Hospital. Cancer, 52: 1728–1735, 1983.

5. Bailey, P., and Murray, H. A. A case of pinealoma with symptoms suggestive of compulsion neurosis. Arch. Neurol. Psychiatry, *19:* 932–945, 1928.
6. Bamberg, M., Metz, K., Alberti, W., *et al.* Endodermal sinus tumor of the pineal region. Metastases through a ventriculoperitoneal shunt. Cancer, *54:* 903–906, 1984.
7. Banerjee, A. K., and Kak, V. K. Pineoblastoma with spontaneous intra and extracranial metastasis. J. Pathol., *114:* 9–12, 1974.
8. Best, P. V. A medulloblastoma-like tumour with melanin formation. J. Pathol., *110:* 109–111, 1973.
9. Bestle, J. Extragonadal endodermal sinus tumours originating in the region of the pineal gland. Acta Pathol. Microbiol. Scand., *74:* 214–222, 1968.
10. Bing, J. F., Globus, J. H., and Simon, H. Pubertas praecox: A survey of the reported cases and verified anatomical findings: With particular reference to tumors of the pineal body. J. Mt. Sinai Hosp. N.Y., *4:* 935–965, 1938.
11. Bjornsson, J., Scheithauer, B. W., and Leech, R. W. Primary intracranial choriocarcinoma: report of a case. Clin. Neuropathol., in press, 1985.
12. Bjornsson, J., Scheithauer, B. W., Okazaki, H., Leech, R. W. Intracranial germ cell tumors: pathobiologic and immunohistochemical aspects of seventy cases. J. Neuropathol. Exp. Neurol., in press, 1985.
13. Bloom, H. J. G. Combined modality therapy for intracranial tumors. Cancer, *35:* 111–120, 1975.
14. Bofin, P. J., and Ebbls, E. A case of medullomyoblastoma. Acta Neuropathol., *2:* 309–311, 1963.
15. Borden, S. IV, Weber, A. L., Toch, R., *et al.* Pineal germinoma: Long-term survival despite hematogenous metastases. Am. J. Dis. Child., *126:* 214–216, 1973.
16. Borit, A. Embryonal carcinoma of the pineal region. J. Pathol., *97:* 165–168, 1969.
17. Borit, A., and Blackwood, W. Pineocytoma with astrocytomatous differentiation. J. Neuropathol. Exp. Neurol., *38:* 253–258, 1979.
18. Borit, A., Blackwood, W., and Miar, W. G. P. The separation of pineocytoma from pineoblastoma. Cancer, *45:* 1408–1418, 1980.
19. Bruton, O. C., Martz, D. C., and Gerard, E. S. Precocious puberty due to secreting chorionepithelioma (teratoma) of the brain. J. Pediatr., *59:* 719–725, 1961.
20. Budde, M. Uber die Genese der Fetalinklusionen. Beitr. Pathol. Anat., *75:* 357, 1926.
21. Castleman, B., and Towne, V. Weekly clinicopathologic exercise. N. Engl. J. Med., *247:* 1036–1040, 1952.
22. Cooper, E. R. A. The human pineal gland and pineal cysts. J. Anat., *67:* 28–46, 1932.
23. Dayan, A. D., Marshall, A. H. E., Miller, A. A., *et al.* Atypical teratomas of the pineal and hypothalamus. J. Pathol. Bacteriol., *92:* 1–28, 1966.
24. DeGirolami, U. Pathology of tumors of the pineal region. In: *Pineal Tumors,* edited by H. Schmidek, pp. 1–19. Masson, New York, 1977.
25. DeGirolami, U., and Schmidek, H. Clinicopathological study of 53 tumors of the pineal region. J. Neurosurg., *39:* 455–462, 1973.
26. DeGirolami, U., and Zvaigzne, O. Modification of the Achucarro-Hortega pineal stain for paraffin-embedded formalin-fixed tissue. Stain Tech., *48:* 48–50, 1973.
27. Donat, J. F., Okazaki, H., Gomez, M. R., *et al.* Pineal tumors: A 53-year experience. Arch. Neurol., *35:* 736–740, 1978.
28. Enriguez, R., Egbert, B., and Bullock, J. Primary malignant melanoma of the nervous system. Pineal involvement in a patient with nevus of ota and multiple pigmented skin nevi. Arch. Pathol., *95:* 392, 1973.
29. Friedman, N. B. Germinoma of the pineal: Its identify with germinoma ("seminoma") of the testis. Cancer Res., *7:* 363–368, 1947.
30. Friedmann, R., and Scheinker, J. Ein Fall von Neuroepithelioma der Zirbeldruse. Monatsschr. Psychiatry Neurol., *89:* 81–96, 1934.

31. Fulton, J. F., and Bailey, P. Tumors of the region of the third ventricle: Their diagnosis and relation to pathological sleep. J. Nerv. Ment. Dis., *69:* 1–25, 1929.
32. Giebel, W. Uber primare Tumoren der Zirbeldruse. Frankfurt Z. Pathol., *25:* 176, 1921.
33. Goldzieher, M. Uber eine Zirbeldrusengeschwulst. Virchows Arch. [Pathol. Anat.], *213:* 353–365, 1913.
34. Halpert, B., Erickson, E. E., and Fields, W. S. Intracranial involvement from carcinoma of the lung. Arch. Pathol., *69:* 93–103, 1960.
35. Hassoun, J., Gambarelli, D., Peragut, J. C., *et al.* Specific ultrastructural markers of human pinealomas: A study of four cases. Acta Neuropathol. (Berl.), *62:* 31–40, 1983.
36. Herrick, M. K., and Rubinstein, L. J. The cytological differentiating potential of pineal parenchymal neoplasms (true pinealomas): A clinicopathological study of 28 tumours. Brain, *102:* 289–320, 1979.
37. Hirtz, M. Lipome de l'encephale. Bull. Soc. Anat. (Paris), *50:* 254–256, 1875.
38. Holness, R. O., and Sangalang, V. E. Myelomatous metastasis to the pineal body. Surg. Neurol., *5:* 97–100, 1976.
39. Hubschnann, O., Kasoff, S., Doniger, D., *et al.* Cavernous hemangioma in the pineal region. Surg. Neurol., *6:* 349–351, 1976.
40. Jakobiec, F. A., Tso, M. O., Zimmerman, L. E., *et al.* Retinoblastoma and intracranial malignancy. Cancer, *39:* 2058–2058, 1977.
41. Jellinger, K. Primary intracranial germ cell tumors. Acta Neuropathol. (Berl.), *25:* 291–306, 1973.
42. Jellinger, K., Minauf, M., Kraus, H., *et al.* Embryonales Carcinoma der Epiphysenregion. Acta Neuropathol. (Berl.), *15:* 176–182, 1970.
43. Jooma, R., and Kendall, B. E. Diagnosis and management of pineal tumors. J. Neurosurg., *58:* 654–665, 1983.
44. Kimura, N., Namiki, T., Wada, T., *et al.* Peritoneal implantation of endodermal sinus tumor of the pineal region via a ventriculoperitoneal shunt. Cytodiagnosis with immunocytochemical demonstration of alpha-fetoprotein. Acta Cytol. (Baltimore), *28:* 143–147, 1984.
45. Kleinman, G., Krishnan, N., Nijensohn, D. Pineal yolk sac tumor cancer, in press, 1985.
46. Kline, K. T., Damjanov, I., Katz, S. M., *et al.* Pineoblastoma: An electron microscopic study. Cancer, *44:* 1692–1699, 1979.
47. Kobayashi, T., Kida, Y., Yoshida, J., *et al.* Brain metastasis of choriocarcinoma. Surg. Neurol., *17:* 395–403, 1982.
48. Leedham, P. W. Primary cerebral rhabdomyosarcoma and the problem of medulloblastoma. J. Neurol. Neurosurg. Psychiatry, *35:* 551–559, 1972.
49. Leiger, J. F., and Wezis, H. A., Jr. Primary cerebellar rhabdomyosarcoma. Case report. J. Neurosurg., *26:* 436–438, 1967.
50. Lerner, A. B., Case, J. D., and Heinzealman, R. V. Structure of melatonin. J. Am. Chem. Soc., *81:* 6084–6085, 1959.
51. Lewis, A. J. Medulloblastoma with striated muscle fibers. Case report. J. Neurosurg., *38:* 642–646, 1973.
52. Markesberry, W. R., Hughes, R. M., and Young, A. B. Ultrastructure of pineal parenchymal neoplasms. Acta Neuropathol. (Berl.), *55:* 143–149, 1981.
53. Marsden, H. B., Birch, J. M., and Swindell, R. Germ cell tumors of childhood: A review of 137 cases. J. Clin. Pathol., *34:* 879–883, 1981.
54. Matsukado, Y., Yokoth, A., and Marubayashi, T. Rhabdomyosarcoma of the brain.

Case report. J. Neurosurg., *43:* 215–221, 1975.

55. McDonnell, D. E. Pineal epidermoid cyst: Its surgical therapy. Surg. Neurol., 7: 387–391, 1977.

56. Min, K-W., Gyorkey, F., and Halpert, B. Primary rhabdomyosarcoma of the cerebrum. Cancer, *35:* 1405–1411, 1975.

57. Mincer, F., Melzer, J., and Botstein, C. Pinealoma. A report of twelve irradiated cases. Cancer, *37:* 2713–2718, 1976.

58. Misugi, K., and Liss, L. Medulloblastoma with cross-striated muscle. A fine structural study. Cancer, *25:* 1279–1285, 1970.

59. Misugi, K., Liss, L., and Bradel, E. J. Electron microscopic study of an ectopic pinealoma. Acta Neuropathol. (Berl.), *9:* 346–356, 1967.

60. Moller, M. The ultrastructure of the human fetal pineal gland. I. Cell types and blood vessels. Cell Tissue Res., *152:* 13–30, 1974.

61. Mostofi, F. K., and Sobin, L. H. Histological typing of testis tumors. In: *International Histologic Classification of Tumors*, No. 16. World Health Organization, Geneva, 1977.

62. Muller, R., and Wohlfart, G. Intracranial teratomas and teratoid tumors. Acta Psychiatr. (Kbh.), *22:* 69, 1947.

63. Murovic, J. A., Ongley, J. P., Parker, J. C., Jr., *et al.* Manifestations and therapeutic considerations in pineal yolk-sac tumors. Case report. J. Neurosurg., *55:* 303–307, 1981.

64. Nakanishi, I., Kawahara, E., Najikawa, K., *et al.* Hyaline globules in yolk-sac tumors. Histochemical, immunohistochemical and electron microscopic studies. Acta Pathol. Jpn., *32:* 733–739, 1982.

65. Nakasu, S., Handa, J., Kozama, F., *et al.* Suprasellar yolk sac tumors in two sisters. Surg. Neurol., *20:* 147–151, 1983.

66. Namba, K., Aschenbrenner, C., Nikpour, M., *et al.* Primary rhabdomyosarcoma of the tentorium with peculiar angiographic findings. Surg. Neurol., *11:* 39–43, 1979.

67. Neuwelt, E. A., Glasberg, M., Frenkel, E., *et al.* Malignant pineal region tumors: A clinico-pathologic study. J. Neurosurg., *51:* 597–607, 1979.

68. Newmann, M. A. Periventricular diffuse pinealoma: Report of a case with clinical features of catatonic schizophrenia. J. Nerv. Ment. Dis., *121:* 193–204, 1955.

69. Nielsen, S. L., and Wilson, C. B. Ultrastructure of a "pineocytoma." J. Neuropathol. Exp. Neurol., *34:* 148–158, 1975.

70. Nishiyama, R. H., Batsakis, J. G., Weaver, D. K., *et al.* Germinal neoplasms of the central nervous system. Arch. Surg., *93:* 342–347, 1966.

71. Norgaard-Pedersen, B., Lindholm, J., Albrechtsen, R., *et al.* Alpha fetoprotein and human chorionic gonadotropin in a patient with a primary intracranial germ cell tumor. Cancer, *41(6):* 2315–2320, 1978.

72. Norris, H. J., Zirkin, H. J., and Benson, W. L. Immature (malignant) teratoma of the ovary: A clinical and pathologic study of 58 cases. Cancer, *37:* 2359–2372, 1976.

73. Olson, J. R., and Abell, M. R. Hemangiopericytoma of the pineal body. J. Neurol. Neurosurg. Psychiatry, *32:* 445–449, 1969.

74. Ortega, P., Malamud, N., and Shimkin, M. B. Metastasis to the pineal body. Arch. Pathol., *52:* 518–528, 1951.

75. Oswald, U., and Hedinger, C. Intrakranielle Kiemzelletumoren (Teratome und Seminome). Virchows Arch. [Pathol. Anat.], *357:* 281–298, 1972.

76. Palmer, P. E., Safaii, H., and Wolfe, H. J. Alpha-1-antitrypsin and alpha fetoprotein markers in endodermal sinus (yolk sac) tumors. Am. J. Clin. Pathol., *65:* 575–582, 1976.

77. Papasozomenos, S., and Shapiro, S. Pineal astrocytoma: Report of a case, confined to the epiphysis, with immunocytochemical and electron microscopic studies. Cancer, *47:* 99–103, 1981.
78. Pasquier, B., Couderc, P., Pasquier, D., *et al.* Primary rhabdomyosarcoma of the central nervous system. Acta Neuropathol., *33:* 333–342, 1975.
79. Ramsey, H. J. Ultrastructure of a pineal tumor. Cancer, *18:* 1014–1025, 1965.
80. Ringertz, N., Nordenstam, H., and Flyger, G. Tumors of the pineal region. J. Neuropathol. Exp. Neurol., *13:* 540–561, 1954.
81. Robertson, H. J. A case of pinealoma in a West African. West Afr. Med. J., *9;* 86–89, 1960.
82. Romshe, C. A., and Sotos, J. F. Intracranial human chorionic gonadotropin-secreting tumor with precocious puberty. J. Pediatr., *86:* 250–252, 1975.
83. Rubin, P., and Kramer, S. Ectopic pinealoma: A radiocurable neuroendocrinologic entity. Radiology, *85:* 512–523, 1965.
84. Rubinstein, L. J. Tumors of the central nervous system. In: *Atlas of Tumor Pathology,* Second Series, Fascicle 6. Armed Forces Institute of Pathology, Washington, D.C., 1972.
85. Rubinstein, L. J. Cytogenetics and differentiation of pineal neoplasms. Hum. Pathol., *12:* 441–448, 1981.
86. Rubinstein, L. J., and Okazaki, H. Gangliogliomatous differentiation in a pineocytoma. J. Pathol., *102:* 27–32, 1970.
87. Russell, D. S. The pinealoma: Its relationship to teratoma. J. Pathol. Bacteriol., *56:* 145–150, 1944.
88. Russell, D. S., and Rubinstein, L. J. *Pathology of Tumors of the Nervous System,* pp. 24–28. Williams & Wilkens, Baltimore, 1977.
89. Sachs, E., Jr., Avman, N., and Fisher, R. G. Meningiomas of pineal region and posterior part of 3rd ventricle. J. Neurosurg., *19:* 325–331, 1962.
90. Sakata, K., Yamada, H., Sakai, N., *et al.* Extraneural metastasis of pineal tumor. Surg. Neurol., *3:* 49–54, 1975.
91. Sambasivian, M., and Nayar, A. Epidermoid cyst of the pineal region. J. Neurol. Neurosurg. Psychiatry, *37:* 1333–1335, 1974.
92. Scully, R. E., Mark, E. J., and McNeely, B. U. Case records of the Massachusetts General Hospital: Weekly Clinicopathologic Exercises. Case 35-1983. N. Engl. J. Med., *309:* 542–549, 1983.
93. Sevitt, S., and Schorstein, J. A case of pineal cyst. Br. Med. J., *2:* 490, 1947.
94. Shuangshoti, S., Piyaratn, P., and Viriyapanich, P. L. Primary rhabdomyosarcoma of cerebellum. Cancer, *22:* 367–371, 1968.
95. Simson, L. R., Lampe, I., and Abell, M. R. Suprasellar germinomas. Cancer, *22:* 533–544, 1968.
96. Sivak, J. G. Historical note: The vertebrate median eye. Vision Res., *14:* 137–140, 1974.
97. Smith, W. T., Hughes, B., and Ermocilla, R. Chemodectoma of the pineal region, with observations on the pineal body and chemoreceptor tissue. J. Pathol. Bacteriol., *92:* 69–76, 1966.
98. Sobel, R. A., Trite, J. E., Nielsen, S. L., *et al.* Pineoblastoma with ganglionic and glial differentiation: Report of two cases. Acta Neuropathol. (Berl.), *55:* 243–246, 1981.
99. Solarski, A., Panke, E. S., and Panke, T. W. Craniopharyngioma in the pineal gland. Arch. Pathol. Lab. Med., *102:* 490–491, 1978.
100. Stefanko, S. Z., and Manschot, W. A. Pinealoblastoma with retinoblastomatous differentiation. Brain, *102:* 321–332, 1979.

101. Stein, B. M. The infratentorial suprasellar approach to pineal lesions. J. Neurosurg., *35:* 197–202, 1971.
102. Steinbok, P., Dolman, C., and Kaan, K. Pineocytomas presenting as subarachnoid hemorrhage. Report of 2 cases. J. Neurosurg., *47:* 776–780, 1977.
103. Tabuchi, K., Yamada, O., and Nishimoto, A. The ultrastructure of pinealomas. Acta Neuropathol. (Berl.), *24:* 117–127, 1973.
104. Takeuchi, J., Handa, H., and Nagata, I. Supracellar germinoma. J. Neurosurg., *49:* 41–48, 1978.
105. Tapp, E., and Huxley, M. The histological appearance of the human pineal gland from puberty to old age. J. Pathol., *108:* 137–144, 1972.
106. Trojanowski, J. Q., Tascos, N. A., and Rorke, L. B. Malignant pineocytoma with prominent papillary features. Cancer, *50:* 1789–1793, 1982.
107. Tso, M. O. M., Fine, B. S., Zimmerman, L. E., *et al.* Photoreceptor elements in retinoblastoma. Arch. Opthalmol., *82:* 57–59, 1969.
108. Wara, W. M., Jenkin, R. D. T., Evans, A., *et al.* Tumors of the pineal and suprasellar region: Childrens Cancer Study Group Treatment Results 1960–1975: A report from Children's Cancer Study Group. Cancer, *43:* 698–701, 1979.
109. Wass, J. A. H., Jones, A. E., Rees, L. H., *et al.* hCGB producing pineal choriocarcinoma. Clin. Endocrinol. (Oxford), *17:* 423–431, 1982.
110. Wilson, E. R., Takei, Y., Bikoff, W. T., *et al.* Abdominal metastases of primary intracranial yolk-sac tumors through ventriculoperitoneal shunts: Report of three cases. Neurosurgery, *5:* 356–364, 1979.
111. Yagashita, S., Itoh, Y., Chiba, Y., *et al.* Primary rhabdomyosarcoma of the cerebrum. An ultrastructural study. Acta Neuropathol., *45:* 111–115, 1979.
112. Yamagami, T., Handa, H., Takeuchi, J., *et al.* Choriocarcinoma arising from the pituitary fossa with extracranial metastasis: A review of the litrature. Surg. Neurol., *19:* 469–480, 1983.
113. Zeitlin, H. Tumors in the region of the pineal body: Clinicopathologic report of 3 cases. Arch. Neurol. Psychiatry, *34:* 567–586, 1935.
114. Zimmerman, B. L., and Tso, M. O. M. Morphologic evidence of photoreceptor differentiation of pinealocytes in the neonatal rat. J. Cell Biol., *66:* 60–75, 1975.
115. Zondek, H., Kaatz, A., and Unger, H. Precocious puberty and chorioepithelioma of the pineal gland with report of a case. J. Endocrinol., *10:* 12–16, 1953.
116. Zulch, K. J. Histological typing of tumors of the central nervous system. In: *International Histologic Classification of Tumors*, No. 21. World Health Organization, Geneva, 1979.
117. Zulch, K. J. Brain tumors: Their biology and pathology, Ed. 2 (American), pp. 240–244, Springer-Verlag, New York, 1965.

19

Shunting and Irradiation of Pineal Tumors

W. RICHARD MARSH, M.D., and EDWARD R. LAWS, JR., M.D.

This chapter will assess the role of cerebrospinal fluid shunting procedures in conjunction with radiotherapy in the treatment of pineal region tumors. The crux of the discussion will be a presentation of a series of patients so managed at the Mayo Clinic between 1950 and 1978. Before proceeding with this, however, let us consider why there is continuing discussion and uncertainty over the optimal therapy for patients with tumors here.

BACKGROUND

Primary pineal tumors are uncommon lesions. In most North American and European series they comprise only 0.4–1% of all primary brain tumors. For unknown reasons, there is a higher incidence in Japan of tumors of the pineal region (3). Here, approximately 4% of all primary intracranial neoplasms occur in the pineal region. This higher incidence is comprised for the most part of the so-called germinoma or pinealoma of the two-cell type pattern. The important point here, however, is that individual clinical experience with these tumors is somewhat limited, except for the most common histologic types, and it becomes very difficult to draw firm conclusions regarding optimal therapy for some of the more uncommon tumors.

As has been pointed out by Dr. Scheithauer, there is a wide spectrum of tumor types encountered in the region. Many series of patients have been presented which "lump" primary pineal tumors, *i.e.*, pineal cell tumors, germ cell tumors, and gliomas of the posterior third ventricle, together with other tumors of the pineal region. These latter include meningioma, dermoids, epidermoids, and metastatic tumors. Certainly, other nonneoplastic conditions may be encountered in the region, most notably arteriovenous malformation of the vein of Galen and arachnoid cysts. Even these have been noted as tumors of the pineal region in some series of patients. It is apparent that before any meaningful discussion of the optimal therapy of these lesions can be made, we need to have a common denominator for discussion. No one would argue the advisability of surgery to remove a benign, encapsulated lesion which is symptomatic and technically removable.

Attempts at surgical excision of these lesions can, however, be problematic. Their central location and relationship to the deep venous system continue to remain a challenge. We are all aware of the early reports in this century of high operative mortality and morbidity following direct operative treatment of these tumors. One has only to peruse series of patients reported from major clinical centers to understand the extent of the problem. Olivecrona and his colleagues endured a 58% surgical case mortality rate among 36 patients subjected to radical surgery. There were only 7 survivors 5–20 years after operation. My predecessors at the Mayo Clinic lost 17 of 34 patients in the first postoperative month, irrespective of treatment, and all 11 suboccipital craniectomies for direct attack on the lesion before 1950 ended fatally (5). Perhaps the most depressing reading that is available are the details of surgery at the Lahey Clinic during the years 1934 to 1952. During this time, the first 32 patients in the series were treated by a number of different approaches, but it appears that only two patients who had the tumor verified by craniotomy achieved a substantial survival period. It is not hard to understand why an attitude of surgical conservatism evolved from this nightmare. The advent of the operating microscope in the last two decades has resulted in a new emphasis on the direct surgical removal of these lesions. It is clear that the refinements of diagnostic radiology, neuroanesthesia, and microneurosurgical techniques have reduced the mortality and morbidity of direct surgery to levels undreamed of earlier in this century (26, 44).

Problems remain, however. While direct surgical treatment is technically feasible, the long-term results of such treatment are less clear. Most current surgical series of patients have not been followed sufficiently long to allow satisfactory comparison to groups of patients treated conservatively in earlier decades. Finally, there is a sizeable proportion of patients who harbor tumors which are not satisfactorily treated by any current modality.

Primary tumors affecting the pineal region may be of glial, pineal, or germ cell origin (17, 18, 20, 22, 35, 58, 62, 65, 68, 72). Although gliomas of the pineal region or quadrigeminal plate may mimick true pineal tumors, their natural history and response to therapy are no different from other supratentorial gliomas. The differential diagnosis of tumors of the pineal region is recorded in Table 19.1. In most cases, excellent radiologic studies can differentiate among primary pineal tumors, cysts, epidermoids, aneurysms, and other nonpineal lesions in the area. The incidence of the various histologic types of primary pineal tumors varies in reported series. Of the true pineal tumors, approximately two-thirds

TABLE 19.1

Tumors of the Pineal Region: Differential Diagnosis

A. Pineal Parenchymal Tumors
   1. Pineocytoma
      a. With neuronal differentiation
      b. With astrocytic differentiation
      c. With neuronal and astrocytic differentiation
   2. Pineoblastoma
      a. With pineocytic differentiation
      b. With retinoblastomatous differentiation
B. Germ Cell Tumors
   1. Germinoma
   2. Embryonal carcinoma
   3. Yolk sac tumor
   4. Choriocarcinoma
   5. Teratoma
      a. Mature
      b. Immature
      c. With malignant transformation
   6. Mixed histology
C. Primary Neuroectodermal Tumors
   1. Astrocytoma
   2. Oligodendroglioma
   3. Ependymoma
   4. Medulloepithelioma
   5. Paraganglioma ("chemodectoma")
   6. Ganglioneuroma
   7. Melanoma
D. Primary Nonneuroectodermal Tumors
   1. Lipoma
   2. Hemangioma
   3. Meningioma
   4. Hemangiopericytoma
   5. Craniopharyngioma
   6. Choroid plexus papilloma
E. Miscellaneous
   1. Pineal cyst
   2. Arachnoid cyst
   3. Epidermoid cyst
   4. Dermoid cyst
   5. Plasma cell leukemia
   6. Metastatic carcinoma
   7. Aneurysm (arteriovenous malformation) vein of Galen

are of germ cell origin. Of these, roughly one-half are germinomas (seminomas) and one-half are teratomas (50% benign, 50% malignant) (7, 30, 63, 64). Aside from tumors of germ cell origin, pineal cell tumors comprise the remaining one-third of the true pineal tumors. These are represented by the pineocytomas and pineoblastomas (22, 33, 40). Long-term survival has commonly followed successful management of germinoma, benign teratoma, and pineocytoma. The more malignant lesions have had a uniformly poor prognosis with current treatment modalities.

Clinically, the age and sex distribution of primary pineal tumors are quite distinctive (9). The mean age at diagnosis is 17 years, and there is a marked male predominance. These tumors are more common in patients of Oriental heritage than in patients of other races (3).

The most frequent presenting symptoms are those of generalized increased intracranial pressure, namely, headache as well as vomiting and drowsiness (11, 18). Visual symptoms are nearly as often noted. These may include blurring of vision and decrease in acuity. Symptoms of hypothalamic dysfunction such as precocious puberty, diabetes insipidus or emaciation are less common, occurring in only 15% of patients (6, 27). The most common neurologic signs of pineal tumors are ophthalmologic, with some abnormality in virtually every case. Papilledema, impairment of pupillary reflexes, and paresis of upward gaze (Parinaud's syndrome) are the most common findings. Other signs, related either to hydrocephalus or local extension of the tumor, may occur. Plain skull x-rays are still valuable in showing abnormal calcifications in the pineal region in roughly one-quarter of patients and signs of increased pressure in a significant portion of the rest (12, 13). Computed tomography (CT) has all but replaced other radiologic procedures as the definitive neuroradiologic procedure for pineal tumors. CT scans show virtually 100% of the tumors. These commonly appear as high-density abnormalities which enhance with contrast (37, 42, 66, 71). The CT scan will indicate the degree of hydrocephalus when present and may also show ependymal seeding or dissemination of tumor in the subarachnoid space. Anterior and posterior extension of the tumor is well demonstrated by axial CT scanning, but the precise relationship of the tumor to the tentorium and the amount of posterior fossa extension is often best shown by imaging the tumor in the sagittal CT plane. The role of magnetic resonance imaging (MRI) in evaluation of these tumors is under investigation. Angiography is occasionally helpful, particularly when surgery is planned. It is useful for revealing the degree of vascularity of the tumor and thus giving us a hint as to its relative malignancy or to mapping the position of the major vessels prior to operation.

Other laboratory tests may be helpful. If cerebrospinal fluid is available, either from the ventricle or the lumbar subarachnoid space, cytologic examination may disclose tumors cells. Radioimmune assays of the cerebrospinal fluid and serum may be performed to detect markers indicative of α-fetoprotein (AFP) or human chorionic gonadotropin

(HCG) (2). It has been shown that certain tumors, such as the chorio-carcinoma of this region, may produce high quantities of AFP and HCG. Furthermore, elevated levels of these biologic markers have also been seen in some of the germinomas but not consistently.

The neurosurgical management of pineal tumors has gone through several phases, as has been eluded to earlier (10, 32, 34, 36, 38, 41, 44, 47, 48, 50, 53, 54, 57, 67, 69, 77, 85, 86). Walter Dandy reported his early experience with a transcallosal approach but was discouraged by high operative mortality (14, 15, 27). Later, Poppen and Marino (43) recom-mended a right occipital transtentorial approach and reported some success with this mode of direct attack. Van Wagenen (67) utilized a right transcortical transventricular approach. In the last 15 years Dr. Stein (62) has popularized the Krause posterior fossa infratentorial supracerebellar approach.

Some of the earliest shunting procedures were performed for hydro-cephalus resulting from pineal tumors. Dr. Dandy had a patient with a pineal tumor and hydrocephalus in whom he passed a red rubber catheter through the aqueduct. In 1948 Dr. Torkildsen (65) reported a series of eight patients treated with ventriculocisternostomy. Three of them were alive and well 7½, 4½, and 2 years after operation. As shunting became more widely and effectively applied in the 1950s with the introduction of the ventriculoatrial and ventriculoperitoneal shunts these, in conjunction with radiotherapy, became the standard treatment for a patient with an inoperable pineal region tumor.

The number of radiosensitive lesions found in the area has been variously estimated at between 60 and 80%. The beneficial effects of radiation on these primary pineal tumors has been recognized for some time. Germinomas, which account for a high proportion of primary pineal tumors, are so radiosensitive that there is no significant difference between the survival of patients irradiated after direct surgery and those receiving radiotherapy alone. The CT scan has given dramatic evidence of the disappearance of many of these lesions following radiotherapy (52, 70). Pineoblastomas and pineocytomas are also sensitive to radiation. Whole brain and spinal axis radiation is commonly recommended in those tumors in which seeding has been documented by myelography or cytology (29). Radiation therapy, either as a primary modality of treat-ment or when given following surgery, can be administered accurately and with safety (4, 8, 19, 23, 28, 39, 42, 45, 46, 49, 55, 56, 61, 66, 68, 71, 72). Virtually every known long-term surviving patient with a primary pineal tumor has been treated with radiation therapy.

Although the results of recent surgical series with the use of the operating microscope are very encouraging, there is still a need for careful evaluation of the direct surgical treatment and more conservative modes of therapy before any firm conclusion can be reached concerning either approach. The following series of patients was compiled in an attempt to fill a portion of that need.

CLINICAL SERIES

This study includes 44 patients seen at the Mayo Clinic between November 1950 and April 1978 (Table 19.2). Patients were diagnosed to have a pineal tumor and treated by radiotherapy and cerebrospinal fluid shunting when hydrocephalus was a problem. Of the group of 44, 32 had both CSF shunting and radiotherapy at the Mayo Clinic. One patient had a shunt placed elsewhere but had radiotherapy at the Mayo Clinic, and 7 patients had radiotherapy at the Mayo Clinic although requiring no CSF shunting procedure.

There were 15 other patients who had both CSF shunting and radiotherapy in other institutions but who were evaluated at our institution during the same time period. These were excluded from the study because most of them were seen at the Mayo Clinic 2–10 years after initial therapy. As will be seen in our primary treated patients, more than 60% of the deaths from disease occurred in our study within 2½ years. Patients who had the same diagnosis but were seen prior to 1950 and also those patients who had direct surgical management therapy have also been excluded from this series.

As is noted in other series, tumors of the pineal area were more common in males, with the highest incidence in the second decade. The age range of our patients was from 1 to 50 years (Table 19.2).

The basis for diagnosis was the clinical history, neurologic examination, and radiographic evaluation. Twenty-five of the 44 patients in this series had CT examinations; 40 had skull radiographs; 17 underwent angiography; and 32 underwent either pneumoencephalography or ventriculography.

TABLE 19.2
Age and Sex Distribution

| Age (yr) | No. of Patients | | |
	Male	Female	Total
1–10	4	2	6
11–20	17	4	21
21–30	5	2	7
31–40	3	1	4
41–50	4	2	6
	33	11	44

Thirty-seven patients underwent CSF shunting prior to radiotherapy; 7 patients without radiographic evidence of hydrocephalus did not require shunts (Table 19.3). Of the 37 patients so-shunted, 18 had Torkildsen shunts, 12 had ventriculoperitoneal shunts, and 7 had ventriculoatrial shunts. The average postoperative hospitalization in these patients was 1 week. Immediate improvement in symptomatology was the usual result of the shunt. Two patients with mental confusion and one with altered consciousness became worse after shunting; these patients were moribund with severe hydrocephalus and disseminated disease upon admission. There were no other operative mortalities from the shunt procedure. None of the patients developed subdural hematoma, intracranial hemorrhage, or seizures. One patient developed a shunt infection 7 months postoperatively and subsequently died at another institution.

Ten of the 37 shunted patients required revision of their shunts because of malfunction during the course of follow-up. Two of these 10 patients required a second revision. Four Torkildsen shunts required revision, with two being converted to a ventriculoperitoneal shunt and two to a ventriculoatrial shunt. One ventriculoatrial shunt required revision 1 day after surgery because of obstruction with tumor cells in a patient with germinoma. Five ventriculoperitoneal shunts required revision 3–33 months after the procedure. Two of these latter required second revisions, including 1 and 13 months, respectively, after the first.

Patients with pinealomas presenting for radiation therapy at the Mayo Clinic were evaluated and treated by many different radiotherapists, and no one uniform treatment policy was incorporated in the planning of the treatment program. Generally, however, radiation therapy was delivered to the pineal region in a dose thought to be adequate for control of the tumor. The tumor dose was in the range of 3500–5000 rads over 3½–5 weeks of treatment. Generally, radiation therapy was delivered to the pineal region in field size ranging from 56 to 300 cm^2, with the majority being treated with an 8 × 8 to 10 × 10 cm field. As with these field sizes, doses ranged from 1850 to 6000 rad (one patient receiving only 650 rad as he was unable to complete his treatment because of a deteriorating condition).

TABLE 19.3

Type of Surgery

Torkildsen (VC shunt)	18
VA shunt	7
VP shunt	12
Total	37

Significant regression of tumor size was demonstrated in five patients who had serial CT examinations following radiation treatment. Several tumors showed a denser, more even pattern of calcification on plain skull x-ray after radiation treatment. In general, tumors with larger size, more amorphous calcification, and contrast enhancement were more likely to show regressive changes with radiation therapy.

RESULTS

The mean survival in this study is 24 years. One-year survival is 80%, 5 years is 70%, 10 years is 64%, and 15 years is 58%. Twenty patients (45%) are alive and well, and 7 (15.5%) are alive with mild residual neurologic deficits (Fig. 19.1).

Of the 17 patients who died, 14 died from their primary disease: three in less than 1 year; eight within 1–4 years; and 1 each after 5, 10, and 20 years. Three patients died of other causes: 1 from a shunt infection 7 months postoperatively; another committed suicide 4 years after initial evaluation; and, the third died from accidental asphyxiation 17 years later.

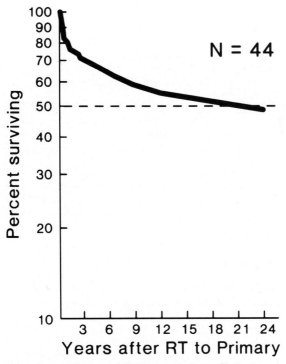

FIG. 19.1. Percent of patients surviving in years after radiation to primary tumor.

Nineteen of the 44 patients (43%) developed recurrences: 4 at the primary site; 4 at other sites in the brain; 2 in the spinal canal; 6 in both the primary site and other brain sites; 2 in other sites in the brain and spinal canal; and 1 in the primary as well as other sites in the brain and spinal canal (Table 19.4). A total of five patients developed spinal axis metastases out of a total of 42 patients who were at risk (two patients having received prophylactic spinal axis irradiation) for an incidence of 11.9%. Of the 19 patients with recurrences, 1 patient had a subsequent craniotomy at another institution, 6 had a second course of radiotherapy, and 3 underwent chemotherapy.

Fifteen patients had histologic diagnoses from later surgery (3 patients) or autopsy (12 patients) (Table 19.5). Most of the deaths in our series occurred within the first 2 years. It is noteworthy that only 1 of the 12 autopsied patients had a truly benign pineal tumor (benign teratoma), and none of these patients with proven histologic diagnosis had a germinoma. There was one patient with a meningioma who lived 24 years.

TABLE 19.4

Site of Recurrence

Pineal area	4
Elsewhere in brain	4
Spinal cord	2
Pineal area and elsewhere in brain	5
Elsewhere in brain and spinal cord	3
Pineal area, elsewhere in brain, and in spinal cord	1
Total recurrence	19

TABLE 19.5

Survival in 15 Patients with Histologic Diagnosis from Autopsy or Surgery[a]

Patient No.	Histologic Diagnosis	Survival Time	Status
3	Pineocytoma	6 yr	Dead
		4.5 yr	Alive and well
		6 mo	Dead
2	Pineocytoma/blastoma	3 yr	Dead
		3 mo	Dead
2	Pineoblastoma	11 yr	Dead
		1 yr	Dead
1	Grade 4 astrocytoma	1 yr	Dead
1	Ependymoma (had craniotomy and RaRx 1 yr later elsewhere)	4 yr	Alive with deficit, 6th cranial nerve
1	Meningioma	24 yr	Dead
N.B.	5 others died, 2 from disease and 3 from other causes, in other institutions; histology could not be obtained.		

[a] RaRx, radiation therapy.

CONCLUSIONS

A dogmatic attitude toward the management of pineal region tumors should be questioned. The crucial point is the differentiation between the various histologic types of tumor that may occur in the area. If the incidence and natural history of these various tumors are considered, several facts seem clear:

1. A high proportion of primary pineal tumors, variously thought to be 60–85%, are either very sensitive to radiation therapy and/or highly malignant.

2. Nearly all long-term survivors had been treated with radiation therapy.

3. CT scanning allows not only more accurate initial diagnosis but also affords the opportunity to closely follow the effects of radiation therapy, shunting, or direct surgery.

Because of these considerations, once a diagnosis of a primary pineal tumor is established, it is our general policy to recommend shunting and radiation therapy as primary treatment (1). We attempt to exclude such pineal region tumors as benign typical teratoma, meningioma, hemangiopericytoma, epidermoid and dermoid tumors, and arachnoidal cysts. If there is doubt regarding this differential diagnosis or if symptoms related to mass effect do not resolve with treatment and the initial lesion on CT scan does not respond to radiotherapy, then direct surgery is undertaken. The particular approach chosen, *i.e.*, whether infratentorial, supracerebellar, or occipital transtentorial, depends on the angiographic demonstration of the venous anatomy and the relation of the lesion to the tentorial notch.

ACKNOWLEDGMENTS

A special thanks to Dr. Eustaquio Abay for his work in the preparation of this paper and to Nancy Holicky for her tireless help in its preparation.

REFERENCES

1. Abay, E. O., Laws, E. R., Jr., Grado, G. L., Bruckman, J. E., Forbes, G. S., Gomez, M. R., and Scott, M. Pineal tumors in children and adolescents—Treatment by CSF shunting and radiotherapy. J. Neurosurg., *55:* 889–895, 1981.
2. Allen, J. C., Nisselbaum, J., Epstein, F., Rosen, G., and Schwartz, M. K. Alphafetoprotein and human chorionic gonadotropin determination in cerebrospinal fluid. J. Neurosurg., *51:* 368–374, 1979.
3. Araki, C., and Matsumoto, S. Statistical re-evaluation of pinealoma and related tumors in Japan. J. Neurosurg., *30:* 146–153, 1969.
4. Backlund, E. O., Rahn, T., and Sarby, B. Treatment of pinealomas by stereotaxic radiation surgery. Acta Radiol. Ther., *13:* 368–376, 1974.
5. Baggenstoss, A. H., and Love, J. G. Pinealomas. Arch. Neurol. Psychiatry, *41:* 1187–1206, 1939.

6. Balagura, S., Shulman, K., and Sobel, E. H. Precocious puberty of cerebral origin. Surg. Neurol., *11:* 315–326, 1979.

7. Bochner, S. J., and Scarff, J. E. Teratoma of the pineal body: Classification of the embryonal tumors of the pineal body: A report of a case of teratoma of the pineal body presenting formed teeth. Arch. Surg., *36:* 303–329, 1938.

8. Bradfield, J. S., and Perez, C. A. Pineal tumors and ectopic pinealomas. Ther. Radiol., *103:* 399–406, 1972.

9. Brodeur, G. M., Howarth, C. B., Pratt, C. B., Caces, J., and Hustu, H. O. Malignant germ cell tumors in 57 children and adolescents. Cancer, *48:* 1890–1898, 1981.

10. Camins, M. B., and Schlesinger, E. B. Treatment of tumors of the posterior part of the third ventricle and the pineal region: A long-term follow-up. Acta Neurochir., *40:* 131–143, 1978.

11. Castleman, B., and McNeely, B. U. Case records of the Massachusetts General Hospital. N. Engl. J. Med., *284:* 1427–1434, 1971.

12. Cole, H. Tumors in the region of the pineal. Clin. Radiol., *22:* 110–117, 1971.

13. Conway, L. W. Stereotaxic diagnosis and treatment of intracranial tumors including an initial experience of cryosurgery for pinealomas. J. Neurosurg., *38:* 453–460, 1973.

14. Dandy, W. E. An operation for the removal of pineal tumors. Surg. Gynecol. Obstet., *33:* 113–119, 1921.

15. Dandy, W. E. Operative experience in cases of pineal tumor. Arch. Surg., *51:* 1–14, 1945.

16. David, M., Vernard-Weik, E., and Dilenge, D. Les tumeurs de la glande pineale. Ann. Endocr. (Paris), *24:* 286–330, 1963.

17. DeGirolami, U., and Schmidek, H. Clinicopathological study of 53 tumors of the pineal region. J. Neurosurg., *39:* 455–462, 1973.

18. Donat, J. F., Okazaki, H., Gomez, M. R., Reagan, T. J., Baker, H. L., Jr., and Laws, E. R., Jr. Pineal tumors. Arch. Neurol., *35:* 736–740, 1978.

19. El-Mahdi, A. M., Phillips, E., and Lott, S. The role of radiation therapy in pinealomas. Radiology, *103:* 407–412, 1972.

20. Glasauer, R. E. An operative approach to pineal tumors. Acta Neurochir., *22:* 177–180, 1970.

21. Globus, J. H. Pinealoma. Arch. Pathol., *31:* 533–568, 1941.

22. Griffin, B. R., Griffin, T. W., Tong, D. Y. K., Russell, A. H., Kurtz, J., Laramore, G. E., and Groudine, M. Pineal region tumors: Results of radiation therapy and indications for elective spinal irradiation. Int. J. Radiation Oncol. Biol. Phys., *7:* 605–608, 1981.

23. Haldeman, K. O. Tumors of the pineal gland. Arch. Neurol. Psychiatry, *18:* 724, 1927.

24. Harris, W., and Cairns, H. Diagnosis and treatment of pineal tumors, with report a case. Lancet, *22:* 3–9, 1932.

25. Herrick, M. K., and Rubinstein, L. J. The cytological differentiating potential of pineal parenchymal neoplasms (true pinealomas). A clinicopathological study of 28 tumors. Brain, *102*(2): 289–320, 1979.

26. Horrax, G. Treatment of tumors of the pineal body: Experience in a series of twenty-two cases. Arch. Neurol. Psychiatry, *64:* 227–242, 1950.

27. Horrax, G., and Bailey, P. Tumors of the pineal body. Arch. Neurol. Psychiatry, *13:* 423–470, 1925.

28. Horsley, V. Tumors of the pineal body: Discussion. Proc. R. Soc. Med., *3*(2): 77, 1910.

29. Hyman, R. A., Loring, M. F., Liebeskind, A. L., Naidich, J. B., and Stein, H. L. Computed tomographic evaluation of therapeutically induced changes in primary and secondary brain tumors. Neuroradiology, *14:* 213–218, 1978.

30. Jamieson, K. G. Excision of pineal tumors. J. Neurosurg., *35:* 550–553, 1971.
31. Jenkin, P. D., Simpson, W. J., and Keen, C. W. Pineal and suprasellar germinomas. Results of radiation treatment. J. Neurosurg., *48:* 99–107, 1978.
32. Juif, J. G., Maitrot, D., Pierson, M., Heldt, N., Buccheit, F., Luckel, J. C. Les tumeurs cerebrales primitive d'origine germinale. Arch. Fr. Pediatr., *34:* 335–346, 1977.
33. Kahn, E. A. Surgical treatment of pineal tumor. Arch. Neurol. Psychiatry, *38:* 883–842, 1937.
34. Kretzschmar, K., Aulich, A., Schindler, E., Lange, S., Grumme, T., and Meese, W. The diagnostic value of CT for radiotherapy of cerebral tumors. Neuroradiology, *14:* 245–250, 1978.
35. Lazar, M. L., and Clark, K. Direct surgical management of masses in the region of the vein of Galen. Surg. Neurol., *2:* 17–21, 1974.
36. Maier, J. G., and Dejong, D. Pineal body tumors. Am. J. Roentgenol. Radium Ther. Nucl. Med., *99:* 826–832, 1967.
37. Mincer, F., Meltzer, J., and Botstein, C. Pinealoma. A report of twelve irradiated cases. Cancer, *37:* 2713–2718, 1976.
38. Neuwelt, E. A., Glasberg, M., Frenkel, E., and Clark, W. K. Malignant pineal region tumors. A clinicopathological study. J. Neurosurg., *51:* 597–607, 1979.
39. Obrador, S., Soto, M., and Gutierrez-Diaz, J. A. Surgical management of tumors of the pineal region. Acta Neurochir. (Wien), *34:* 159–171, 1976.
40. Onoyama, Y., Ono, K., Nakajima, T., Hiraoka, M., and Abe, M. Radiation therapy of pineal tumors. Radiology, *130:* 757–760, 1979.
41. Page, L. K. The infratentorial-supracerebellar exposure of tumors in the pineal area. Neurosurgery, *1:* 36–40, 1977.
42. Pertuiset, B., Visot, A., and Metzger, J. Diagnosis of pinealoblastomas by positive response to cobalt-therapy. Acta Neurochir. (Wien), *34:* 151–152, 1976.
43. Poppen, J. L., and Marino, R. Pinealomas and tumors of the posterior portion of the third ventricle. J. Neurosurg., *28:* 357–364, 1968.
44. Rand, R. W., and Lemmen. L. J. Tumors of the posterior portion of the third ventricle. J. Neurosurg., *10:* 1–18, 1953.
45. Rao, Y. T. R., Medini, E., Haselow, R. E., Jones, T. K., and Levitt, S. H. Pineal and ectopic pineal tumors: The role of radiation therapy. Cancer, *48:* 708–713, 1981.
46. Ray, P., Olson, M. H., Sarivar, M., Wright, A. E., Wu, J., and Allam, A. A. Pinealoma: Analysis of treatment and failure. Proceedings of the American Society of Therapeutic Radiologists. Int. J. Radiat. Oncol. Biol. Phys. (Suppl.), *1:* 144, 1976.
47. Reid, W. S., and Clark, W. K. Comparisons of the infratentorial and transtentorial approaches to the pineal region. Neurosurgery, *3:* 1–8, 1978.
48. Ringertz, N., Nordenstam, H., and Flyger, G. Tumors of the pineal region. J. Neuropathol. Exp. Neurol., *13:* 540–561, 1954.
49. Rubin, P., and Kramer, S. Ectopic pinealoma: A radiocurable, neuroendocrinologic entity. Radiology, *85:* 512–523, 1965.
50. Rubenstein, L. J. Tumors of the central nervous system. In: *Atlas of Tumor Pathology,* Fascicle 6. Armed Forces Institute of Pathology, Washington, D.C., 1972.
51. Rubenstein, L. J. Cytogenesis and differentiation of pineal neoplasms. Hum. Pathol., *12:* 441–448, 1981.
52. Russel, D. S. The pinealoma: Its relationship to teratoma. J. Pathol. Bacteriol., *56:* 145–150, 1944.
53. Russel, D. S., and Sachs, E. Pinealoma. A clinicopathologic study of 7 cases with a review of literature. Arch. Pathol., *35:* 869–888, 1943.
54. Salazar, O. M., Castro-Vita, H., Bakos, R. S., Feldstein, M. L., Keller, B., and Rubin,

P. Radiation therapy for tumors of the pineal region. Int. J. Radiat. Oncol. Biol. Phys., *5:* 491–499, 1979.

55. Sano, K. Diagnosis and treatment of tumors in the pineal region. Acta Neurochir. (Wien), *34:* 153–157, 1976.

56. Sano, K. Pinealomas in children. Child's Brain, *2:* 62–72, 1976.

57. Sano, K., and Mitsutani, M. Pinealoma (germinoma) treated by direct surgery and postoperative irradiation. Child's Brain, *8:* 81–97, 1981.

58. Sharan, V. M. Management of pineal tumors by radiation therapy and CT scanning (meeting abstract). Int. J. Radiat. Oncol. Biol. Phys., *2*(2): 154, 1978.

59. Sheline, G. E. Radiation therapy of tumors of the central nervous system in childhood. Cancer, *35:* 957–964, 1975.

60. Smith, N. J., El-Mahdi, A. M., Constable, W. C. Results of irradiation of tumors in the region of the pineal body. Acta Radiol. Ther. Phys. Biol., *15:* 17–22, 1976.

61. Spiegel, A. M., DiChiro, G., Gorden, P., Ommaya, A. K., Kolins, J., and Pomeroy, T. C. Diagnosis of radiosensitive hypothalamic tumors without craniotomy. Endocrine and neuroradiologic studies of intracranial atypical teratomas. Ann. Intern. Med., *85:* 290–293, 1976.

62. Stein, B. M. supracerebellar-infratentorial approach to pineal tumors. Surg. Neurol., *11*(5): 331–337, 1979.

63. Sung, D., II, Harisiadis, L., and Chang, C. H. Midline pineal tumors and suprasellar germinomas: highly curable by irradiation. Radiology, *128:* 745–751, 1978.

64. Suzuki, J., and Iwabachi, T. Surgical removal of pineal tumors (pinealomas and teratomas). J. Neurosurg., *23:* 565–571, 1965.

65. Torkildsen, A. A new palliative operation in cases of inoperable occlusion of the Sylvian aqueduct. Acta Chir. Scand., *82:* 117–124, 1939.

66. Tucker, W. G., Leong, A. S. Y., and McCulloch, G. A. J. Tumors of the pineal region— Neuroradiological aspects. Australas. Radiol., *21:* 313–324, 1977.

67. Van Wagenen, W. P. A surgical approach for the removal of certain pineal tumors. Surg. Gynecol. Obstet., *53:* 216–220, 1931.

68. Wara, W. M., Fellows, C. F., Sheline, G. E., Wilson, C. B., and Townsend, J. J. Radiation therapy for pineal tumors and suprasellar germinomas. Radiology, *124:* 221–223, 1977.

69. Wilson, C. B. Diagnosis and surgical treatment of childhood brain tumors. Cancer, *35:* 950–956, 1975.

70. Wood, J. H., Zimmerman, R. A., Bruce, D. A., Bilaniuk, L. T., Norris, D. G., and Schut, L. Assessment and management of pineal-region and related tumors. Surg. Neurol., *16:* 192–210, 1981.

71. Zimmerman, R. A., Bilaniuk, L. T., Wood, J. H., Bruce, D. A., and Schut, L. Computed tomography of pineal, parapineal, and histologically related tumors. Radiology, *137:* 669–677, 1980.

72. Zulch, K. J. *Brain Tumors: Their Biology and Pathology*, Ed. 2. Springer-Verlag, Berlin, 1965, pp. 326.

CHAPTER

20

An Update on the Surgical Treatment of Malignant Pineal Region Tumors

EDWARD A. NEUWELT, M.D.

INTRODUCTION

It is the purpose of this communication to review the experience with malignant pineal region tumors at both the University of Texas Southwestern Medical School between 1972 and 1980 and the more recent experience of the author at the Oregon Health Sciences University. More specifically, our purpose is: (*a*) to show that surgical exploration and biopsy of these lesions can be safe when the operating microscope is used; (*b*) to show that even malignant pineal tumors are often surprisingly well encapsulated, permitting gross total excision; (*c*) to demonstrate the lack of criteria to make an accurate histological diagnosis on the basis of neuroradiological studies; (*d*) to point out the clinical importance of the tumor markers associated with these tumors, particularly the β subunit of human chorionic gonadotropin and α-fetoprotein (AFP); (*e*) to relate ultrastructural and immunopathological studies of these tumors; and (*f*) to demonstrate the role that chemotherapy can play in the treatment of these tumors, particularly when a histological diagnosis is available. The initial eight patients in this series have been reported previously (27).

CLINICAL MATERIAL AND METHODS

Thirty-four patients with pineal region lesions have been treated in this series (Table 20.1). Twenty-nine of these patients have undergone direct surgical tumor exploration. Of these 34 patients, 15 had primary malignant pineal tumors, of which 13 were explored surgically. These 15 malignant pineal tumors are the basis of this report (Table 20.2). One patient with metastatic adenocarcinoma and three patients with glioma involving the pulvinar have been excluded from this surgical series of malignant pineal region tumors.

Immunological studies were carried out on fresh aliquot specimens of three resected tumors. Identification of surface immunoglobulin (SIG), and erythrocyte rosetting was recognized by methods involving separated cells isolated from the tumor by gentle teasing (26).

TABLE 20.1

Pineal Region Lesions Seen at the University of Texas Southwestern Medical School from 1972 to 1981 and the Oregon Health Sciences University from 1981 to 1984

Lesions	No. of Cases	
Benign, operative		
Meningiomas	2	
Epidermoid cyst	1	
Cystic astrocytoma–superior vermis	1	
Thrombosed vein of Galen aneurysm	1	
Vein of Galen aneurysm	1	
Hematoma of splenium–cryptic arterio-venous malformation	1	
Cysticercosis–quadrigeminal cistern	1	
Dermoid cysts	3	
Teratoma	1	
Malignant, operative		
Thalamic gliomas	3	
Metastatic adenocarcinoma	1	
Ependymoma–posterior 3rd ventricle	1	
Germinomas	2	
Germinoma + astrocytoma	1	Primary
Pineocytomas	2	Malignant
Pineoblastoma	3	Pineal
Pineoblastoma + astrocytoma[a]	3	Tumors
Embryonal cell	1	($n = 15$)
Malignant, nonoperative		
Germinoma	1	
Pineoblastoma	1	
Unknown	3	
Total	34	

[a] Two cases were predominantly pineoblastoma with areas of well-differentiated astrocytoma; the other case was vice versa.

SURGICAL TECHNIQUE

Currently there are two major techniques advocated for exploration of the pineal region—the transtentorial (24) and the infratentorial supracerebellar. We prefer to use the Jamieson modification of Poppen's occipital transtentorial approach. Stein supports an infratentorial supracerebellar approach (24).

In using the transtentorial approach, the patient is placed in the semisitting position. The head is flexed and stabilized in 3-point fixation with a Mayfield head-holder. Children under 2 years of age are taped to a cerebellar headrest in the semisitting position or are positioned prone. A right occipital scalp flap is hinged inferiorly (Fig. 20.1*A*) and fashioned so that a generous bone flap can be removed, exposing the sagittal sinus medially and the torcular herophili and transverse sinus inferiorly. The

TABLE 20.2
Clinical Course in 15 Patients with Malignant Primary Pineal Tumors

Case No.	Patient's Initials	Histological Diagnosis	Shunt	Occipital Transtentorial Craniotomy	Radiation	Chemotherapy	Outcome
1	P.M.	Germinoma	VP	Subtotal decompression	Craniospinal	−	Alive and well; tumor-free after 7 yr
2	J.T.	Germinoma	VP		Craniospinal	+	Alive and well; tumor-free after 5 yr
3	D.K.	Germinoma	VP	Subtotal decompression	None	−	Died 1 yr postop, received laetrile only post-op
4	R.M.	Embryonal cell	VP	Gross total excision	Craniospinal	−	Died of spinal metastases
5	Q.A.	Pineocytoma	VP	Gross total excision	Craniocervical	−	Alive and well; tumor-free after 5 yr
6	R.G.	Pineocytoma	VP	Gross total excision	Craniospinal	−	Alive and well; tumor-free after 6 yr
7	R.M.	Pineoblastoma	VP		Cranial only	−	Died of spinal metastases
8	S.W.	Pineoblastoma + astrocytoma	VP	Gross total excision	Craniospinal	−	Alive and well; tumor-free after 5 yr
9	W.K.	Astrocytoma + pineoblastoma	VP	Gross total excision	Cranial only	−	Alive and well; tumor-free after 2 yr
10	P.H.	Pineoblastoma	VP	Biopsy	Cranial	+	Died of metastatic renal carcinoma 1 yr following pineal surgery (*i.e.*, of a 2nd primary)
11	T.N.	Pineoblastoma	VP	Gross total excision	Craniospinal	−	Alive and well; tumor-free after 18 mo
12	S.S.	Pineoblastoma + astrocytoma	VP	Gross total excision	None	+	Alive and well; CT scan recurrence at 8 mo
13	E.G.	Pineoblastoma	VP	Biopsy	Craniospinal	+	Died 1 yr postop
14	R.J.	Malignant ependymoma	VP	Gross total excision	Cranial only	−	Alive and well; tumor-free after 12 yr
15	G.S.	Germinoma + astrocytoma	VP	Gross total excision	Cranial only	−	Alive and well; tumor-free after 5 mo

craniotomy is generous laterally and superiorly to prevent entrapping the occipital lobe with the retractor. The dura is opened in a stellate fashion. The occipital lobe is then retracted superiorly and laterally, exposing the tentorium, falx, and straight sinus (Fig. 20.1B). It is rare to be hampered by bridging veins between the occipital lobe and the sagittal sinus, but veins are frequently noted from the inferior aspect of the occipital lobe to the transverse sinus. The tentorium is then incised about 1.0 cm from the torcular herophili, and the incision is extended just lateral to the straight sinus anteriorly up to and including the tentorial incisura. The medial edge of the divided tentorium is retracted with sutures, exposing the dense arachnoid covering the deep venous system. The thickened milky-appearing arachnoid is then opened sharply, starting inferiorly. The resulting exposure (Fig. 20.1C) demonstrates the quadrigeminal plate, the superior vermis, the splenium, and the major veins draining into the straight sinus (i.e., the internal cerebral veins, the basilar veins of Rosenthal, the vein of Galen and the precentral cerebellar vein). Aside from the precentral cerebral vein, which is routinely sacrificed in the exposure of pineal lesions, compromise of the other veins can result in major morbidity and mortality. Indeed, the greatest risk in surgically exposing the pineal region is damaging the vein of Galen, basilar veins of Rosenthal, or internal cerebral veins.

Careful microdissection is required to dissect the major draining veins from the tumor capsule. With the use of the operating microscope, safe dissection has been possible with avoidance of the major veins in all our cases. In some cases well-encapsulated tumors can be removed without prior internal decompression. If necessary, the capsule is opened sharply, and the tumor is debulked with tumor forceps, suction, and any available automated dissection device, such as the Cavitron ultrasonic surgical aspirator. After complete tumor resection, the entire third ventricle can be visualized, as the posterior wall is now open.

SELECTED CASE REPORTS

Case 1 (P.M.). This 17-year-old boy presented with Parinaud's syndrome, headaches, and papilledema. A pneumoencephalogram and angiogram revealed a tumor in the pineal region, which was confirmed by computed tomographic (CT) scan (Fig. 20.2A). His symptoms were transiently relieved by a ventriculoperitoneal (VP) shunt, but progressive headaches, increasing limitation of upward gaze, and lethargy precipitated a subtotal decompression via an occipital transtentorial approach. Pathological examination of the tumor revealed a pineal germinoma. Postoperative myelography was normal, and he was treated with radiation therapy (Table 20.3). Serial CT scans revealed progressive disap-

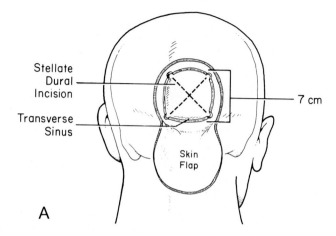

Stellate
Dural
Incision

Transverse
Sinus

7 cm

Skin
Flap

A

FIG. 20.1. Occipital transtentorial approach to pineal region tumors. (*A*) Skin flap, bone flap, and dural incision. A large bone flap and dural incision is important to prevent injury to the occipital lobe. (*B*) Retraction of occipital lobe superolaterally and section of the tentorium just lateral to the straight sinus from the torcular to the incisura. (*C*) Exposure of the pineal tumor and the surrounding large draining venous system.

pearance of the tumor, and 18 months after surgery, he was free of tumor (Fig. 20.2*B*). He is currently alive and well 7 years postoperatively.

Case 2 (J.T.). This 16-year-old boy had presented at another institution 3½ years previously with headaches, a sixth-nerve palsy, and diabetes insipidus. Metrizamide ventriculography and CT scans demonstrated two lesions involving the anterior and posterior third ventricles, respectively. A ventriculoperitoneal (VP) shunt was placed and, on the presumptive diagnosis of germinoma, craniospinal irradiation was given (Table 20.3). The patient's symptoms resolved, although the diabetes insipidus persisted in a mild form, and he returned to school.

He noted a protuberant abdomen 2½ years after his initial presentation. Chest film revealed elevation of the right hemidiaphragm and a large pleural effusion. Panmyelography was normal. The CSF cytology was normal. Cranial CT and metrizamide ventriculography were normal, except for a large pineal calcification. A CT scan of the abdomen demonstrated massive intraperitoneal and retroperitoneal tumor involvement, as well as beaded tumor nodules along the thoracic portion of the VP shunt and on the superior surface of the diaphragm. Laboratory investigation revealed a serum HCG level of 67 ng/ml (normal is less than 3 ng/ml). Biopsy revealed a massive tumor filling the abdominal cavity which, on histological study, was found to be a germinoma.

The patient was started on multiagent systemic chemotherapy with

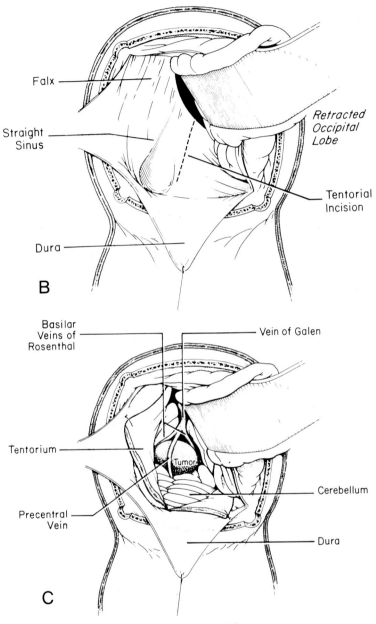

Falx

Straight Sinus

Dura

B

Retracted Occipital Lobe

Tentorial Incision

Basilar Veins of Rosenthal

Tentorium

Precentral Vein

C

Vein of Galen

Tumor

Cerebellum

Dura

FIG. 20.1*B* and *C*

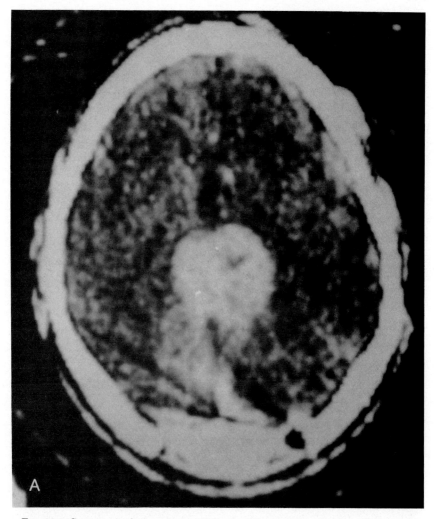

FIG. 20.2. Computerized tomography (CT) scan following the administration of paren-teral iodinated contrast agent showing a pineal germinoma (Case 3, P.M.). (A) After occipital transtentorial craniotomy and biopsy. (B) Following the completion of cranial irradiation.

cis-platinum, bleomycin, and vinblastine (13). Excellent cytocellular re-duction was achieved and, after 4 courses of chemotherapy, his serum HCG returned to normal, and he had achieved a complete remission with no evident tumor by all measurable criteria. His stable condition has persisted for 5 years. His VP shunt has been removed.

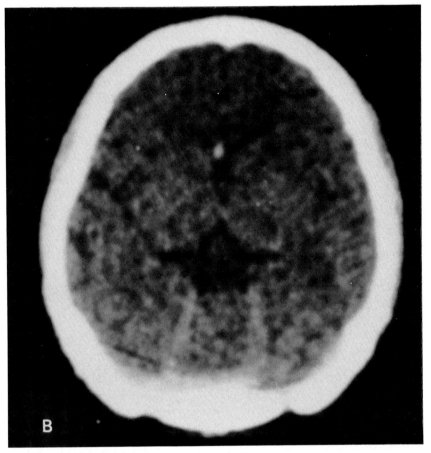

FIG. 20.2*B*

Case 3 (D.K.). This 16-year-old boy presented with Parinaud's syndrome and mild right-sided weakness. A CT scan revealed a massive pineal region lesion which enhanced markedly with iodinated contrast administration. Angiography revealed that the tumor was relatively avascular. The patient underwent an occipital transtentorial exploration of this lesion. A subtotal decompression was performed, and the histological diagnosis was a germinoma, as revealed by a diffuse proliferation of large cells against a background of small round cells with a lymphocytic appearance. Immunopathological studies performed on an aliquot revealed that the majority of the small cells could be classified as T-lymphocytes by virtue of their ability to form rosettes with sheep red

TABLE 20.3

Details of Radiation Therapy of Patients with Primary Malignant Pineal Tumors

Case No.[a]	Patient's Initials	Cranial Irradiation		Spinal Dose
		Port	Dose	
1	P.M.	Whole head, boost to pineal	4000 rad 1000 rad	4000 rad
2	J.T.	Whole head, boost to pineal	3800 rad 1000 rad	2500 rad
4	R.M.	Whole head, boost to pineal	4000 rad 1500 rad	4000 rad (cervical only)
5	Q.A.	Whole head, boost to pineal	4000 rad 1000 rad	4300 rad
6	R.G.	Whole head, boost to tumor	5000 rad	2700 rad
7	R.M.	Whole head, boost to tumor	5000 rad 1500 rad	2250 rad[b]
8	S.W.	Whole head	4000 rad	3400 rad
9	W.K.	6×6 cm tumor, port	5000 rad	none
10	P.H.	Cranial	5000 rad	
11	T.N.	Whole head, boost to tumor	4000 rad 1500 rad	4000 rad
13	E.G.	Whole head, boost to tumor	4500 rad 900 rad	4000 rad
14	R.J.	7×7 cm tumor port	5000 rad	None
15	G.S.	Whole head, boost to tumor	4000 rad 1500 rad	None

[a] Cases 3 and 12 did not receive radiation therapy.
[b] Spinal irradiation given 1 yr after cranial irradiation when patient presented with quadriplegia. Patient died before planned dose of 4000 rad to spinal canal could be given.

blood cells. A small proportion of the lymphocytes were found to have surface immunoglobulins indicative of B-lymphocytes (26). Serum and cerebrospinal fluid (CSF) levels of human chorionic gonadotropin (HCG) and α-fetoprotein were undetectable. The patient's parents refused postoperative radiotherapy, and the patient received laetrile, as prescribed by an outside physician, and he died while on this drug.

Case 5 (Q.A.). This 23-year-old woman presented with severe progressive headaches. On physical examination, she was lethargic, had anisocoria, decreased upward gaze, and bilateral ptosis. Her initial CT scan revealed moderate hydrocephalus and an enhancing mass in the pineal region. The levels of α-fetoprotein and of the β subunit of HCG (β-HCG) in the serum and CSF were normal. The patient underwent a VP shunt with marked resolution of her headache and lethargy. Two weeks later, she underwent an occipital transtentorial exploration of her pineal region. A well-encapsulated, well-demarcated tumor was totally excised microsurgically. Microscopic examination of the tumor revealed nests, sheets, and rosettes of neoplastic pineal cells. Mitoses and focal necrosis were also present. This neoplasm was believed to be a pineocytoma. The patient developed a posterior fossa epidural clot 48 hours postoperatively which was evacuated. Her recovery was excellent, her shunt was removed, and she then received craniospinal radiotherapy. She is alive and well without evidence of recurrence 5 years postoperatively (Table 20.3).

Case 6 (R.G.). This 58-year-old man presented with Parinaud's syndrome and ataxia. A CT scan revealed a well-circumscribed spherical 3-cm mass in the pineal region (Fig. 20.3A–C). Angiography confirmed a vascular pineal-region mass. A VP shunt was inserted which relieved him of his headaches. Two weeks later the lesion was entirely removed via an occipital transtentorial craniotomy.

Microscopic examination of the tumor revealed a repetitious pattern of interlacing columns and rosettes of differentiating pineal cells. Occasional Homer Wright pseudorosettes were present. The neoplasm was thought to have a degree of differentiation consistent with a pineocytoma.

Postoperatively, radiation was given (Table 20.3). All neurological abnormalities cleared. Repeat CT scan and metrizamide myelography 18 months postoperatively revealed no evidence of tumor recurrence (Fig. 20.3D). The patient continues to do well 6 years postoperatively.

Case 7 (R.M.). This 23-year-old woman presented to another institution with limitation of upward gaze and papilledema. A CT scan revealed an enhancing tumor of the pineal region, pineal calcification, and hydrocephalus. A VP shunt was inserted with excellent resolution of her signs and symptoms. She then received cranial radiotherapy (Table 20.3).

Ten months after radiotherapy, she developed back pain and progressive motor and sensory symptoms in all 4 extremities. The symptoms progressed over 2 months until she was essentially quadriplegic. She was transferred to our service. A myelogram done via C1-2 puncture revealed a complete block at the C2-3 level. Radiotherapy to her entire spinal axis was begun immediately. Cytological examination of the CSF revealed the presence of malignant CSF cells. The patient became septic and died 15 days following admission.

Post-mortem examination revealed a 1-cm mass in the pineal region which on microscopic examination contained viable tumor despite a normal CT scan just prior to her death. Tumor filled the subarachnoid space from C-2 to C-7. Microscopic examination of the tumor showed sheets of small cells with round-to-oval nuclei and scanty cytoplasm. Homer Wright rosettes were present. Electron microscopy showed mem-

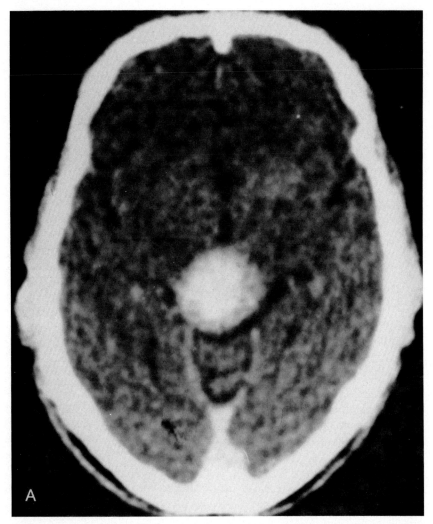

FIG. 20.3. Computerized tomography scans following administration of parenteral io-
thalamate, showing a pineocytoma (Case 6, R.G.). (A) Transverse cut. (B) Sagittal cut. (C)
Coronal cut. The ventricular catheter can be seen as a small high density just above the
tumor mass. (D) Transverse scan done in the immediate postoperative period demonstrating absence of any evidence of residual tumor.

brane-bound vesicles within most cell processes, which may represent
secretory granules. A diagnosis of pineoblastoma was made.

Case 8 (S.W.). This 38-year-old woman presented with papilledema,
titubation of the head, and no other focal neurological abnormalities. A
CT scan revealed a 3- to 4-cm spherical mass in the pineal region with

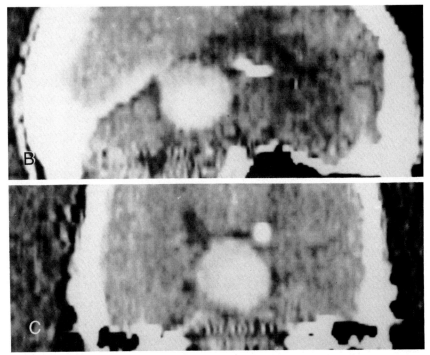

FIG. 20.3*B* and *C*

multiple calcifications; enhancement was seen with intravenous iodinated contrast agent (Fig. 20.4*A*–*C*). Marked hydrocephalus was also noted. Angiography confirmed a pineal region mass. A VP shunt was inserted which markedly decreased her head-bobbing. Search for tumor markers (β-HCG and α-fetoprotein) in the serum, and CSF was negative. An occipital transtentorial resection of her tumor was performed. The lesion was well-circumscribed; a very definitive capsule permitted gross total surgical resection. Microscopic examination of the tumor revealed a small primitive neuroectodermal neoplasm with prominent pseudorosette formation and focal areas of glial differentiation. There was one prominent region of pilocytic astrocytoma with dense glial processes and Rosenthal's fibers. This tumor was diagnosed as a pineoblastoma with associated pilocytic astrocytoma. The postoperative course was uneventful, her shunt was removed, and she was given prophylactic craniospinal irradiation (Fig. 20.4*D*). She is alive and well 5 years postoperatively with no evidence of recurrence (Table 20.2).

Case 14 (R.J.). This 12-year-old girl presented with severe headaches and dystonic movements of her head and neck. Four-vessel cerebral

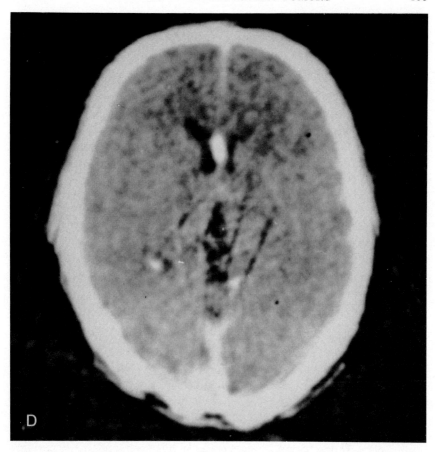

FIG. 20.3D

angiography revealed marked hydrocephalus but no evidence of tumor. Ventriculography showed a large tumor arising from the ependymal wall of the right posterior third ventricle. A VP shunt was inserted, and radiation therapy initiated to the tumor bed (Table 20.3). Three months after treatment, angiography and ventriculography revealed a progressive increase in tumor size. The pineal region was explored via an occipital transtentorial approach; the tumor was located anterior to the vein of Galen and between the two basilar veins of Rosenthal. It had a well-defined capsule permitting total piecemeal tumor resection. Postoperatively, she had Parinaud's syndrome but no other deficits. Although shunt revision was needed, the patient has continued to be well 12 years later. Histological examination of the tissue revealed a vascular glial stroma with perivascular pseudorosettes and papillomatous configurations; focal areas of necrosis were present. The histological diagnosis was anaplastic ependymoma.

SUMMARY OF CASES

Fourteen patients showed enhancing pineal region tumors on CT scan, and the diagnosis in the other patient was made by angiography and ventriculography. There was no accurate correlation of radiological appearance and tumor histology. Indeed, several of the cases clinically and radiologically (i.e., Case 6, R.G., Fig. 20.3; Case 8, S.W., Fig. 20.4) could have been a pineal region meningioma (see Figs. 20.5 and 20.6).

The initial therapeutic step in all 15 patients was insertion of a VP shunt. In 12 cases this was followed by direct surgical exploration (usually 7–10 days later) and postoperative irradiation (Tables 20.2 and 20.3). In one case, irradiation preceded surgery, and in the other 2 cases, radiation therapy only was given. One patient (Case 12, S.S.) was not irradiated due to her age (6 months). The ports and doses of radiation are summarized in Table 20.3.

Complete gross microsurgical excision of well-encapsulated tumors was possible in 9 of 13 patients who underwent definitive surgical exploration. Subtotal excision only was possible in 2 of the other patients. In the remaining 2 patients who had pineal germinomas, a less aggressive subtotal excision was done because of the known radiosensitivity of this tumor. Postoperative CT scans confirmed these results. The operative complications were: three patients developed a persistent homonymous hemianopsia (several patients had transient field defects); one patient had a mild transient hemiparesis; one an epidural hematoma of the posterior fossa; one patient had an epidural hygroma; and, many patients had a postoperative increase in their Parinaud's syndrome which was usually transient. Tissue obtained at surgery or autopsy revealed that three of these lesions were germinomas, 1 was an embryonal cell tumor, 4 were pineoblastomas, 4 were mixed tumors (pineoblastomas + astrocytoma, germinoma + astrocytoma), 2 were pineocytomas, and 1 was an anaplastic ependymoma.

The 2 patients treated with a shunt and radiation therapy but without craniotomy both developed metastases outside their radiation ports. One of the patients who developed metastases (Case 2, J.T.) had a germinoma which secreted HCG. His massive metastatic tumor burden totally disappeared with chemotherapy. Ten other patients were evaluated for tumor markers (HCG and α-fetoprotein) in their serum and CSF but none were found.

One patient (Case 7, R.M.), who developed spinal metastases from her

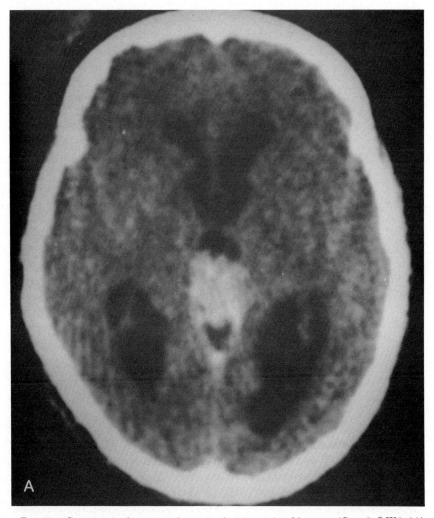

FIG. 20.4. Computerized tomography scans showing a pineoblastoma (Case 8, S.W.). (A) Enhanced transverse section. (B) Coronal section (unenhanced) showing tumor calcification. (C) Enhanced sagittal section. (D) Normal enhanced CT scan (transverse section) 3 years postoperatively and after radiotherapy.

pineoblastoma, was initially treated with a shunt and cranial radiation. Despite complete tumor regression by CT scan, she seeded her unirradiated spinal canal with tumor. Interestingly, at post-mortem examination, she had 1 cm of residual viable tumor in the pineal region which was not apparent on her enhanced CT scan done 2 weeks earlier.

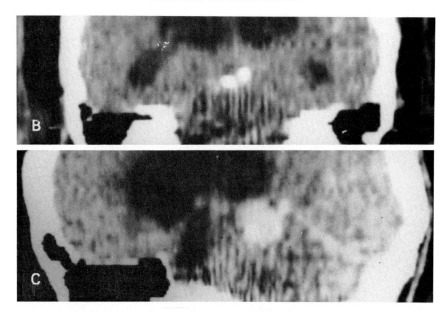

FIG. 20.4B and C

In summary, 9 patients appear to be in complete remission; one has evidence of recurrence by CT scan; and 5 patients died. One patient (Case 1, D.K.) with a germinoma received Laetrile only postoperatively (against our advice) and died; Case 4 (R.M.) with embryonal cell cancer died with spinal metastases despite craniospinal irradiation. Case 7 (R.M.) died from spinal seeding of her pineoblastoma 10 months after VP shunt and empiric cranial irradiation. Case 10 (P.H.) died 1 year postoperatively of a second neoplasm (clear cell carcinoma of the kidney). Patient E.G. (Case 13) died of progressive disease one year postoperatively. His tumor progressed 3 months after radiation, and he transiently responded to chemotherapy with methotrexate, Cytoxan, and procarbazine in association with osmotic blood-brain barrier opening (25, 28), before succumbing to his tumor.

DISCUSSION

The Role of Surgery

An important aspect of the present series is its deviation from some of the classic tenets of therapeutic intervention in pineal region tumors. In the past, radiotherapy has been the generally accepted primary treatment for pineal tumors. Schmidek's extensive review (40) of therapy led him

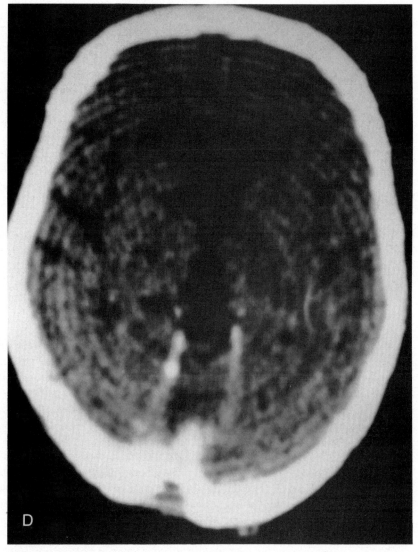

FIG. 20.4D

to conclude that "the mortality and morbidity associated with surgery of the pineal region would confirm the impression that primary excision of these lesions at the time they are diagnosed is not warranted." He stated that a small fraction (10–15%) with classical neurodiagnostic criteria of benignity merited consideration for surgical resection, but that for most pineal region tumors, primary removal was associated with a 25–70% mortality (6–8, 14, 15, 20, 32–34, 37). Similarly, Donat *et al.* (12) reviewed 53 years of experience at the Mayo Clinic and concluded that surgery should be reserved for tumors that are radioresistant or that progress after radiotherapy. Another basis for concern regarding operative attack on the tumor was expressed by Jenkins *et al.* (17), who suggested that surgical intervention increased the risk of distant subarachnoid metastases. Two of their 10 patients whose pineal germinomas were biopsied and treated with only cranial irradiation developed meningeal seeding.

An alternative view was expressed by Jamieson (16), who advocated primary surgical exploration of all pineal region tumors. In his series of nine cases, successful complete excision of four germinomas and two pineocytomas was performed with "minimal morbidity." One postoperative death occurred in a patient in whom biopsy only was attempted, and four patients with invasive or ectopic lesions were treated nonoperatively. Stein (45) has also advocated that surgery precede a decision regarding radiotherapy. However, in spite of these exceptions, the prevailing attitude has been the use of radiotherapy as the initial therapeutic modality for all pineal region tumors, except for those with clearly benign features on CT scan, that is, lesions with mixed fat and CSF density indicative of the presence of an epidermoid tumor, dermoid, or teratoma.

Of the 34 patients (Table 20.1) with pineal region lesions seen over the past 12 years, 28 have undergone microsurgical exploration, and 1 patient had a needle biopsy. The occipital transtentorial approach was used in 24 cases and the infratentorial approach in four cases. These approaches have been described and compared previously (36). The operative microscope has provided the major therapeutic advance and with it, the risk of injury to the large venous structures in this region can be reduced. There has been only one operative death, and that was a patient with metastatic adenocarcinoma. Morbidity has been minimal in the overall series of 29 procedures. We have not had any persistent visual field deficits since 1978, possibly because of the increased size of the bone flap, which gives more room to retract the occipital lobe. Surgery has been relatively safe and has allowed gross total removal in some cases.

This experience provides evidence that a wide variety of lesions in the pineal region can be microsurgically excised. In those circumstances where excision is not possible, the operative approach has provided tissue for histological examination which has been helpful in planning appropriate postoperative therapy. It is of further interest that in the patients with known histology, 19 of 31 (61%) lesions were malignant (in 3 of the 34 cases, the histology is unknown). This is in marked contrast to Schmidek's calculation (40) that 85–90% of pineal region lesions are

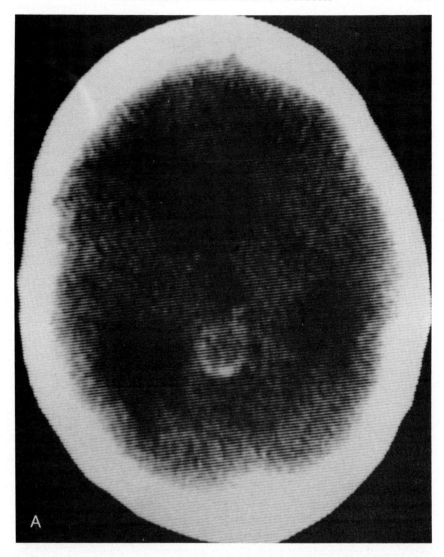

FIG. 20.5. Tentorial meningioma in a 56-year-old female which has the appearance of a pineal tumor prior to tumor resection. (A) Unenhanced transverse-cut CT scan which shows a partially calcified pineal region mass. (B) The mass enhances markedly after intravenous contrast administration. (C) True coronal enhanced CT scan. (D) Venous phase lateral angiogram shows no evidence of a blush typical of a meningioma.

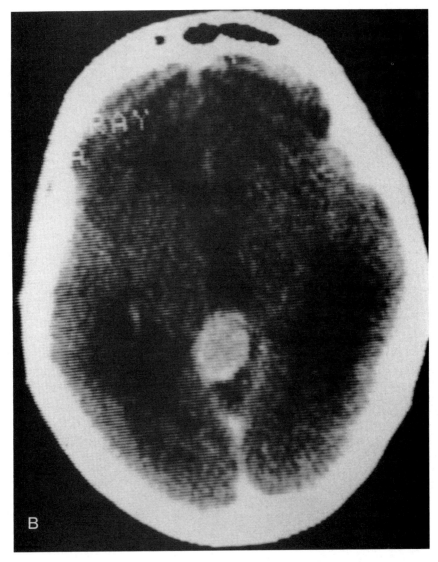

Fig. 20.5*B*

malignant. In 9 patients in whom gross complete excision of a malignant tumor was possible, there have only been 2 recurrences with a follow-up of up to 11 years.

Since benign lesions are more radioresistant, their relative frequency is of importance in the strategy of therapy. Empiric radiation in a benign

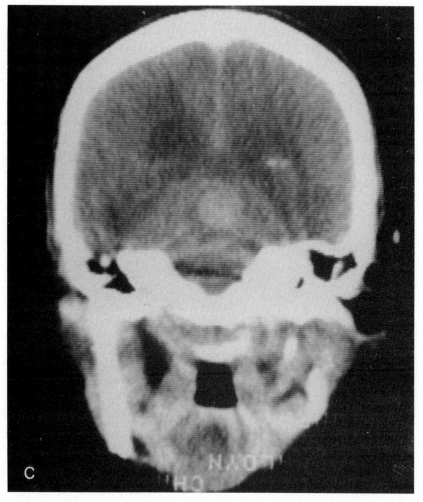

FIG. 20.5C

lesion not only risks radiation damage to the central nervous system parenchyma but also increases scarring of the thick arachnoid which encases the pineal and the deep venous system. These factors increase the difficulty and risks of subsequent surgery. It is also interesting that only one of the 15 surgically treated malignant primary tumors of the pineal region have developed metastases, whereas two of our nonoperative cases have done so.

These data from our clinical experience strongly support the impor-

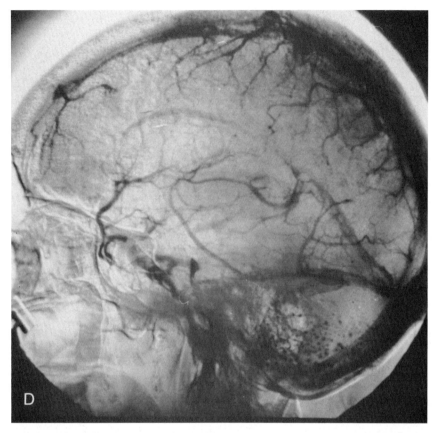

FIG. 20.5D

tance of surgical exploration and biopsy or excision as the initial therapeutic modality in pineal region tumors. Indeed, these results, at least
initially, are better than those achieved with radiotherapy alone and
provide a more rational approach for the application of other therapeutic
modalities, such as chemotherapy, which in the past has not been
available nor tried (24). Stereotactic biopsy is another alternative, but
the limited tissue sample and the risk of damage to the deep veins
surrounding pineal lesions must be considered with stereotactic biopsy.

Neuroradiological Studies

Although it has been stated that a number of pineal region tumors can
be identified neuroradiologically as either benign or malignant (40), this

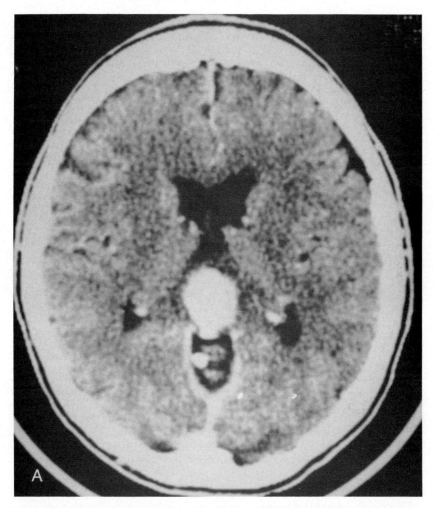

FIG. 20.6. Falcotentorial meningioma in a 60-year-old female which has the appearance of a pineal region tumor prior to tumor resection. (*A*) Transverse-cut enhanced CT scan showing a pineal region enhancing mass. (*B*) Coronal rreconstruction of the tumor illustrated in *A*. (*C*) Venous phase angiogram showing no evidence of a typical "menigioma" blush. At surgery, the tumor was attached to the anterior aspect of the vein of the Galen and *above* the internal cerebral veins (*arrowheads*). This location would have made excision from a suboccipital supratentorial approach difficult but was straightforward from an occipital transtentorial approach.

was not substantiated in the series of pineal tumors at our institution (Table 20.2) nor in another similar-sized series (44). In addition, no consistent neuroradiological criteria for the excisability of pineal tumors was detected. This topic is examined in more detail elsewhere (24).

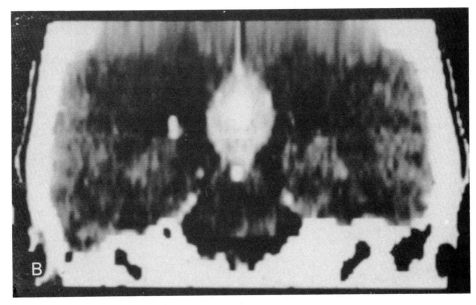

FIG. 20.6B

Pathological Studies

The pathological diagnoses of the 15 malignant primary pineal tumors are as follows: 3 germinomas, 2 pineocytomas, 4 pineoblastomas, 3 pineoblastoma + astrocytoma, one astrocytoma + germinoma, and one anaplastic ependymoma. The classification of pineal tumors has been described previously (40). Although most series consider the germinoma to be the most common pineal tumor (9, 40), there have been other series (5), including our own, in which tumors of the pineal parenchymal cells (pineoblastoma and pineocytoma) were more common.

The diagnosis of the 3 pure germinomas was straightforward, as these tumors are composed of two distinct cell populations: (a) large rounded germ cells with prominent, rounded, vesicular nuclei; and (b) clusters of cells of lymphoid appearance. The pathological evaluation of our one patient (Case 15) whose tumor was a mixture of germinoma and astrocytoma has been reviewed (24).

The microscopic picture of the well-differentiated pineocytoma is quite distinctive and resembles the normal pineal gland. Mitotic figures, necrosis, and hemorrhage are not usually present. The 2 pineocytomas in this series are less well differentiated and more closely resemble the lobular structure of the embryonal pineal gland. Cells within the lobules are more rounded and have less cytoplasm than in the better differen-

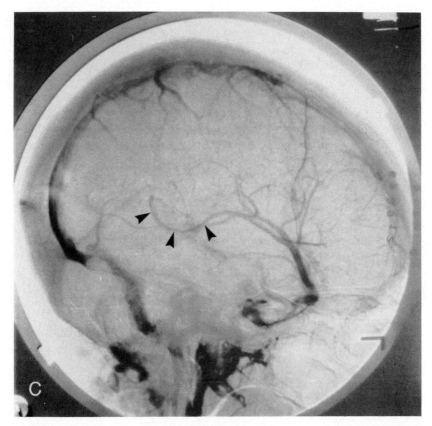

FIG. 20.6C

tiated pineocytomas. One of our cases also had a significant degree of mitotic activity and necrosis.

Our seven pineoblastomas were composed of dense cellular aggregates of small rounded or oval cells with scanty cytoplasm and are indistinguishable from primitive neuroectodermal tumors in other locations. Three of the cases showed a prominent focus of differentiation toward astrocytoma. In 2 of the cases, the tumor was primarily pineoblastoma with small areas of astrocytoma, whereas the third case was primarily a low grade astrocytoma. Although previously reported in a medulloblastoma, these cases, to our knowledge, are unique.

Electron microscopy was performed in several cases of pineal parenchymal cell tumors. Prior reports in the literature include one published case (31) and one abstract (23), reporting the ultrastructure of the pineocytoma. Our cases (27) showed similar findings, with numerous cell processes, often rich in microtubules, resembling neuronal processes, and an overall similarity to the normal adult pineal gland. The pineoblastomas in this series are the first, to our knowledge, to have their ultrastructure reported (27). They also had some features resembling normal pineal gland; however, overall there was even more of a resemblance to the undifferentiated cells of the medulloblastoma. One of the tumors contained membrane-bound vesicles that may represent secretory granules. A more detailed review of the ultrastructure of the pineocytoma and pineoblastoma has been published (24).

Immunopathological evaluation of the germinoma from Case 1 revealed that 81% of the "small cells" formed rosettes with sheep red blood cells, as is characteristic of T-lymphocytes. The remainder of the "small cells" appear to be B-lymphocytes, as evidenced by the presence of surface immunoglobulins. The details of our immunopathological study of this pineal germinoma have been reported (26). Similar studies on a pineocytoma (from Case 5) and a pineoblastoma (from Case 8) were negative for B- and T-cell markers. These immunological studies corroborate the morphological impression at the light and electron microscope level that the "small cells" in germinomas are lymphocytes. The predominance of T-lymphocytes in this pineal germinoma is analogous to the predominance of T-lymphocytes in the perivascular spaces of malignant gliomas (43). The presence of lymphoid cells in tumors of the central nervous system (CNS) may have pathogenic significance (26).

Tumor Markers

The most important marker of pineal germinomas appears to be the β chain of human chorionic gonadotropin (β-HCG). Elevated β-HCG has been reported in a number of patients with this tumor (10, 19, 38, 41), and its plasma level correlates with tumor growth or regression. Unfortunately, it is not secreted by all germinomas and indeed is not necessarily associated with a malignant tumor (Dr. Mike Edwards, Univ. of California, San Francisco, personal communication). Only one of our three patients with a germinoma in this series whose serum HCG was assayed had increased plasma levels (Case 2). As expected, when the tumor regressed following the administration of chemotherapy, the plasma level of HCG returned to normal.

The carcinoembryonic antigen (CEA) and the α-fetoprotein (AFP) have also been reported to be secreted by germ-cell tumors. Lee et al. (21) reported increased levels at α-fetoprotein in serum and CSF in a patient with an endodermal sinus tumor of the pineal region. At present, there are no known markers of nongerminomatous pineal tumors, although melatonin (29) and luteinizing hormone-releasing hormone have been suggested as possible candidates (41, 49, 50). Preoperative evaluation of melatonin was carried out in two of our patients with pineal tumors (cases 9 and 15, Table 20.2). One patient had a normal pattern of plasma melatonin levels, and the other patient had no evidence of any melatonin. The importance of tumor markers in pineal germ cell tumors has been reviewed recently (24).

Role of Radiotherapy

Except for a 6-month-old patient who was felt to be too young and another patient who refused all therapy except for laetrile, all patients with malignant tumors were treated with postoperative radiotherapy regardless of whether a complete surgical excision was accomplished. The incidence of meningeal seeding can be as high as 57% with malignant pineal tumors (46). Pineal germinomas seem to have the greatest propensity for meningeal seeding (46). Brady (4) recommends a dose of 4000 rad to the entire craniospinal axis with a 1000- to 1500-rad boost to the tumor bed in subtotally resected tumors. A lesser dose is associated with an increased recurrence rate. For instance, Sung et al. (46) reported intracranial relapses in 14 of 27 patients with midline pineal tumors treated with 3800–4500 rad, but only 2 of 30 midline pineal tumors recurred after doses of 5000–5500 rad.

Not all radiotherapists advocate prophylactic spinal irradiation (42). Wara et al. (48) reviewed the experience at the University of California at San Francisco over a 25-year period. None of 19 patients developed spinal seeding. They advocated CSF cytology following cranial irradiation to screen for meningeal seeding. However, Sung et al. (46) only obtained a positive CSF cytology in 3 of 12 patients with meningeal metastases. Periodic myelography and/or body CT scan plus periodic CSF cytology might be an alternative to prophylactic spinal radiation (24).

Metastases

Two of the three patients with metastases in this series did not undergo surgical exploration of the pineal region. They were initially treated elsewhere with VP shunts and irradiation. The shunted but not operated patient (case 7, Table 20.2) with meningeal seeding and resultant quadriplegia was given only cranial irradiation, which resulted in a complete cranial remission as shown by CT scan. In retrospect, spinal irradiation may have averted or delayed the meningeal seeding.

The one patient who developed postoperative CSF seeding had an embryonal cell tumor. In this patient a well-encapsulated spherical embryonal cell carcinoma of the pineal gland that was 4 cm in diameter was grossly excised without complication. The serum and CSF were evaluated for the presence of α-fetoprotein by radioimmunoassay, and no increased levels were observed. Similarly, no increased levels of the β chain of human chorionic gonadotropin were seen in serum. The absence of α-fetoprotein in serum and CSF is contrary to the results of Allen *et al.* (1). Postoperatively the patient received whole head (5800 rad) and cervical spine (4000 rad) irradiation. An attempt to initiate chemotherapy was made (*cis*-platinum, bleomycin, and vinblastine), but the patient did not tolerate the regimen due to intractable nausea and vomiting. The patient developed recurrent tumor, initially in the spine, and then died. In retrospect, this recurrence may have been prevented or delayed if total craniospinal irradiation had been given.

Nineteen embryonal cell pineal tumors reported previously have recently been reviewed (2). As the authors point out, this malignancy is relatively radioresistant, and most patients survive only a few months. Our case is important since it was possible to grossly excise this radioresistant tumor. Having a histological diagnosis has also given us the opportunity to give postoperative chemotherapy. Embryonal carcinoma of the testes is highly sensitive to chemotherapy with *cis*-platinum, bleomycin, and vinblastine. These drugs may well have access to any microscopic foci of residual tumor since there is no blood-brain barrier in the pineal gland.

One patient (Case 2, J.T.) with a germinoma was treated with craniospinal irradiation which resulted in a complete CNS tumor remission, but he developed massive peritoneal metastases, probably secondary to his VP shunt. Extraneural metastasis is very rare with pineal tumors. Of the 8 known cases reviewed by Sakata *et al.* (39), all were either typical teratomas or germinomas, and all appeared to disseminate by a hematogenous route, as evidenced by pulmonary metastases in all 8 cases. Only one of these patients had a VP shunt, and his metastases were to the lung, urinary bladder, and pancreas. Therefore, our case appears to be relatively unique. Although the use of a filter in this boy's shunt may have prevented his peritoneal metastases, the increased incidence of shunt obstruction when filters are used probably outweighs their prophylactic value in patients with pineal tumors. However, as has been done in this series, the shunt should be removed after the tumor burden has been minimized.

Chemotherapy

Another therapeutic modality is now available that increases and expands the approach to pineal region tumors. Histologically, the pineal germinoma is identical to the seminoma of the testes, a tumor which is highly responsive to chemotherapy. A complete remission rate with testicular seminomas of 82% in response to bleomycin, vinblastine, and *cis*-platinum has been reported (13). The response of the massive tumor burden of case 2 to this regimen is, therefore, not surprising, although his cell burden was greater than that of most patients so treated. We have observed fatal pulmonary fibrosis in two of our patients which almost certainly was the result of the use of bleomycin. Therefore, we feel that this drug should not be used as a first line agent in intracranial germ cell tumors and that VP-16-213 be used in its place (24).

There have been a few previous reports of the use of chemotherapy with pineal tumors. Sakata *et al.* (39) used bleomycin without success to treat an embryonal cell pineal tumor that metastasized to the spinal canal and to extraneural organs. On the other hand, de Tribolet and Barrelet (11) treated a patient with a large pineal region tumor and malignant cells in the CSF with a combination of daunorubicin, vincristine, and bleomycin. There was a dramatic decrease in tumor size shown by CT scan over a 3-month period. The absence of a blood-brain barrier in the pineal gland may contribute to the sensitivity of this tumor to systemic chemotherapy (35). Borden *et al.* (3) have also demonstrated objective tumor regression of a pulmonary metastasis from a pineal germinoma with a combination of chlorambucil, methotrexate, and dactinomycin. There is no evidence that pineal tumors of glial origin are sensitive to chemotherapy. In fact, glial tumors are well known to be poorly responsive to conventional chemotherapy. Again, this interest in a new treatment modality adds another strong basis for a specific tissue diagnosis in planning therapy in patients with pineal tumors. The chemotherapy of pineal tumors is discussed further elsewhere (24).

Prognosis

The prognosis in pineal region tumors with shunting procedures and radiotherapy without a tissue diagnosis has been fairly well established. For instance, Camins and Schlesinger (5) reported a 64% survival in a series of 50 cases of pineal region tumors with a mean follow-up period for the survivors of more than 10 years. However, the median survival of their 18 patients who died was only 2 months. The tumor type, heterogeneity, the ability to completely remove some tumors with microsurgery, and the exciting vistas of alternative therapeutic modalities (chemotherapy and immunotherapy) pose new and strong biases in favor of an aggressive initial surgical approach to pineal region tumors.

SUMMARY

Our current pineal region tumor series (*n* = 34) now spans 11 years and currently includes 15 patients with malignant pineal region tumors, only 3 of whom had pure germinomas. Complete gross microsurgical excision of well-encapsulated tumors was possible in 9 of 13 patients (69%) who underwent definitive surgical exploration. Subtotal excision only was possible in 2 of the other patients. In the remaining 2 patients who had pineal germinomas, a less aggressive subtotal excision was done because of the known radiosensitivity of this tumor. Four of the operative patients had a tumor of mixed histology with benign and malignant components, emphasizing the need for adequate tissue sampling (Table 20.2). Eleven of the 13 surgical patients received postoperative craniospinal radiation; a 6-month-old girl who had a gross total excision of a pineoblastoma was too young to be irradiated. Ten of the patients continue to do well up to 12 years postoperatively. In view of the fact that only 3 of the 15 patients had pure germinomas, these results appear to be better than those reported with shunting and radiotherapy. Only one of our surgical patients developed postoperative metastases, an embryonal cell tumor that spread to the spinal canal. In the 34 patients in this series with lesions of the pineal region, surgical exploration was associated with only one death (a patient with metastatic adenocarcinoma). As is common with the occipital transtentorial approach, a postoperative hemanopsia is common but usually transient. The wide exposure of this approach, however, may be responsible for the greater proportion of complete gross excisions of malignant pineal tumors using other approaches (24). We have also shown the importance of tumor markers and that germinomas are very sensitive to chemotherapy. Thus, microsurgery for pineal tumors provides a viable potential for complete gross tumor extirpation *even with malignant lesions,* and/or adequate tissue for diagnosis which is necessary in appropriate therapeutic planning for radiotherapy and/or chemotherapy. The traditional therapeutic approach of empiric radiotherapy without a tissue diagnosis for pineal lesions may no longer be acceptable.

ACKNOWLEDGMENTS

We would like to express our gratitude to Drs. Joel Kirkpatrick, Mark Glasberg, Nathan Blank, and Colin Buchan, and to the Armed Forces Institute of Pathology for their consultations on the cases described. Major portions of the material in this chapter have been published previously in our recent monograph entitled *The Diagnosis and Treatment of Pineal Region Tumors* (24) and are reprinted with permission. The reader is referred to this source for additional material, including the bibliography.

REFERENCES

1. Allen, J. C., Nisselbaum, J., Epstein, F., *et al.* Alphafetoprotein and human chorionic gonadotropin determination in cerebrospinal fluid. An aid to the diagnosis and management of intracranial germ cell tumors. J. Neurosurg., *51:* 368–374, 1979.
2. Arita, N., Ushio, N., Abekura, M., *et al.* Embryonal carcinoma with teratomatous elements in the region of the pineal gland. Surg. Neurol., *9:* 198–202, 1978.

3. Borden, S., IV, Weber, A. L., Toch, R., and Wang, C. C. Pineal germinoma. Am. J. Dis. Child., *126:* 214–216, 1973.

4. Brady, L. W. The role of radiation therapy. In: *Pineal Tumors,* edited by H. H. Schmidek, pp. 127–132. Masson, New York, 1977.

5. Camins, M. B., and Schlesinger, E. B. Treatment of tumours of the posterior part of the third ventricle and the pineal region: A long-term follow-up. Acta Neurochir., *40:* 131–143, 1978.

6. Cummins, F. M., Taveras, J. N., and Schlesinger, E. B. Treatment of gliomas of the third ventricle and pinealomas. Neurology, *10:* 1031–1036, 1960.

7. Dandy, W. E. *Benign Tumors in the Third Ventricle of the Brain: Diagnosis and Treatment.* Charles C Thomas, Springfield, Ill., 1933.

8. Davidoff, L. M. Some considerations in the therapy of pineal tumors. Bull. N.Y. Acad. Med., *43:* 537–561, 1967.

9. DeGirolami, U., and Schmidek, H. Clinicopathological study of 53 tumors of the pineal region. J. Neurosurg., *39:* 455–462, 1973.

10. Demura, R., Demura, H., Shizume, K., Kubo, O., and Kitamura, K. A female case of the HCG-producing ectopic pinealoma associated with precocious puberty. Endocrinol. Jap., *23:* 215–219, 1976.

11. deTribolet, N., and Barrelet, L. Successful chemotherapy of pinealoma. Lancet, *12:* 1228–1229, 1977.

12. Donat, J. F., Okazaki, H., Gomez, M. R., Reagan, T. J., Baker, H. L., and Laws, E. R. Pineal tumors. Arch. Neurol., *35:* 736–740, 1978.

13. Einhorn, L. H. Combination chemotherapy of disseminated testicular carcinoma with *cis*-diamminedichloroplatinum, vinblastine, and bleomycin (PVB): An update. In: *Proceedings of the American Association of Clinical Oncology* edited by S. Weinhouse. Washington, D.C. New York, American Cancer Society, 1978 p 308.

14. Horrax, G. Treatment of tumors of the pineal body. Experience in a series of twenty-two cases. Arch. Neurol. Psychiatry, *64:* 227–242, 1950.

15. Horrax, G., and Daniels, J. T. The conservative treatment of pineal tumors. Surg. Clin. North Am., *22:* 649–659, 1942.

16. Jamieson, K. G. Excision of pineal tumors. J. Neurosurg., *35:* 550–553, 1971.

17. Jenkins, R. D. T., Simpson, W. J. K., and Keen, C. W. Pineal and suprasellar germinomas: Results of radiation treatment. J. Neurosurg., *48:* 99–107, 1978.

18. Krabbe, K. H. Histologische und Embryologische Untersuchungen uber die Zirbeldruse des Mechen. Anat. Hefte, *54:* 187–319, 1916.

19. Kubo, O., Yamasaki, N., Kamijo, Y., Amano, K., Kitamura, K., and Demura, R. Human chorionic gonadotropin produced by ectopic pinealoma in a girl with precocious puberty. J. Neurosurg., *47:* 101–105, 1977.

20. Kunicki, A. Operative experiences in 8 cases of pineal tumors. J. Neurosurg., *17:* 815–823, 1960.

21. Lee, S. H., Sundararesan, N., Jereb, B., *et al.* Endodermal sinus tumor of the pineal region: A case report. Neurosurgery, *3:* 407–411, 1978.

22. Mincer, F., Meltzer, J., and Botstein, C. Pinealoma. A report of twelve irradiated cases. Cancer, *37:* 2713–2718, 1976.

23. Nakazato, Y., Ishida, Y., and Kawabuchi, J. Ganglioneuroblastic differentiation in a pineocytoma. In: *Eighth International Congress of Neuropathology,* Abstract 255.

24. Neuwelt, E. A. (ed.). *The Diagnosis and Treatment of Pineal Region Tumors,* Williams & Wilkins Press, Baltimore, 1984.

25. Neuwelt, E. A., Balaban, E., Diehl, J., Hill, S., and Frenkel, E. Successful treatment of primary central nervous system lymphomas with chemotherapy after osmotic blood-brain barrier opening. Neurosurgery, *12:* 662–671, 1983.

26. Neuwelt, E. A., and Clark, W. K. *Clinical Aspects of Neuroimmunology.* Williams & Wilkins, Baltimore, 1978.
27. Neuwelt, E. A., Glasberg, M., Frenkel, E., and Clark, W. K. Malignant pineal region tumors: A clinico-pathological study. J. Neurosurg., 51:597–607, 1979.
28. Neuwelt, E. A., and Lewy, A. Disappearance of plasma melatonin after removal of a neoplastic pineal gland. N. Engl. J. Med., *308:* 1132–1135, 1983.
29. Neuwelt, E. A., and Smith, R. G. Presence of lymphocyte membrane surface markers on "small cells" in a pineal germinoma. Ann. Neurol., *6:* 133–136, 1979.
30. Neuwelt, E. A., Specht, H. D., Howieson, J., Haines, J. E., Bennett, M. J., Hill, S. A., and Frenkel, E. P. Osmotic blood-brain barrier modification: Clinical documentation by enhanced CT scanning and/or radionuclide brain scanning. Am. J. Neuroradiol., *4:* 907–913, 1983.
31. Nielsen, S. L., and Wilson, C. B. Ultrastructure of a "pineocytoma." J. Neuropathol. Exp. Neurol., *34:* 148–158, 1975.
32. Olivercrona, H. Acoustic tumors. J. Neurosurg., *26:* 6–13, 1967.
33. Poppen, J. L., and Marino, R., Jr. Pinealomas and tumors of the posterior portion of the third ventricle. J. Neurosurg., *28:* 357–364, 1968.
34. Rand, R. W., and Lemmen, L. J. Tumors of the posterior portion of the third ventricle. J. Neurosurg., *10:* 1–18, 1953.
35. Rapoport, S. I. Blood-brain barrier in physiology and medicine. Raven Press, New York, 1976, pp. 77–78.
36. Reid, W. S., and Clark, W. K. Comparison of the infratentorial and transtentorial approaches to the pineal region. Neurosurgery, *3:* 1–8, 1978.
37. Ringertz, N., Nordenstam, H., and Flyger, G. Tumors of the pineal region. J. Neuropathol. Exp. Neurol., *13:* 540–561, 1954.
38. Romshe, C. A., and Sotos, J. F. Intracranial human chorionic gonadotropin-secreting tumor with precocious puberty. J. Pediatr., *86:* 250–252, 1975.
39. Sakata, K., Yamada, H., Sakai, N., Hosono, Y., Kawasako, T., and Sasaoka, I. Extraneural metastasis of pineal tumor. Surg. Neurol., *3:* 49–54, 1975.
40. Schmidek, H. H. (ed.). *Pineal Tumors,* pp. 1–138. Masson, New York, 1977.
41. Scully, R. E., Galdabini, J. J., and McNeely, B. U. Case records of the Massachusetts General Hospital (Case 38-1975). N. Engl. J. Med., *293:* 653–660, 1975.
42. Smith, N. J., El-Mahdi, A. M., and Constable, W. C. Results of irradiation of tumors in the region of the pineal body. Acta Radiol. Ther. Phys. Biol., *15:* 17–22, 1976.
43. Stavrou, D., Anzil, A. P., Wiedenback, W., *et al.* Immunofluorescence study of lymphocytic infiltration in gliomas. Identification of T-lymphocytes. J. Neurol. Sci., *33:* 275–282, 1977.
44. Stein, B. Personal communication, 1979.
45. Stein, B. M. The infratentorial supracerebellar approach to pineal lesions. J. Neurosurg., *35:* 197–202, 1971.
46. Sung, D., Harisiadis, L., and Chang, C. H. Midline pineal tumors and suprasellar germinomas: Highly curable by radiation. Radiology, *128:* 745–751, 1978.
47. Suzuki, J., and Iwabuchi, T. Surgical removal of pineal tumors (pinealomas and teratomas). J. Neurosurg., *23:* 565–571, 1965.
48. Wara, W. M., Fellows, C. F., Sheline, G. E., Wilson, C. B., and Townsend, J. J. Radiation therapy for pineal tumors and suprasellar germinomas. Radiology, *124:* 221–223, 1977.
49. Wurtman, R. J., and Moskowitz, M. A. The pineal organ (part I). N. Engl. J. Med., *296:* 1329–1333, 1977.
50. Wurtman, R. J., and Moskowitz, M. A. The pineal organ (part II). N. Engl. J. Med., *296:* 1383–1386, 1977.

CHAPTER
21

Intracranial Germ Cell Tumors

KINTOMO TAKAKURA, M.D., D.M.SC.

INTRODUCTION

Intracranial germ cell tumors have attracted considerable attention during the past few years. The reasons for this include: (*a*) improved diagnostic imaging of tumors in the pineal and suprasellar regions; (*b*) the histopathological polymorphism and tumor marker production; and (*c*) the increased survival rate with multimodal treatment including microsurgical removal, radiotherapy, and chemotherapy.

Intracranial germ cell tumors are potentially curable in many cases, with malignant germ cell tumors being the most refractory to treatment. Intracranial germ cell tumors are composed of a variety of histologically different types. Since the nomenclature of these tumors has not yet been unified, I have categorized them into three types: germinoma (two-cell pattern pinealoma), mature teratoma (benign), and immature teratoma (malignant, including choriocarcinoma, endodermal sinus tumor, embryonal carcinoma *etc.*). It is also well realized that mixed types of tumor are often present and demonstrate complicated pathological and clinical features.

Intracranial germ cell tumors are now easily diagnosed by computed tomographic (CT) scanning and magnetic resonance imaging (MRI). MRI is especially useful for revealing the anatomical structure of those tumors mainly located in the central axis of the brain and gives us some insight into the pathological diagnosis and determination of surgical approaches. Pathophysiology of functioning germ cell tumors which produce human chorionic gonadotropin (HCG), α-fetoprotein (AFP), or carcinoembryonic antigen (CEA) has gradually been clarified. These functioning tumors are invariably malignant and require multimodal treatment. One of the most prominent characteristics of intracranial germ cell tumors is the influence of endocrine factors on their growth.

Intracranial germ cell tumors are more common in Japan than in North America or Europe. In this chapter, our experience with these tumors and long-term follow-up in 130 cases are reviewed.

DIAGNOSIS WITH MAGNETIC RESONANCE IMAGING (MRI)

Although CT scanning has greatly improved the detection of intracranial germ cell tumors, MRI has provided better visualization of the three-dimensional anatomical structure of tumors located in the central axis of the brain. The location and the extension of the tumor inside the third ventricle can be clearly visualized by MRI. This is particularly helpful in selecting the best surgical approach to tumors in the region of the pineal body. As well, the setting of the field for radiotherapy can be determined with greater accuracy.

The MRI examples shown in this paper were taken by Siemens Magnetom H15 in our hospital. The magnetic field strength used was 0.35 Tesla (maximum 1.5 Tesla). Typical MRI appearance of pineal germinoma are shown in Figures 21.1 and 21.2. In Figure 21.1, the tumor is well demarcated and has a homogeneous signal intensity except a tiny calcified spot with low p (proton density) at the anterior upper portion of the tumor. The anatomical relationships of the compressed cerebellum, the brain stem, and the extension of the tumor inside the posterior part of the third ventricle are well visualized. Figure 21.2 demonstrates a

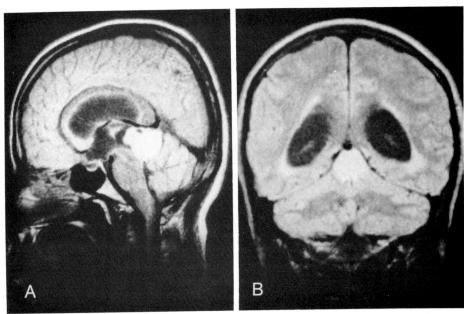

FIG. 21.1. MRI of a pineal germinoma with a tiny calcification in the anterior upper portion of the tumor. (A) Sagittal view. (B) Coronal view. (Courtesy of Dr. Isao Hayakawa of the Bokuto Municipal Hospital.)

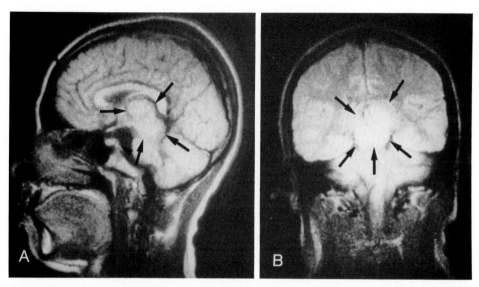

FIG. 21.2. (A and B) MRI of pineal germinoma extending to the anterior part of the third ventricle.

larger germinoma. The tumor is extending anteriorly to the infundibular recess and upward to the fornix.

For comparison, Figure 21.3 shows the CT scan and MRI of a metastatic tumor from renal clear cell carcinoma. CT scan revealed an oval-shaped enhanced mass located slightly toward the right side of the pineal region. The MRI figure demonstrates a round tumor with inhomogeneous intensity, surrounded by irregular-shaped brain edema with high p. The extension of the edema is easily seen. One of the characteristic features of metastatic brain tumor is marked brain edema surrounding a rather well-demarcated tumor. The irregular intensity inside the tumor correlates well with the inhomogeneity of metastatic tumor tissue containing necrosis, bleeding, cyst, and tumor tissue with various vascularities.

Malignant lymphoma can develop in the pineal region. Typically it presents as a "plow-shaped" enhanced mass lesion in the pineal region that is often accompanied by multiple tumors in other intracranial locations, especially near the central axis. Figure 21.4 demonstrates CT scans and the MRI of a malignant lymphoma. The sagittal MRI section was taken at the plain 2 cm lateral from the midline. The extension of marked edema surrounding the malignant lymphoma in the pineal region and the left parietal lobe were well visualized.

Differential diagnosis of various tumors in the pineal region by CT scan was reported in a previous study (24).

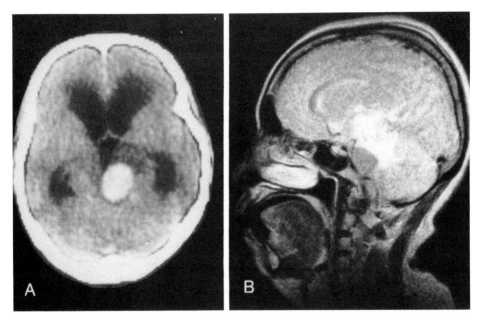

FIG. 21.3. Metastatic renal cell carcinoma in pineal region. (*A*) CT scan with contrast enhancement. (*B*) MRI. Brain edema is noted surrounding the tumor.

ENDOCRINE FACTORS CONTROLLING THE DEVELOPMENT OF INTRACRANIAL GERM CELL TUMORS

Intracranial germ cell tumors are common brain tumors in Japan, constituting 12.7% of all verified brain tumors in children (3). About 60% of germ cell tumors are germinomas. These tumors develop more commonly in males than females. Age and sex distribution of 434 cases of germinoma accumulated by the Japanese Brain Tumor Registry (3) is shown in Figure 21.5. In our series of 80 cases of germinoma, the male:female sex ratio was 64:16. Although the total male:female ratio of germinoma is 3:1 (327:107) (3), the ratio varies with the patient's age. There is no sex difference in children whose ages are under 10 years old. In puberty from 10 to 14 years old, the male:female ratio was 2:1 (82:38) and 5.5:1 in adult patients whose ages range from 15 to 40 years.

In cases of mature and immature teratoma, a more distinct male predominance is noted. In 50 teratomas in our series, 40 cases were male. There was no sex difference in the incidence of cases of suprasellar mature or immature teratomas (Fig. 21.6). In contrast, we have not had a female with a pineal teratoma (Fig. 21.7).

Most cases of immature teratoma producing HCG and/or AFP have been seen in males. In our series of 19 functioning tumors, 17 cases were

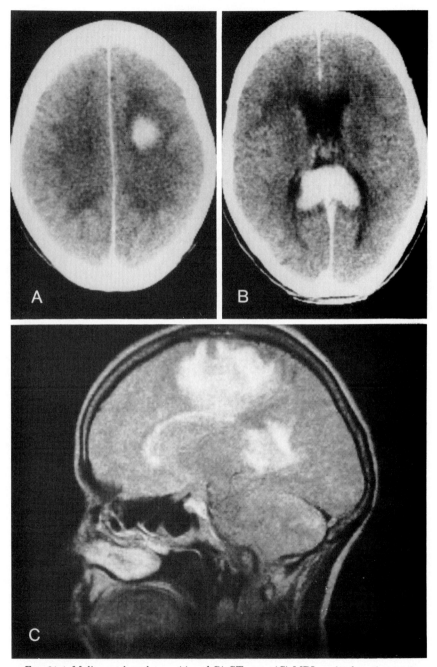

FIG. 21.4. Malignant lymphoma. (*A* and *B*) CT scan. (*C*) MRI, sagittal section, at 2 cm from the midline.

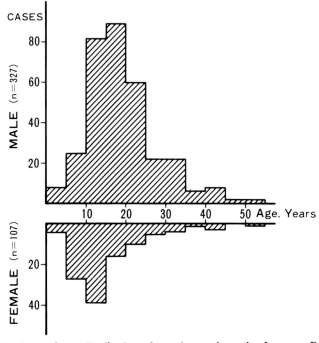

FIG. 21.5. Age and sex distribution of germinoma from the Japanese Brain Tumor Registry (3).

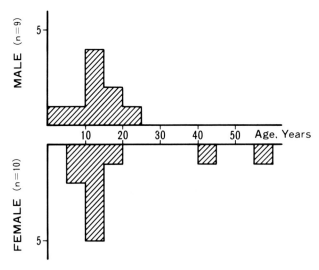

FIG. 21.6. Age and sex distribution of mature and immature teratoma in the suprasellar region. (Cases are from the University of Tokyo.)

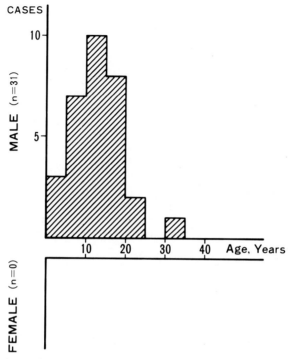

FIG. 21.7. Age and sex distribution of mature and immature teratoma in the pineal region. (Cases are from the University of Tokyo.)

male. Fatal recurrence, metastases, or dissemination of the tumor have occurred only in male cases. The distinct male predominance after puberty strongly suggests endocrine control of development and growth of intracranial germ cell tumors. Although the effect of hormonal steroids, such as testosterone or estradiol, on the pathogenesis and growth of germ cell tumors has not been studied on the cellular level, hormonal treatment of immature teratoma may prove beneficial in the future.

FUNCTIONING GERM CELL TUMORS

Functioning germ cell tumors were found in 19 cases (7 HCG, 7 AFP, and 5 HCG- and AFP-producing tumors) in our clinic. The prognosis of these patients depends on the biological tumor marker producing function of the tumor. Among 5 cases demonstrating maximal serum HCG level of more than 1000 IU/liter, 4 died within 4 years after initial treatment, while all 7 cases having maximal serum HCG level of less than 1000 IU/liter are still alive 2–20 years later. On the other hand, all 3 cases demonstrating maximal serum AFP level of more than 10,000 ng/ml died within 4 years after initial treatment whereas in 9 cases with AFP level of less than 10,000 ng/ml, 7 are still alive 1–5 years later. Both HCG- and AFP-producing tumors are essentially malignant and require adequate radiotherapy and chemotherapy. The recurrence of these functioning tumors must always be kept in mind. The following case reports suggest that inadequate treatment failed to prevent recurrence.

Case 1. A Case of Inadequate Radiotherapy: K.G., a 16-year-old boy (TU-83143). The patient complained of headache, nausea, vomiting and decreasing visual acuity in July 1983 at the age of 16. Bilateral choked discs and Parinaud's symptom were noted at the time of admission. CT scan (Fig. 21.8A) revealed an oval tumor mass and marked hydrocephalus. Serum AFP was 206 ng/ml, but serum HCG and CEA were both within normal limits. Ventriculoperitoneal (VP) shunting was performed on August 17. CSF-AFP was 86.5 ng/ml, and CSF-HCG was 62 IU/liter. CSF-CEA was again within normal limits. Since local radiotherapy (20 Gray (Gy)) did not decrease the size of the tumor (Fig. 21.8B), the tumor was macroscopically removed via the right occipital transtentorial approach on October 18, 1983. The histological diagnosis was mature teratoma. The postoperative course was uneventful. CT scan taken on December 22, 1983 (Fig. 21.8C) revealed no residual tumor mass, and hydrocephalus was improved. One year later, however, a CT scan taken on November 19, 1984 (Fig. 21.8D) demonstrated the recurrence of an egg-sized tumor situated slightly to the right of its primary pineal location. Serum AFP, HCG, and CEA were all within normal limits. Radiotherapy of the pineal region (22 Gy) as well as whole brain (20 Gy) and chemotherapy with vincristine and ACNU was given and was followed by moderate reduction in tumor size. This case provides important information about the recurrence of functioning germ cell tumors. First, macroscopically total removal of the tumor does not mean complete cure. Second, the measurement of serum tumor markers AFP, HCG, and CEA does not always detect the recurrence of the tumor, and thus follow-up with CT scan or MRI is indispensable. Third, a full course of radiotherapy, both to the tumor as well as to the whole brain, with suitable chemotherapy might be required for preventing the recurrence of functioning tumor, even though the histological examination did not detect immature cells in the surgically removed specimen.

Case 2. A Case of Very Late Recurrence: S.S., a 15-Year-Old-Boy (TU 64533). The patient complained of decreased visual acuity in 1964 at the age of 15. At the time of admission, bitemporal hemianopsia and diabetes insipidus were noted. Pneumoencephalography and angiography revealed a tumor mass in the suprasellar region. Craniotomy and biopsy were performed. Postoperative local radiotherapy (40 Gy) im-

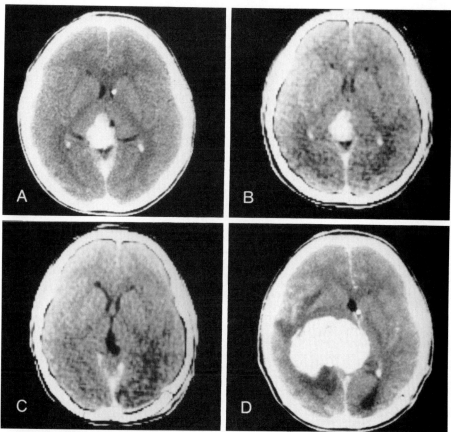

FIG. 21.8. Case 1. CT scans of a pineal functioning teratoma in a 16-year-old boy (HCG-and AFP-producing tumor). (A) Before treatment. (B) After the "diagnostic radiotherapy." (C) After surgical removal. (D) Recurrence of the tumor at 13 months after the surgical removal.

proved his visual acuity and normalized his visual field. He had no complaints during the 18-year period after the radiotherapy. Routine follow-up CT scan subsequently revealed a tiny contrast-enhancing mass in the suprasellar region in May 1982 at the age of 32 (Fig. 21.9A). The following year, he began to complain again of decreasing visual acuity and narrowing visual field. CT scan revealed further enlargement of the tumor (Fig. 21.9B). The serum HCG level was 170 IU/liter in June 1983. Since the recurrence of the suprasellar tumor was evident, radiotherapy (50 Gy) was locally given. His vision had returned to normal by September 1983. A CT scan showed the disappearance of the tumor (Fig. 21.9C). Serum HCG level decreased to less than 1 IU/liter. Since then he has

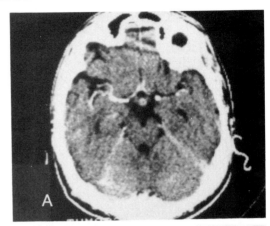

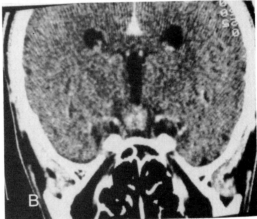

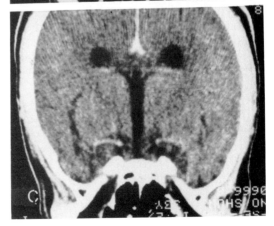

FIG. 21.9. Case 2. CT scans of late recurrence of suprasellar HCG-producing tumor in a 15-year-old boy. (A) The CT scan taken at the age of 33 in May 1982 18 years after radiotherapy. A tiny enhanced mass is visible in the suprasellar region. (B) In June 1983, the patient complained of decreasing visual acuity and narrowing visual field. The enlargement of the tumor was noted. Serum HCG was 170 IU/liter. (C) September 1983. After the second course of radiation therapy, the tumor disappeared. Serum HCG was less than 1 IU/liter. (Courtesy of Dr. Tetsuo Wakao of the Yamanashi Central Hospital.)

maintained good health and returned to his job. Although serum HCG could not be assayed in 1964, it was presumed that the primary tumor contained a choriocarcinoma component. This case recurred 18 years after initial treatment and indicates the difficulty of complete cure of immature teratoma.

Immunohistochemical studies have revealed that all HCG-producing tumors contained histologically a choriocarcinoma component and all AFP-producing tumors have an endodermal sinus tumor component. CEA-producing tumors are less frequent than HCG- or AFP-producing tumors. We had only two cases of CEA-producing tumors. HCG- or AFP-producing tumor cells are located in the parenchyme of the tumor, while CEA producing cells line only the surface of epithelial tumor cells.

Functioning tumors with very active HCG or AFP production invariably are clinically malignant. These tumors often disseminate intrathecally throughout the subarachnoid space and metastasize to extracranial organs such as the lung, liver, and retroperitoneal region. A case of HCG-producing tumor demonstrating a fulminant course was previously reported (24).

Recent chemotherapy using a combination of cisplatinum, vinblastine, and bleomycin (PVB therapy) has resulted in excellent tumor suppressive effect (13, 16, 17). Using multiple-drug therapy it may be possible to prevent the recurrence of many malignant functioning germ cell tumors.

TREATMENT AND RESULTS

The outcome of treatment for intracranial germ cell tumors largely differs according to the histological type of tumor (Fig. 21.10).

Germinoma is quite sensitive and responds well to radiotherapy. The 10-year survival rate of our 79 cases of germinoma was 71.8%. In those cases of germinoma, 49 tumors were located in the pineal region, 22 in the suprasellar region, and 8 in other regions such as frontal lobe or basal ganglia. No surgical mortality occurred in the group with suprasellar region tumors. The survival rate of the suprasellar tumors was best of all in intracranial germ cell tumors, that is, 90.9% at 5 years and 84.4% at 10 years after initial treatment. On the contrary, the survival rate of pineal region germinoma was 65.0% at 5 years and 10 years after the initial treatment (Fig. 21.11). However, the present data include all pineal region germinoma cases treating during the past 20 years. The mortality and morbidity of surgical intervention during the initial 10-year period was much higher than in the last 10 years. The lower surgical survival rate of the pineal region tumors, as opposed to that of the suprasellar region tumors, was attributed partly to the greater difficulty in exposing and removing tumors in the former location. Although total removal of pineal region germinoma is often difficult, the recent improvements in

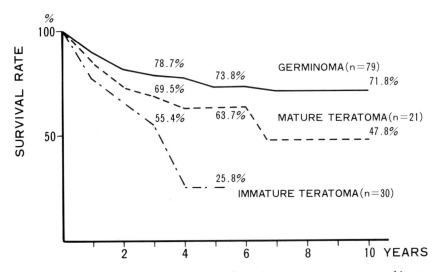

FIG. 21.10. Survival curves of the intracranial germinoma, mature teratoma, and immature teratoma. (Cases are from the University of Tokyo.)

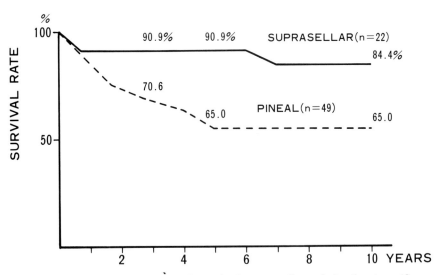

FIG. 21.11. Survival curves of germinoma in the suprasellar and pineal regions. (Cases are from the University of Tokyo.)

microsurgical technique have helped to reduce the postoperative mortality to 0% in the last 5 years. Since our data clearly show that postsurgical radiotherapy almost completely suppressed recurrence, the moderately extensive removal of the tumor avoiding damage to any adjacent brain tissue is recommended for pineal region germinoma, rather than an attempt at radical removal of the tumor. In cases of suprasellar germinoma, the tumor often invades an optic nerve or chiasm, and it becomes a limiting factor for the total removal of the tumor.

In cases of mature teratoma, radiotherapy and chemotherapy are less effective, and a greater emphasis is placed upon surgical removal. The outcome depends largely on the size of the tumor and the extension of the tumor to the adjacent brain tissue. The tumor is usually encapsulated and well demarcated within the third ventricle. The tumor can be totally removed through a frontal or occipital transcallosal, or transinfratentorial-supracerebellar approach (9–11, 18, 19, 21, 27). In our series, the survival rate of the mature teratoma was 63.7% at 5 years and 47.8% at 10 years after the surgery (Figure 21.10). The lower survival rate of mature teratoma compared to that of germinoma is mainly due to postsurgical morbidity and radiosensitivity. However, the mortality and morbidity for mature teratomas has also decreased definitely in recent cases and the overall outcome has improved.

Mature teratomas often contain a portion of immature teratomatous components. A case previously presented (case 1) was initially diagnosed histologically as mature teratoma, but the tumor marker study revealed the presence of HCG- and AFP-producing tumor cells. This case clearly indicates that the tumor contained a component of choriocarcinoma and endodermal sinus tumor, even though the surgically removed portion of specimen did not demonstrate those tumor cells. We have to realize that there are limitations with respect to histological examination, since some parts of the tumor are unavailable or difficult to fully examine.

Thirty cases of immature teratoma were treated. Among them, 19 cases were functioning tumors producing HCG and/or AFP. Since the tumor markers could not be assayed in the early days, the percentage of functioning tumors in immature teratoma might be expected to be higher than in the current study. The outcome of those tumors was poor, and the survival rate was 25.8% at 5 years after the initial treatment (Fig. 21.10). A definite factor influencing the prognosis is the biological function producing AHC or AFP. Tumors producing abundant marker proteins or polypeptides are biologically active, grow rapidly, and metastasize through CSF and to remote organs as described earlier.

DISCUSSION

Our therapeutic schedule for intracranial germ cell tumors differs with the location of the tumor. For suprasellar tumors, surgical removal and histological verification are performed as the initial step. In germinoma, simple radiotherapy is given. In cases of functioning tumor, chemotherapy using vincristine and ACNU (23) is given concomitantly with radio-therapy.

For pineal region tumors, radiotherapy with rather small doses of 20 Gy is given as the initial treatment. We call this method "diagnostic radiation." If the tumor is a germinoma, almost all of the tumor disappears on the CT scan during this radiotherapy. Hydrocephalus due to compression of aqueduct by tumor is generally ameliorated without VP shunting. VP shunting is necessary only when there is a danger that extensive hydrocephalus will induce herniation. When the size of the tumor is extensively reduced during the 20 Gy of radiation, the radio-therapy is continued up to 40 Gy to the pineal region, and 20 Gy is given to the whole brain. The total dose of radiation is reduced according to the age of the patient. When the size of the tumor is not reduced by diagnostic radiotherapy, the tumor is not considered a germinoma and is removed surgically. When a tumor marker is detected in the serum, the amount of the marker is always reduced by 20 Gy of radiation, or surgical removal of the tumor is carried out.

Postoperative radiotherapy concomitant with chemotherapy is advis-able for the immature teratoma. Radiotherapy should be given also to the whole brain and spinal cord in cases of immature teratoma, that is, in a manner similar to that of the treatment of medulloblastoma.

The outcome of radiotherapy for intracranial germ cell tumors has been described by various authors (1, 2, 5, 8, 12, 15, 20, 22, 25, 26). Sung et al. (22) reported the best 10-year survival rate for intracranial germi-noma by radiotherapy (65%), whereas our results revealed a 10-year survival rate for all germinoma of 71.8%. For suprasellar germinoma, the 10-year survival rate was 84.4%, and no deaths have been encountered in the last 10 years. A cure for suprasellar germinoma can thus be expected in the majority of cases.

In general, the morbidity is higher for surgery in the pineal region, as opposed to the suprasellar region. As described previously, a course of so-called "diagnostic radiation" is often given as the initial approach to tumors of the pineal body. In contrast, germ cell tumors in other sites cannot be diagnosed before histological verification of the tumor, unless the tumor is functioning. Consequently, these tumors are usually ap-proached surgically prior to making a decision regarding radiotherapy or chemotherapy.

Several authors have reported the effectiveness of cisplatinum for treating immature teratoma (14, 16, 17). Matsutani et al. (14) treated five cases of intracranial immature teratoma by combined chemotherapy using cisplatinum, vinblastine, and bleomycin (PVB therapy), and they observed tumor suppression in all patients. In a case of endodermal sinus tumor with a choriocarcinoma component, the tumor disappeared on the CT scan without radiotherapy, and a serum AFP level of 6700 ng/ml before treatment returned to a normal level. The rate of effectiveness of PVB therapy on the extragonadal germ cell tumors has ranged from 71 to 100% (4, 6, 7, 13). A limiting factor of cisplatinum administration is its side effect on renal function. The outcome of PVB therapy for immature teratoma is now under investigation in our phase II study.

CONCLUSIONS

We categorize germ cell tumors into three groups: germinoma, mature teratoma, and immature teratoma. Immature teratoma is mostly functioning tumor producing HCG, AFP, or CEA. Germinoma and mature teratoma have become curable diseases using microsurgical and radiotherapeutic approaches. Improved chemotherapeutic regimens are needed to limit the recurrence of malignant teratomas. Endocrine factors controlling the development of these tumors should be elucidated.

ACKNOWLEDGMENT

This work was supported by Cancer Research Grant 59-22 from the Ministry of Health and Welfare. The cooperation of Drs. Masao Matsutani, Tsukasa Sasaki, Shu Kobayashi, Isao Hayakawa, and Tetso Wakao is greatly appreciated. MRI and CT scans were supplied by Dr. Tohru Machida and Prof. Masahiro Iio of the Department of Radiology, the University of Tokyo. I thank Miss Haruko Ichimura for the preparation of this manuscript.

REFERENCES

1. Bradfield, J. S., and Perez, C. A. Pineal tumors and ectopic pinealomas. Analysis of treatment and failures. Radiology, 103: 399–406, 1972.
2. Camins, M. B., and Schlesinger, E. B. Treatment of tumours of the posterior part of the third ventricle and the pineal region: A long-term follow-up. Acta Neurochir., 40: 131–143, 1978.
3. Committee of the Japanese Brain Tumor Registry: All Japan Brain Tumor Registry, vol. 5, 1984.
4. Danoff, B., and Sheline, G. E. Radiotherapy of pineal tumors. In Diagnosis and Treatment of Pineal Region Tumors, edited by E. A. Neuwelt, pp. 300–308. Williams & Wilkins, Baltimore, 1984.
5. Daugaard, G., Rorth, M., and Hansen, H. H. Therapy of extragonadal germ cell tumors. Eur. J. Cancer Oncol., 19: 895–899, 1983.
6. Funes, H. C., Mendez, M., Alonso, E., Ouiben, R., Manãs, A., and Mendiola, C. Mediastinal germ cell tumors treated with Cis Platin, Bleomycin and Vinblastine (PVB). Proc. Am. Assoc. Cancer Res., 22: 474, 1981.
7. Hainsworth, J. D., Einhorn, L. H., Williams, S. D., Stewart, M., and Greco, A. Advanced extragonadal germ cell tumors—Successful treatment with combination chemotherapy. Ann. Intern. Med., 97: 7–11, 1982.
8. Jenkin, R. D. T., Simpson, W. J. K., and Keen C. W. Pineal and suprasellar germinomas. Results of radiation treatment. J. Neurosurg., 48: 99–107, 1978.
9. Kahn, E. A. Surgical treatment of pineal tumors. Arch. Neurol. Psychiatry, 38: 833–842, 1937.

10. Krause, F. Operative Freilegung der Vierhügel Nebst Beobachtungen über Hirndruck und Dekompreesion. Zentralbl. Chir., *53:* 2812–2819, 1926.
11. Lapras, C. Surgical therapy of pineal region tumors. In: *Diagnosis and Treatment of Pineal Region Tumors*, edited by E. A. Neuwelt, pp. 289–299. Williams & Wilkins, Baltimore, 1984.
12. Laws, E. R., Abay, III, E. O., Forbes, G. S., Grado, G. L., Bruckman, J. E., and Scott, M. Conservative management of pineal tumors—Mayo Clinic experience. In: *Diagnosis and Treatment of Pineal Region Tumors*, edited by E. A. Neuwelt, pp. 323–331. Williams & Wilkins, Baltimore, 1984.
13. Matsutani, M. Treatment of germ cell tumor. In: *Brain Tumor, Surgery MOOK (Jpn.)*, edited by K. Takakura, pp. 200–208. Kanehara Publ. Tokyo, 1984.
14. Matsutani, M., Sano, K., Takakura, K., and Seto, K. Intracranial germ cell tumor. Neurosurgeons (Jpn.), *3:* 83–100, 1984.
15. Mincer, F., Meltzer, J., and Bostein, C. Pinealoma. Cancer, *37:* 2713–2718, 1976.
16. Neuwelt, E. A., and Frenkel E. P. Germinomas and other pineal tumors: Chemotherapeutic responses. In: *Diagnosis and Treatment of Pineal Region Tumors*, edited by E. A. Neuwelt, pp. 332–343. Williams & Wilkins, Baltimore, 1984.
17. Neuwelt, E. A., Frenkel E. P., and Smith, R. G. Suprasellar germinomas (ectopic pinealomas): Aspects of immunological characterization and successful chemotherapeutic responses in recurrent disease. Neurosurgery, *7:* 352–358, 1980.
18. Sano, K. Pineal region tumors: Problems in pathology and treatment. Clin. Neurosurg., *30:* 59–91, 1982.
19. Sano, K., and Matsutani, M. Pinealoma (germinoma) treated by direct surgery and postoperative irradiation. A long-term follow up. Child's Brain, *8:* 81–97, 1981.
20. Smith, N. J., El-Mahdi, A. M., and Constable, W. C. Results of irradiation of tumors in the region of the pineal body. Acta Radiol. Ther. Phys. Biol., *15:* 17–22, 1976.
21. Stein, B. M. The infratentorial supracerebellar approach to pineal lesions. J. Neurosurg., *35:* 197–202, 1971.
22. Sung, D. H., Harisiadis, L., and Chang, C. H. Midline pineal tumors and suprasellar germinomas: Highly curable by irradiation. Radiology, *128:* 745–751, 1978.
23. Takakura, K. Synchronized chemo-radiotherapy for brain tumors. Prog. Nerv. Res. (Jpn.), *26:* 105–112, 1982.
24. Takakura, K. Nonsurgical pineal tumor therapy—The Japanese experience. In: *Diagnosis and Treatment of Pineal Region Tumors*, pp. 309–322. Williams & Wilkins, Baltimore, 1984.
25. Wara, W. M., Fellows, C. F., Sheline, G. E., Wilson, C. B., and Townsend, J. J. Radiation therapy for pineal tumors and suprasellar germinomas. Radiology *124:* 221–223, 1977.
26. Wara, W. M., Jenkin, D. T. Evans, A., Ertel, I., Hittle, R., Ortega, J., and Wilson, C. B. Tumors of the pineal and suprasellar region. Children's Cancer Study Group Treatment Results, 1960–1975. Cancer, *43:* 698–701, 1979.
27. Zapletal, B. Ein neuer operativer Zugang zum Gebiet der Incisura Tentorii. Zentralbl. Neurochir., *16:* 64–69, 1956.

Therapeutic Modalities for Pineal Region Tumors

BENNETT M. STEIN, M.D., and MICHAEL R. FETELL, M.D.

For many years, until the mid 1970s (and in some circles, even today), the therapy of pineal region tumors consisted of ventricular shunting and radiation therapy. Sparse data were available about the histological type of tumors being treated, and reports generally lumped nonverified cases in with a few verified cases. Results in larger series of cases treated by radiotherapy demonstrate that, compared to other forms of brain cancer, pineal region tumors carry a moderately good prognosis, with 5-year survivals in the 60–80% range and 10-year survivals approximately 60% (17, 23).

However, we submit that today the treatment of pineal region tumors should involve three principles: (a) the control of hydrocephalus, which is almost always associated with tumors in this region; (b) the total resection of benign encapsulated tumors of the pineal region; and (c) the histological identification of nonresectable tumors and adjunctive treatment with radiation or chemotherapy. We consider the foundation of therapy to be surgical exploration and identification of the nature of the tumors, of which there are a great variety (5, 19). By means of ancillary testing, one must then determine the extent of the tumor, whether or not it has spread locally within the third ventricle and into surrounding structures, or whether it has seeded throughout the CSF pathways, especially to the spinal cord.

Indeed, a variety of surgical approaches have been developed for exposing and resecting benign tumors of the pineal region (Fig. 22.1) (22). In addition, therapeutic regimes consisting of combinations of radiation and various chemotherapeutic agents tested on small numbers of pineal tumors and more widely on similar tumors involving the gonads have provided a rational treatment plan for nonresectable pineal region tumors (2, 3, 17).

This approach to tumors of the pineal region has resulted in a much higher cure rate, decreased surgical mortality and morbidity, and in-

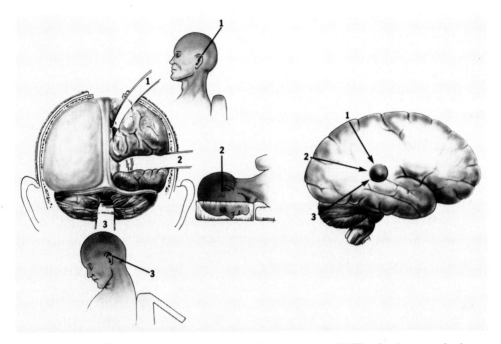

FIG. 22.1. The primary approaches to pineal region tumors. (*1*) The classic approach of Dandy. (*2*) The approach recommended by Poppen is either medial or under the occipital lobe. (*3*) Posterior fossa approach of Krause is depicted. The routes are equidistant from the pineal and differ only in the portions of the brain retracted and the relationship of the route to the pineal gland and the deep venous system.

creased longevity for those individuals who have recurrence of tumor at a distance from therapy.

CONTROL OF HYDROCEPHALUS

In addition to the syndrome of Parinaud (Fig. 22.2) and ataxia, the most common clinical finding in pineal region tumors is the presence of raised intracranial pressure presenting with papilledema, headache, and vomiting due to obstruction of the aqueduct and subsequent hydrocephalus. In many instances, the relief of hydrocephalus by various shunting procedures will result in the reversal of most of the neurological abnormalities seen in the early stage of these tumors. Furthermore, the control of hydrocephalus and the relief of raised intracranial pressure are absolutely mandatory prior to or during an operative procedure on tumors in this region since, by any route, the exposure is limited and the brain must be relaxed. However, a shunt may disseminate malignant tumor

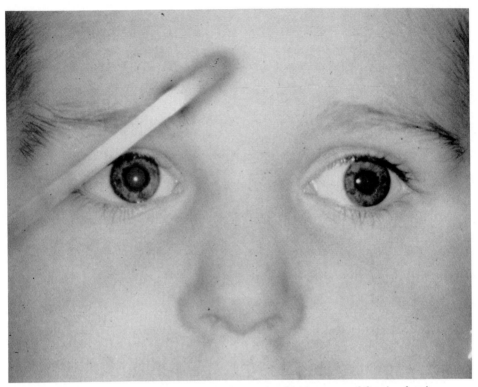

Fig. 22.2. Failure of upward gaze frequently associated with tumors of the pineal region.

cells into the peritoneal cavity (11). Although the potential for seeding of malignant tumors through a nonfiltered shunt is always present, from a practical standpoint this is uncommon. Our approach to hydrocephalus has been to decompress the ventricular system, either before or during the preliminaries of surgery. The timing depends on the acuteness of the situation and the need to proceed with definitive operation on the pineal tumor. In many instances, we receive patients who have already had ventricular shunting procedures, usually of the ventriculoperitoneal variety, without identification of the tumor. In these situations, the ventricles have been thoroughly decompressed, often for many weeks, and exposure presents no problem at the time of the definitive operation. On the other hand, we see another group of patients who are in the acute stages of ventricular obstruction. In these patients we prefer to control the hydrocephalus at the time of surgery by insertion of a ventriculostomy and release of the CSF, since shunts inserted before surgery may be occluded by air or blood at operation, and uncontrolled ventricular drainage with the patient in the sitting position may lead to cortical collapse. The ventricular drain may be converted to a ventriculoperitoneal shunt after 1 or 2 days of ventricular drainage. Despite the concern about seedling of a malignant tumor via the shunt system, we have not inserted filters in the shunt since these tend to occlude rapidly.

SURGERY FOR RESECTION OF BENIGN TUMORS OF THE PINEAL REGION

Since the early surgical efforts of Dandy (4), surgery on pineal region tumors has now become commom place. Dandy's approach was a parafalx, parietal lobe route through the posterior aspect of the corpus callosum to reach the pineal tumor through or around the deep venous plexus that is so often associated with the dorsal aspect of these tumors. He was severely limited by the lack of adequate lighting and the operating microscope. His mortality rate was high, and the probability of successfully removing benign tumors was low. Following this initial attempt, a number of reports entered the literature, recommending other approaches to the pineal region, including a paraoccipital lobe-supratentorial approach (15, 18), a transventricular approach (24), and a suboccipital-infratentorial approach (10, 22). We prefer the posterior fossa approach for the following reasons: (a) the patient may be operated on in the sitting position, a comfortable position for the surgeon and a position in which gravity assists retraction by dropping the cerebellum away from the tentorium; (b) these tumors are generally central and of modest size and are best approached by a midline or central route; (c) the tumors invariably lie ventral to the deep venous system, and even in malignant tumors the invasion of these veins is via the dorsal aspect of the tumor; therefore, the bulk of the tumor is almost always below this critical venous system; and (d) retraction of the parietal or occipital lobes results frequently in neurological deficits related to these structures such as contralateral sensory loss, hemiparesis, and visual field defects. In some cases, these defects may be serious and permanent. In the suboccipital exposure, cerebellar defects have been minimal and usually temporary. Deficits related to the dorsal midbrain or tectum are often in proportion to the degree of dissection carried out between the tumor and these structures and will be present regardless of which exposure is utilized. It is for these reasons, we have favored the posterior fossa approach to these lesions.

Description of Posterior Fossa Surgery for Pineal Tumors

This approach was originally described by Krause in 1926 (10). He had partial success from three operations via this route. This was a considerable accomplishment on his part since the lighting and magnification of the present day microscope were not available at that time. The operating microscope has made this route and operation feasible with low mortality and morbidity.

The operation is carried out in the sitting-slouch position, with the head flexed forward and the body in "C" configuration (Fig. 22.3). The head is held rigidly by a pin vise type of headholder. The tentorium should be horizontal and parallel to the floor for maximum ease of exposure. A midline incision is carried out, followed by a modest craniectomy extending above the lateral sinuses, torcular region, and laterally as far as possible, extending inferiorly to above but not including the foramen magnum. The ventricles should be decompressed. Mannitol may be added to improve exposure. The dura is opened in a cruciate fashion to expose the dorsal surface of the cerebellum maximally. All veins bridging the cerebellum and the tentorium are cauterized and divided as the cerebellum drops by gravity. Modest retraction over protective substances on the dorsal surface of the cerebellum is required. The operating microscope is brought into the field and, using long instruments and microdissection techniques, the precentral cerebellar vein is divided, and

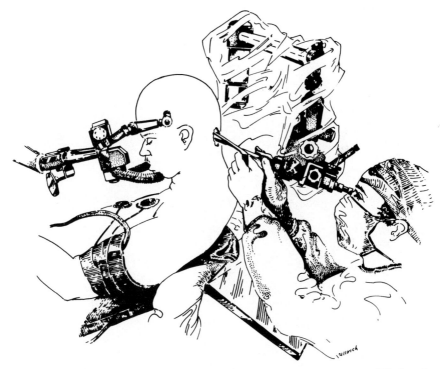

FIG. 22.3. The sitting-slouch position in which the patient occupies a "C"-shaped configuration with the surgeon working behind with the operating microscope.

the arachnoid over the area of the tumor and the anterior portion of the cerebellum is opened widely. The arteries in this region are primarily the posterior choroidals which can be cauterized and divided without concern. The deep venous system invariably lies above the tumor, and injury to it must be guarded against (16). At this point of the exposure, the surgeon can determine whether or not the tumor is encapsulated and proceed accordingly. For tumors which infiltrate, our policy has been to do a decompressive biopsy. For those tumors which are well encapsulated, total removal is accomplished in a piecemeal fashion. Various curets, scissors, cauteries (all extra long), and the long curved extension of the Cavitron are used to remove these tumors, which can vary considerably in their consistency and attachment to surrounding structures (Fig. 22.4). In benign encapsulated tumors, the strongest attachment is usually to the tela choroidea. Minor attachments to both medial thalamic regions and the tectum of the midbrain may be encountered. These are cauterized and divided in standard microsurgical fashion. After the tumor surgery, the dura is closed. The patient is kept in a sitting position postoperatively. Ventricular drainage or a preexisting shunt will keep the ventricles decompressed in the postoperative period. CT scans with and without contrast are performed at an expedient point in the postoperative course.

A CT scan-guided stereostatic biopsy technique may be employed for

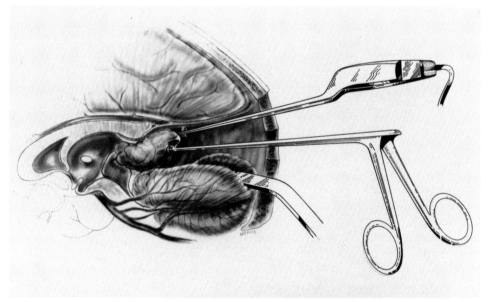

FIG. 22.4. The posterior fossa approach to pineal region tumors and the utilization of especially designed long instruments.

the diagnosis of pineal region tumors. This can save the patient the rigors of a formal craniotomy, and in a small series of patients has been safe. One must be certain that the lesion is not highly vascular, which can be determined by a prebiopsy angiogram. An issue which must be raised, however, is related to the amount of material obtained at the time of biopsy. Because of the wide variety of histological tumor types in this region and the difficulty encountered in making an accurate diagnosis even by an experienced pathologist, it is often necessary to obtain more tissue from these tumors than would be required from tumors found elsewhere in the central nervous system. The possibility of error on a small biopsy is, therefore, proportionately increased, which is a major problem with this technique. Further evaluation of larger series of cases managed by this technique must be available before it can be widely recommended.

SURGICAL IDENTIFICATION OF MALIGNANT TUMORS AND CONTROL BY RADIATION AND/OR CHEMOTHERAPY

In those tumors which are found at the time of surgery to be malignant and invasive, a modest removal is carried out, depending on the vascularity of the tumor. Specimens are sent for frozen section and for light and electron microscopy as well as immunohistochemical studies. Radical removal of a malignant vascular tumor should not be attempted, as it may result in a fatal intraoperative or postoperative hemorrhage. At the very least, severe damage to the surrounding critical structures may ensue.

COMBINED SURGICAL AND OTHER THERAPEUTIC ENDEAVORS

Basic to all therapeutic endeavors is the knowledge of what is being treated. Nomenclature referable to pineal region tumors has been in a state of confusion over the years with overlapping and elaborate terminology (5, 20). The categorization that we have followed and which appears to be popular in most reports on large series of pineal tumors is as follows: (*a*) *Germ cell tumors,* including germinoma, teratoma, dermoid, epidermoid, choriocarcinoma, endodermal sinus tumor, and embryonal carcinoma. Within this category there is a full spectrum of tumor activity from the most benign to the most malignant. (*b*) *Pineal cell tumors,* including pineocytoma and pineoblastoma. The pineocytoma may behave in either benign or malignant fashion. Rubinstein *et al.* (9, 20) believe that a subcategory of pineocytomas with gangliogliomatous elements are more slowly growing and have a benign course (9, 20). In our series, pineocytomas were associated with the highest incidence of preoperative hemorrhage, and two of the patients died immediately postoperatively due to intratumoral and subarachnoid hemorrhage. (c) *Supporting cell tumors,* including astrocytoma (either cystic or solid), ependymoma, oligodendroglioma, meningioma (19), as well as a miscellaneous group (including sarcomas). (d) *Nonneoplastic lesions include arachnoidal cyst, granuloma, and atrioventricular malformation (AVM).*

With the sophistication of microneurosurgical techniques, operative mortality and morbidity have been reduced to acceptable levels. In our experience, the mortality has been three patients of 80 operated on for pineal region tumors. These three patients died of immediate postoperative hemorrhage into malignant tumors, on which only a biopsy was performed. The long-term morbidity has been negligible in terms of extraocular movement disorders, cerebellar disorders, and other neurological deficits of a permanent nature. However, benign tumors may be removed with low morbidity, sparing the patient the side effects of unnecessary radiation and/or chemotherapy. In addition, nonneoplastic lesions such as granulomas (25) and arteriovenous malformations may be appropriately treated. Tumors in the benign category which are considered resectable have accounted for approximately 30% of our cases. These include the following: teratoma, dermoid, epidermoid, some pineocytomas, some astrocytomas, meningioma, ependymoma, and a miscellaneous group including colloid cyst and choroid plexus papilloma, as well as simple cysts. Surgery also permits the debulking of some mixed germ cell tumors in which the majority of the tissue is well differentiated teratoma with small, often microscopic elements of choriocarcinoma, endodermal sinus tumor, or embryonal carcinoma. Following radical removal of tumors, temporary disturbances of extraocular movement have been severe at times; prolonged lethargy has been rare; and the troublesome but benign "posterior fossa syndrome" has been frequent.

Radiation therapy has been effective in certain tumors and should be given to the whole brain with a dosage of approximately 4000 rads and a boost to the pineal and third ventricular regions (where seeding is frequent) of an additional 1500 rad through parallel opposing ports (23).

Whether or not to give prophylactic spinal radiation therapy is controversial (17, 23). Second only to medulloblastomas, malignant pineal region tumors show a propensity to seed the subarachnoid space. Seeding is most frequent with germinomas; however, other nongerminomatous germ cell tumors and pineal cell origin malignancies have also been documented to seed (9). Part of the reason for the high incidence of seeding relates to the location of pineal region tumors directly within a subarachnoid cistern with ready access to the spinal fluid pathways. The trend now is to stage patients after diagnosis with CT and myelography for tumor outside the primary site. In addition, spinal fluid cytology from both the lumbar fluid and ventricular fluid and the biological markers α-

fetoprotein (AFP) and β-human chorionic gonadotropin (B-HCG) may provide clues to the presence of otherwise asymptomatic tumor (7, 12, 14). Spinal radiation therapy may then be administered when there are documented spinal metastases or when the probability of seeding based upon marker studies is high. Judicious use of radiation therapy has the dual advantages of averting vertebral growth problems in children and improving future tolerance for chemotherapy if needed.

Biological markers (AFP and β-HCG) have been most useful in alerting us to the presence of more malignant elements in mixed germ cell tumors. β-HCG is elevated in CSF in all choriocarcinomas and some, but not all, germinomas and embryonal carcinomas. In two germinoma cases with elevated AFP levels in CSF and serum, coexistent embryonal carcinoma was found upon further sectioning of the surgical biopsy specimen.

Recent advances in chemotherapy have dramatically improved the prognosis of patients with testicular cancer, the leading cause of cancer-related death in males from 29 to 35 years of age (2). Most testicular cancers are of germ cell origin and consist of seminomas, well-differentiated teratomas, and teratocarcinomas (teratoma with embryonal carcinoma). Seminomas are radiosensitive tumors, and the standard treatment for nonmetastatic seminoma is orchiectomy and local radiation therapy. For metastatic seminoma, and for all patients with teratocarcinoma, multimodality chemotherapy offers an 80–90% chance of cure. The most widely used regimen is that of Einhorn and Donahue (6), consisting of vinblastine, bleomycin, and cisplatinum.

The same array of germ cell tumors seen in the testes is seen in the pineal region. Central nervous system germinomas are identical histologically to germinomas occurring elsewhere in the body, such as testicular seminomas or ovarian dysgerminomas (20). Teratomas and teratocarcinomas of the pineal region are also analogous to their gonadal counterparts. Hence, with pineal region germ cell tumors, there is a good rationale for employing a similar treatment plan to that which has proven so successful in the treatment of testicular cancer.

Beginning in 1973, isolated case reports documented response of germinomas to various forms of chemotherapy (1, 3, 7, 8, 13, 14, 21). In one case, quite dramatic regression of tumor was documented (21). In all instances, chemotherapy has been used for recurrent tumor, *i.e.*, for tumor that has failed radiation therapy. Although chemotherapy might be as effective as radiation therapy in the initial preoperative treatment of germinomas, this has not yet been formally tried.

SUMMARY

Since there is no radiographic test that can definitely predict the histology of a pineal tumor, we believe all patients should be treated first with a surgical approach to the tumor. This usually is accomplished by the supracerebellar-suboccipital route. Hydrocephalus is best treated at the time of surgery with ventricular drainage. Sometimes, surgery can decompress the CSF obstruction, and the need for a shunt can be averted following surgery; if not, the ventricular drain is converted to a shunt several days later.

If a pineal tumor is found to be benign and encapsulated, it is removed by surgery, and the patient requires no additional therapy. Meningiomas, cysts, and low grade cystic astrocytomas all fall into this category.

Some germ cell tumors are well differentiated and can also be grossly excised, but one must exercise caution in assuming that the entire tumor is benign. Many seemingly well-differentiated teratomas contain admixtures, sometimes microscopic, of more malignant elements. Careful pathological evaluation of the operative specimen and analysis of biological markers (AFP and β-HCG) can alert the clinician to the presence of malignant tumor. With germinomas, radiation therapy is initially effective, and chemotherapy has a proven role in treating recurrences. Spinal radiotherapy is withheld unless there is a strong suspicion of spinal seeding. Tumors of pineal cell origin are radiosensitive and should be treated with radiation therapy. Because these tumors are rare, there is little data to date to justify one particular form of chemotherapy over another for recurrent pineal cell malignancies. Likewise, whether chemotherapy is preferable to radiation therapy in the initial treatment of nongerminomatous germ cell malignancies is as yet unclear.

REFERENCES

1. Allen, J. C., and Helson L. High-dose cyclophosphamide chemotherapy for recurrent CNS tumors in children. J. Neurosurg., 44: 749–756, 1981.
2. Anderson, T., Waldman, T. A., Javadpour, N., et al. NIH Conference: Testicular germ Cell Neoplasms: Recent Advances in Diagnosis and Therapy. Ann. Int. Med., 90: 373–385, 1979.
3. Borden, S., Weber, A. L., Toch, R., et al. Pineal germinoma long-term survival despite hematogenous metastases. Am. J. Dis. Child., 126: 214–216, 1973.
4. Dandy, W. E. Operative experience in cases of pineal tumor. Arch. Surg., 33: 19–46, 1936.
5. DeGirolami, U., and Schmidek, H. Clinicopathological study of 53 tumors of the pineal region. J. Neurosurg., 39: 455–462, 1973.
6. Einhorn, L. H., and Donohue, J. Cis-diamine dichloroplatinum, vinblastine, and bleomycin combination chemotherapy in disseminated testicular cancer. Ann. Int. Med., 87: 293–298, 1977.
7. Gindhart, T. D., and Tsukahara, Y. C. Cytologic diagnosis of pineal germinoma in cerebrospinal fluid and sputum. Acta Cytol., 23: 341–346, 1979.
8. Ginsberg, S., Kirshner, J., Reich, S., et al. Systemic chemotherapy for a primary germ cell tumor of the brain: A pharmaco-kinetic study. Cancer Treat. Rep., 65: 477–483, 1981.
9. Herrick, M. K., and Rubinstein, L. J. The cytological differentiating potential of pineal parenchymal neoplasms (the pinealomas). A clinicopathological study of 28 tumors. Brain, 102: 321–332, 1979.

10. Krause, F. Operative Frielegung der vierhugen, nebst Beobachtungen uber hirndruck und dekompression. Zentralbl. Chir., *53:* 2812–2819, 1926.

11. Kun, L. E., Tang, T. T., Sty, Jr., *et al.* Primary cerebral germinoma and ventriculoperitoneal shunt metastases. Cancer, *48:* 213–216, 1981.

12. Neuwelt, E. A., Frenkel, E. P., and Smith, R. G. Suprasellar germinomas (ectopia pinealomas): Aspects of immunological characterization and successful chemotherapeutic responses in recurrent disease. Neurosurgery,*7:* 352–358, 1980.

13. Neuwelt, E. A., Ginsberg, M., and Frenkel, E. P., *et al.* Malignant pineal region tumors. A clinico-pathological study. J. Neurosurg., *57:* 597–607, 1979.

14. Ono, N., Takeda, F., Uki, J., *et al.* A suprasellar embryonal carcinoma producing alphafetoprotein and human chorionic gonadotropin: Treated with combined chemotherapy followed by radiotherapy. Surg. Neurol., *18:* 435–443, 1983.

15. Poppen, J. L., The right occipital approach to a pinealoma. J. Neurosurg., *25:* 706–710, 1966.

16. Quest, D. O., and Kleriga, E. Microsurgical anatomy of the pineal region. Neurosurgery, *6:* 385–390, 1979.

17. Rao, Y. T. R., Medini, E., Haselow, R. E. *et al.* Pineal and ectopic pineal tumors: The role of radiation therapy. Cancer, *48:* 708–713, 1981.

18. Reid W. S., and Clark, K. Comparison of the infratentorial and transtentorial approaches to the pineal region. Neurosurgery, *3:* 1–8, 1978.

19. Rozario, R., Adelman, L., Prager, R. J., and Stein, B. M.: Meningiomas of the pineal region and third ventricle. Neurosurgery, *5:* 489–495, 1979.

20. Rubinstein, L. F. Cytogenesis and differentiation of pineal neoplasms. Hum. Pathol., *12:* 441–448, 1981.

21. Seigal, T., Pfeffer, R., Catane, R., *et al.* Successful chemotherapy of recurrent intracranial germinoma with spinal metastases. Neurology, *33:* 631–633, 1983.

22. Stein, B. M. Supracerebellar Approach for Pineal Region Neoplasms. In: *Operative Neurosurgical Techniques,* edited by H. Schmidek and W. Sweet, Vol. 1 pp. 599–607. Grune & Stratton, New York, 1982.

23. Sung, D., Harisiadis, L., and Chang, C. H. Midline pineal tumors and suprasellar germinomas: Highly curable by irradiation. Radiology, *128:* 745–751, 1978.

24. Van Wagenen, W. P. A surgical approach for the removal of certain pineal tumors. Report of a case. Surg. Gynecol. Obstet., *53:* 216–220, 1931.

25. Whittle, I. R., Allsop, J. L., and Besser, M. Tuberculoma mimicking a pinealoma. J. Neurosurg., *59:* 875–878, 1983.

VI

Orbital Tumors

23

Neuro-Ophthalmology of Orbital Tumors

NEIL R. MILLER, M.D.

Tumors that originate in, or invade, the orbit produce symptoms and signs by compression, infiltration, and/or infarction of the orbital structures. In some cases, they may act simply as mass lesions, producing only proptosis and generalized limitation of eye movement. Most tumors, however, eventually produce neuro-ophthalmologic symptoms and signs through their effects on the optic nerve, the ocular motor nerves, the orbital branches of the ophthalmic division of the trigeminal nerve and, rarely, the nerve supply to the iris sphincter and dilator muscles.

GENERAL CONSIDERATIONS

Proptosis

Most orbital tumors produce some proptosis, although the degree of proptosis is not always impressive and may be overlooked during the initial examination (Fig. 23.1). Optic nerve sheath meningiomas, which take up little room within the orbit, usually produce minimal proptosis. Similarly, vascular tumors, which have a soft consistency, may become quite large before they produce significant proptosis. On the other hand, gliomas that involve the orbital portion of the optic nerve usually produce more impressive protusion of the eye, as do firm tumors such as neurinomas and tumors of the lacrimal gland. Tumors located within the extraocular muscle cone (e.g., hemangioma, optic nerve glioma, meningioma) are more likely to produce axial proptosis—the eye is pushed directly forward, while tumors outside the muscle cone (dermoid cyst, neurinoma, lacrimal gland tumor) tend to push the eye out or in a direction opposite that of the lesion. Thus, both the amount and the direction of proptosis may be helpful in identifying the nature of an orbital process.

Although proptosis is usually caused by orbital processes, lesions outside the orbit, particularly those in the cavernous sinus, may impair venous outflow from the orbit and produce proptosis. In such cases, however, other signs of cavernous sinus disease are usually present, and the use of computed tomography or magnetic resonance imaging is sufficient to allow the correct diagnosis (Fig. 23.2).

Optic Neuropathy

Tumors within the orbit may compress the optic nerve, producing one of three classic syndromes. In some cases, there is progressive visual loss associated with proptosis and swelling of the optic disc. Many patients, however, retain good visual acuity despite substantial optic disc swelling. This is particularly true in patients with optic nerve gliomas (35) and optic nerve sheath meningiomas (28, 34) (Fig. 23.3). Other tumors that may produce a similar picture are hamartomas (hemangioma, lymphangioma), choristomas (dermoid cyst), and malignant neoplasms (carci-

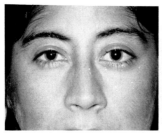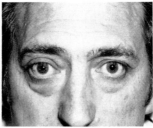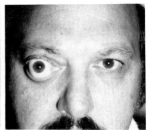

FIG. 23.1. Proptosis in three patients with orbital tumors. (*Left*) Mild left proptosis was initially overlooked when the patient presented with complaints of blurred vision in her left eye. She was found to have an optic nerve sheath meningioma. (*Center*) Moderate right proptosis in a patient with no visual complaints but with a mildly swollen right optic disc. Computed tomographic scan demonstrated a mass that was found to be a lymphangioma. (*Right*) Marked right proptosis in a patient with slowly progressive protrusion of the right eye for 7 years. The patient had a large hemangioma.

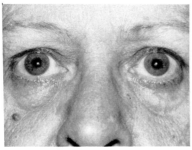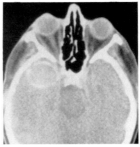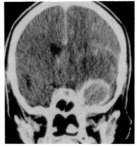

FIG. 23.2. Pseudo-orbital syndrome in a 56-year-old woman who presented with mild right proptosis and ophthalmoparesis. (*Left*) The right eye is proptotic and slightly higher than the left eye. The patient was initially thought to have an orbital mass, but computed tomographic (CT) scanning (*center and right*) demonstrated a large, well-circumscribed mass with a calcified rim that was found to represent a giant intracranial aneurysm.

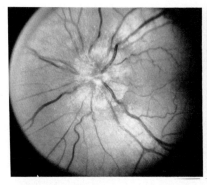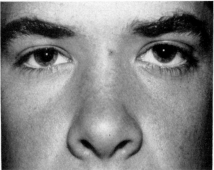

FIG. 23.3. (*Left*) Left optic disc swelling in a 35-year-old man with vague visual complaints but 20/20 vision. The patient was found to have an optic nerve sheath meningioma involving the orbital and intracanalicular portions of the nerve. (*Right*) The left eye is only minimally proptotic.

noma, lymphoma, sarcoma, and multiple myeloma) (6). In such patients, careful testing of color vision may reveal subtle defects even when visual acuity is thought to be normal. There may occasionally be an afferent pupillary defect. The visual field of the involved eye generally shows only enlargement of the blind spot, although slight peripheral field constriction may also be present. When other signs of orbital disease (proptosis, limitation of ocular motility, orbital congestion) are absent, these patients may be thought to have unilateral "papilledema" from increased intracranial pressure. Nevertheless, while it is obvious that patients with slowly progressive unilateral, visual loss and proptosis associated with optic disc swelling should undergo evaluation for a possible orbital tumor, patients with "isolated" optic disc swelling without visual loss should also undergo such an evaluation as well, particularly when they have no systemic or neurologic symptoms or signs suggestive of increased intracranial pressure (19). The most common cause of unilateral optic disc swelling without visual loss is orbital disease.

A second form of presentation of orbital tumors is that of unilateral transient visual loss (3, 31). The visual loss occurs only in certain positions of gaze and immediately clears when the direction of gaze is changed. It has been assumed that either direct pressure on the optic nerve or interruption of blood supply is the explanation for this phenomenon.

Finally, in many patients with chronic compression of the intraorbital (and intracanalicular) portion of the optic nerve, a specific clinical triad develops: (*a*) loss of vision; (*b*) optic disc swelling that resolves into optic atrophy; and (*c*) the appearance of optociliary shunt veins (Fig. 23.4). Optociliary shunt veins are vessels that overlie the optic disc and shunt

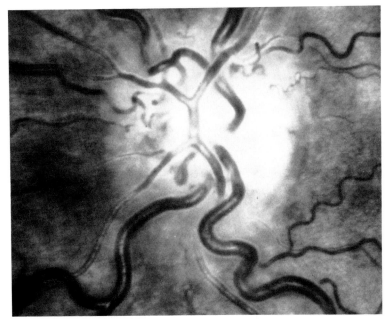

FIG. 23.4. Optociliary shunt veins in a patient with a left optic nerve sheath meningioma. The patient had vision of 3/200 in the eye.

blood between the retinal and choroidal venous circulations (Fig. 23.5). The common denominator in patients with this triad appears to be prolonged compression of the optic nerve with gradual compression and obstruction of the central retinal vein. The normal route of retinal venous blood flow is through the central retinal vein directly to the cavernous sinus. Chronic obstruction of the central retinal vein presumably results in dilation of a previously existing system that shunts blood to the choroid, allowing it to leave the eye via the vortex veins. These veins drain directly into the superior and inferior ophthalmic veins that anastomose with the facial and angular veins and with the pterygoid venous plexus. Thus, an outlet is provided for retinal venous blood other than via the central retinal vein to the cavernous sinus. This clinical picture has been described most frequently in patients with spheno-orbital meningiomas (1, 4, 36), but it may also occur in patients with optic nerve gliomas (7, 9), as well as in patients with other types of chronic optic nerve compression (19).

Ocular Motor Nerve Paresis

All three of the ocular motor nerves enter the orbit through the superior orbital fissure. Each of these nerves may be damaged by enlarging orbital

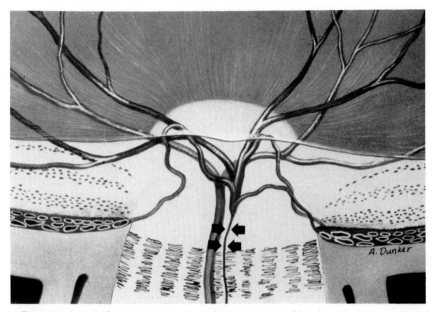

FIG. 23.5. Artist's drawing of optociliary shunt veins caused by chronic compression and occlusion of the central retinal vein (*arrows*). In this setting, venous blood is shunted from the retinal to the choroidal venous circulation.

tumors, resulting in varying degrees of diplopia. Patients may complain of double vision that is horizontal, vertical, or both. Such patients usually have some degree of proptosis, but this is by no means always the case. Tumors that are located at the orbital apex may involve the ocular motor nerves early, before they are large enough to produce proptosis. Thus, such patients may present with a partial oculomotor nerve, abducens nerve or, rarely, a trochlear nerve paresis. The ophthalmoparesis that is produced by orbital tumors is indistinguishable from that produced by intracranial lesions. The appropriate diagnosis can only be made clinically by the presence of other signs of orbital disease (20). Often, it is made only when computed tomography (CT) or magnetic resonance imaging (MRI) are performed (Fig. 23.6). The most common orbital tumor that produces diplopia is metastatic carcinoma or lymphoma, although optic nerve gliomas, neurinomas, hemangiomas, and lymphangiomas can also produce it.

It is important to realize that since some orbital tumors may infiltrate or compress one or more of the extraocular muscles, preventing them from functioning properly, the diplopia produced by orbital tumors may be neurogenic or myogenic and is occasionally a combination of both. In such cases, several tests may be used to determine whether a mechanical

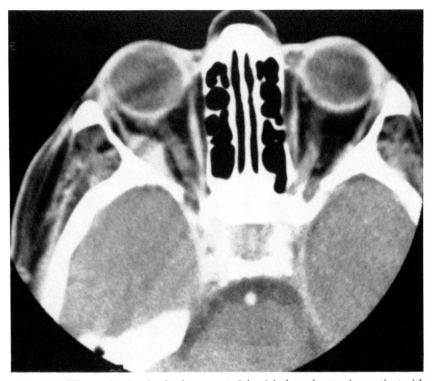

FIG. 23.6. CT scan showing focal enlargement of the right lateral rectus in a patient with diplopia and right abduction weakness. The patient was found to have metastatic tumor within the muscle. (Courtesy of Dr. C. Citrin.)

restriction of ocular motion is present. Mechanical limitation can be inferred if intraocular pressure increases substantially when the patient attempts to look in the direction of gaze limitation (24, 27, 37). The intraocular pressure measurements are most easily performed using a pneumatic tonometer (27), although any instrument may be used.

Mechanical limitation of motion can also be detected with forced duction (or traction) testing. In such tests, an attempt is made to move the eye forcibly in the direction(s) of gaze limitation (Fig. 23.7). As described by Jaensch (11), this test is performed as follows. The cornea is anesthetized using several drops of a topical anesthetic such as pro-paracaine or tetracaine hydrochloride. The conjunctiva is further anes-thetized by holding a cotton swab or cotton-tipped applicator soaked with 5–10% cocaine against it for about 30 seconds. The conjunctiva is then grasped with a fine-toothed forceps near the limbus on the side opposite the direction in which the eye is to be moved. The patient is

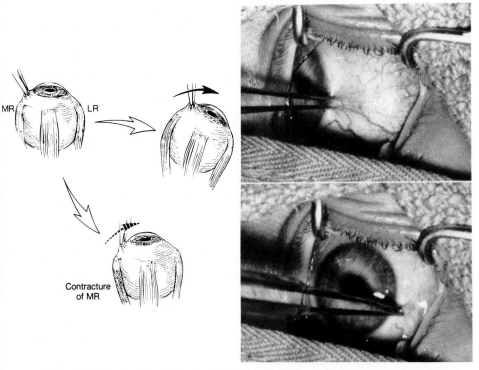

FIG. 23.7. The forced duction test. (*Left*) Artist's drawing showing possible results. (*Right*) The forced duction test performed in a patient with limitation of adduction. Note that the eye can easily be moved completely to the nose. Thus, there is no mechanical limitation of adduction. *LR*, lateral rectus muscle; *MR*, medial rectus muscle.

instructed to try to look in the direction of limitation, and an attempt is made to move the eye in that direction (*i.e.*, opposite that in which mechanical restriction is suspected). If no resistance is encountered, the motility defect is not restrictive; however, if resistance is encountered, then mechanical restriction does exist. In some patients, particularly those who are cooperative and have substantial limitation of movement, the forced duction test can be performed simply by asking the patient to look in the direction of limitation and then attempting to move the eye by placing a cotton-tipped applicator stick against the eye on the opposite side just posterior to the limbus (29).

Pain

As a general rule, neoplasms that involve the orbit are not painful; however, when pain is present, the tumors are likely to be malignant (5, 15, 17, 30). Tumors that spread to the orbit from the paranasal sinuses are usually associated with late pain. In some cases, however, pain may be the earliest sign of a tumor involving the orbital apex and cavernous sinus. The pain is severe, continuous, and associated with facial dysesthesia. It has been described as chronic, burning, and intermittently stabbing, and it involves one or more divisions of the trigeminal nerve. When this type of pain is present, it is evidence of intraneural infiltration by neoplastic cells, usually from basal cell, squamous cell, or nasopharyngeal carcinoma (2, 14, 23, 30). When the pain is combined with involvement of one or more ocular motor nerves, one can confidently predict neural infiltration within the cavernous sinus (2, 22, 23, 30, 32, 33).

Pupillary Abnormalities

Since both parasympathetic and sympathetic nerve pathways pass through the superior orbital fissure to reach the eye, it is theoretically possible that patients with an orbital tumor could develop either a Horner's syndrome from damage to the oculosympathetic pathway that supplies the iris dilator muscle or a tonic pupil from damage to the ciliary ganglion or short ciliary nerves that supply the iris sphincter muscle. In fact, such abnormalities rarely occur in isolation, probably because tumors that produce them are usually so extensive that they produce oculomotor nerve palsy with pupillary involvement as well. Thus, if there is separate damage to either the sympathetic or parasympathetic fibers, it is usually masked by the oculomotor nerve palsy.

SPECIFIC ORBITAL TUMORS

Because of the many technical advances in orbital surgery, most orbital tumors, even those located in the superior orbit, are outside the province of the neurosurgeon. Such lesions can be more easily and safely managed by the ophthalmic surgeon using any one of a number of approaches, particularly the lateral orbitotomy (21). Nevertheless, there are several tumors that remain of concern to the neurosurgeon.

Neurinoma

Neurinomas may arise from branches of the ocular motor or trigeminal nerves. They usually arise intracranially, often within the cavernous sinus. Thus, when they involve the orbit it is usually by extension through the superior orbital fissure. In such cases, a craniotomy or a combined orbitotomy-craniotomy approach is used.

Optic Nerve Glioma

Optic nerve gliomas account for about 3% of all orbital tumors (25). Seventy-five percent of cases of optic nerve glioma present in the first incidence is from 2 to 6 years of age. Females appear to be affected slightly more often than males. It seems clear that there is a relationship between optic nerve (and chiasmal) gliomas and neurofibromatosis. Among reports of optic nerve glioma, the incidence of neurofibromatosis varies from 12 to 38% (16). The clinical presentation of optic nerve gliomas falls into two patterns, depending on whether the tumor is largely orbital or intracranial. While patients with optic nerve gliomas that are primarily intracranial usually present with monocular loss of vision associated with a normal or pale optic disc, patients with intraorbital optic nerve gliomas usually present with strabismus, proptosis, and optic disc swelling. Pain is unusual. Visual field defects are variable and range from central scotomas to peripheral constriction. With the increasing use of screening CT scanning and MRI in patients with neurofibromatosis, more and more patients are being identified with radiologic evidence of optic nerve glioma but without any significant visual complaints.

The clinical diagnosis of optic nerve glioma can be confirmed using either CT scanning or MRI. Within the orbit, the tumor is seen as a fusiform enlargement of the optic nerve that is often, but not invariably, associated with enlargement of the optic canal (Fig. 23.8) (13). In view of the excellent imaging techniques currently available, biopsy of such lesions simply to establish the diagnosis is unnecessary.

The management of optic nerve gliomas remains one of the most controversial topics involving ophthalmologists, neurologists, and neurosurgeons. It has been the practice of many physicians to recommend an attempt at complete removal of the tumor as soon as it is diagnosed in an effort to prevent its spread to adjacent structures such as the optic chiasm, opposite optic nerve, and the hypothalamus. In recent years, however, it has been suggested that these tumors have a self-limited growth pattern and behave more like benign hamartomas than true neoplasms (8). If this was the case, there would certainly be no need to excise them immediately, particularly if there were still vision remaining in the involved eye. It has been our experience that, indeed, many of these lesions show no clinical or radiologic evidence of growth over many years; however, some tumors clearly possess the ability to expand and spread to adjacent structures (18). For this reason, we recommend that once a diagnosis of optic nerve glioma is made with relative certainty, the patient be followed closely with respect to both clinical and radiologic parameters. If and when useful vision is lost or there is evidence of tumor growth, we would recommend surgical excision via either a transcranial route or a combined transcranial-orbital procedure (12).

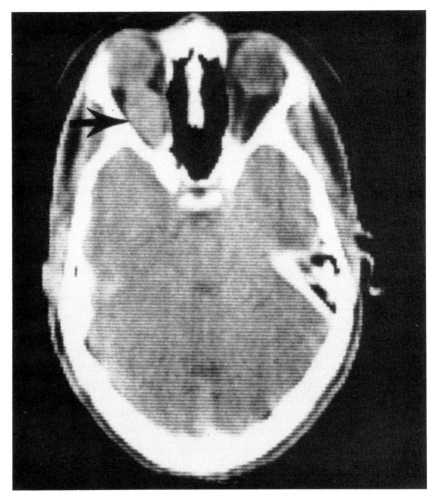

FIG. 23.8. CT scan showing fusiform enlargement of the right optic nerve in a young boy with moderately reduced visual acuity. At surgery, the patient was found to have an optic nerve glioma that extended through the optic canal.

While most optic nerve gliomas are benign, malignant optic nerve gliomas do exist (10). They usually occur in middle-aged males, producing progressive visual loss often associated with pain. These tumors are highly invasive and extend along the subpial portion of the nerve, compromising its blood supply. The tumor may progress toward the globe, where it produces swelling of the optic disc and subsequent occlusion of the central retinal vein and artery. At the same time, the tumor extends to involve the chiasm, the opposite optic nerve, and the hypothalamus. The course is rapid. Most patients are completely blind within 2–4 months, and all die within 6–9 months. There is presently no surgical or radiotherapeutic treatment for this lesion.

Meningiomas

Meningiomas of the orbit may be primary, originating from the sheath of the intraorbital or intracanalicular optic nerve, or secondary, originating along the sphenoid wing or in the basofrontal region and subsequently invading the orbit through bone or foramina (1). Secondary meningiomas are much more common than primary intraorbital meningiomas and are usually managed by a combined craniotomy-orbitotomy approach.

In any large series, intraorbital optic nerve sheath meningiomas comprise about 5–7% of primary orbital tumors (26). They occur more often in females than males and usually present in the fourth and fifth decades of life. Patients with optic nerve sheath meningiomas that originate in the orbit usually complain initially of a vague feeling that their vision is abnormal. When such patients are evaluated, they may be found to have normal visual acuity associated with optic disc swelling (28, 34). While some of these patients can be shown to have color vision defects and/or an afferent pupillary defect, some have virtually no clinical visual abnormalities at all. In such patients, the diagnosis is made only after a CT scan or MRI is obtained. Using such techniques, the orbital optic nerve can be seen to be diffusely thickened (Fig. 23.9) (13). When coronal views of the nerve are obtained, the nerve can often be seen to be surrounded by the tumor.

Because these tumors are virtually always located within the subdural space of the optic nerve (between the dura and the pia-arachnoid) and are wrapped completely around the optic nerve at the time of diagnosis, they cannot be removed without sacrificing vision (Figs. 23.10 and 23.11). Thus, as with optic nerve gliomas, the optimum management of patients with optic nerve sheath meningiomas has not been determined. If there is no evidence of intracranial extension, the patient can be followed until he or she loses vision, at which time the nerve and tumor can be removed together. Some physicians, however, suggest immediate surgery in the hope that intracranial extension can be prevented. We have decompressed the optic canal and opened the intracanalicular dural sheath in several patients with optic nerve sheath meningiomas. In all patients, the progression of visual loss has been stopped over a period of follow-up ranging from 3 to 7 years. The effect of this procedure on subsequent intracranial spread of tumor, however, is not clear. The value of radiotherapy in optic nerve sheath meningiomas has not been determined.

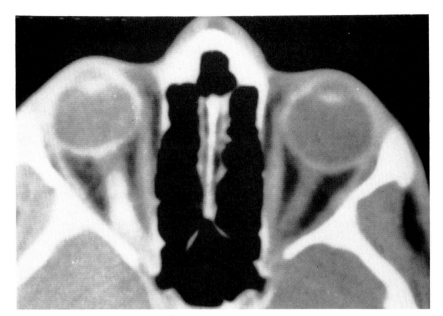

FIG. 23.9. CT scan showing a diffusely enlarged intraorbital optic nerve with calcification in its posterior portion. Although the patient had 20/25 vision in the eye, he demanded removal of the nerve, which was found to be surrounded by an optic nerve sheath meningioma.

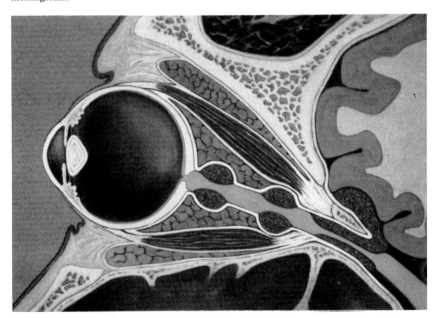

FIG. 23.10. Artist's drawing depicting sites of origin of optic nerve sheath meningiomas. Note that meningiomas which involve the intraorbital portion of the optic nerve are located between the optic nerve dural sheath and the pia-arachnoid. They surround the nerve and cannot be removed without sacrificing all vision. (Courtesy of Dr. M. Alper.)

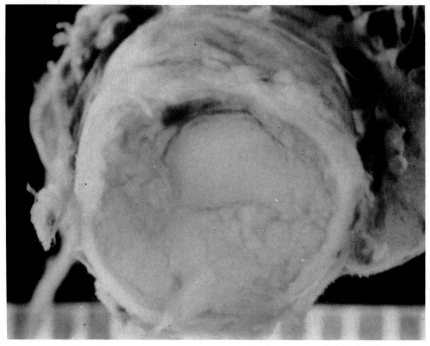

FIG. 23.11. Cross-section of optic nerve sheath meningioma involving the intraorbital portion of the optic nerve. Note that the meningioma completely surrounds the nerve and is located between the dural sheath and the pia-arachnoid of the nerve.

REFERENCES

1. Alper, M. G. Management of primary optic nerve meningiomas. J. Clin. Neuro-ophthalmol., *1:* 101–117, 1981.
2. Ballantyne, A. J., McCarten, A. B., and Ibanez, M. L. The extension of cancer of the head and neck through peripheral nerves. Am. J. Surg., *106:* 651–667, 1963.
3. Brown, G. C., and Shields, J. A. Amaurosis fugax secondary to presumed cavernous hemangioma of the orbit. Ann. Ophthalmol., *13:* 1205–1209, 1981.
4. Frisen, L., Hoyt, W. F., and Tengroth, B. M. Optociliary veins, disc pallor and visual loss. Acta Ophthalmol., *51:* 241–249, 1973.
5. Grinberg, M. A., and Levy, N. S. Malignant neurilemoma of the supraorbital nerve. Am. J. Ophthalmol., *78:* 489–492, 1974.
6. Harris, G. J. Bilateral blindness due to orbital lymphoma. Ann. Ophthalmol., *13:* 427–430, 1981.
7. Henkind, P., and Benjamin, J. V. Vascular anomalies and neoplasms of the optic nerve head. Trans. Ophthalmol. Soc. U.K., *96:* 418–423, 1976.
8. Hoyt, W. F., and Baghdassarian, S. A. Optic glioma of childhood: Natural history and rationale for conservative management. Br. J. Ophthalmol., *53:* 793–798, 1969.
9. Hoyt, W. F., and Beeston, D. *The Ocular Fundus in Neurologic Disease.* C.V. Mosby, St. Louis, 1966.
10. Hoyt, W. F., Meshel, L. G., Lessell, S., Schatz, N. J., and Suckling, R. Malignant optic gliomas of adulthood. Brain, *96:* 121–132, 1973.

11. Jaensch, P. A. Paresen der schragen heber. Albrecht von Graefes Arch. Klin. Ophthalmol., *121:* 113–125, 1929.
12. Jain, N. S. Two-stage intracranial and orbital operation for glioma of the optic nerve. Br. J. Ophthalmol., *45:* 54–58, 1961.
13. Jakobiec, F. A., Depot, M. J., Kennerdell, J. S., Shults, W. T., Anderson, R. L., Alper, M. E., Citrin, C. M., Housepian, E. M., and Trokel, S. L. Combined clinical and computed tomographic diagnosis of orbital glioma and meningioma. Ophthalmology, *91:* 137–155, 1984.
14. Jefferson, G. Concerning injuries, aneurysms and tumors involving the cavernous sinus. Trans. Ophthalmol. Soc. U.K., *73:* 117–152, 1953.
15. Jones, I. S., Jakobiec, F. A., and Nolan, B. Patient examination and introduction to orbital disease. In: *Diseases of the Orbit*, edited by I. S. Jones and F. A. Jakobiec, p. 29. Harper & Row, Hagerstown, Md., 1979.
16. Manschot, W. A. Primary tumors of the optic nerve in von Recklinghausen's disease. Am. J. Ophthalmol., *37:* 15–36, 1954.
17. McDonald, W. I. Pain around the eye: Inflammatory and neoplastic causes. Trans. Ophthalmol. Soc. U.K., *100:* 260–262, 1980.
18. McDonnell, P., and Miller, N. R. Chiasmatic extension of optic nerve glioma. Arch. Ophthalmol., *101:* 1412–1415, 1983.
19. Miller, N. R. *Walsh and Hoyt's Clinical Neuro-Ophthalmology*, Ed. 4, Vol. 1, pp. 249–253. Williams & Wilkins, Baltimore, 1982.
20. Miller, N. R. *Walsh and Hoyt's Clinical Neuro-Ophthalmology*, Ed. 4, Vol. 2, pp. 652–784. Williams & Wilkins, Baltimore, 1985.
21. Miller, N. R., and Iliff, W. J. Surgery of the orbit. In: *Ophthalmic Surgery*, Ed. 4, edited by T. A. Rice, and R. G. Michels, and W. J. Stark, pp. 383–398. C.V. Mosby, St. Louis, 1984.
22. Mohs, F. E., and Lathrop, T. G. Modes of spread of cancer of the skin. Arch. Dermatol., *66:* 427–439, 1952.
23. Moore, C. E., Hoyt, W. F., and North, J. B. Painful ophthalmoplegia following treated squamous cell carcinoma of the forehead: Orbital apex involvement from centripetal spread via the supraorbital nerve. Med. J. Aust., *1:* 657–659, 1976.
24. Reader, A. L., III. Normal variations of intraocular pressure on vertical gaze. Ophthalmology, *89:* 1084–1087, 1982.
25. Reese, A. B. *Tumors of the Eye.* Hoeber, New York, 1963.
26. Reese, A. B. Expanding lesions of the orbit. Trans. Ophthalmol. Soc. U.K., *91:* 85–104, 1971.
27. Saunders, R. A., Helveston, E. M., and Ellis, F. D. Differential intraocular pressure in strabismus diagnosis. Ophthalmology, *87:* 59–70, 1981.
28. Sibony, P. A., Krauss, H. R., Kennerdell, J. S., Maroon, J. C., and Slamovits, T. L. Optic nerve sheath meningiomas: Clinical manifestations. Ophthalmology (Suppl.): 66, 1983.
29. Smith, J. L. The office forced duction test. Ophthalmic Surg., *6:* 62–63, 1975.
30. Trobe, J. D., Hood, C. I., Parsons, J. T., and Quisling, R. G. Intracranial spread of squamous carcinoma along the trigeminal nerve. Arch. Ophthalmol., *100:* 608–611, 1982.
31. Unsold, R., and Hoyt, W. F. Blickinduzierte monokulare Obskurationen bei orbitalem Haemangiom. Klin. Monatsbl. Augenheilkd., *174:* 715–721, 1979.
32. Unsold, R., Safran, A. B., Safran, E., and Hoyt, W. F. Metastatic infiltration of nerves in the cavernous sinus. Arch. Neurol., *37:* 59–61, 1980.

33. Willis, R. A. *The Spread of Tumors in the Human Body,* pp. 124–127. C.V. Mosby, St. Louis, 1952.
34. Wright, J. E., Call, N. B., and Liaricos, S. Primary optic nerve meningioma. Br. J. Ophthalmol., *64:* 553–558, 1980.
35. Wright, J. E., McDonald, W. I., and Call, N. B. Management of optic nerve gliomas. Br. J. Ophthalmol., *64:* 545–552, 1980.
36. Zakka, K. A., Summerer, R. W., Yee, R. D., Foos, R. Y., and Kim, J. Opticociliary veins in a primary optic nerve sheath meningioma. Am. J. Ophthalmol., *87:* 91–95, 1979.
37. Zappia, R. J., Winkelman, J. Z., and Gay, A. J. Intraocular pressure changes in normal subjects and the adhesive muscle syndrome. Am. J. Ophthalmol., *71:* 880–883, 1971.

24

Radiologic Evaluation of Orbital Tumors

GLENN FORBES, M.D.

Radiologic examination is a key step in the evaluation of orbital tumors. It not only may lead to the definitive diagnosis when classic findings are demonstrated but also may result in exclusion of many other conditions that might be considered in the clinical examination. With known tumors, it defines the anatomic extent of the mass and the integrity of the adjacent structures. The specific information gained from the different examinations varies, with a relatively low yield from the plain skull films to a high yield from late-generation, high-resolution computed tomographic (CT scan).

Before the advent of computer-processed examinations, radiologic evaluation of the orbit depended on indirect findings from plain films, plain film tomography and, in some cases, pneumoencephalography and angiography. During the past decade, CT scanning has been established as the key imaging method in orbital diagnosis (16). The accessibility and ease of examination, combined with the high level of information returned, quickly earned favor for the new technique. Advances in displaying images in multiple projections and increased resolution with late-generation scanners further refined the examination and established CT both as a preferred screening diagnostic tool and as the definitive imaging study for orbital lesions. With CT, orbital masses can be excluded confidently. The diagnosis and detailed anatomic extent of other lesions, including tumor, inflammatory and endocrine changes, and injuries due to trauma, can usually be obtained. Because CT is dominant in the imaging of orbital tumors, the main emphasis of this chapter will be on this method. Near the end of the chapter, the place of plain films, the future of magnetic resonance (MRI) scanning, and the more limited contribution of arterial and venous angiography will be discussed.

The radiographic examination is customarily used to evaluate orbital pain, proptosis, diplopia, or change in visual acuity (5). Although any of these symptoms can be associated with tumor, more commonly an inflammatory, infectious, or underlying endocrine problem is expected to be a cause of the clinical symptoms (13). In this regard, the imaging study, particularly CT, may also be extremely useful in determining the kind of problem, in excluding tumor, and in evaluating potential sinus or intracranial extension of the orbital lesion. In trauma, the extent of possible hemorrhage, fractures, and sinus and intracranial involvement can be evaluated. Plain radiographs are helpful in assessing most injuries due to trauma but are generally disappointing for the study of masses or inflammatory conditions of the orbit. Special plain radiographs, such as views of the optic canal and plain film tomography, may demonstrate subtle bony changes or secondary signs of orbital, particularly optic canal, masses. Seldom, if ever, would such primary pathologic abnormalities not be shown to be of equal or better advantage with CT of good quality. Low cost, accessibility, and determination of the extent of fractures in cases of trauma help to maintain the usefulness of plain radiography in orbital examination.

Carotid arteriography is occasionally used to evaluate the periorbital extent of known extra-axial lesions that may involve the sinuses or parasellar region. It is particularly used with tumors, such as sphenoid meningiomas, that are characteristically quite vascular and frequently invade the orbit. Arteriography is definitive for the diagnostic evaluation of dural arteriovenous fistulas that may arise in or extend into the orbit and that must be differentiated from true neoplasms. The use of arteriography for the common orbital masses is otherwise limited. Orbital venography has largely been replaced by CT in most situations, although it is still occasionally used in inflammatory conditions and venous abnormalities, such as angiomas and varices. Ultrasonography is also used for evaluation of some orbital masses and lesions, particularly in the region of the globe and anterior compartments.

COMPUTED TOMOGRAPHY

Orbital CT has been an evolutionary process, since technical advances have continually improved the examination. The first CT orbital images in the mid-1970s were relatively crude by today's standards; nevertheless, their introduction brought about a major change in the radiologic evaluation of the orbit because of the many limitations of standard roentgenography in orbital disease (2, 4, 18, 30, 34, 40, 41, 56). Orbital masses that previously had been undetectable on plain films and had required venography or arteriography for diagnosis were accessible with noninvasive CT. As CT images improved, findings relating to more specific orbital disease were reported (9, 19, 20, 25, 39, 54, 55). Additional information, including the anatomic location and compartment of orbital masses, involvement of various intraorbital structures, and extension of pathologic change into periorbital regions, such as sinuses and the intracranial compartment, could be routinely obtained. The widespread accessibility of CT in most medium and large hospitals and refinements in image display, including multiplane reformatted imaging and high-resolution, thin-section scanning, further established CT as the mainstay of orbital imaging for tumors.

TECHNIQUE OF COMPUTED TOMOGRAPHY SCANNING

The standard head CT examination must be modified in several ways for proper imaging of the orbit (14). The modifications include the use of thinner and occasionally overlapping slices, a different reference angle in the axial plane, and the addition of coronal and, occasionally, sagittal or reformatted projections. The orbit may be studied separately or as an additional part of a CT examination of the head.

The CT study of the orbit with a late-generation scanner consists of thin coronal and axial cuts. The axial slices are within 1–5 mm at 0° to −10° from the orbitomeatal base line. The thicker slices offer good image contrast and field size and acceptable spatial resolution. The thinner slices, from 1 to 1.5 mm, offer less volume averaging, better spatial resolution, and superior reformatted displays but lose some image contrast, take longer, and place greater heat-loading demands on the x-ray tube. Coronal views are an integral part of the orbital evaluation and may be either direct coronal scans combining gantry tilt with head extension or reformatted coronal views from thin axial scans.

The CT orbital study can be obtained in one of two ways. In the first method, direct axial scans of about 5 mm are immediately followed by direct coronal scans of 5 mm with the patient's head extended 65° to avoid molar artifacts. From 15 to 20 slices are made during a 25- to 30-minute examination. The second method involves scanning of the orbit in the axial plane only; about 25 contiguous 1- or 1.5-mm slices are made with reformatting techniques to obtain coronal, sagittal, and oblique imaging displays. Slices 5 mm thick are made at 400 mA and 3 milliseconds (576 views); 1- or 1.5-mm slices are made at 400–600 mA, and for a 25-slice examination, approximately 1 minute is required for each slice for scanning, reconstruction, and tube cooling.

The direct 5-mm axial and direct coronal study provides new imaging data in the coronal plane and is slightly faster to perform. The thin (1–1.5 mm) axial study achieves higher limits of anatomic definition with less volume-averaging of small structures and can be used in patients who are uncomfortable with head extension. This examination, however, requires good patient cooperation for steady positioning of the head and places a higher heat-loading demand on the x-ray tube because of the high milliampere exposures. We use both techniques interchangeably, preferring the thin-slice scanning and reformatting, particularly for optic nerve lesions and the question of small masses.

Multiplane reformatted imaging may be used to best advantage with very thin (1–1.5 mm) section scanning; greater appreciation of the relative anatomy of orbital lesions can be achieved, and the relationship of lesions to other intraorbital structures becomes more evident. The reformatted images are generally displayed in the coronal and off-axis sagittal planes along the course of the optic nerve and require a complete lack of movement by the patient during the examination and some extra time by the radiologist or technician afterward for the reconstruction of good images. Although morphologic features may be clarified in the viewing of the different displays, no real diagnostic scanning data are obtained.

Intravenously administered contrast material is widely used with orbital CT and is particularly useful in the evaluation of tumors. Many tumors show enhancement in contrast to the surrounding tissues, and some lesions, notably meningiomas, hemangiomas, and arteriovenous malformations, can be specifically characterized by their marked degree of contrast enhancement. Between 20 and 42 gm of iodine are customarily injected or infused, depending on the patient's age and renal status; we prefer to infuse 42 gm over 2–3 minutes in patients under age 65 with no history of kidney disease.

The lens of the eye is one of the parts of the body that is sensitive to radiation. A risk of cataract formation is thought to be present in direct exposures of 100 R or more. However, the dose for the orbital CT examination—from 3.5 to 5 R for either a combined axial and coronal study or a thin axial slice study—is considered well within acceptable limits (15). This amount is slightly higher than that for plain radiography of the skull and orbit but is less than that received during multiple-exposure plain-film tomography or angiography, which may produce eye entrance doses of 10 R or more.

ANATOMIC CONSIDERATIONS FOR RADIOLOGIC EXAMINATION

For purposes of CT imaging, the orbit may be considered to be made up of several anatomic compartments, and lesions are often first characterized by their respective locations. Because the globe is more accessible by clinical examination and ultrasound, more emphasis is placed on the retrobulbar area with the CT study. The ocular muscles attach to the globe at its periphery and extend posteriorly to the apex of the orbit. In a simplified fashion, they are often thought of as passing in superior, inferior, medial, and lateral rectus groups in terms of imaging. The reason is that the levator palpebrae averages in with the superior rectus in both

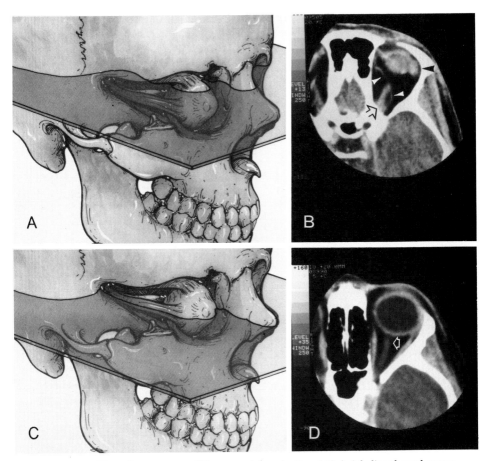

FIG. 24.1. Normal anatomy on CT scan, axial projection. (*A*) Axial slice through upper portion of orbit. (*B*) Axial CT slice corresponding to that in *A* shows lacrimal gland (*black arrowhead*), superior ophthalmic vein (*white arrowheads*), and part of superior rectus and levator group (*open black arrow*). (*C*) Axial slice through middle of orbit. (*D*) Axial CT slice corresponding to that in *C* shows optic nerve (*arrow*). (*E*) Axial slice through lower portion of orbit. (*F*) Axial CT slice corresponding to that in *E* shows part of inferior rectus muscle group (*arrow*). (Reproduced with permission from: G. Forbes (14).)

transverse and coronal scans, and the oblique muscles cut across the standard imaging planes and, unlike the other rectus groups, are not customarily demonstrated in their entirety in any one scan. A cone is thus formed, with the globe as a base and the orbital apex as a point; this formation is appropriately referred to as the "muscle cone." The

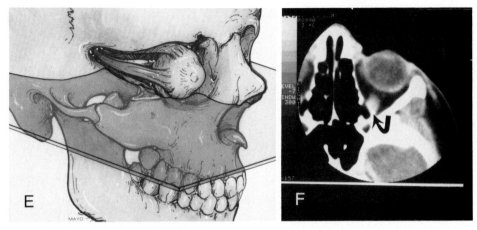

FIG. 24.1*E* and *F*

muscles are generally isodense in CT imaging, although they show slight contrast enhancement on intravenous contrast studies because of their vascularity (Figs. 24.1 and 24.2).

Within the cone, the optic nerve runs from the apex toward the posterior center of the globe and forms a parallel axis within the center of the muscle cone. The nerve has a slightly undulating course, and very thin CT slices can be sectioned obliquely at different levels; the result is an alternating fat-thin appearance, which should be recognized as a normal occurrence of partial volume averaging (38, 53). This recognition is of particular importance in making subtle judgments of optic nerve enlargement from potential optic nerve gliomas. The optic nerve is encircled by the ophthalmic artery, which passes with the nerve through the optic canal until the artery bifurcates into ethmoidal and lacrimal branches just behind the globe (Fig. 24.3).

The superior ophthalmic vein is another prominent vessel that is often visualized in contrast studies; it courses laterally along the upper margin of the cone before dividing into medial and lateral tributaries above and behind the globe. Considerable fat fills the remaining spaces in the orbit, both within and outside the muscle cone, and it is this fat that in CT imaging gives the excellent contrast in the soft tissue structures of the muscles, nerves, and vessels.

Although all of the components of the muscle cone converge toward a point at the apex, the different structures pass through various foramina to leave the orbit. The optic nerve and ophthalmic artery pass through the optic canal, which is the uppermost orbital foramen, and the ocular

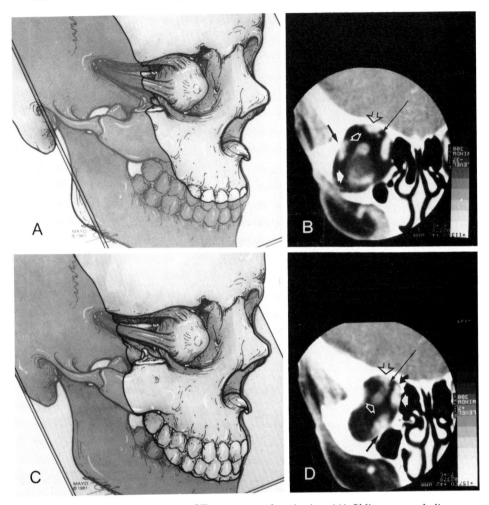

FIG. 24.2. Normal anatomy on CT scan, coronal projection. (*A*) Oblique coronal slice
tilted to miss most dental fillings to avoid artifacts. (*B*) Coronal CT slice corresponding to
that in *A* shows superior rectus and levator group (*open black arrow*), superior ophthalmic
vein (*long, thin black arrow*), lateral rectus (*black arrow*), optic nerve (*open white arrow*),
and part of back of globe (*white arrow*). (*C*) Oblique coronal slice through posterior portion
of orbit. (Figures 24.2*A–C* reproduced with permission from: G. Forbes (14).) (*D*) Coronal
CT slice corresponding to that in *C* shows superior rectus and levator group (*open black
arrow*), superior ophthalmic vein (*long, thin black arrow*), superior oblique muscle (*curved
black arrow*), inferior rectus group (*black arrow*), medial rectus group (*white arrow*), and
optic nerve (*open white arrow*).

motor nerves (cranial nerves III, IV, and VI), the ophthalmic division of
cranial nerve V, and the superior ophthalmic vein pass through the
superior orbital fissure. Because these two adjacent foramina are separated by only a thin strut of bone almost in the axial plane, they may be

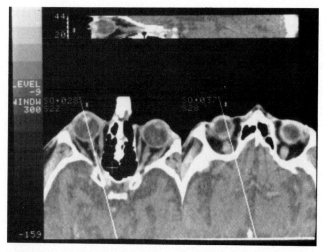

FIG. 24.3. Undulating optic nerve anatomy. Optic nerve undulates in and out of transverse scanning plane on CT and thus may normally appear slightly "thicker" or "thinner" in different segments. This concept is important to recognize when one considers possible optic nerve enlargement due to glioma.

difficult to differentiate on the axial projection, although the superior orbital fissure is seen to extend lateral to the optic canal on axial projections. The orbit is separated from the ethmoid sinus by the medial orbital wall, from the maxillary sinus below by the orbital floor, and from the frontal sinus and anterior fossa above by the orbital roof.

All of these orbital structures are measured in millimeters; therefore, this is one of the main areas in which the effect of volume-averaging on image projections must always be kept in mind. Volume-averaging has already been referred to in the imaging of the optic nerve from thin axial cuts, but similar volume-averaging of superior and inferior muscle groups, along with the optic nerve on high or low axial cuts, may also affect the appearance on the scan of the size of the nerve. Volume-averaging of the orbital roof or floor with orbital structures makes the assessment of a lesion in the most superior and inferior regions extremely difficult, and for this reason, the coronal views are considered very helpful, and even mandatory by some, in completing a thorough CT study of the orbit.

RADIOGRAPHIC PATHOLOGY

A properly designed CT examination may be used as both a screening and a definitive examination for masses in the orbit. More than 95% of surgically proved orbital tumors are detected with the use of such techniques (15, 16). Considerable information about the size, quadrant location, relation to muscle cone and other structures and, frequently, the

TABLE 24.1

Features of Common Orbital Tumors

Lesion	Clinical Features	Radiographic Computed Tomography
Optic nerve tumor	Vision impaired early (scotoma or blindness) before prominent proptosis or diplopia Association with neurofibromatosis Gliomas in younger age group Meningiomas in older age group	Thickened fusiform or lobulated nerve Contrast enhancement tracking along course of nerve in meningiomas May appear as mass in orbital apex
Hemangioma	Most frequent benign tumor Common pediatric tumor Marked proptosis Visual acuity often unimpaired Occasional stress proptosis	Large, lobulated, high-density mass Marked contrast enhancement Phleboliths possible Potential intracranial extension Valsalva or jugular compression may accentuate or demonstrate lesion
Lacrimal gland tumor	Easily palpated Specific diagnosis often clinically suspected Frequently dermoid cysts	Superior temporal quadrant Low density due to dermoid fat May have calcific deposits
Neurofibroma	Benign; often slow progression Frequent recurrence Prominent proptosis and diplopia with unimpaired vision frequent	Well-demarcated mass May occur anywhere in orbit Bone expansion of orbit wall common Calcified capsule may be present
Lymphoma	Older age group Aggressive destructive process Pain and periorbital edema may be present	Irregular, poorly defined soft tissue density Isodensity or high density May encase globe as infiltrative density May extend outside orbit Bone destruction more frequent
Metastases	Usually secondary to known tumor but occasionally presenting lesion Carcinoma from breast, kidney, lung, and colon most frequent	Bone destruction frequent Occasional calcification in mass

nature of the lesion are obtained. The purpose of CT is to detect the mass and to define these anatomic relationships (Table 24.1). The density and margins of the mass and the potential calcification, bone expansion, and intracranial extension are assessed. Most of the tumors demonstrated radiographically will be associated with unilateral proptosis and, often, with diplopia. Visual acuity in the affected eye may remain surprisingly intact, even with large lesions, except for optic nerve tumors, in which blindness or field defects precede other symptoms.

OPTIC NERVE TUMORS, INCLUDING OPTIC NERVE GLIOMAS, PRIMARY OPTIC SHEATH MENINGIOMAS, AND ORBITAL MENINGIOMAS

Before the advent of computer-processed examinations, radiologic evaluation of the optic nerve depended on indirect findings from plain films, optic foramen views, or tomograms and, in some cases, angiography. The optic nerve itself was not imaged unless pneumoencephalography was performed, and then only the intracranial part of the optic chiasm was demonstrated. By imaging the optic nerve directly, CT provided a new phase for tumor detection. CT is now commonly accepted as the definitive method for examination of the optic nerve (6, 42).

The two tumors of primary interest because of frequency and clinical significance are optic nerve gliomas and primary intraorbital optic nerve meningiomas (Table 24.2). These two lesions need to be assessed by definitive radiographic techniques because clinical findings of blindness, central scotomata, and field defects may be caused by other lesions, such as optic nerve atrophy, optic neuritis, and demyelinating plaques of multiple sclerosis that are not always easy to differentiate from the tumors. Optic nerve imaging of high quality should be used to definitively either diagnose or exclude the glioma or meningioma as the cause of the

TABLE 24.2
Radiographic Characteristics of the Two Major Intraorbital Optic Nerve Tumors

	Glioma	Meningioma
Plain films and optic canal views	Enlarged canal	Normal-sized canal
	Adjacent bone normal	Hyperostosis
Computed tomography		
Nerve enlargement	Fusiform, lobulated	Eccentric apical segment
Calcification	Uncommon	Common
Contrast enhancement	Occasional	Very frequent
Density	Isodense	High density, railroad tracking
Chiasm	Frequently enlarged	Usually unaffected

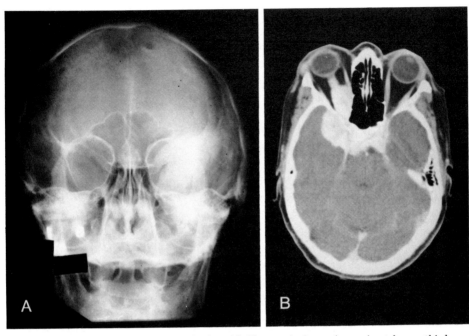

Fig. 24.4. Orbital involvement of sphenoid ridge meningioma. Approximately one-third of sphenoid ridge meningiomas involve the orbit. (A) Large tumors may produce the familiar dense, reactive sclerosis easily recognizable on plain skull films. (B) Thickened bone or tumor tissue, or both, may extend into orbit and cause proptosis and optic nerve compression.

clinical problem and to direct the further diagnostic workup or therapy accordingly. Optic chiasm gliomas and sphenoid ridge meningiomas frequently extend into the orbit through the optic canal, although their origin lies outside the orbit. They are easily recognized with standard head CT scanning because the main component of tumor lies outside the orbit (Fig. 24.4). The chiasm gliomas may be confined to the chiasm or may extend into one or both optic nerves (42). Fifteen percent of intracranial meningiomas occur along the greater sphenoid ridge, and one-third of these have tumor tissue or produce bony hyperostosis that extends into the orbit and causes vision problems and proptosis. These lesions are to be differentiated from true primary optic nerve sheath meningiomas, which constitute only 1–2% of all intracranial meningiomas (28, 31).

The *optic nerve gliomas* arise from glial cells, most commonly, astrocytes, and less commonly, oligodendrocytes. They may affect any part of the visual pathway from the nerve fiber layer of the retina through the optic nerve and chiasm. Most often, they become manifest in the first decade of life and have an increased incidence in patients with neurofibromatosis (8, 33). Histologically, most of these tumors are of low-grade malignancy (grades 1 or 2). The histologic picture may vary from a predominantly fibrillar pattern to one that is microcystic. Rosenthal fibers—eosinophilic bodies formed from the cytoplasm of degenerating cells—are a frequent finding. As the tumor grows, the meninges undergo reactive proliferation and thereby contribute to the increased size of the nerve. Gliomas occurring in adults have been reported to be more aggressive and of higher grade malignancy than those occurring in young patients (45).

Primary intraorbital meningiomas arise from arachnoid cells situated along the sheath; rarely, they arise from ectopic arachnoid cells within the muscle cone or the walls of the periorbita (28, 31, 49). Histologically, the cells of the orbital meningioma are usually of the meningotheliomatous type but occasionally are transitional. This tumor most often occurs in adult patients but can be seen in young patients with neurofibromatosis. There is an increased incidence in women (22, 48).

Other conditions that should be considered in the differential diagnosis of optic nerve tumors include optic neuritis, optic nerve meningoceles, optic nerve atrophy, and drusen (Table 24.3). Optic neuritis is often associated with demyelinating diseases, such as multiple sclerosis (26). Meningoceles may not cause significant field defects or blindness. Drusen are hyaline bodies of uncertain origin that often calcify, can often be

TABLE 24.3

Other Occasional Nontumorous Causes of Optic Nerve Enlargement

Condition	Comment	Reference No.
Optic neuritis	Idiopathic or with demyelinating disease	42
Graves' ophthalmopathy	Advanced disease with other changes already present in muscles and fat	50, 51, 59
Increased intracranial pressure	Bilateral	3, 7, 17, 23, 32
Inflammatory pseudotumor	Advanced disease with other orbital changes	13
Sarcoidosis	Disk edema in 5%; optic nerve involvement rare	44

seen funduscopically, and appear at the junction of the optic nerve and globe (52). Optic nerve enlargement may be seen in advanced cases of Graves' ophthalmopathy after widespread extraocular muscle enlargement has occurred (51). Similar enlargement, along with other findings of the inflammatory infiltrate, has been seen in cases of pseudotumor (50).

Plain skull films often show indirect findings of optic nerve tumors, and occasionally the appearance is specific for the tumor type. In a recent review, my colleagues and I noted abnormal findings in 33% of patients with proven optic nerve tumors, with the appearance indicative of the tumor in 23% (47). Gliomas most often produce erosion of the anterior clinoid processes or chiasmatic sulcus. Erosion was found in 10 of 22 (45%) optic and chiasm gliomas by Savoiardo et al. (42). Erosion is associated with the intracranial extension of these lesions. Conversely, intraorbital meningiomas may cause hyperostosis of the anterior clinoid process and optic canal that can be detected on the plain skull films. Tumor calcification is less commonly seen on the plain films unless the mass is neglected and becomes quite large. In most cases, the information gained from plain films is best obtained from the lateral view.

Optic foramen views are much more helpful in evaluating both intraorbital gliomas and intraorbital meningiomas. Widened foramina are seen with gliomas, and normal-sized foramina with hyperostosis of the surrounding bone are seen with optic nerve meningiomas. Such changes may be seen in up to three-fourths of the gliomas with optic canal views and in 90% with optic canal complex motion tomography (42). Caution should be exercised in interpreting widened foramina in patients with neurofibromatosis because of bony dysplastic changes. Strother et al. (46), using complex motion tomography, demonstrated the hyperostosis of the canalicular meningiomas in 10 of 10 surgically proved cases. Optic canal tomography has been used with considerably less frequency with the advent of detailed CT examinations of the optic nerve (Fig. 24.5).

Most patients do not undergo invasive arteriography unless the presence of unusually large or extensive tumors is suggested. In patients who do undergo arteriography, findings characteristic of the lesion are frequently demonstrated. In our series, 12 of 15 (80%) had abnormal signs of displacement of the ophthalmic or supraclinoid internal carotid arteries, arterial encasement, or tumor stain (Fig. 24.6) (47).

Byrd et al. (6) reported abnormal findings in three-fourths of angiograms performed in children with proven optic nerve gliomas. Angiography is also useful in the diagnosis of intraorbital and intracanalicular meningiomas.

Although early-generation CT proved valuable in evaluating most

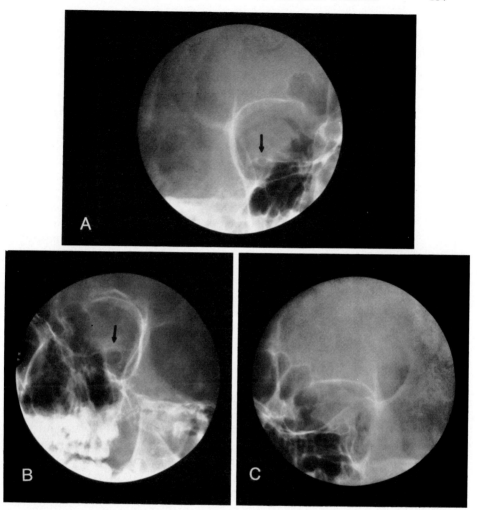

FIG. 24.5. Optic canal normal, enlarged, and sclerotic. Normal-sized optic canal (*A, arrow*) should be compared with enlarged canal (*B, arrow*). Uniform enlargement with normal surrounding bone is very characteristic of optic nerve glioma. Normal-sized canal with surrounding sclerosis (*C*) is similarly characteristic of meningioma involving optic canal.

orbital masses, definitive imaging diagnosis of the optic nerve tumors awaited the development of high-resolution, thin-slice scanning of the late-generation units. In almost all series reported, late-generation orbit scans have been positive in cases of tissue-proved optic nerve tumors. We believe that CT obtaining ultrathin, high-resolution slices of 1–1.5

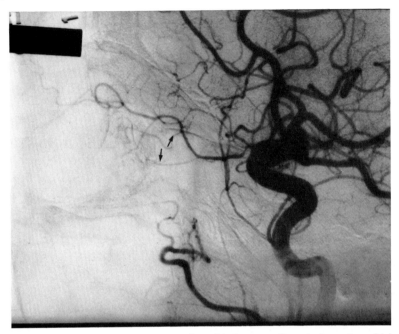

Fig. 24.6. Arteriographic displacement by orbital tumor. On arteriography, which is infrequently used for orbital mass diagnosis, some large tumors may produce splaying of ethmoidal and lacrimal branches of ophthalmic artery (*arrows*). Patient had large optic nerve glioma. Generally, cerebral arteriogram is relegated to evaluation of potential intracranial extension and orbital arteriovenous malformations.

mm is the current procedure of choice for suspected intraorbital meningiomas and both intraorbital and chiasm optic nerve gliomas. This examination can often be definitive for diagnosing an optic nerve tumor and excluding other types of intraorbital neoplasms not arising from the optic nerve. The anatomic position of the tumor and the extent of involvement among the globe, optic canal, and intracranial compartment can also be assessed. With ultrathin slices in the range of 1–1.5 mm and multiplanar reformatting, mistakes caused by partial volume effect in determining the caliber and the course of the nerve can be minimized.

The classic appearance of an optic nerve glioma is fusiform enlargement of the entire nerve from the canal to the back of the globe (Fig. 24.7). The enlargement may be irregular and even multilobulated, involving one or both nerves and the chiasm. The tumor usually is isodense, and some larger lesions show minimal degrees of contrast enhancement, varying between 20 and 25% in reported series (47). Calcification is not customarily seen, being reported in only 1 of 22 cases before surgery or

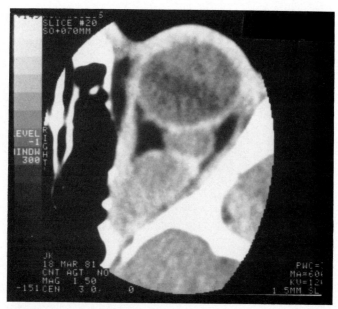

FIG. 24.7. Optic nerve glioma. Enlarged lobulated nerve is very apparent, extending from apex to back of globe. Note isodense appearance in contrast to higher-density sheath meningiomas in Figure 24.9. (Reproduced with permission from: G. Forbes (14).)

radiation in the series of Savoiardo *et al.* (42). Both contrast enhancement and calcification are much more frequently seen in optic nerve meningiomas, as described below, than in gliomas, and this difference is often a helpful distinguishing point. Expansion of the optic canal may be appreciated if wide window settings for bone detail are used. Metrizamide cisternography has been used to aid in evaluating the extent of tumor involvement of the chiasm (10).

Key points to notice during evaluation are the uniform density of the enlarged nerve, the relative lack of obvious proptosis, and the degree of invasion into the chiasm or extension into the opposite nerve. Because the tumor involves the nerve tissue itself, the density pattern produced is more uniform than that of the meningiomas, which first affect the sheath outlining the lower density nerve. The lack of proptosis is due to the customarily early onset of blindness with these tumors; most other tumors, because of their bulky orbital mass, are manifested by proptosis and diplopia before optic nerve compression occurs. The extent of the tumor should be correlated with clinical field testing, since gliomas, in particular, may be associated with a wide variety of degrees of invasion in the anterior optic pathways (Fig. 24.7).

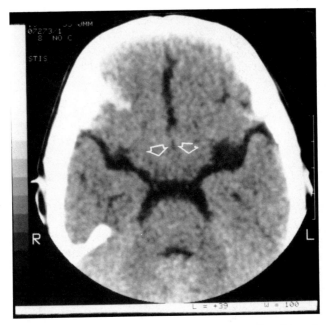

FIG. 24.8. Optic chiasm glioma. Anterior portion of suprasellar cistern is filled with oblong, enlarged chiasm (*arrows*) representing tumor.

When the glioma involves the chiasm, the size may increase enough to produce enlargement on CT. The tumor is seen as a sausage-shaped mass in the anterior suprasellar cistern or, if large enough, total filling of the suprasellar cistern by a soft tissue mass (Fig. 24.8). In advanced cases, marked contrast enhancement and, less frequently, calcification on CT may occur within the enlarged chiasm. Although coronal views may seem ideal for this problem, computer artifacts from teeth may obscure the area, and the transverse slices may best demonstrate the problem. If either the chiasmatic sulcus or the sella is enlarged on plain skull films in a patient with known or suspected optic nerve glioma, involvement of the chiasm may usually be presumed. In earlier times, fractional pneumoencephalography was used to evaluate the chiasm, but this has given way to reliance on high-resolution CT. If a subtle small change needs to be documented, CT may be enhanced with contrast medium introduced intrathecally by spinal puncture before the examination.

The classic appearance of an intraorbital optic nerve meningioma is segmental uniform thickening of the nerve, usually beginning in the apical region (Fig. 24.9). The tumor is frequently hyperdense and is further enhanced by intravenous injection of contrast medium. Tumor

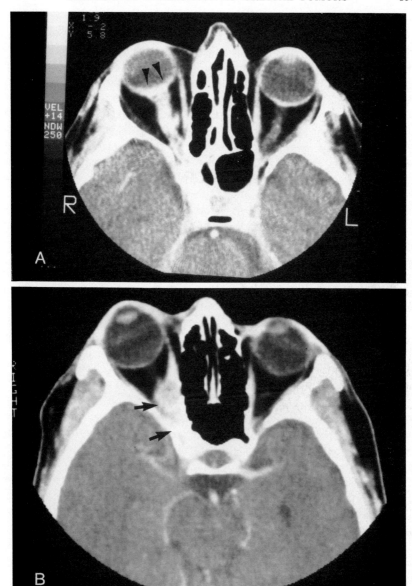

FIG. 24.9. Optic nerve sheath meningioma. (A) Sheath meningioma produces character-istic thickening and increased density along course of nerve. Note thickening along back of globe at point of nerve attachment; this indicates tumor infiltration into choroid (arrow-heads). (B) In another patient, meningioma is confined to optic canal and apex of orbit (arrows).

enhancement has been between 80 and 100% in reported cases (36, 47). Calcification is often seen and is much more common than in the gliomas. Very thin sectioning may produce a railroad track appearance that is due to the denser tumor margins surrounding the nerve; this appearance may be helpful in differentiating meningioma from glioma (36). Optic canal enlargement may be demonstrated occasionally, although a more frequent bone change is hyperostosis in the canal and around the anterior clinoid process and lesser sphenoid wing. This finding also helps differentiate meningioma from glioma. Hyperostosis is often described in CT studies and was detected in all cases in a series, described earlier, that was evaluated with complex motion tomography. Small needle biopsy of these meningiomas and gliomas has been performed with CT guidance (12).

Other nontumorous conditions should be considered when an enlarged optic nerve is radiographically assessed. Several infiltrative disorders can produce thickening of the perineural tissues, but they are seldom seen without corresponding changes to suggest the true diagnosis. One notable exception is the lobulated enlargement of one or both optic nerves due to pseudomeningocele. These are dilated extensions of the subarachnoid intracranial space along the course of the nerves into the orbit. Continuity of the intracranial subarachnoid space along the optic nerve sheath frequently occurs in normal persons without ophthalmologic symptoms, and this condition may predispose to the development of meningoceles in some patients (17, 32). Meningoceles may or may not be associated with field defects and are relatively rare (Fig. 24.10).

Other causes of enlargement, such as Graves' ophthalmopathy and pseudotumor, are associated with characteristic changes in the orbital muscles or fat (50, 51). The role of late-generation CT in differentiating the focal optic neuritis of demyelinating disease from more clearly defined lesions remains to be established. Much of this difficulty lies in the lack of uniform acceptance of clinical criteria for determining the true underlying pathologic condition. Several uncommon optic nerve lesions associated with sarcoidosis, tuberculosis, and toxoplasmosis have been reported (27, 44). Bilateral enlargement due to increased intracranial pressure and the small calcific deposits of optic nerve drusen are other well-recognized nonneoplastic conditions with characteristic radiographic findings (3, 7, 23).

For the diagnostic workup, plain skull films occasionally show findings but are frequently negative in cases of intraorbital optic nerve tumor. Plain film optic foramen views are much more helpful for both gliomas and meningiomas and deserve mention because of their simplicity and low cost. Complex motion optic canal tomography has gradually been replaced by CT. Angiography may be quite useful in selected cases in

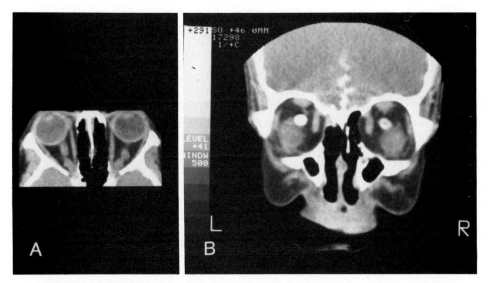

FIG. 24.10. Optic nerve meningoceles. (A) With meningoceles, irregular, lobulated appearance along course of both optic nerves may be seen. (B) Meningoceles are isodense and more irregular than most gliomas or meningiomas. Fluid collections may also become lobulated and are sometimes referred to as "optic nerve subdural hygromas." A possible mechanism of meningoceles and hygromas is episodic increased intracranial pressure. Free communication of intracranial subarachnoid space along optic nerves is normal variant, well known to neuroradiologists, that can be demonstrated in up to one-third of ophthalmologically asymptomatic patients during course of metrizamide cisternograpy.

which very large lesions or intracranial extension is suspected. Late-generation CT with special techniques for optimal optic nerve visualization has become the definitive imaging examination for evaluation of optic nerve tumors.

ANGIOMAS, INCLUDING HEMANGIOMAS, LYMPHANGIOMAS, VENOUS MALFORMATIONS, AND ARTERIOVENOUS MALFORMATIONS

The vascular angiomas, the most common of the orbital tumors, include cavernous hemangiomas, lymphangiomas, and venous malformations. They are the most common benign orbital tumors in the pediatric age group and are also seen frequently in adults. The lesions are often large and have both intraconal and extraconal components. Because of the large size, most patients have marked proptosis and diplopia, and the role of CT is to characterize the mass as an angioma, to suggest the particular subtype, and to delineate the extent of the mass, including possible intracranial extension (Fig. 24.11).

The cavernous hemangiomas are histologically composed of large vas-

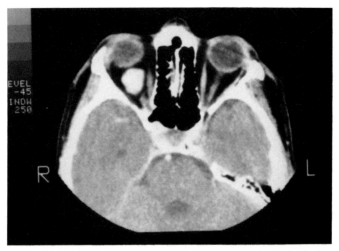

FIG. 24.11. Hemangioma. Well-circumscribed lesion of extremely high density lying within muscle cone is characteristic of vascular hemangioma. This lesion produced optic nerve compression in a middle-aged man.

cular channels lined by endothelial cells. Radiographic contrast material pools in these spaces, frequently producing marked contrast enhancement. The mass is usually of high density to begin with, so that the final attenuation of the mass on a contrast examination may range up to 80–100 Hounsfield units. Davis *et al.* (11) found enhancement in 18 of 18 cavernous hemangiomas. Forbes *et al.* (15) reported that 22 of 24 angiomas had high attenuation on precontrast scans and that all 18 of 18 postcontrast scans showed enhancement. Encapsulation of the tumors, which occurs frequently, sharply demarcates the border of the mass from the surrounding fatty tissue. Arteriography may show a slightly dense stain relating to the pooling of contrast material in the capillary spaces. However, the lack of direct venous shunting usually results in a normal-sized ophthalmic artery unless the lesion is exceptionally large.

Lymphangiomas are composed of clear fluid channels and lymphoid follicles, and the contrast enhancement is not quite as frequent or as intense. In the same series, Davis *et al.* (11) noted enhancement in half the lymphangiomas; the precontrast density was similar to that of hemangiomas. A more infiltrative and less encapsulated mass has been described as a common finding with lymphangiomas, and it is not unusual on CT to see a more irregular, lobulated mass, although this is a weak finding in the attempt to differentiate the mass from a hemangioma.

Venous malformations or varices may simulate hemangiomas, with the additional finding of increased size and prominence when a scan is performed after contrast enhancement during jugular compression or a Valsalva maneuver. Because of the dilated venous space communicating with the large draining jugular venous system, a significant increase in intrathoracic pressure or jugular vein pressure often is directly transmitted to the varix, which increases in size on the CT image. Although a Valsalva maneuver or direct jugular compression during scanning is the most productive measure to take, sometimes simple hyperextension of the head during coronal scanning produces the same result. Direct orbital venography may be used to confirm the presence of a varix, although this procedure has been less frequently used since the advent of high-resolution CT (Figs. 24.12 and 24.13).

Phleboliths are characteristically found in relation to orbital angiomas. The small, round, dense calcifications should be easily distinguishable from irregular calcifications that may occur with other types of tumors. In our experience, only small shotgun pellets may exactly mimic the phleboliths of an angioma, and the history of trauma should differentiate these from foreign bodies (Fig. 24.14).

The angioma may occur outside or within the muscle cone, and a combination of the axial and coronal views may be necessary to assess this relationship. The angioma does not customarily arise from the orbital apex, but a large lesion can extend into this region. Davis et al. (11) reported that 22% of hemangiomas and two of seven lymphangiomas extended into the orbital apex on CT. Although an occasional vascular angioma can be seen in this area, stronger consideration of an optic nerve tumor should be given to the presence of a small, dense apical mass. Intracranial extension may occur through the orbital roof or through one of the orbital foramina, such as the optic canal or the superior orbital fissure. Extension is seen on CT as dense enhanced tissue within the intracranial compartment. Intracranial extension does not necessarily correlate with radiographic bony changes seen on plain films. Thinning or expansion of the bony orbital wall may occur from chronic pressure of an angioma confined to the orbit, whereas a soft component of the tumor may extend through an orbital foramen into the intracranial space without enlarging the bone margins. High-resolution CT with contrast enhancement is the best technique for determining intracranial extension (Fig. 24.15 and 24.16).

MALIGNANT NEOPLASMS, INCLUDING LYMPHOMA, METASTASES, AND SINUS TUMORS EXTENDING INTO THE ORBIT

Malignant tumors may arise directly within the orbit, extend into the orbit from a sinus origin, or spread to the orbit as metastases from

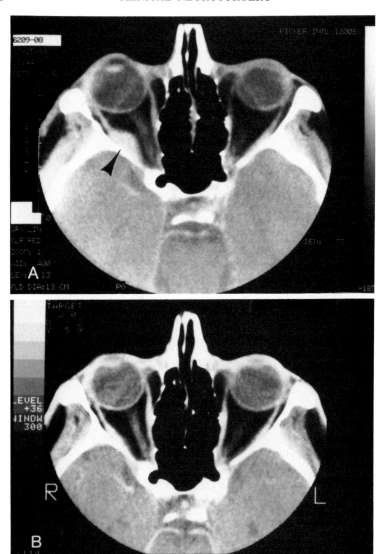

FIG. 24.12. Venous varix with bleeding. (A) After acute onset of pain and limited ocular motion, scan in 58-year-old man showed small, discrete, high-density mass (*arrowhead*) representing hematoma along lateral rectus sheath. (B) Seven days later, hematoma had resorbed and transverse scan was negative. (C) At same setting, however, patient's head was hyperextended for coronal scanning after intravenous injection of contrast material. Increased orbital venous pressure enlarged varix and caused mass (*arrowhead*) to reappear.

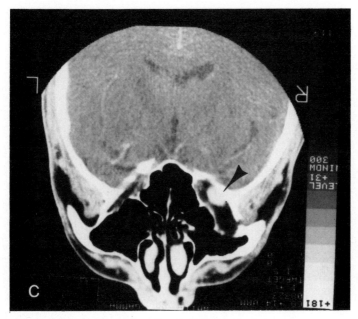

FIG. 24.12C

hematogenous dissemination. The most common forms representing these groups are lymphoma, sinus carcinoma, and metastatic carcinoma from breast, lung, kidney, or gastrointestinal tract. Less common malignant tumors include osteogenic sarcoma, malignant dermoid and cystic adenocarcinomas of the lacrimal gland, and the rhabdomyosarcomas and retinoblastoma of childhood. Intraorbital esthesioneuroblastoma is considered by some to be a locally invasive tumor of indolent but relentless progression.

The key radiographic feature of the malignant tumor is a tendency toward bone destruction. Whereas benign disease may produce a soft tissue mass that occasionally expands and thins the orbital walls, the malignant tumor often destroys any bony margins as it invades adjacent anatomic spaces. Whether on CT or plain films, this radiographic appearance of masses extending across anatomic compartments and destroying intervening bony walls strongly suggests malignant neoplasm. In these cases, both diagnosis and definition of extension into sinus or intracranial areas are the goals of the radiologic examination (15, 16).

Lymphoma is a common lesion that may be classified as primary in the orbit or secondary in the orbit from systemic body disease (35). It is generally considered to be malignant in all forms and primarily affects

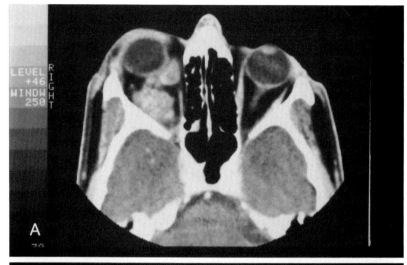

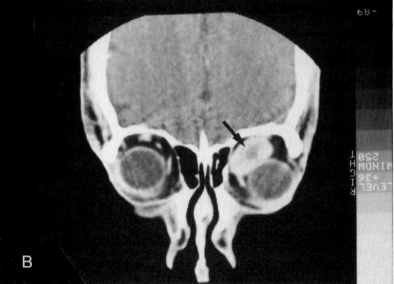

FIG. 24.13. Large lobulated hemangioma with clot. (*A*) Axial projection demonstrates extensively lobulated, high-density mass sometimes seen with this lesion. (*B*) Coronal view demonstrates contrast enhancement around low-density region in anterior portion of mass, which represents blood clot found at surgery (*arrow*).

older age groups, particularly persons in the fifth through the seventh decades. It may have a varied radiographic appearance, including presentation as an isolated intraorbital mass or as a diffuse infiltrative lesion in the retrobulbar space. The customary finding is a large, lobulated soft

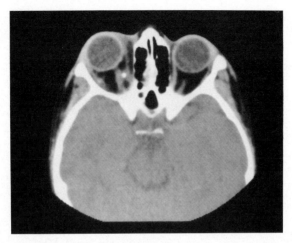

FIG. 24.14. Hemangioma phlebolith. Phlebolith is seen as tiny dense calcification with or without associated soft tissue mass.

tissue component with poorly defined margins that is either isodense or of high density and that is moderately enhanced on CT after intravenous administration of contrast material. Occasionally, lymphoma, by arising or extending into the globe, produces an enlarged, dense globe with normal retrobulbar structures. Generally, the common findings are poorly defined increased retrobulbar density and lack of differentiation of orbital structures, such as rectus muscles and optic nerve (Fig. 24.17).

The pattern of malignant lymphoma can be difficult to differentiate from that of inflammatory pseudotumor. Generally, more aggressive bony destructive changes suggest malignant lymphoma, although pseudotumor can occasionally erode through bone. Although less dramatic response to steroid therapy and aggressive radiographic changes point toward lymphoma, sometimes only open biopsy achieves the final differentiation of these two processes.

Metastasis to the orbit, a frequent occurrence in late advanced stages of disease, may also occur early, even as a lesion from an unknown primary. Some authors report that 7–45% of orbital neoplasms are due to metastasis in late stages. In an earlier comprehensive study, however, Albert *et al.* (1) found five metastatic orbital tumors and five choroid metastatic tumors in a series of 213 adults with general metastatic disease. Orbital lesions have been found to be metastases from breast, lung, kidney, and colon carcinomas. Although tissue biopsy is not often performed, CT may still be widely used to confirm suspected orbital metastasis in a patient with known tumor (Fig. 24.18).

As in other malignant conditions, the metastatic orbital tumor fre-

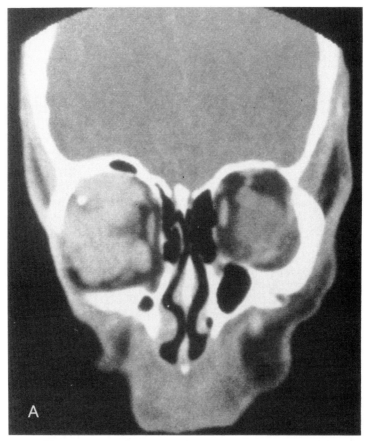

FIG. 24.15. Hemangioma with intracranial extension. (*A*) Extremely bulky mass with characteristic phlebolith entirely fills orbital space. (*B*) Coronal slice through level of optic canal and superior orbital fissure also demonstrates extension of angioma through foramina into intracranial compartment. (Reproduced with permission from: G. S. Forbes *et al.* (15).)

quently causes erosion or destruction of bony orbital walls identifiable on plain films, plain film tomography, or CT. The soft tissue mass may be enhanced by contrast material and not uncommonly shows calcification on a precontrast scan. In our series, intracranial extension was seen more frequently with metastases than with other tumors, except meningiomas.

Carcinoma may extend directly into the orbit from an adjacent sinus (sinus adenocarcinoma) or from the skin (basal cell carcinoma). These lesions usually cause ophthalmologic symptoms similar to those of the primary orbital tumors. In many patients, the tumor diagnosis and

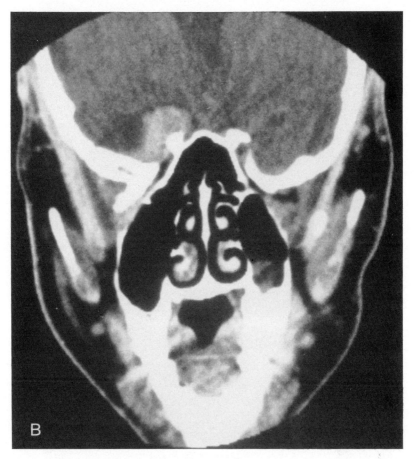

Fig. 24.15*B*

extraorbital origin have already been established, and plain film tomography or CT is used to evaluate the degree of orbital extension. Patients with early symptoms, such as diplopia or proptosis, may be scanned to document orbital invasion from a known sinus tumor; in such cases, the rectus muscle sheath is frequently involved without encroachment on the optic nerve. Orbital invasion with proptosis has been noted in 5% of patients with nasopharyngeal carcinomas, whereas as many as 25% of such patients may have a lesion of the motor nerve of the eye, the trigeminal nerve, or the last four bulbar nerves. Extension into the medial compartment of the orbit is characteristic of sinus carcinoma, and the sinus soft tissue mass is usually readily visible. Carcinomas

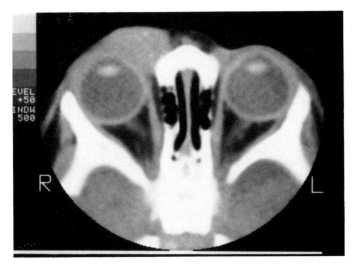

FIG. 24.16. Pediatric periorbital hemangioma. Large, bulky soft tissue mass involves only anterior periorbital tissues. CT scan excludes posterior extension into retrobulbar compartment.

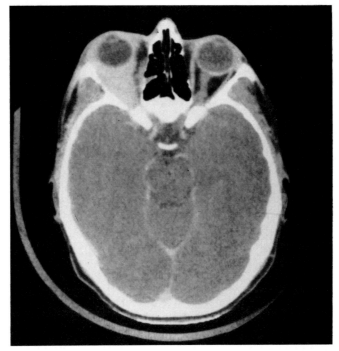

FIG. 24.17. Lymphoma. Extensive infiltrative process has encased globe, filling orbit without causing significant proptosis. This phenomenon occasionally occurs with orbital lymphoma but is quite uncharacteristic of other orbital neoplasms, which usually produce marked proptosis.

502

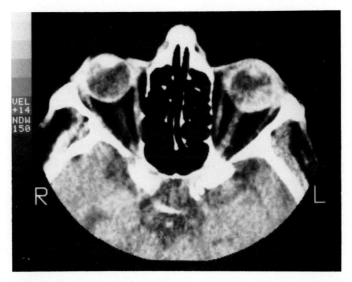

FIG. 24.18. Tumor within globe. High-density mass fills posterior portion of globe and produces thickening of sclera at attachment of lateral rectus muscle (metastasis from bronchogenic lung carcinoma).

produce more positive findings of bone destruction on plain radiographs than other tumors. Contrast enhancement of the carcinoma on CT is also frequent in intraorbital extension.

Basal cell carcinomas of the skin may impinge on the globe or invade the orbit. Thickening of the periorbital tissues is easily identified and corresponds to the obvious clinical condition. CT may be useful in defining the extent of the intraorbital component, particularly in the retrobulbar region. Advanced cases may also produce bone destruction, and unlike other tumors, basal cell mass may be associated with enophthalmos, which can be seen on CT.

Several rare malignant neoplasms are occasionally seen in both the adult orbit and the pediatric orbit (29). Esthesioneuroblastoma, a locally invasive tumor with an insidious progressive course, arises from germinal rest cells along the olfactory tract in young and middle-aged adults. The mass more commonly involves the cribriform plate and ethmoid sinus, with frequent sinus-intracranial segments, but may extend into the orbit and, rarely, may even appear to have most of its bulk anatomically within the orbit. In one of the largest series reported, Shah and Feghali (43) found orbital involvement in 11 of 31 patients (35%). Calcification within the mass and bone destruction are common radiographic findings. Surgical resection with or without follow-up radiation treatment is consid-

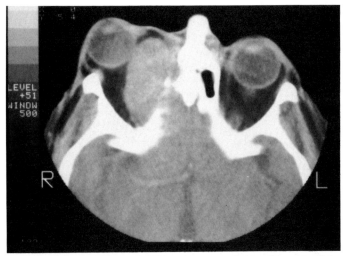

FIG. 24.19. Esthesioneuroblastoma. This rare tumor is usually confined to olfactory groove and cribriform plate region, but in advanced cases such as this, it may grow off midline to invade orbit in superior medial quadrant. High density, scattered calcification, and bone destruction are characteristic.

ered necessary for the best possible management of these difficult lesions (Fig. 24.19).

Neuroblastoma, a malignant condition in the pediatric age range, infiltrates the extracranial tissues and bone and, at the skull base, may extend into the extraconal component of the orbit. In this region, the lesion generally is not surgical and is easily recognized by its characteristic radiographic appearance on CT. Linear high-density deposits extend along the lateral extraconal margins of both orbits, and a lytic pattern of the orbital wall is invariably seen on special window settings on the scans. This appearance indicates widespread dissemination of the process along the meningeal tissues (Fig. 24.20).

Retinoblastoma, on the other hand, is a well-demarcated mass which, when confined to the orbit, requires surgical removal to prevent further progression. If the lesion extends into the intracranial compartment, survival is poor. Anatomic assessment of this tumor is readily made from the CT examination, since the tumor is dense, sharply outlined, and frequently calcified. It usually occurs in black infants and is detected from the clinical examination (Fig. 24.21).

MISCELLANEOUS TUMORS, INCLUDING NEUROFIBROMA, LACRIMAL GLAND CYST, AND DERMOID

Neurofibromas arise from the sheath cells of small intraorbital muscular nerves and may occur singly as isolated lesions or may be associated

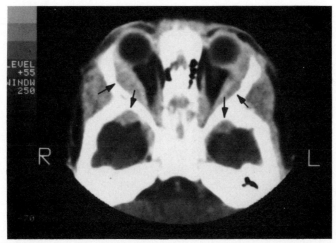

FIG. 24.20. Neuroblastoma. Orbital involvement with this neoplasm produces a characteristic CT picture of infiltrating soft tissue masses along lateral extraconal margins of both orbits and anterior margins of middle fossa (*arrows*). Bone window settings may also demonstrate mottled lytic pattern of sphenoid bone from tumor destruction.

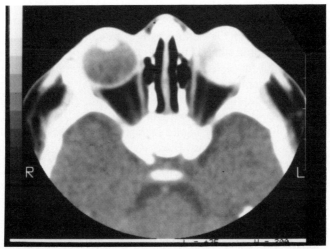

FIG. 24.21. Retinoblastoma. This ocular tumor produces dense picture on CT scan because large amount of calcium is present. Confinement to globe, as in this case, is a good sign; extension of tumor to retrobulbar compartment carries poor prognosis.

with neurofibromatosis. In patients with neurofibromatosis, however, an orbital tumor is more likely to be an optic nerve glioma or meningioma, as previously described. The fibromas are encapsulated tumors that radiographically are round or oval-shaped masses well demarcated from

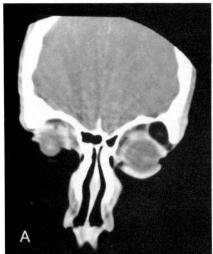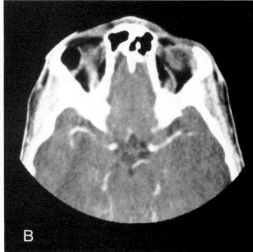

FIG. 24.22. Dermoid cyst. This fatty cyst is seen as low-density mass occasionally filled with some cellular debris. It usually is found in the region of the lacrimal gland and may cause expansion of superior-temporal bony orbit wall, as in this case. (*A*) Coronal view. (*B*) Axial view.

surrounding tissues and frequently calcified. Bone wall expansion from longstanding pressure of the benign tumor may occur.

Lacrimal gland tumors arise in the superior temporal quadrant of the orbit at the lacrimal fossa. The term is sometimes loosely used to include lesions that arise from the lacrimal gland itself or any mass arising in this region. These include benign cysts, dermoids, and a rare malignant tumor, cystic adenocarcinoma (Fig. 24.22) (24).

The radiographic character of the lacrimal gland mass is usually quite characteristic in the diagnosis of these lesions. The benign, well-marginated tumors may have fatty elements mixed with calcific deposits. The fat gives a low-density appearance to the ground substance, which may measure below 0 in Hounsfield attenuation units on CT. Because the lesions are slow-growing, bony expansion of the superolateral wall is common. Since the anterior location facilitates clinical diagnosis, CT is used to evaluate soft tissue retrobulbar extension and bony roof intracranial expansion. The rare malignant lesions are hyperdense, are enhanced by contrast medium, extend into the temporal periorbital tissues, and have a poor prognosis.

As part of the orbital tumor diagnostic workup, nonorbital lesions need to be identified. This is most easily done if the common nonorbital lesions are remembered during the radiographic evaluation. Benign mucoceles and pyoceles may on occasion extend from their sinus origin into the orbit. When extension occurs, the center of the lesion is still usually identified to lie within the sinus, and telltale associated findings of inflammatory membrane thickening are often seen. The masses are well demarcated and often calcified, and the bone change is expansion or local erosion (Figs. 14.23–14.25).

Other tumors arising from the base of the skull and the infratemporal regions may involve the orbit. Involvement usually is from advanced progression of a large, aggressive lesion. In these cases, the radiographic evaluation is more often directed toward intracranial extension and vascular anatomy, with orbital involvement as a secondary complication. Tumors such as fibrosarcomas and vascular lesions such as angiofibromas would be included in this group.

TECHNIQUES OTHER THAN COMPUTED TOMOGRAPHY

Although CT offers a thorough evaluation of the orbital mass in most cases, a few circumstances continue to benefit from the complementary use of other radiographic techniques. The plain films are positive in 50–69% of proved orbital tumors, but this rate is lower when findings are

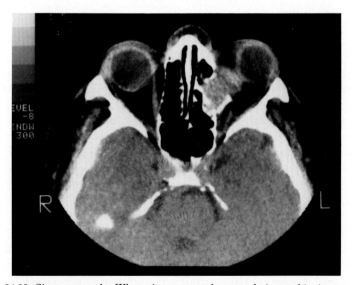

FIG. 24.23. Sinus mucocele. When sinus mucocele expands into orbit, it causes mass effect, proptosis, and occasional optic nerve compression similar to that of orbit neoplasm. Its sinus origin usually is apparent with extension through sinus-orbital wall and radiographic density higher than that of orbital fat, sinus air, and ocular fluid.

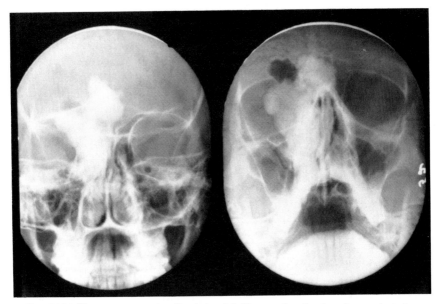

FIG. 24.24. Sinus osteoma extending into orbit. Dense sclerotic, sharply marginated mass characteristic of bony osteoma usually is well seen on plain films. Although usually confined to sinuses, occasionally it may extend into orbit.

used to indicate tumor type. In this situation, the incidence of characteristic findings is between 30 and 40%, which is a more accurate reflection of the value of the plain radiograph. In our earlier series, 46% of plain radiographs were positive, and 37% were indicative or diagnostic of the orbital tumor. The highest rate of information return is from optic nerve tumors, as has been described previously, in which enlargement of the optic foramen or sclerosis of the adjacent bone is quite characteristic of the glioma or sheath meningioma. Coronal plain film tomograms can be useful to assess the integrity of the orbital roof when a question of tumor extension into the anterior intracranial fossa is raised. Other uses of the plain films generally are related to trauma and periorbital lesions (37, 57, 58).

Angiography is not often used in the evaluation of primary orbital masses. Its principal role is in detecting small vascular malformations, such as dural arteriovenous malformations, that may mimic vascular masses on CT. When arteriography is performed in a patient with an orbital tumor, one may see stretching of lacrimal and ethmoidal branches of the ophthalmic artery, effacement of the choroidal blush at the back of the globe, and a faint vascular stain within the mass. The magnification

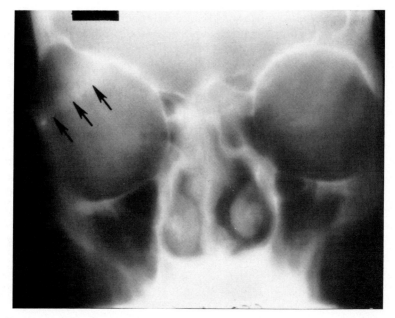

FIG. 24.25. Orbital roof expansion from bone cyst. Benign, slowly enlarging process produced enlargement of superior-lateral orbit by expanding bony margin rather than destroying it. At surgery, hematic cyst from old trauma was found.

subtraction technique is used to derive the most information from the intra-arterial injections of contrast medium. Although the ophthalmic artery arises directly from the internal carotid, either common carotid injections or a complementary selective external carotid artery injection should be done, since dural lesions and anatomic variants of meningeal-ophthalmic artery origins may be missed from selective internal carotid injections.

Orbital venography has largely been replaced by high-resolution CT, although it may still be used in a few selected instances. In this technique, contrast material is injected through a small forehead vein cannulated with a pediatric scalp vein needle. With a forehead compression band in place, the contrast material is driven retrograde into the orbital veins for filling. Although sensitive to pathologic change, the examination lacks specificity, since many lesions, including tumor, benign mass, inflammation, endocrine disease, and granulomatous disease can cause occlusions and abnormal venous filling. The examination may still occasionally be used when a question of granulomatous disease or cavernous sinus disease is raised and CT findings are negative or indeterminate.

Magnetic resonance imaging (MRI) is being introduced in major medical centers as a complementary and potentially alternative scanning examination for various head and neck problems, including those affecting the orbit. Early experience with orbital imaging suggests that this method may lend itself very well to orbital problems because of a high degree of sensitivity for fat tissue and changes of hydration within soft tissue and the lack of ionizing radiation (21). Another advantage is its ability to produce different projections in transverse, coronal, and sagittal planes without the need to move the patient or to perform time-consuming off-line computer analysis. The early scanners offer lower spatial resolution than late-generation CT, although preliminary investigative work at very high field strengths and with specially adapted surface detector coils for the orbit suggests that clinical orbital scanning resolution could equal or exceed high-resolution CT. Over the next few years, investigation of several such technical developments and of the economic questions, since the technique is expensive, will be of considerable interest for orbital tumor diagnosis.

In MRI, the information needed for an image is produced by the stimulation of tissue within a strong magnetic field by radiowave pulses at specific frequencies. The applied energy is absorbed by the hydrogen protons, which precess in the magnetic field because of their nuclear magnetic moments. As the excess energy is emitted, it creates a signal that is detected and analyzed by computer techniques similar to those used in a CT system. Changing the pulse sequences of the radio transmission forms different types of images that provide information based on different characteristics of the tissue. The marked differences of proton density and macromolecular environment or orbital fat and muscle result in excellent contrast between these types of structures in magnetic resonance images. It is likely that most orbital masses demonstrated on CT will also be seen on MRI. The important question is whether MRI can further characterize orbital tumor type and location at acceptable costs. Finding the answer will require study of larger clinical groups over the next few years.

REFERENCES

1. Albert, D. M., Rubenstein, R. A., and Scheie, H. G. Tumor metastasis to the eye. Part I. Incidence in 213 adult patients with generalized malignancy. Am. J. Ophthalmol., 63: 723, 1967.
2. Baker, H. L., Jr., Kearns, T. P., Campbell, J. K., et al. Computerized transaxial tomography in neuro-ophthalmology. Am. J. Ophthalmol., 78: 285, 1974.
3. Behrens, M. M. Neuro-ophthalmic aspects of orbital disease. In: Diseases of the Orbit, edited by I. S. Jones and F. A. Jakobiec, pp. 105–122. Harper & Row, Hagerstown, MD., 1979.

4. Bergström, K. Computer tomography of the orbits. Acta Radiol. [Suppl.] (Stockh.), *346:* 155, 1975.
5. Bullock, L. J., and Reeves, R. J. Unilateral exophthalmos: Roentgenographic aspects. A.J.R., *82:* 290, 1959.
6. Byrd, S. E., Harwood-Nash, D. C., Fitz, C. R., *et al.* Computed tomography of intraorbital optic nerve gliomas in children. Radiology, *129:* 73, 1978.
7. Cabanis, E. A., Salvolini, U., Rodallec, A., *et al.* Computed tomography of the optic nerve. Part II. Size and shape modifications in papilledema. J. Comput. Assist. Tomogr., *2:* 150, 1978.
8. Chutorian, A. M., Schwartz, J. F., Evans, R. A., *et al.* Optic gliomas in children. Neurology (Minneap.), *14:* 83, 1964.
9. Dallow, R. L., Momose, K. J., Weber, A. L., *et al.* Comparison of ultrasonography, computerized tomography (EMI scan), and radiographic techniques in evaluation of exophthalmos. Trans. Am. Acad. Ophthalmol. Otolaryngol., *81:* 305, 1976.
10. Daniels, D. L., Haughton, V. M., Williams, A. L., *et al.* Computed tomography of the optic chiasm. Radiology, *137:* 123, 1980.
11. Davis, K. R., Hesselink, J. R., Dallow, R. L., *et al.* CT and ultrasound in the diagnosis of cavernous hemangioma and lymphangioma of the orbit. CT, *4:* 98, 1980.
12. Dubois, P. J., Kennerdell, J. S., Rosenbaum, A. E., *et al.* Computed tomographic localization for fine needle aspiration biopsy of orbital tumors. Radiology, *131:* 149, 1979.
13. Enzmann, D., Donaldson, S. S., Marshall, W. H., *et al.* Computed tomography in orbital pseudotumor (idiopathic orbital inflammation). Radiology, *120:* 597, 1976.
14. Forbes, G. Computed tomography of the orbit. Radiol. Clin. North. Am., *20:* 37, 1982.
15. Forbes, G. S., Earnest, F. IV, and Waller, R. R. Computed tomography of orbital tumors, including late-generation scanning techniques. Radiology, *142:* 387, 1982.
16. Forbes, G. S., Sheedy, P. F., II, and Waller, R. R. Orbital tumors evaluated by computed tomography. Radiology, *136:* 101, 1980.
17. Fox, A. J., Debrun, G., Vinuela, F., *et al.* Intrathecal metrizamide enhancement of the optic nerve sheath. J. Comput. Assist. Tomogr., *3:* 653, 1979.
18. Gawler, J., Sanders, M. D., Bull, J. W. D., *et al.* Computer assisted tomography in orbital disease. Br. J. Ophthalmol., *58:* 571, 1974.
19. Gonzalez, C. F., Grossman, C. B., and Palacios, E. *Computed Brain and Orbital Tomography: Technique and Interpretation.* John Wiley & Sons, New York, 1976.
20. Gyldensted, C., Lester, J., and Fledelius, H. Computed tomography of orbital lesions: A radiological study of 144 cases. Neuroradiology, *13:* 141, 1977.
21. Han, J. S., Benson, J. E., Bonstelle, C. T., *et al.* Magnetic resonance imaging of the orbit: A preliminary experience. Radiology, *150:* 755, 1984.
22. Henderson, J. W., and Campbell, R. J. Primary intraorbital meningioma with intraocular extension. Mayo Clin. Proc., *52:* 504, 1977.
23. Henderson, J. W., and Farrow, G. M. The individual tumors: Clinical features, pathology, and management. In: *Orbital Tumors,* pp. 77–614. W.B. Saunders, Philadelphia, 1973.
24. Hesselink, J. R., Davis, K. R., Dallow, R. L., *et al.* Computed tomography of masses in the lacrimal gland region. Radiology, *131:* 143, 1979.
25. Hilal, S. K., and Trokel, S. L. Computerized tomography of the orbit using thin sections. Semin. Roentgenol., *12:* 137, 1977.
26. Howard, C. W., Osher, R. H., and Tomsak, R. L. Computed tomographic features in optic neuritis. Am. J. Ophthalmol., *89:* 699, 1980.
27. Jacoby, C. G., Go, R. T., and Beren, R. A. Cranial CT of neurofibromatosis. AJR, *135:* 553, 1980.

28. Karp, L. A., Zimmerman, L. E., Borit, A., *et al.* Primary intraorbital meningiomas. Arch. Ophthalmol., *91:* 24, 1974.
29. Lallemand, D. P., Brasch, R. C. Char, D. H., *et al.* Orbital tumors in children: Characterization by computed tomography. Radiology, *151:* 85, 1984.
30. Leone, C. R., Jr., and Wilson, F. C. Computerized axial tomography of the orbit. Ophthalmic Surg., *7:* 34, 1976.
31. Macmichael, I. M., and Cullen, J. F. Primary intraorbital meningioma. Br. J. Ophthalmol., *53:* 169, 1969.
32. Manelfe, C., Pasquini, U., and Bank, W. O. Metrizamide demonstration of the subarachnoid space surrounding the optic nerves. J. Comput. Assist. Tomogr., *2:* 545, 1978.
33. Marshall, D. Glioma of the optic nerve: As a manifestation of von Recklinghausen's disease. Am. J. Ophthalmol., *37:* 15, 1954.
34. Momose, K. J., New, P. F. J., Grove, A. S., Jr., *et al.* The use of computed tomography in ophthalmology. Radiology, *115:* 361, 1975.
35. Morgan, G. Lymphocytic tumours of the orbit. Mod. Probl. Ophthalmol., *14:* 355, 1975.
36. Peyster, R. G., Hoover, E. D., Hershey, B. L., *et al.* High-resolution CT of lesions of the optic nerve. AJNR, *4:* 169, 1983.
37. Pfeiffer, R. L. Roentgenography of exophthalmos with notes on the roentgen ray in ophthalmology. Am. J. Ophthalmol., *26:* 724, 816, 1943.
38. Salvolini, U., Cabanis, E. A., Rodallec, A., *et al.* Computed tomography of the optic nerve. Part I. Normal results. J. Comput. Assist. Tomogr., *2:* 141, 1978.
39. Salvolini, U., Menichelli, F., and Pasquini, U. Computer assisted tomography in 90 cases of exophthalmos. J. Comput. Assist. Tomogr., *1:* 81, 1977.
40. Sanders, M. D. Computer-assisted tomography (EMI scan) in orbital and neuro-ophthalmologic diagnosis. Trans. Pac. Coast Otoophthalmol. Soc., *56:* 17, 1975.
41. Sanders, M. D., and Gawler, J. Computerized tomographic scanning (EMI scan) in neuro-ophthalmology. Trans. Ophthalmol. Soc. U.K., *95:* 237, 1975.
42. Savoiardo, M., Harwood-Nash, D. C., Tadmor, R., *et al.* Gliomas of the intracranial anterior optic pathways in children: The role of computed tomography, angiography, pneumoencephalography, and radionuclide brain scanning. Radiology, *138:* 601, 1981.
43. Shah, J. P., and Feghali, J. Esthesioneuroblastoma. Cancer, *33:* 154, 1983.
44. Som, P. M., Sacher, M., Weitzner, I., Jr., *et al.* Sarcoidosis of the optic nerve. J. Comput. Assist. Tomogr., *6:* 614, 1982.
45. Spoor, T. C., Kennerdell, J. S., Martinez, A. J., *et al.* Malignant gliomas of the optic nerve pathways. Am. J. Ophthalmol., *89:* 284, 1980.
46. Strother, C. M., Hoyt, W. F., Appen, R. E., *et al.* Meningiomatous changes in the optic canal: A polytomographic study. Radiology, *135:* 109, 1980.
47. Swenson, S. A., Forbes, G. S., Younge, B. R., *et al.* Radiologic evaluation of tumors of the optic nerve. AJNR, *3:* 319, 1982.
48. Takahashi, M., Lombardi, G., Passerini, A., *et al.* Primary intraorbital meningiomas: A roentgenologic study. Neuroradiology, *5:* 95, 1973.
49. Tan, K. K., and Lim, A. S. M. Primary extradural intra-orbital meningioma in a Chinese girl. Br. J. Ophthalmol., *49:* 377, 1965.
50. Trokel, S. L., Hilal, S. K. Recognition and differential diagnosis of enlarged extraocular muscles in computed tomography. Am. J. Ophthalmol., *87:* 503, 1979.
51. Trokel, S. L., and Jakobiec, F. A., Correlation of CT scanning and pathologic features of ophthalmic Graves' disease. Ophthalmology, *88:* 553, 1981.
52. Turner, R. M., Gutman, I., Hilal, S. K., *et al.* CT of drusen bodies and other calcific lesions of the optic nerve: case report and differential diagnosis. AJNR, *4:* 175, 1983.

53. Unsöld, R., DeGroot, J., and Newton, T. H. Images of the optic nerve: Anatomic-CT correlation. AJNR, *1:* 317, 1980.
54. Weinstein, M. A., Berlin, A. J., Jr., and Duchesneau, P. M. High resolution computed tomography of the orbit with the Ohio Nuclear Delta head scanner. AJR, *127:* 175, 1976.
55. Wende, S., Aulich, A., Nover, A., *et al.* Computed tomography of orbital lesions: A cooperative study of 210 cases. Neuroradiology, *13:* 123, 1977.
56. Wright, J. E., Lloyd, G. A. S., and Ambrose, J. Computerized axial tomography in the detection of orbital space-occupying lesions. Am. J. Ophthalmol., *80:* 78, 1975.
57. Zizmor, J. Recent trends in the roentgenographic diagnosis of orbital tumors. Trans. Am. Acad. Ophthalmol. Otolaryngol., *70:* 579, 1966.
58. Zizmor, J., Fasano, C. V., Smith, B., *et al.* Roentgenographic diagnosis of unilateral exophthalmos. J.A.M.A., *197:* 343, 1966.
59. Healy, J. F., and Rosenkrantz, H. Enlargement of the optic nerve sheath complex in thyroid ophthalmopathy. CT, *5:* 8, 1981.

25

Neurosurgical Involvement in Tumors of the Orbit

DONLIN M. LONG, M.D.

In 1921 Dandy (6) explored a patient with a bilateral progressive optic neuropathy and found bilateral meningiomas of the optic canals with small intracranial extensions. Twenty years later, his monograph *Orbital Tumors* described his experience with 31 patients harboring a variety of diseases. He came to the conclusion that intracranial exploration of the orbit was superior to the traditional lateral approach and recommended radical surgery for orbital tumors. In spite of Dandy's example, neurosurgical involvement with tumors of the orbit has remained limited. Housepian *et al.* (9, 10) has written extensively about the treatment of optic gliomas. Maroon and Kennerdell (19, 22) have described a team approach between Neurosurgery and Ophthalmology for diagnosis and treatment of orbital tumors, but the writings in the neurosurgical literature are generally sparse. Most commonly, orbital masses do not involve the canal or the intracranial space (Table 25.1). Maroon and Kennerdell (21, 22) have detailed the lateral and medial approaches to the orbit recently. The intracranial approach for decompression (Table 25.2) of the optic canal and exploration of the canal and orbit via the intracranial approach holds the greatest interest for the neurosurgeon.

TABLE 25.1

Orbital and Periorbital Masses—Differential

Diagnosis (in order of descending frequency)
1. Inflammation—nonspecific
2. Metastatic tumors
3. Meningiomas
4. Dermoids
5. Hemangiomas
6. Lacrimal gland tumors
7. Optic gliomas
8. Neurofibromas, fibrous dysplasia, and other tumors of orbital structures occur with about the same frequency.
9. Aneurysms of ophthalmic area
10. Carotid dolichoectasia

TABLE 25.2

Results of Transcranial Canalicular Decompression for Nontraumatic Compressive Optic Neuropathy

1922–1984, 29 cases
  Meningioma–15
  Fibrous Dysplasia–7
  Dolichoectasia–5
  Hemangioma–2
Results:
  33% improved
  33% stabilized
  33% worsened by surgery

Johns Hopkins Series 1977 to 1984
  Meningioma–6:2 bilateral
  Dolichoectasia–2:1 bilateral
  Hemangioma–1
  Bony Compression–1
  Unknown cause of visual loss–2
Results
  Immediate: 66.7% improved
           26.6% stabilized
            6.7% worsened by surgery
           93.3% improved or stabilized
  At 34 mos: 66.7% improved
           13.3% stable
           13.3% deteriorated
            6.7% worsened by surgery
           80% remained improved or stable

TUMORS OF THE ORBIT

For surgical purposes, the tumors may be divided into three groups: those that are wholly within the orbit; those that involve the optic canal and orbital cone; and those in the orbital area which also have significant intracranial extensions. In some instances, these latter tumors originate in the canal and extend intracranially (16). More commonly, there is a canalicular extension of a tumor originating inside the skull (6).

TUMORS WITHIN THE ORBIT

The most common lesion to be found in the orbit is the nonspecific inflammation often associated with thyroid disease (11). Other frequent lesions are metastatic tumor, hemangioma, invasive carcinoma and, less frequently, optic glioma and orbital meningioma (1, 7, 8, 11, 12, 20, 23, 27, 31, 32). In spite of Dr. Dandy's preference, it is now obvious that lesions which are entirely within the orbit and which do not extend posteriorly into the cone, can be most conveniently removed by the lateral or medial approach (25). Neurosurgeons are not commonly involved in such procedures, except in those places where there are teams of specialists dedicated to the treatment of lesions in and around the orbit (9, 10, 13, 22).

TUMORS OF THE ORBITAL CONE

The most common tumors of this region are optic sheath meningiomas (1, 28, 31). Hemangiomas of the canal are sometimes found (Fig. 25.1). Optic gliomas may be isolated to this region. Of course, any of the more commonly occurring orbital tumors may extend posteriorly and involve the cone and canal.

INTRACRANIAL TUMORS WITH CANALICULAR AND ORBITAL EXTENSIONS

The most common tumor is the meningioma (6, 19). Soft tissue may invade the canal and expand into the orbit. Enplaque meningiomas may thicken the bone and compress the optic canal or produce an orbital mass. This may be from direct tumor involvement or simple exostosis. Fibrous dysplasia commonly involves the posterior portion of the orbit and the sphenoid wing. Ectasia of the carotid artery and aneurysms of the osseous portion of the carotid or the ophthalmic artery can compress the optic nerve and extend into the canal (16). Invasive carcinoma may extend intracranially (2, 29, 30).

DIAGNOSIS OF POSTERIORLY PLACED ORBITAL AND CANALICULAR LESIONS

The principal symptom of the posteriorly placed tumors is progressive painless visual loss (Fig. 25.2). Acuity and fields will be equally involved. The field deficits are irregular and unpredictable. Pain is an uncommon symptom occurring most frequently when the tumor also involves the Gasserian ganglion or its branches (30). The extraocular cranial nerves are sometimes affected by the tumor, and if the orbital mass is large, proptosis may occur (27). Of course, when the intracranial extension is substantial, then other neurological signs may appear, depending on the location of the tumor. Abnormalities of eye movement may be related to the orbital mass on a mechanical basis, as well as from nerve dysfunction. The cardinal clinical features which most commonly should lead to the diagnosis are proptosis and limitation of motion for purely orbital tumors and painless progression visual loss for the posteriorly placed lesions.

DIAGNOSTIC STUDIES

Computerized axial tomography (CT) has virtually eliminated every other diagnostic procedure (5, 14, 18, 26). When an orbital tumor is suspected, the CT scan can be utilized to define the entire orbit, the

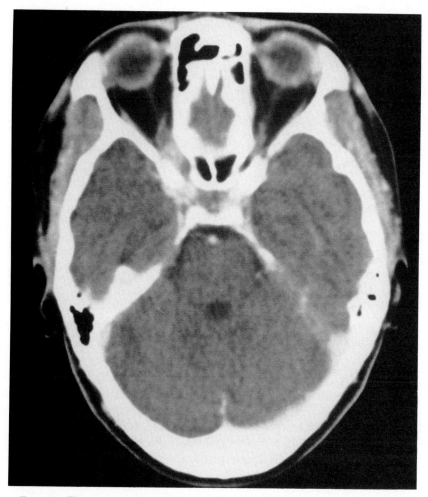

FIG. 25.1. There is an enhancing mass occupying the orbital cone and the orbital canal on the left side. By the time the patient was operated on, vision had deteriorated to light perception only. At surgery the optic nerve was exposed; the roof of the canal was drilled away using a left subfrontal approach; and an angioma of the canal beneath the nerve was discovered. The decompression did not afford any change in vision.

canal, and the surrounding intracranial structures of interest. The late model, high quality scans will demonstrate an abnormality virtually all of the time. Plain x-rays are redundant. Pneumosinus dilatans has a peculiar association with optic sheath meningioma which must be remembered. It also can occur with planum and tuberculum meningiomas which are more obvious. When the CT scan does not clearly demonstrate

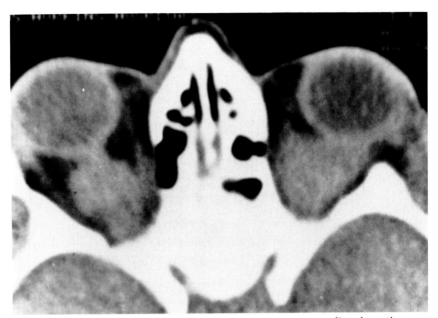

FIG. 25.2. This scan demonstrates large posterior masses surrounding the optic nerves bilaterally. The diagnosis proved to be nonspecific inflammatory disease.

an abnormality, a contrast cisternogram can be very helpful. Even tiny intracranial extensions and abnormalities can be demonstrated in this way (26). In the event all of the studies are normal and a thorough screening has failed to reveal a toxic metabolic or degenerative process, intracranial exploration of the chiasm and optic canals is still warranted (25). Needle biopsy can be an alternative in purely orbital lesions (17).

THE SURGICAL APPROACHES

Medial and Lateral Approaches to the Orbit

These are standard operations well described in the literature and routine to ophthalmological surgeons (3). The recent reviews by Maroon and Kennerdell (19, 22) provide an extensive review of these procedures.

The Intracranial Approach to Orbit Tumors

The selection of the bone flap and the approach will depend upon the location of the lesion and what is to be accomplished (4, 9, 10). If bilateral orbital exploration and decompression of the canals are required, then a coronal skin incision to allow a bifrontal bone flap is best. When the problem is unilateral but the lesion is largely within the orbit, it is better to utilize a subfrontal approach on the side of the abnormality (15). This can easily be accomplished with a unilateral skin incision, but if there is any doubt, a coronal skin incision should be employed, and then a unilateral frontal flap should be raised. For unilateral exploration of posteriorly placed lesions, whether unilateral or bilateral, the pterional approach affords an excellent exposure and is the first choice. After the induction of general anesthesia, the patient is placed supine, with the head turned away from the lesion about 30°, and then the table is turned with the patient firmly held in position until the zygoma is nearly parallel to the floor. Skeletal fixation headrest will provide stability during the delicate drilling to be done. A concealed unilateral question mark flap is made behind the hairline, and a single burr hole is placed in the keyhole at the base of the zygomatic process of the frontal bone. A power drill is then used to cut a flap based upon the temporalis muscle. There is no need to have an extensive temporal exposure, but the flap will expose the anterior 3 cm of the temporal lobe, the Sylvian fissure, and the frontal lobe. The key is to be low on the frontal lobe so that most of the sphenoid wing can be removed. The dura is then opened along the base, and the frontal lobe is retracted upward. Spinal drainage may be utilized but is not necessary if one takes the time to remove cerebrospinal fluid during the exposure. As soon as the optic nerve is visualized, self-retaining retractors are put in place, and the arachnoid around the optic nerve and carotid artery is removed so that the frontal lobe can be gradually elevated, exposing the anterior margin of the chiasm, both optic nerves, and both carotid arteries. The frontal retractor is then placed directly over the exposed optic nerve and as deep as it will go without risking any impingement upon the nerve. This will allow a thorough exploration of the chiasmal area. Once it is certain that there is no intracranial problem that needs attention, or the intracranial extension of the orbital abnormality is defined, the ipsilateral orbital canal can be opened. The first 5–10 mm of the canal are fibrous only, and a significant amount of nerve can be exposed simply by opening this band. An arachnoid knife is an excellent tool for doing that, and it is quite simple to open the canal in the midline to bone without injuring the nerve as long as adequate magnification is employed. The dural incision is then carried in the midportion of the canal well over onto the orbit, and the dura covering the canal and orbit is scraped away exposing bare bone. A second incision from medial to lateral margins of the canal is made, and the dura is scraped away there so that the margin of the canal is well defined. Bony removal is best carried out with a high speed gas-driven drill. Drills capable of 90,000 rpm have little torque and make it possible to have exquisite control. The surgeon can drill to dura beneath since the optic sheath is reasonably thick, but it is also possible to drill a very thin rim of bone which can then be removed with a small curette. This bone should be virtually paper thin so that no significant force is required. The entire optic canal is opened from medial to lateral, and the bony removal is extended with the drill until it is clear that the orbit has been reached. Then removal of the orbital roof, if indicated, can be carried out with standard rongeurs since there is virtually no risk of injury to the eye by compression. If decompression is all that is required, then the procedure can be terminated at this point. However, if there is a concern about a sheath meningioma, or a hemangioma, or an optic glioma, then the optic sheath must be carefully opened under high magnification, taking great care to avoid injury to the nerve. The bony portion of the procedure may be much more difficult in fibrous dysplasia, wherein the bone can be very vascular and very thick, or with meningioma involvement, wherein bleeding is even a greater problem. Hyperostotic bone secondary to meningioma is usually not vascular but is very hard and requires careful drilling.

It is probably not possible to totally remove most sheath meningiomas at this time. Whether laser techniques will make this feasible remains to be seen, but at present decompression and removal of exophytic tumor is the best that can be done for most cases. There is an occasional meningioma outside the sheath which can be removed safely, but those which are within the sheath can only be removed when the anatomical relationships are particularly favorable.

When the lesion occupies the posterior portion of the orbit, the situation is more difficult. It may be necessary to open the annulus in order to obtain removal of a tumor. This should be done superiorly in the midline of the optic nerve. If adequate eye movement is to be obtained, it is extremely important that the ends of the divided annulus be identified, tagged so that they are not lost, and then reapproximated with fine sutures in exact anatomical relationships. Otherwise, a significant muscular imbalance may occur. It is also important in closing the annulus to avoid any constriction of the optic nerve.

Tumors which are in the orbit may be exposed from above very well. The location can be ascertained from the CT scan, and sonography may also be useful. In order to expose these tumors, the periorbita is opened over the expected location of the mass. The orbital fat herniates through any incision and makes exploration of the orbit very difficult. Small self-retaining retractors of the type described by Maroon and Kennerdell (22) are very helpful in controlling the orbital fat. Cottonoid pledgets which cover the fat may be utilized with hand-held retractors as well. The entire orbit can easily be exposed and explored from above.

Before any neurosurgeon enters the orbit from above, a thorough understanding of the intraorbital relationships should be renewed. Because of the herniating fat, structures are difficult to identify and easy to damage. Our team approach, which leaves the intracranial and optic canal procedures to the neurosurgeon and the orbit surgery to the ophthalmologist, with both being present through the entire procedure, has been extremely successful in utilizing the talents of both surgeons.

The majority of tumors of the orbit which are approached intracranially do not present significant technical problems, and no special techniques are required. There is one situation in which an important difficult judgment must be made. This is when an optic nerve glioma or sheath meningioma is discovered in the face of normal or functional vision. The optic nerve glioma or meningioma can be identified with reasonable certainty on CT scanning alone, so the decision for treatment is usually made before a surgical procedure is undertaken. Our general practice is to defer surgery and follow the patient with regular evaluations of vision and CT estimation of tumor size as long as the glioma is intraorbital and confined to one nerve. Definitive resection is carried out when unilateral vision fails. We use the same guidelines when an optic nerve glioma or meningioma is encountered during orbital exploration. If the patient has functional vision and the lesion is clearly limited to one nerve, we do not remove the tumor but decompress only. If vision is seriously impaired, then the entire tumor, with adequate margins, is removed in order to eliminate any chance of chiasmal spread (12, 24).

The radical surgical techniques required for removal of invasive nasopharyngeal malignancies which have reached the orbit are well described. The neurosurgeon's role is to provide an estimation of intracranial spread, to then obtain an intracranial bony resection which will circumscribe the tumor and, often, to divide the optic nerve and control the ophthalmic artery safely. This is a problem different from that of purely orbital tumors and has been adequately described elsewhere.

SUMMARY

The neurosurgeon has a great deal to offer in the therapy of orbital tumors. Dr. Dandy's supposition that all orbital tumors could be approached by the intracranial route is certainly correct, but technical advances have made the medial and lateral approaches to the orbit more useful for most tumors which are confined to the orbit (22, 25). For those which involve the posterior orbit and canal and have intracranial extensions, the intracranial approach is excellent. Since Dandy's first description of the procedure in 1922, there have been 29 patient reports concerning the results of transcranial canalicular decompression for nontraumatic causes. The most common diagnosis was meningioma (15), and other tumor diagnoses were fibrous dysplasia (7) and hemangioma (2). One-third of the patients were improved; one-third had vision stabilized; and one-third were made worse by surgery. Modern techniques with the microscope and high speed drill have greatly improved these results. Our own experience in the decompression of 15 canals in 11 patients is as follows. There were six patients with meningioma, and two were bilateral. Three patients were found to have a vascular dolichoectasis and one patient had an hemangioma, and in two patients no compression was identified. Immediately postoperatively, two-thirds of the patients were improved, and only one eye (representing 6.7% of the nerves decompressed) was worsened. This resulted from an attempt to totally remove an adherent sheath meningioma. Long-term follow-up median 34 months has demonstrated maintenance of these gains. Eighty percent of the patients have improved or remained stable. These data indicate that the procedure described can be done safely without major risk of visual loss. The neurosurgeon should play an increasingly important role in the evaluation and therapy of posteriorly placed orbital tumors and unexplained compressive optic neuropathy.

REFERENCES

1. Alper, M. G. Management of primary optic nerve meningiomas. J. Clin. Neuro-ophthalmol., 1: 101–117, 1981.
2. Ballantyne, A. J., McCarten, A. B., and Ibanez, M. L. The extension of cancer of the head and neck through peripheral nerves. Am. J. Surg., 106: 651–667, 1963.
3. Berke, R. N. A modified Krönlein operation. Trans. Am. Ophthalmol. Soc., 51: 193–231, 1953.
4. Brihaye, J. Neurosurgical approaches to orbital tumours. In Advances and Technical Standards in Neurosurgery, Vol. 3, edited by H. Krayenbühl, pp. 103–121. Springer-Verlag, New York, 1976.
5. Char, D. H., and Norman, D. The use of computer tomography and ultrasonography in the evaluation of orbital masses. Surv. Ophthalmol., 27: 49–63, 1982.
6. Dandy, W. E. Results following the transcranial operative attack. In: Orbital Tumors, pp. 161–164. Oskar Piest, New York, 1941.
7. Grinberg, M. A., and Levy, N. S. Malignant neurilemoma of the supraorbital nerve. Am. J. Ophthalmol., 78: 489–492, 1974.
8. Harris, G. J. Bilateral blindness due to orbital lymphoma. Ann. Ophthalmol., 13: 427–430, 1981.
9. Housepian, E. M. Intraorbital tumors. In: Operative Neurosurgical Techniques, Vol. 1, edited by H. H. Schmidek and W. H. Sweet, pp. 227–244. Grune & Stratton, New York, 1982.
10. Housepian, E. M., Trokel, S. L., Jakobiec, F. O., et al. Tumors of the orbit. In: Neurological Surgery, Ed. 2, Vol. 5, edited by J. R. Youmans, pp. 3024–3064, Philadelphia, W.B. Saunders, 1982.
11. Hoyt, W. F., and Bashdassarian, S. A. Optic glioma of childhood: Natural history and rationale for conservative management. Br. J. Ophthalmol., 53: 793–798, 1969.
12. Hoyt, W. F., Meshel, L. G., Lessell, S., Schatz, N. J., and Sucklins, R. Malignant optic gliomas of childhood. Brain, 96: 121–132, 1973.

13. Jain, N. S. Two-stage intracranial and orbital operation for gliomas of the optic nerve. Br. J. Ophthalmol., *45:* 54–58, 1961.

14. Jakobiec, F. A., Depot, M. J., Kennerdell, J. S., Shults, W. T., Anderson, R. L., Alper, M. D., Citrin, C. M., Housepian, E. M., and Trokel, S. L. Combined clinical and computed tomographic diagnosis of orbital glioma and meningioma. Ophthalmology, *91:* 137–155, 1984.

15. Jane, J. A., Park, T. S., Pobereskin, L. H., *et al.* The supraorbital approach: Technical note. Neurosurgery, *11:* 537–542, 1982.

16. Jefferson, G. Concerning injuries, aneurysms and tumors involving the cavernous sinus. Trans. Ophthalmol. Soc. U.K., *73:* 117–152, 1953.

17. Kennerdell, J. S., Dubois, P. J., Dekker, A., *et al.* CT-guided fine needle aspiration biopsy of orbital optic nerve tumors. Ophthalmology, *87:* 491–496, 1980.

18. Kennerdell, J. S., and Ghoshhajra, K. Computed tomographic scanning of orbital tumors. Int. Ophthalmol. Clin., *22(4):* 99–131, 1982.

19. Kennerdell, J. S., and Maroon, J. C. Microsurgical approach to intraorbital tumors. Technique and instrumentation. Arch. Ophthalmol., *94:* 1333–1336, 1976.

20. Manschot, W. A. Primary tumors of the optic nerve in von Recklinghausen's disease. Am. J. Ophthalmol., *37:* 15–36, 1954.

21. Mark, L. E., Kennerdell, J. S., and Maroon, J. D., *et al.* Microsurgical removal of a primary intraorbital meningioma. Am. J. Ophthalmol., *86:* 704–709, 1978.

22. Maroon, J. C., and Kennerdell, J. S. Lateral microsurgical approach to intraorbital tumors. J. Neurosurg., *44:* 556–561, 1976.

23. McDonald, W. I. Pain around the eye: Inflammatory and neoplastic causes. Trans. Ophthalmol. Soc. U.K., *100:* 260–262, 1980.

24. McDonnell, P., and Miller, N. R. Chiasmatic extension of optic nerve glioma. Arch. Ophthalmol., *101:* 1412–1415, 1983.

25. Miller, N. R., and Iliff, W. J. Surgery of the orbit. In *Ophthalmic Surgery*, Ed. 4, edited by T. A. Rice, R. G. Michels, and W. J. Stark. pp. 383–398. C.V. Mosby, St. Louis, 1984.

26. Peyster, R. G., Hoover, E. D., and Hershey, B. L., *et al.* High resolution CT of lesions of the optic nerve. A.J.N.R., *4:* 169–174, 1983.

27. Reese, A. B. Expanding lesions of the orbit. Trans. Ophthalmol. Soc. U.K., *91:* 85–104, 1971.

28. Sibony, P. A., Krauss, H. R., Kennerdell, J. S., Maroon, J. C., and Slamovits, T. L. Optic nerve sheath meningiomas. Clinical manifestations. Ophthalmology (Suppl.): 66, 1983.

29. Trobe, J. D., Hood, C. I., Parsons, J. T., and Quislins, R. G. Intracranial spread of squamous carcinoma along with trigeminal nerve. Arch. Ophthalmol., *100:* 608–611, 1982.

30. Unsold, R., Safran, A. B., Safran, E., and Hoyt, W. F. Metastatic infiltration of nerves in the cavernous sinus. Arch. Neurol., *37:* 59–61, 1980.

31. Wright, J. E., Call, N. B., and Liaricos, S. Primary optic nerve meningioma. Br. J. Ophthalmol., *64:* 553–558, 1980.

32. Wright, J. E., McDonald, W. I., and Call, N. B. Management of optic nerve gliomas. Br. J. Ophthalmol., *64:* 545–552, 1980.

VII

Hydrocephalus

The Investigation of Hydrocephalus by Computed Tomography

DAVID G. McLONE, M.D., Ph.D., and THOMAS P. NAIDICH, M.D.

Hydrocephalus is nearly always associated with increased ventricular size. However, the precise relationships among the degree of ventriculomegaly, intracranial pressure, CSF pulse pressure, daily production of CSF, absorptive capacity for CSF, and patency of CSF flow ways remain both complex and obscure. From the often puzzling experimental data, there emerge two unifying themes that likely explain some of the clinical phenomena demonstrated by computed tomography. These are (a) the relative magnitude of the endoventricular pressure needed to activate CSF absorption vs. that needed to distend the ventricle, and (b) the amplitude of the CSF pulse pressure (20).

"ACTIVATION" PRESSURE AND "YIELD" PRESSURE

Experimental data suggest that resorption of CSF is zero, until CSF pressure exceeds a critical "opening" or "threshold" pressure. Above opening pressure, resorption of CSF increases nearly linearly with increasing pressure (27). Similarly, in experimental animals with obstructive hydrocephalus, the compensatory resorption of CSF by "alternate pathways" may not begin until ventricular pressure exceeds the "threshold" pressure that "activates" the compensatory pathways (24). Thereafter, the pressure necessary to *maintain* compensatory flow may decrease below the initial "activation pressure," even though the rate of compensatory flow remains high or increases. The compensatory pathways appear to divert the CSF to the lymphatic system of the neck (18).

Experimental data in man and animals also suggest that the degree of ventricular dilatation depends, in part, on the distensibility (compliance) of the brain, dura, and calvarium that surround and support the ventricle (1, 4, 7, 8, 10, 12, 15–17, 19, 24–31). Greater distensibility of the ventricular walls (*i.e.*, low yield pressure) is associated with more rapid ventricular enlargement, earlier cessation of ventricular enlargement, larger final ventricular size, more rapid decline in intraventricular pressure, and lower final pressure after compensation (4). Greater rigidity of the ventricular walls (*i.e.*, high yield pressure) is associated with slower

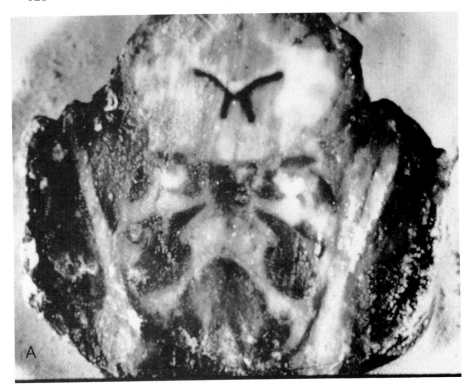

FIG. 26.1. Role of the skull and dura. Experimental feline hydrocephalus. Coronal sections. (*A*) Normal control. (*B*) Intact skull and dura. Kaolin-induced hydrocephalus compensated at enlarged ventricular size. (*C*) Skull and dura resected prior to instillation of kaolin. Marked, bilateral, nearly symmetrical ventriculomegaly attenuates the cerebral mantles. (*D*) Skull and dura resected unilaterally. Consequent asymmetrical ventriculomegaly and mantle attenuation. (Figs. *C* and *D* reproduced with permission from G. M. Hochwald *et al.* (12).)

ventricular enlargement, smaller final ventricular size, later decline in intraventricular pressure, and higher final pressure after compensation (4).

Taken together, these findings indicate that ventricular size may be determined, in part, by the relative magnitudes of the "activation" and "yield" pressures. Furthermore, the relative magnitude of these pressures will likely change over time as hydrocephalus distends the brain, the compensatory mechanisms are established, and the initially high intraventricular pressure falls toward normal. Simplistically, when the yield pressure necessary to distend the ventricle is lower than that needed to activate compensatory resorption of CSF by alternate pathways, the ventricles dilate remarkably, driving the brain, dura, and skull outward.

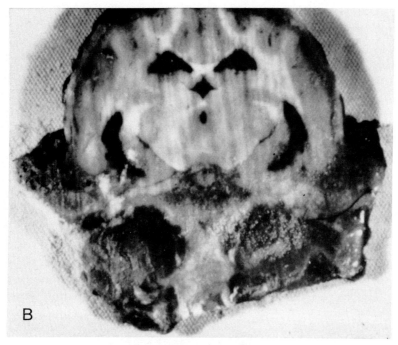

FIG. 26.1*B*

The structural changes induced then increase ventricular distensibility, so the lowered endoventricular pressure maintains the larger ventricular volume achieved (4).

In elegant experiments, Hochwald *et al.* (11, 12) demonstrated that the integrity of the skull and dura is a major factor in determining ventricular size (Fig. 26.1). These authors induced hydrocephalus in cats by injecting the sclerosing agent kaolin into the basal cisterns. Otherwise, normal cats responded to the kaolin by modest ventricular dilatation, mantle attenuation, and clinical signs of elevated pressure. Over time, the ventricular size stabilized, and the cats appeared clinically to have compensated hydrocephalus. Removal of the skull and dura from such compensated cats caused renewed progression of hydrocephalus with progression ventricular dilatation and progressive mantle attenuation. Removal of the skull and dura only unilaterally caused ventricular dilatation and mantle attenuation only on the side ipsilateral to the craniectomy-durectomy. Cats from which the skull and dura were re-sected prior to injection of kaolin did not stabilize their ventricular size, did not exhibit clinical compensation, and manifested progressive ventricular dilatation.

Clinical observation suggests that the cat, in which yield pressure is

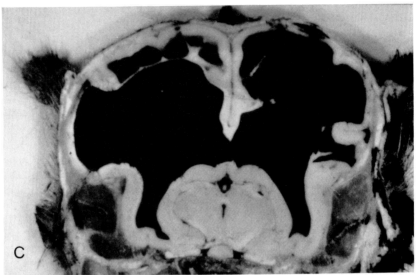

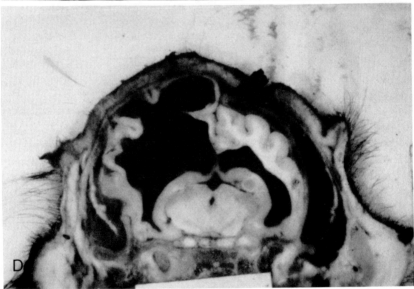

FIG. 26.1C and D

lowered by removal of the skull and dura, is a valid model for the human
neonate, in whom the sutures and fontanelles are open and mobile.
Common experience indicates that hydrocephalic infants with open
sutures and fontanelles usually exhibit far larger ventricles than do
children in whom hydrocephalus develops after the sutures close (Fig.

26.2). Infants with large encephaloceles typically exhibit greater dilatation of the portions of the ventricles and cisterns situated outside the calvarium than of those situated within. Hydrocephalic patients with focal brain damage, durectomy, or craniectomy that focally reduces ventricular yield pressure typically exhibit focally greater dilatation of the ventricles at that site. Thus, post-traumatic hydrocephalus is usually most marked at the site of trauma and/or surgical intervention. Post-meningitic hydrocephalus is usually greatest at the site(s) of concomitant encephalomalacia. Since most patients with hydrocephalus have greatest dilatation of the atria (21, 22), CT demonstration of hydrocephalus with greater dilatation of the frontal horns than of the atria suggests concomitant frontal encephalomalacia (Fig. 26.3).

Conversely, patients in whom severe cranial suture pansynostosis creates an exceedingly rigid skull with high yield pressure may exhibit deceptively little ventricular dilatation despite markedly elevated endoventricular pressure (Fig. 26.4) (22). Subsequent craniofacial reconstructions reduce yield pressure and may lead to remarkable ventricular

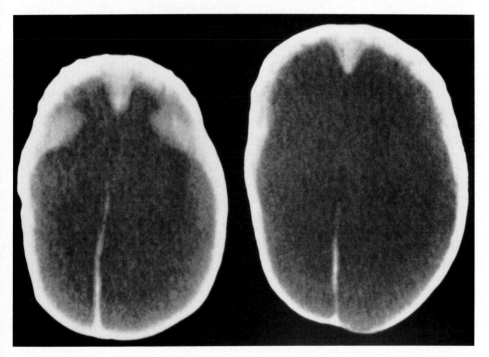

FIG. 26.2. (*A* and *B*) Very severe hydrocephalus. Patient, a 9-day-old girl, with congenital hydrocephalus, patent sutures, and open fontanelles. CT reveals large head, thin mantle, and bulging of brain and mantle at the fontanelle.

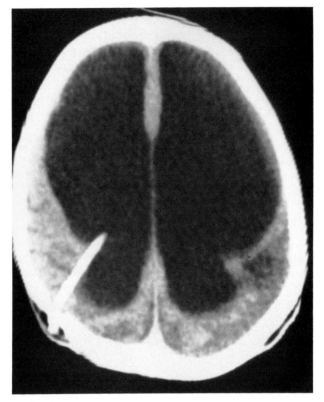

FIG. 26.3. Hydrocephalus following tuberculous meningitis. Post-mortem revealed encephalomalacia. Frontal mantle was reduced to fibrotic membranes less than 1 mm thick.

dilatation which is greatest at the site(s) of maximal release. Since shunting these ventricles after the craniofacial reconstruction may lead to ventricular collapse and "jumbling" of the calvarial fragments, it is our deliberate practice to shunt even mildly dilated ventricles prior to undertaking reconstruction procedures in these patients (22).

CSF PULSE PRESSURE

The systolic-diastolic variations of arterial pressure are transmitted to the CSF in damped form by the cerebral vasculature and the choroid plexus. The pressure waves generated by this CSF pulse appear to keep the ventricles open. In hydrocephalic animals, surgical resection of the choroid plexus from one lateral ventricle causes reduced size of that lateral ventricle (2). Prior resection of one choroid plexus (2) or prior ligation of the anterior choroidal artery to that ventricle (32) prevents later dilatation of the ventricle when hydrocephalus is induced experi-

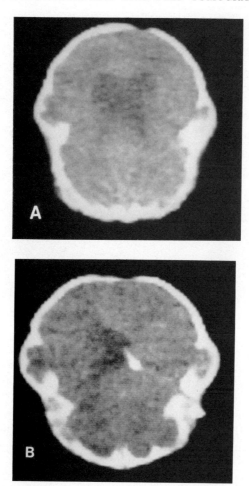

FIG. 26.4. Severe cranial pansynostosis. (A) Age, 3 days. Modest ventriculomegaly despite extremely high endoventricular pressure at shunt insertion. (B) Age, 7 days. Reduced ventricular size following shunt diversion of CSF. (C) Age, 3 months, following stage 1 craniodural release. Malfunction of the shunt is now associated with marked ventriculomegaly that is greatest at the sites of maximal release.

mentally. Measurements document lower CSF pulse pressure on the side of the arterial ligation (smaller ventricle) and increased difference between left and right ventricular pulse pressures as the mean CSF pressure rises (32).

In a classic experiment, DiRocco et al. (3) proved that a threefold increase in the amplitude of the CSF pulse pressure will cause rapid and substantial ventricular dilatation, even though the mean CSF pressure

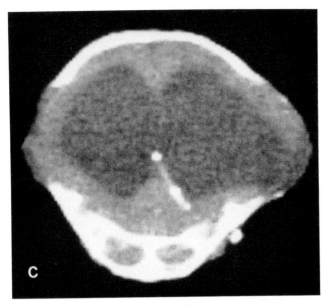

FIG. 26.4C

is kept normal, and all CSF flow ways are patent (Fig. 26.5). These scientists placed balloon catheters into the lateral ventricles of normal sheep and gaited rhythmic expansion and contraction of the balloon to the electrocardiogram. The balloon expanded in synchrony with the systolic pulse wave to augment the CSF pulse pressure threefold without changing mean CSF pressure. Within 3–8 hours, the lateral ventricles dilated. The ependyma became attenuated and separated from the underlying brain, and the brain became pathologically indistinguishable from that seen with "obstructive" hydrocephalus. Repetition of the experiment after obstruction of the ipsilateral foramen caused unilateral ventriculomegaly.

Since the volume and the arterial flow of the choroid plexus increase in patients with choroid plexus papilloma, it is possible that augmentation of the CSF pulse wave contributes to the hydrocephalus seen in such patients (27).

In vivo, the amplitude of the CSF pulse wave represents a balance between the force created by entry of arterial blood and the damping of that force by the simultaneous exit of venous blood and of CSF. The ventricular dilatation observed clinically in patients with patent CSF flow ways, but impaired egress of CSF or of venous blood is believed to result from the consequent increase in CSF pulse pressure. Since the

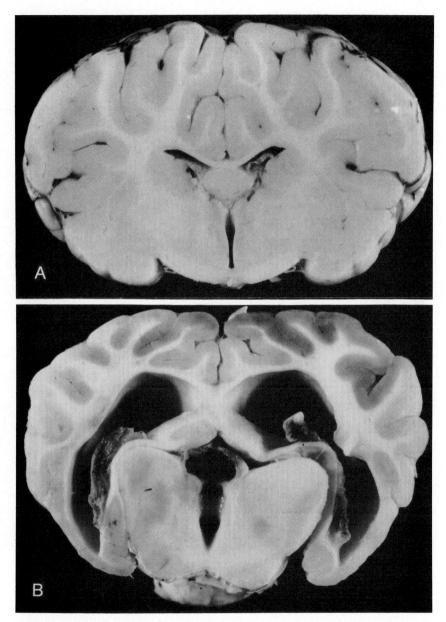

FIG. 26.5. Role of the CSF pulse pressure. Coronal sections of sheep brains. (A) Normal control. (B) Ventriculomegaly results from the increased amplitude of endoventricular CSF pulse pressure achieved by balloon augmentation.

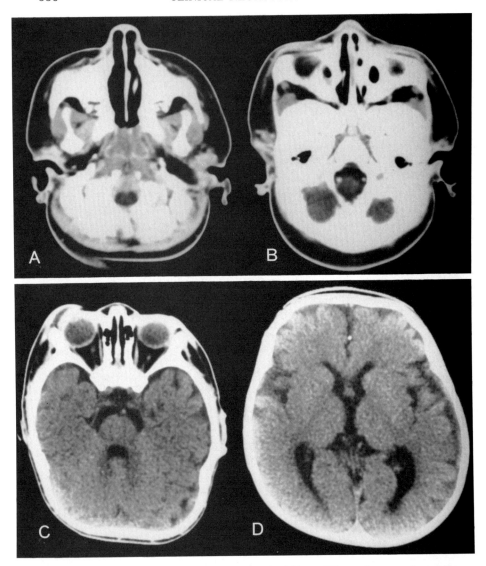

FIG. 26.6. (A–F) Achondroplasia in a 5-month-old boy. CT reveals narrowing of the foramen magnum, dilatation of the fourth, third, and lateral ventricles, and prominence of the subarachnoid cisterns.

amplitude of CSF pulse pressure rises rapidly, perhaps exponentially, with increasing mean intracranial pressure (10), a vicious cycle may ensue. Thus, patients with open cranial sutures and (*a*) bilateral jugular vein thrombosis, (*b*) superior vena cava obstruction, or (*c*) palliative cardiac procedures such as right pulmonary artery to superior vena cava

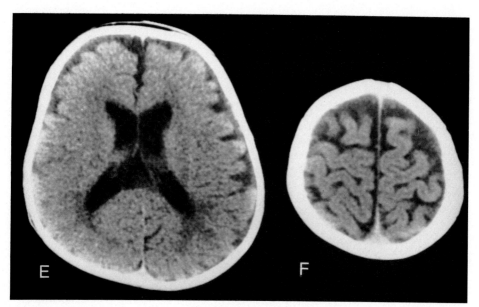

FIG. 26.6*E* and *F*

anastomoses (23) may develop ventricular dilatation, possibly on the basis of increased CSF pulse pressure. Patients with high-flow arteriovenous malformations may have ventricular dilatation on a similar basis.

As first described by Dandy, patients with achondroplasia commonly exhibit dilated ventricles and cisterns (Fig. 26.6) (9). In at least some of these patients, there is obstruction to venous outflow and elevated sagittal sinus pressure (9). This may result in elevated CSF pulse pressure in addition to elevation of the threshold pressure for CSF resorption.

Older patients with rigid "pipestem" basilar arteries or with aneurysms of the basilar tip also exhibit ventricular dilatation without obstruction to CSF flow ways (5, 6). Increased amplitude of CSF pulse pressure resulting from loss of the elastic damping of the pulse wave by the artery likely accounts for this ventricular dilatation.

Conversely, in animals and patients with lateral ventricular shunt catheters, the shunt-containing ventricle is often smaller than the contralateral ventricle, despite patent CSF flow ways (13, 14). Measurements of mean CSF pressure and of CSF pulse pressure show that the mean pressure is equal bilaterally but the pulse pressure is damped on the side of the shunt (13). Instantaneous egress of CSF via the shunt damps the CSF pulse pressure unilaterally, causing the smaller ventricular size.

By reference to these two mechanisms, (*a*) the relative magnitudes of activation and yield pressures, and (*b*) the amplitude of the CSF pulse pressure, it is possible to understand some of the changes observed daily on CT scans of our patients.

REFERENCES

1. Avezaat, J. J., Van Eijndhoven, J. H. M., and Wyper, D. J. Cerebrospinal fluid pulse pressure and intracranial volume-pressure relationships. J. Neurol. Neurosurg. Psychiatry, *42:* 687–700, 1979.
2. Bering, E. A. Circulation of the cerebrospinal fluid: Demonstration of the choroid plexuses as the generator of the force for flow of fluid and ventricular enlargement. J. Neurosurg., *19:* 405–413, 1962.
3. DiRocco, C., DiTrapani, G., Pettorossi, V. E., and Caldarelli, M. On the pathology of experimental hydrocephalus induced by artificial increase in endoventricular CSF pulse pressure. Child's Brain, *5:* 81–95, 1979.
4. Drapkin, A. J., and Sahar, A. Experimental hydrocephalus: Cerebrospinal fluid dynamics and ventricular distensibility during early stages. Child's Brain, *4:* 278–288, 1978.
5. Ekbom, K., and Greitz, T. Syndrome of hydrocephalus caused by saccular aneurysm of the basilar artery. Acta Neurochir., *24:* 71–77, 1971.
6. Ekbom, K., Greitz, T., and Kugelberg, E. Hydrocephalus due to ectasia of the basilar artery. J. Neurol. Sci., *8:* 465–477, 1969.
7. Ekstedt, J. CSF hydrodynamic studies in man. Normal hydrodynamic variables related to CSF pressure and flow. J. Neurol. Neurosurg. Psychiatry, *41:* 345–353, 1978.
8. Fridén, H. G., and Ekstedt, J. Volume/pressure relationship of the cerebrospinal space in humans. Neurosurgery, *13:* 351–366, 1983.
9. Friedman, W. A., and Mickle, J. P. Hydrocephalus in achondroplasia: A possible mechanism. Neurosurgery, *7:* 150–153, 1980.
10. Guinane, J. E. Cerebrospinal fluid pulse pressure and brain compliance in adult cats. Neurology, *25:* 559–564, 1975.
11. Hochwald, G. M., Epstein, F., Malhan, C., and Ransohoff, J. The relationship of compensated to decompensated hydrocephalus in the cat. J. Neurosurg., *39:* 694–697, 1973.
12. Hochwald, G. M., Epstein, F., Malhan, C., *et al.* The role of the skull and dura in experimental feline hydrocephalus. Dev. Med. Child Neurol., (Suppl.), *27:* 65–69, 1972.
13. Kaufman, B., Weiss, M. H., Young, H. F., *et al.* Effects of prolonged cerebrospinal fluid shunting on the skull and brain. J. Neurosurg., *38:* 288–297, 1973.
14. Linder, M., Diehl, J. L., and Sklar, F. H. Significance of post shunt ventricular asymmetries. J. Neurosurg., *55:* 183–186, 1981.
15. Lorenzo, A. V., Page, L. K., and Watters, G. V. Relationship between cerebrospinal fluid formation, absorption, and pressure in human hydrocephalus. Brain, *93:* 679–692, 1970.
16. Marmarou, A., Shulman, K., and LaMorgese, J. Compartmental analysis of compliance and outflow resistance of the cerebrospinal fluid system. J. Neurosurg., *43:* 523–534, 1975.
17. Marmarou, A., Shulman, K., and Rosende, R. A nonlinear analysis of the cerebrospinal fluid system and intracranial pressure dynamics. J. Neurosurg., *48:* 332–344, 1978.
18. McComb, J. G. Recent research into the nature of cerebrospinal fluid formation and absorption. J. Neurosurg., *59:* 369–383, 1983.
19. McComb, J. G., Davson, H., Hyman, S., and Weiss, M. H. Cerebrospinal fluid drainage as influenced by ventricular pressure in the rabbit. J. Neurosurg., *56:* 790–797, 1982.
20. Naidich, T. P. Pediatric hydrocephalus. I. Pathophysiologic basis for radiologic findings from weekly update. *Neurology/Neurosurgery,* 1984.

21. Naidich, T. P., Epstein, F., Lin, J. P., *et al.* Evaluation of pediatric hydrocephalus by computed tomography. Radiology, *119:* 337–345, 1976.

22. Naidich, T. P., Schott, L. H., and Baron, R. L. Computed tomography in evaluation of hydrocephalus. Radiol. Clin. North Am., *20:* 143–167, 1982.

23. Rosman, N. P., and Shands, K. N. Hydrocephalus caused by increased intracranial venous pressure: A clinicopathological study. Ann. Neurol., *3:* 445–450, 1978.

24. Sahar, A., Hochwald, G. M., Sadik, A. R., and Ransohoff, J. Cerebrospinal fluid absorption: In animals with experimental obstructive hydrocephalus. Arch. Neurol., *21:* 638–644, 1969.

25. Sato, K., Fuchinoue, T., and Yahagi, Y. CSF pulse wave changes in cases with normal pressure hydrocephalus. In: *Intracranial Pressure II*, edited by M. Lundberg, U. Ponten, and M. Brock, pp. 133–136. Springer-Verlag, New York, 1975.

26. Sklar, F. H., Beyer, C. W., and Clark, W. K. Physiological features of the pressure/volume function of brain elasticity in man. J. Neurosurg., *53:* 166–172, 1980.

27. Sklar, F. H., Beyer, C. W., Diehl, J. T., and Clark, W. K. Significance of the so-called absorptive reserve in communicating hydrocephalus: A preliminary report. Neurosurgery, *8:* 525–529, 1981.

28. Sklar, F. H., Diehl, J. T., Peyer, C. W., and Clark, W. K. Brain elasticity changes with ventriculomegaly. J. Neurosurg., *53:* 173–179, 1980.

29. Sklar, F. H., and Elashvili, I. The pressure/volume function of brain elasticity: Physiological considerations and clinical applications. J. Neurosurg., *47:* 670–679, 1977.

30. Sklar, F. H., Beyer, C. W., Ramanathan, M., *et al.* Servo-controlled lumbar infusions: A clinical tool for the determination of CSF dynamics as a function of pressure. Neurosurgery, *3:* 170–175, 1978.

31. Sklar, F. H., Beyer, C. W., Ramanathan, M., and Clark, W. K. Servo-controlled lumbar infusions in children: A quantitative approach to the problem of arrested hydrocephalus. J. Neurosurg., *52:* 87–98, 1980.

32. Wilson, C. B., Bertan, V. Interruption of the anterior choroidal artery in experimental hydrocephalus. Arch. Neurol., *17:* 614–619, 1967.

27

Magnetic Resonance Imaging *vs.* Computed Tomography: Advantages and Disadvantages

FRANKLIN EARNEST, IV, M.D., HILLIER L. BAKER, JR., M.D.,
DAVID B. KISPERT, M.D., and EDWARD R. LAWS, JR., M.D.

INTRODUCTION

Computed tomography (CT) has proved an accurate, cost-effective imaging modality since its introduction in 1972. CT quickly replaced pneumoencephalography for diagnosis of intracranial disorders and has reduced the use of plain film examinations of the head. Magnetic resonance imaging (MRI) has evolved as another method of imaging, employing the resonance phenomena exhibited by paramagnetic nucleons, particularly hydrogen, in a gradient magnetic field (9, 10, 17). MRI has several distinct advantages over x-ray-computed tomography. MRI avoids exposure to ionizing radiation, produces no artifacts referable to bone, and permits direct axial, sagittal, and coronal imaging.

Although early reports have suggested the sensitivity of MRI in the detection of brain and spinal cord lesions, comparative experience with existing modalities, particularly computed tomography, has been limited (2–4, 6, 7, 14, 20). MRI studies (788 of them), obtained for suspected diseases of the head or spine, were compared with other radiologic examinations. Sixty-two MRI examinations from this group demonstrated abnormalities not apparent on CT examination, and 11 CT examinations demonstrated abnormalities not apparent on MRI. These examinations were reviewed and correlated with clinical or surgical diagnosis, as well as the anatomic area examined, to determine sources of diagnostic error associated with each technique.

METHODS

The MRI examinations in this study were performed on a 0.15-Tesla, 4-coil, resistive magnetic resonance imager (Picker International) with a resonant frequency of 6.5 MHz. This system employs selective irradiation for slice determination, with nominal slice thicknesses of 5, 10, and 20 mm.

Partial saturation spin-echo (PSSE) images (1) employed a 90–180° pulse sequence with echo times (TE) of 40 milliseconds and repetition times (TR) of 200–650 milliseconds. Free induction decay (FID) images employed a sequence of repetitive 90° pulses with repetition times of 200–500 milliseconds. These sequences provide good spatial resolution and high contrast at tissue-fluid interfaces and were frequently used to image basal cisterns, the foramen magnum, and spinal cord.

Inversion recovery (IR) images employed (1) a 180–90° pulse sequence with inversion times (TI) of 400 milliseconds for normal brain and up to 800 milliseconds for evaluation of some pathologic lesions (particularly tumors), with repetition times (TR) of 2000 milliseconds. A refocusing 180° pulse was added in later IR sequences. Inversion recovery images provide good delineation of fat and cerebral white matter.

Spin-echo (SE) images (1) were obtained using a 90–180° pulse sequence with echo times (TE) of 60–120 milliseconds and repetition times (TR) of 2000 milliseconds. Spin-echo images provide good grey-white matter discrimination and exhibit excellent sensitivity to pathology (19).

Early studies used back-projection reconstruction with single-slice acquisition displayed on a 128 × 128 matrix, interpolated to 256 × 256. Later studies employed a multislice technique, using phase encoded or two-dimensional Fourier transform (2-DFT) reconstruction, routinely acquired on a 128 × 256 matrix, interpolated to 256 × 256.

Routine intracranial examinations obtained with a 30-cm head coil most commonly used a multislice spin-echo technique (TE 60 milliseconds, TR 2000 milliseconds), acquiring eight adjacent 10-mm slices with two averages, for a total acquisition time of 8.5 minutes and a processing time of 30 seconds/slice. Examinations of the spine, using a body coil (50 × 30 cm), commonly employed from 4 to 8 averages, at similar repetition times, requiring from 17 to 34 minutes for data acquisition.

Patients were questioned regarding pregnancy and the presence of aneurysm clips or a cardiac pacemaker, and informed consent was obtained prior to examination.

CT examinations, performed on GE 8800 (320 × 320 matrix) or GE 9800 (512 × 512 matrix) scanners, or recent CT examinations performed on comparable equipment from other institutions, were used for comparison.

MRI examinations (a total of 788) of the head or spine obtained in 772 patients were reviewed and compared with available radiologic examinations, particularly CT examinations. CT examinations were considered comparative studies if recently obtained on late-generation CT equipment. (Lesions associated with cerebral infarction were only compared if MR and CT examinations were obtained within 24 hours of each other.) Sixty-two patients had abnormal magnetic resonance (MR) examinations and normal CT examinations. Eleven patients had abnormal CT examinations and normal MRI examinations. These examinations were correlated with clinical or surgical diagnosis and, often, subsequent imaging studies. Based on this correlation and subsequent follow-up, the cases were classified into four groups: (a) false-positive CT examinations; (b) false-negative CT examinations; (c) false-positive MR examinations; and (d) false-negative MR examinations. Examinations in each group were reviewed again to determine possible sources of diagnostic error and to compare the relative advantages and disadvantages of each modality.

RESULTS

Five negative MR examinations from a total of 778 MR examinations (0.6%) of the head or spine reviewed in this study were classified as having false-positive CT examinations (Table 27.1). These errors, frequently due to bone artifact, lacked appropriate clinical findings, and MR failed to confirm the presence of an abnormality. CT artifacts most often appeared in the posterior fossa between the petrous bones (Fig. 27.1) or along the floor of the posterior or middle cranial fossa (Fig. 27.2).

Fifty-nine of 778 MR examinations (7.5%) were positive and were associated with a contemporary negative CT examination. Based upon positive MR studies in association with appropriate clinical and/or laboratory findings (Table 27.1), these CT studies were regarded as false-negative. Forty-nine of these patients had clinical findings and MR lesions attributable to multiple sclerosis, and six patients had typical findings of Chiari malformation, associated with hydromyelia (Fig. 27.3) in three cases. Two of the patients had vascular lesions, one due to lateral

TABLE 27.1

Computed Tomography

5 False-Positive Examinations:
5/788 (0.6%)

No. of exams	Errors or Undetected Lesions
3	Bone artifact, posterior fossa
1	Bone artifact, middle fossa
1	Misinterpretation of prominent jugular bulb

59 False-Negative Examinations:
59/788 (7.5%)

No. of exams	Errors or Undetected Lesions
49	Multiple sclerosis
6	Chiari malformation
2	Vascular disease (lateral sinus thrombosis, cerebellar infarction)
1	Astrocytoma (medulla)
1	Temporal lobe seizures (perivascular edema)

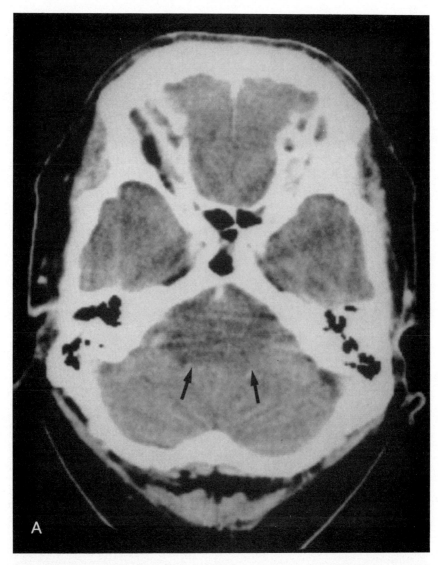

FIG. 27.1. Contrast-enhanced CT image (*A*) through the pons suggested the presence of a low attenuation mass lesion (*arrows*). A midline sagittal inversion recovery MR image (*b*) through the brain stem demonstrated no abnormality.

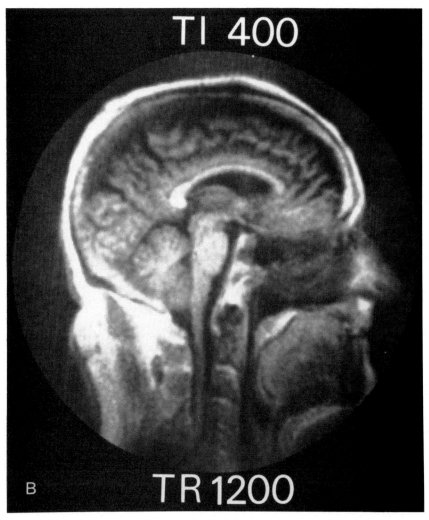

FIG. 27.1*B*

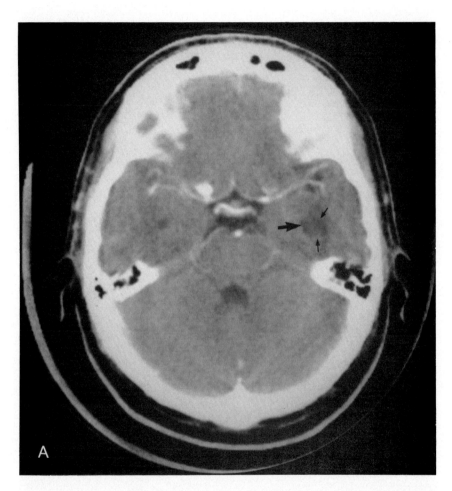

FIG. 27.2. Contrast-enhanced CT image (*A*) demonstrated a well-circumscribed area of low attenuation in the left temporal lobe (*arrows*). (*B*) Coronal inversion recovery MR image through the temporal lobes demonstrated no abnormality.

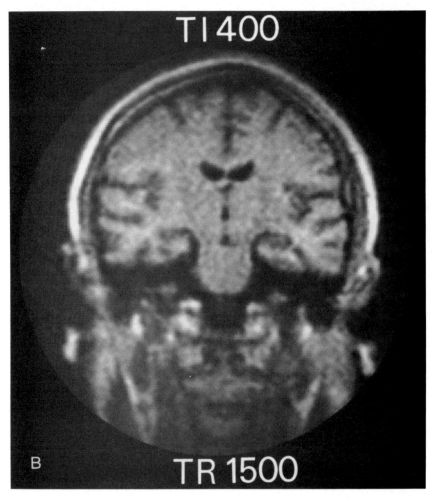

Fig. 27.2*B*

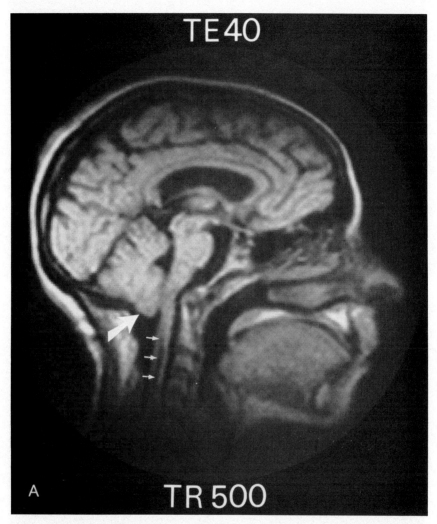

FIG. 27.3. Midline sagittal saturation recovery MR image of the head (*A*) demonstrated a Chiari malformation (adult form) with tonsillar herniation (*large arrow*) and associated hydromyelia (*small arrows*). Midline, sagittal, partial saturation spin-echo MR image of the thoracic cord (*B*), demonstrated that the hydromyelia (*arrows*) extended throughout the thoracic spinal cord.

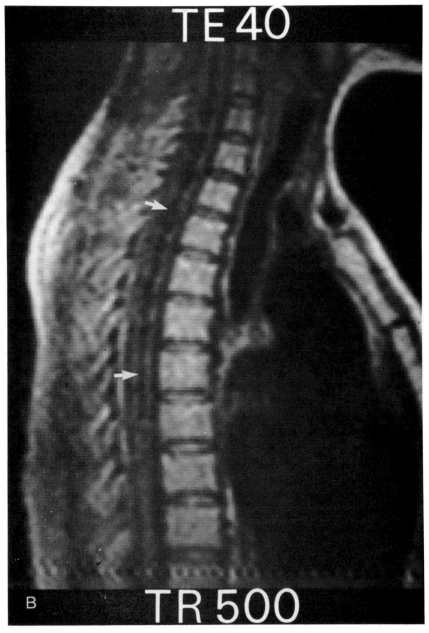

Fig. 27.3B

sinus thrombosis and one due to cerebellar infarction. One patient had a small astrocytoma arising from the posterior surface of the medulla that was undetected on two previous CT examinations, one using intravenous contrast and the other using intrathecal contrast in the basal cisterns (Fig. 27.4). One patient with a longstanding right temporal lobe seizure disorder had numerous negative CT examinations. A coronal MR examination of the head revealed increased signal arising from the right temporal pole (Fig. 27.5). Subsequent temporal lobectomy demonstrated a focal perivascular edema, but no neoplasm was found.

Three of 778 MR examinations (0.4%) were classified as false-positive MR studies (Table 27.2). In one patient, cerebral atrophy present on IR images was not substantiated on SE images or CT examination. One patient felt to have an extra-axial mass at the foramen magnum on MR had subsequent conventional complex motion tomography and CT demonstrating bony asymmetry of the foramen magnum (Fig. 27.6). Another patient had the central artifact projected over the midbrain on SE images misinterpreted as a lesion, which was unsubstantiated by IR images or CT.

Six of 778 MR examinations (0.8%) were classified as false-negative studies (Table 27.2). In three of these examinations, MR failed to detect disc herniations, which were well demonstrated on postmyelographic metrizamide CT examinations (Fig. 27.7). Two patients had lesions of the brain stem without mass effect, one densely calcified, which were undetected on MR images obtained in multiple planes through the lesions (Figs. 27.8 and 27.9). One patient had cerebellar degeneration and atrophy missed on SE images of the head that were well demonstrated on previous CT studies (Fig. 27.10).

These errors, classified by anatomic location, are listed in Table 27.3. CT errors were most often related to white matter lesions of the cerebral hemispheres in patients clinically felt to have demyelinating diseases and to beam hardening or streak artifacts referable to bone about the skull base, posterior fossa, and foramen magnum. MR errors involved evaluation of the spinal epidural space, atrophy of the cerebral and cerebellar cortex, and several lesions in the brain stem.

DISCUSSION

The strength of the signal depicted in proton magnetic resonance images depends on four parameters (13). First is the concentration of mobile hydrogen nuclei, or nuclear spin density, of tissues. This concentration varies little in biologic soft tissues; therefore, variation of nuclear spin density does not appear to be the primary determinant of contrast differences between soft tissues (15).

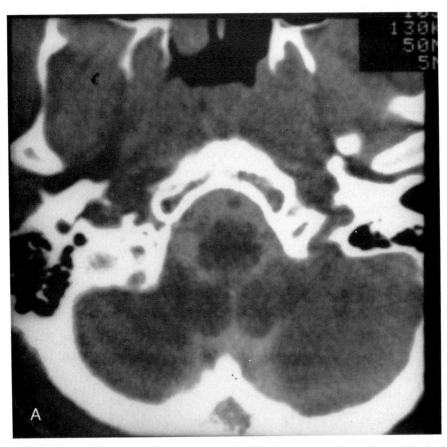

FIG. 27.4. A metrizamide CT cisternogram (*A*) failed to demonstrate an abnormality in this 32-year-old man with medullary signs. A small, low grade astrocytoma (*arrow*), demonstrated by axial spin-echo MR examinations (*B*), was surgically removed.

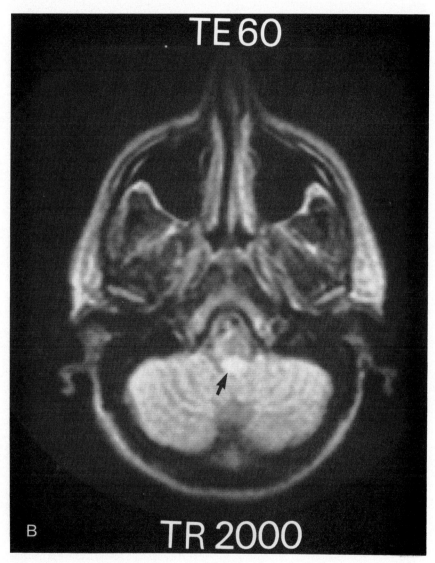

FIG. 27.4*B*

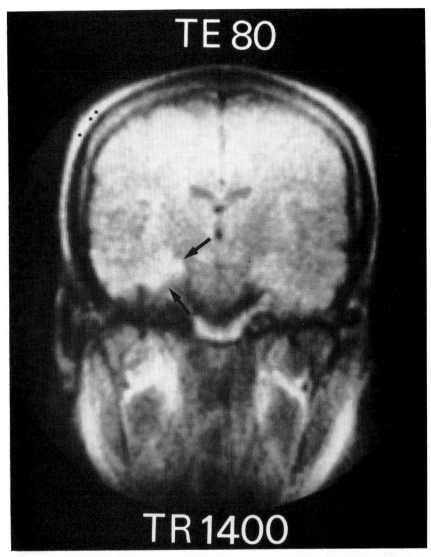

FIG. 27.5. MR examination demonstrated increased signal on a coronal, spin-echo image of the temporal lobes (*arrows*) in a woman with temporal lobe seizures. Previous CT examinations were normal. Perivascular edema was verified histologically after temporal lobectomy. No neoplasm was identified.

TABLE 27.2

Magnetic Resonance Imaging

3 False-Positive Examinations: 3/788 (0.4%)	
No. of exams	Errors or Undetected Lesions
1	Atrophy overestimated on IR images
1	Asymmetry of foramen magnum called mass
1	MR artifact misinterpreted as a lesion
6 False-Negative Examinations: 6/778 (0.8%)	
No. of exams	Errors or Undetected Lesions
3	Disc herniations (C6, L4, L5)
2	Indeterminate brain stem lesions, Ca^{2+} (?thrombosed vascular malformations)
1	Atrophy missed on SE images

Spin-lattice (T1) and spin-spin (T2) relaxation times are two parameters largely responsible for the relative differences in signal intensity within different soft tissues (15). T1 represents the exponential time constant of energy dissipation to adjacent molecules in the so-called lattice, a term describing the organization of the chemical milieu about the resonant nucleon. T2 is an exponential time constant describing the loss of phase coherence between adjacent nucleons, which is a measure of local inhomogeneities in the magnetic field on a molecular level. These parameters seem sensitive to the state of water in biologic tissues. Although the precise changes represented by alterations in relaxation times are not well understood, it is believed to be a relative shift in the proportion of bound water to free water, with the latter increasing in and around many pathologic processes, including inflammatory, ischemic, and neoplastic lesions (13, 15).

The last parameter significantly influencing signal strength is flow. Fluids passing through the sensitive plane of the MRI slice can be seen to have either increased or decreased signal strength, depending on the radiofrequency (RF) pulse sequence used and the velocity of flow through the imaging plane. These properties can be employed to both detect and measure flow (8).

Magnetic resonance imaging sequence must be carefully selected to avoid potential interpretive errors. Each sequence can be useful in a particular setting to answer a specific clinical question. Spin-echo images with relatively long repetition times provide a sensitive technique for detecting most lesions within the brain and spinal cord (19). Although there are few instances where MR findings have been specific, the sensitivity of MR using SE sequences was well demonstrated in the large

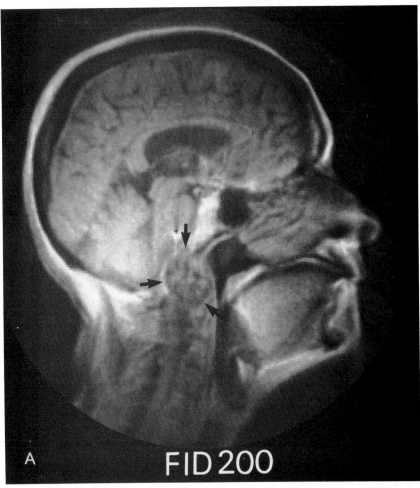

FIG. 27.6. Midline sagittal free induction decay MR image (A) in an elderly woman with rheumatoid arthritis suggested a mass (arrows) involving the skull base anterior to the foramen magnum. An axial MR image (B) verified this abnormality (arrows) and was accompanied by possible displacement of the medulla (curved arrow). Axial CT examination (C) and plain films of the craniovertebral junction demonstrated asymmetry of the foramen magnum (arrows) and rotatory subluxation at the atlantooccipital articulation. No mass was identified.

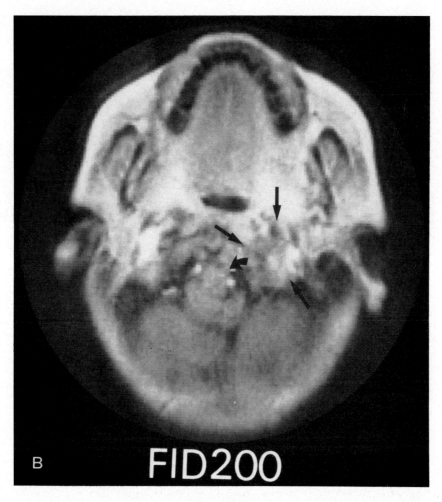

Fig. 27.6*B*

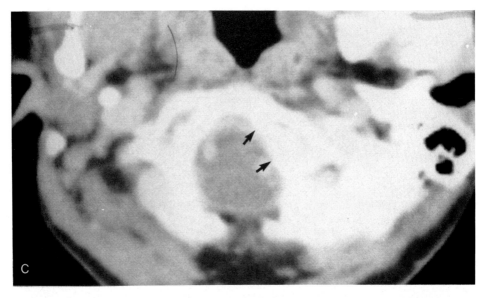

FIG. 27.6C

group of patients with multiple sclerosis in this study and in previous reports (11, 18, 19). Because of this high sensitivity, SE sequences have been employed as survey or screening examinations. Images acquired using PSSE or FID sequences with short repetition times show little relative contrast between soft tissues, but the resultant suppression of signal from cerebrospinal fluid (long T1 relaxation time) provides excellent delineation of the soft tissue-fluid interfaces about the ventricular system, and intracranial and intraspinal subarachnoid spaces. Sequences with short repetition times permit a greater number of averages to be obtained at each data point without the penalty of prolonged examination times, thus increasing the signal-to-noise ratio and improving resolution. These sequences are useful in evaluating patients with Chiari malformation, hydrosyringomyelia, and atrophy or focal enlargement of the brain or spinal cord (16). We have obtained a midline sagittal PSSE image as a part of our routine screening head examination.

IR sequences have been used both to depict white matter lesions and to investigate the internal structure of neoplastic lesions using long inversion times. The findings of prolonged T2 and short T1 relaxation times within a lesion have been associated with hemorrhage (7), and this paradoxical change represents an MR finding specific for hemorrhage.

This study demonstrates a greater sensitivity of MR in the evaluation of the brain. CT examinations in this study were erroneous in over 8% of cases for indicating the presence or absence of intracranial or intra-

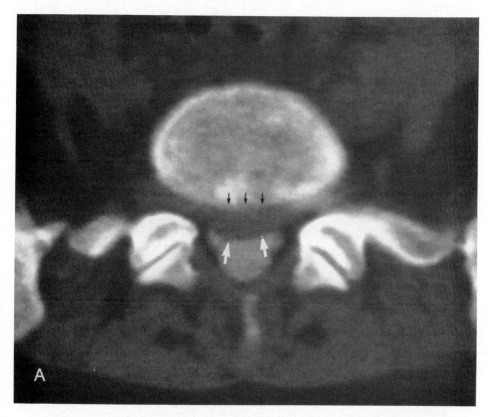

FIG. 27.7. A metrizamide-enhanced axial CT image just below the lumbosacral interspace (*A*) revealed a large, midline disc herniation (*white arrows*), displacing the opacified dural sac from the posterior margin of the vertebral body (*small arrows*). Midline sagittal saturation recovery MR image of the lower lumbar spine (*B*) failed to demonstrate this lesion.

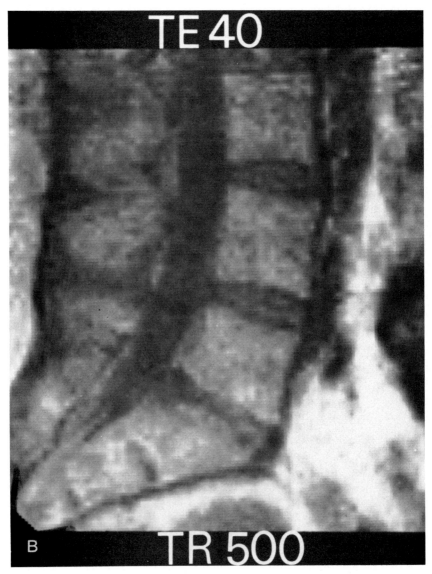

FIG. 27.7B

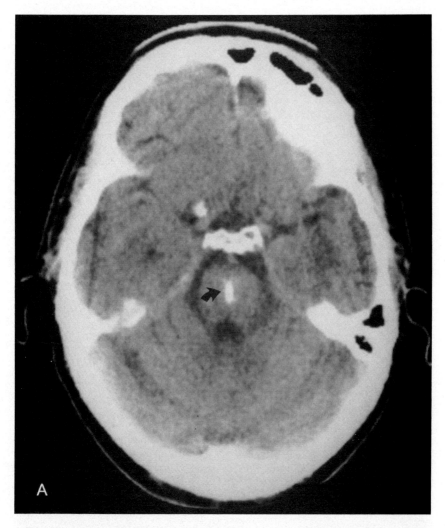

FIG. 27.8. An unenhanced, axial CT image (*A*) revealed a calcified mass in the upper pons (*curved arrow*). Slight enhancement was noted anteriorly (*B*) after administering contrast intravenously. Axial inversion recovery MR image through the upper pons (*C*) demonstrated symmetric pontine atrophy, but the calcified lesion could not be detected. Vertebral angiography demonstrated no abnormality.

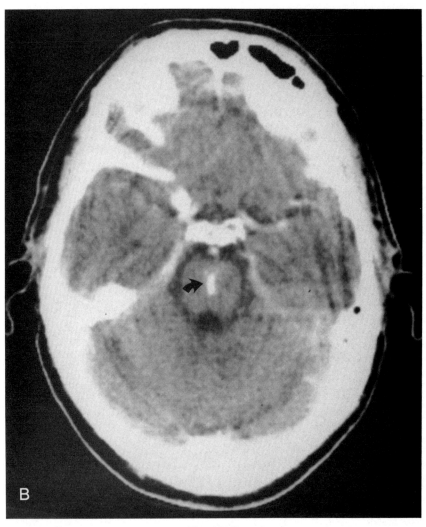

FIG. 27.8*B*

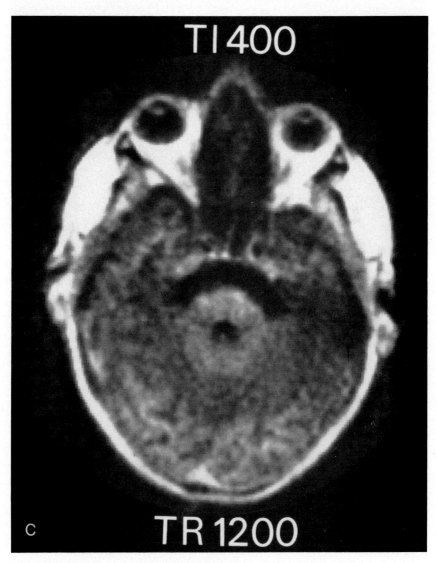

FIG. 27.8*C*

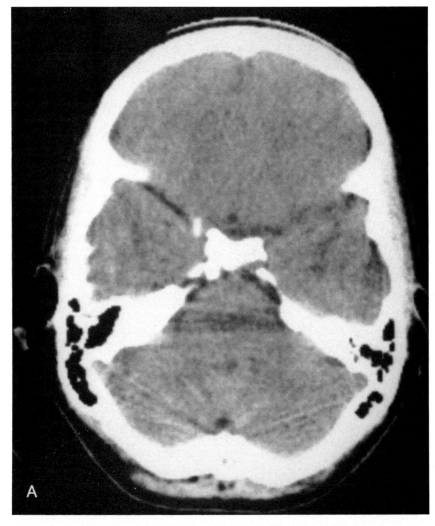

FIG. 27.9. Axial CT images through the pons before (A) and after (B) contrast enhancement demonstrated a small area of pathologic contrast enhancement (arrow). Vertebral angiography demonstrated no abnormality. Spin-echo MR examination of the pons in axial (C) and coronal (D) planes failed to demonstrate this lesion.

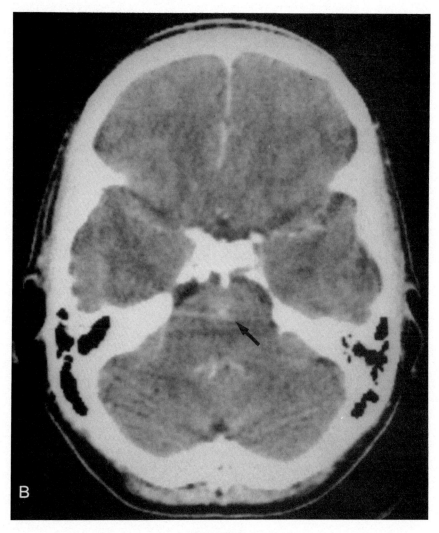

B

Fig. 27.9*B*

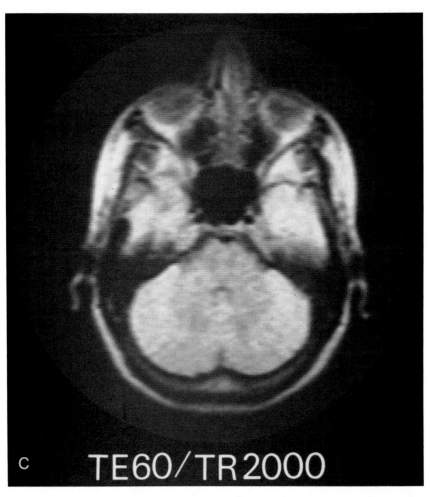

FIG. 27.9C

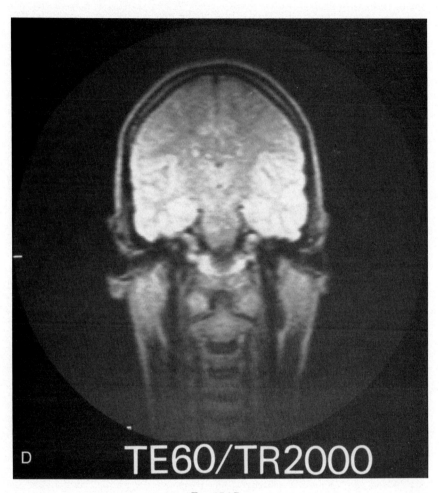

FIG. 27.9*D*

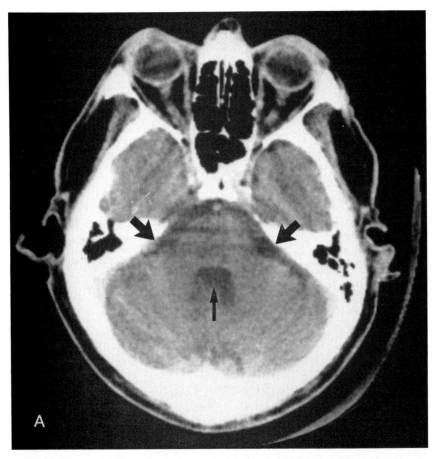

FIG. 27.10. An axial CT image through the posterior fossa (A) demonstrated enlargement of the cerebellopontine angle cisterns (*large arrows*), enlargement of the 4th ventricle (*small arrow*), and prominence of the cerebellar folia in an older man with cerebellar signs and presumed primary cerebellar degeneration. CT images through the cerebral hemispheres showed little cerebral atrophy (B). Midline sagittal saturation recovery MR image (C) shows enlargement of the 4th ventricle, but coronal spin-echo examination of the cerebellum failed to demonstrate cerebellar atrophy (D).

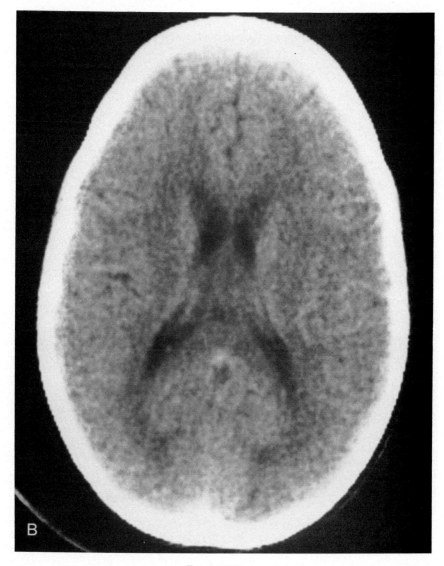

Fig. 27.10*B*

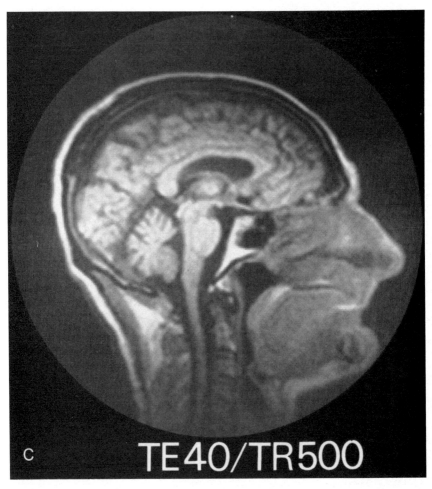

FIG. 27.10C

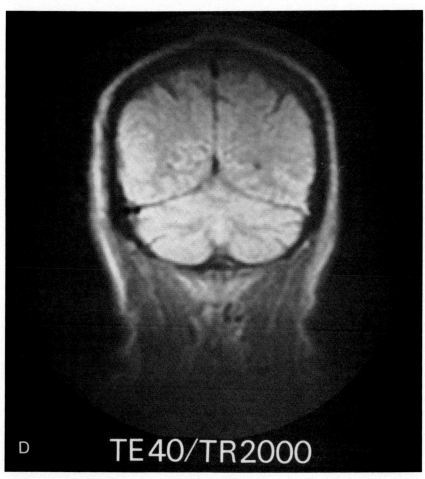

Fig. 27.10*D*

TABLE 27.3

Errors by Anatomic Location

Computed Tomography: 64/788 (8.1%)	
No. of exams	Location
49	White matter of cerebrum, cerebellum, and brain stem
13	Posterior fossa, foramen magnum
2	Middle fossa
Magnetic Resonance Imaging: 9/788 (1.1%)	
No. of exams	Location
3	Spine, epidural
3	Brain stem (Ca^{2+}, thrombus, artifact)
2	Cerebral, cerebellar cortex
1	Foramen magnum

spinal disease. The most common deficiency of CT was in the detection of small white matter lesions associated with multiple sclerosis. Previous studies have indicated the utility of MR in evaluation of such patients (11, 18). Although our studies of the spinal cord in patients thought to have myelopathy due to demyelinating disease have rarely demonstrated lesions within the spinal cord, examination of the brain has frequently demonstrated periventricular lesions associated with multiple sclerosis. Misinterpretation of beam hardening artifacts, associated with the bony structures of the posterior fossa, foramen magnum, and spine, has proved to be the second most frequent error associated with CT.

MRI shows great promise in early and accurate detection of cerebral ischemia and edema (5, 7, 20). Previous studies have emphasized the value of MRI in the delineation of brain stem and cerebellar infarction. Few studies have specified the temporal relationship between the MR and CT examinations compared in cerebral infarction. We have noted superior detection and delineation of cerebral infarction on MR studies obtained one or more days after a negative CT examination. Further clinical evaluation of MR in early stroke is needed.

False-positive MR examinations were related to interpretive errors and were found in only 3 of 778 examinations. These errors were associated with artifact, unusual bony anatomy, or the evaluation of atrophy with inappropriate MR sequences which failed to optimize contrast between brain and cerebrospinal fluid, and these errors will hopefully be reduced with greater experience. The skull base and other bony structures will probably remain an occasional source of error in MR interpretation.

In reviewing the false-negative MR examinations, it was apparent that the MR equipment and techniques used in this study failed to identify lumbar or cervical disc herniation in the few patients referred for comparative examination. Similar difficulties have been previously reported by Modic and co-workers (12). CT has the advantage of fine spatial resolution in the examination of high contrast interfaces (soft tissue/ bone/fat) and the ability to obtain oblique angles in the plane of the intervertebral space. The development and use of similar oblique image acquisition with MR may facilitate the diagnosis of disc herniation in the future.

Calcified lesions which are missed may represent a more difficult problem for MR imaging (3, 4, 7, 14, 20). Cortical hamartomas in patients with tuberous sclerosis were better demonstrated by MR than CT, but diagnostic periventricular calcifications were not demonstrated at all. We have now examined four lesions in the brain stem, with increased CT attenuation, which have been poorly demonstrated or undetected by PSSE, IR, and single-echo pulse sequence techniques. These lesions demonstrated CT attenuation values which varied from slightly greater than those of brain to high attenuation values associated with dense calcification. Vertebral angiography in these patients has demonstrated no angiographic abnormality. We have made a presumptive diagnosis of thrombosed vascular malformation, and these patients are being followed. We have previously noted a signal intensity in thrombus which is similar to that of normal brain (4, 9), and we suspect that thrombosed vascular malformations may be difficult to detect, especially using single-echo MR sequences. Multiecho sequences should detect lesions which were undetected using single-echo data acquisition.

Magnetic resonance imaging of the brain and spinal cord was superior to CT in lesion detection and was associated with fewer false-positive examinations attributable to artifact. It should be used as a screening examination in patients with suspected abnormalities of the central nervous system, unless contraindicated due to the presence of a cardiac pacemaker or intracranial aneurysm clips or pregnancy. Patients who are unable to remain immobile for MR examination should be examined by CT.

Lesions associated with calcification, thrombus, or adjacent to the skull base may be missed or incompletely evaluated by MR (3, 14). The use of MR in the initial evaluation of epidural disease, particularly disc herniation, is probably limited at this time.

SUMMARY

Magnetic resonance imaging (MRI) of the head and spine exceeds the sensitivity of computed tomography (CT) in detecting parenchymal lesions of the brain and spinal cord. MRI should be employed as a screening examination, particularly in patients suspected of having demyelinating diseases. CT continues to be the imaging technique of choice in evaluation of trauma, accurately depicting bony abnormalities and intracranial hemorrhage in evaluation of the spinal column and suspected disc herniation and in uncooperative patients.

REFERENCES

1. Axel, L., Margulis, A. R., and Meaney, T. F. Glossary of NMR Terms. American College of Radiology, 1983.
2. Bradley, W. G., Jr., Waluch, V., Yadley, R. A., and Wycoff, R. R. Comparion of CT and MR in 400 patients with suspected disease of the brain and cervical spinal cord. Radiology, 152: 695–702, 1984.
3. Brant-Zawadzki, M., Badami, J. P., Mills, C. M., Norman, D., and Newton, T. H. Primary intracranial tumor imaging: A comparison of magnetic resonance and CT. Radiology, 150 (2): 435–440, 1984.
4. Brant-Zawadzki, M., Davis, P. L., Crooks, L. E., Mills, C. M., Norman, D., Newton, T. H., Sheldon, P., and Kaufman, L. NMR demonstration of cerebral abnormalities: Comparison with CT. A.J.R., 140(5): 847–854, 1983.
5. Buonanno, F. S., Pykett, I. L., Brady, T. J., Vielma, J., Burt, C. T., Goldman, M. R., Hinshaw, W. S., Pohost, G. M., and Kistler, J. P. Proton NMR imaging in experimental ischemic infarction. Stroke 14(2): 178–184, 1983.
6. Bydder, G. M., Steiner, R. E., Thomas, D. J., Marshall, J., Gilderdale, D. J., and Young, I. R. Nuclear magnetic resonance imaging of the posterior fossa: 50 cases. Clin. Radiol, 34(2): 173–188, 1983.
7. Bydder, G. M., Steiner, R. E., Young, I. R., Hall, A. S., Thomas, D. J., Marshall, J., Pallis, C. A., and Legg, N. J. Clinical NMR imaging of the brain: 140 cases. A.J.R., 139(2): 215–236, 1982.
8. Crooks, L. E., Mills, C. M., Davis, P. L., Brant-Zawadzki, Hoenninger, J., Arakawa, M., Watts, J., and Kaufman, L. Visualization of cerebral and vascular abnormalities by NMR imaging. The effects of imaging parameters on contrast. Radiology, 144: 843–852, 1982.
9. Doyle, F. H., Gore, J. C., Pennock, J. M., Bydder, G. M., Orr, J. S., Steiner, R. E., Young, I. R., Burl, M., Clow, H., Gilderdale, D. J., Bailes, D. R., and Walters, P. E. Imaging of the brain by nuclear magnetic resonance. Lancet, 2(8237): 53–57, 1981.
10. Holland, G. N., Moore, W. S., and Hawkes, R. C. Nuclear magnetic resonance tomography of the brain. J. Comput. Assist. Tomogr., 4(1): 1–3, 1980.
11. Lukes, S. A., Crooks, L. E., Aminoff, M. J., Kaufman, L., Panitch, H. S., Mills, C., and Norman, D. Nuclear magnetic resonance imaging in multiple sclerosis. Ann. Neurol., 13(6): 592–601, 1983.
12. Modic, M. T., Weinstein, M. A., Pavlicek, W., Starnes, D. L., Duchesneau, P. M., Boumphrey, F., and Hardy, R. J., Jr. Nuclear magnetic resonance imaging of the spine. Radiology, 148(3): 757–762, 1983.
13. Pykett, I. L., Newhouse, J. H., Buonanno, F. S., Brady, T. J., Goldman, M. R., Kistler, J. P., and Pohost, G. M. Principles of nuclear magnetic resonance imaging (review). Radiology, 143(1): 157–168, 1982.
14. Randell, C. P., Collins, A. G., Young, I. R., Haywood, R., Thomas, D. J., McDonnell, M. J., Orr, J. S., Bydder, G. M., and Steiner, R. E. Nuclear magnetic resonance imaging of posterior fossa tumors. A.J.R., 141(3): 489–496, 1983.
15. Wehrli, F. W., MacFall, J. R., Shutts, D., Breger, R., and Herfkens, R. J. Mechanisms of contrast in NMR imaging. J. Comput. Assist. Tomogr., 8(3): 369–380, 1984.

16. Yeates, A., Brant-Zawadzki, M., Norman, D., Kaufman, L., Crooks, L. E., and Newton, T. H. Nuclear magnetic resonance imaging of syringomyelia. A.J.N.R., *4*(3): 234–237, 1983.

17. Young, I. R., Burl, M., Clark, G. J., Hall, A. S., Pasmore, T., Collins, A. G., Smith, D. T., Orr, J. S., Bydder, G. M., Doyle, F. H., Greenspan, R. H., and Steiner, R. E. Magnetic resonance properties of hydrogen: Imaging the posterior fossa. A.J.R., *137*(5): 895–901, 1981.

18. Young, I. R., Hall, A. S., Pallis, C. A., Legg, N. J., Bydder, G. M., and Steiner, R. E. Nuclear magnetic resonance imaging of the brain in multiple sclerosis. Lancet, *2*(8255): 1063–1066, 1981.

19. Young, I. R., Randell, C. P., Kaplan, P. W., James, A., Bydder, G. M., and Steiner, R. E. Nuclear magnetic resonance imaging in white matter disease of the brain using spin-echo sequences. J. Comput. Assist. Tomogr., *7*(2): 290–294, 1983.

20. Zimmerman, R. A., Bilaniuk, L. T., Goldberg, H. I., Grossman, R. I., Levine, R. S., Lynch, R., Edelstein, W., Bottomley, P., and Redington, R. Cerebral NMR imaging: Early results with a 0.12 T resistive system. A.J.R., *141*(6): 1187–1193, 1983.

Ultrasonic Diagnosis of Fetal and Neonatal Hydrocephalus

MICHAEL L. MANCO-JOHNSON, M.D., and
DOLORES H. PRETORIUS, M.D.

Diagnostic ultrasound imaging capability has improved dramatically since the 1970s. With the advent of grey scale, real-time, high frequency, portable systems, ultrasound has become the primary diagnostic modality in evaluating the neonatal brain and the only imaging modality successful in imaging the fetal brain routinely. Neurosurgeons trained during the days of A-mode echoencephalography still remember the bad name ultrasound achieved in the attempt to demonstrate the midline echo and determine if there was a midline shift. One must forget those archaic times and realize we are now talking about cross-sectional imaging of the brain in multiple projections, with high resolution ultrasound resulting in images which parallel the detail seen with computed tomography (CT).

The diagnosis of hydrocephalus, whether in the fetus or neonate, is dependent upon a firm understanding of normal brain anatomy and developmental changes. We will begin with the evaluation of the fetus and then extend this into the neonate.

With modern equipment, fetal intracranial anatomy can be visualized in great detail and at a relatively early gestational age. At 14–15 weeks gestation (menstrual age) the lateral ventricles can be identified. At this time they are relatively large, occupying most of the cerebral hemisphere. The choroid plexus nearly fills the ventricle (Fig. 28.1). With advancing gestation the ventricles decrease in size relative to the cerebral hemisphere. This is felt to represent the rapid growth of the diencephalon (including the lateral ventricles) in the early 15–18 weeks of gestation and then later catch-up growth of the telencephalon (cerebral hemispheres) after 20 weeks.

Comparison of the width of the lateral ventricle to the width of the hemisphere is a reproducible and relatively easy measurement made best on an axial scan through the body of the lateral ventricles. The lateral walls of the lateral ventricles are identified as parallel lines, equidistant from the interhemispheric fissure on the axial scan (Fig. 28.2). The medial walls of the lateral ventricles are occasionally identified. An

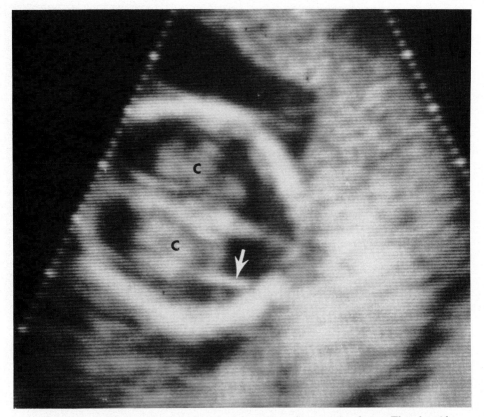

FIG. 28.1. Axial scan through fetal brain at 14 weeks gestational age. The choroid plexuses (*C*) are echogenic and nearly fill the lateral ventricles bilaterally. The lateral wall of the lateral ventricle is denoted by the *arrow*.

echogenic structure is usually identified within the lateral ventricles which is the choroid plexus. The choroid plexus is particularly prominent earlier in gestation and becomes less prominent as the fetus reaches term; this prominence (during 8–22 weeks) may be due to glycogen deposits within the choroid which may be necessary to provide an extra energy source for brain development (6). A range of normal ventricular measurements has been identified by several authors by relating ventricular width to hemispheric width (7, 15, 16). In our department, the lateral ventricular width (LVW) is measured from the middle of the midline echo to the lateral wall of the lateral ventricle at the point where the ventricular walls parallel the midline (Fig. 28.2). The hemispheric width (HW) is taken on the same scan from the middle of the midline echo to the inner table of the calvarium. The LVW-HW ratio (LVR) is calculated

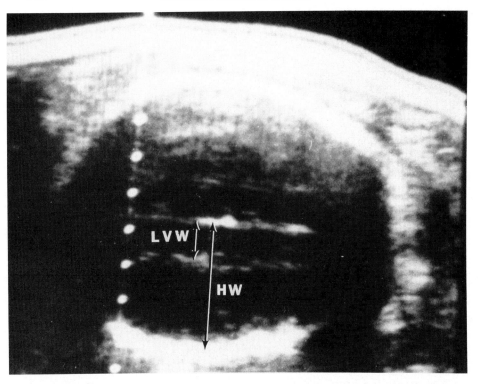

FIG. 28.2. Axial scan through the fetal brain of a 31-week gestation at the level of the lateral ventricles. The bright linear echo in the middle of the skull arises from the intrahemispheric fissure, and the lateral ventricular width (*LVW*) is measured from the midline echo to the lateral wall of the lateral ventricle. The hemispheric width (*HW*) is measured from the midline echo to the inner table of the skull. The lateral ventricular ratio is determined by dividing the LVW by the HW.

and compared to a table of values developed in our department from a study of 196 normal fetuses (Fig 28.3) (19). The LVR is much higher early in pregnancy, reaching as high as 0.71 (average 0.56) at about 15 weeks gestational age; the ratio gradually decreases to an average of 0.28 at term. This gradual decrease in the LVR is consistent with the rapid growth of the cerebral hemispheres that occurs as pregnancy proceeds. The ventricles appear to reach their maximum normal dimension of 1.1 cm by 25 weeks, and after that time there is only growth of the cerebral hemispheres (telencephalon) which increases the fetal biparietal diameter. As such, the ratio of ventricle to brain diameter decreases rapidly from 16 to 22 weeks. This growth relationship has also been observed by neuroanatomists (22, 26).

The lateral ventricles are visualized quite rostrally in the fetal calvar-

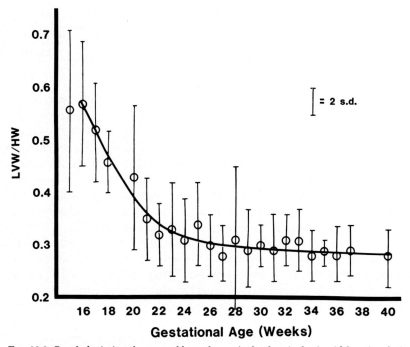

FIG. 28.3. Graph depicting the normal lateral ventricular-hemispheric width ratio relative to gestational age. Bars indicate two standard deviations above the mean. (Reproduced with permission from: M. L. Johnson *et al.* (17).)

ium, and as the scan plane is moved more toward the base of the fetal skull, the paired thalami are seen on either side of the third ventricle. At this level the middle cerebral arteries can be seen bilaterally pulsating in the insulas, which later become the Sylvian fissures. The frontal and temporal horns of the lateral ventricles are also imaged in this axial plane. The cavum septi pellucidi is a fluid-filled structure in the midline located between the frontal horns and the anterior border of the thalami. It is present in all normal fetuses and most newborns and should not be mistaken for the third ventricle (16).

Inferior to this plane the cerebral peduncles are identified as heart-shaped echo-poor structures in the midline surrounded by dense echoes. The tentorium is seen posteriorly as well as the cerebellar hemispheres. The basilar artery can be seen pulsating in the interpeduncular cistern anterior to the cerebral peduncles. The posterior cerebral arteries are seen as they course around the midbrain in the ambient cistern. On real-time ultrasound, these vessels are easily seen, as well as the circle of Willis and its tributaries. The vessels act as very good anatomic landmarks and are reproducibly imaged in the fetus (16).

DIAGNOSIS OF HYDROCEPHALUS

Hydrocephalus is cerebral ventricular dilatation due to increased intracranial pressure. The incidence of this abnormality is estimated at between 0.5 and 1.8 per 1000 births (30). In considering the diagnosis and management of this disorder it is essential to note that ventricular dilatation is a physical sign and not a disease. It can be produced by a wide range of diseases (3, 14, 25). In some cases the ventricles are large due to loss of brain tissue or failure of brain tissue to grow normally in the absence of pressure. Cerebrospinal fluid (CSF) hypertension can occasionally be caused by tumors of the choroid plexus causing an excessive rate of fluid production. More commonly, hydrocephalus is due to obstruction of CSF circulation or failure of absorption at the arachnoid granulations. Since the cerebral aqueduct is the narrowest point in the circulation path, it is not surprising that partial or complete obstruction at this site is one of the most common causes of congenital hydrocephalus. A small but important minority of these cases are inherited as single gene disorders, either X-linked or autosomal recessive. Chromosomal anomalies such as trisomies, deletions and imbalanced translocations are associated with aqueductal stenosis. Congenital infections such as cytomegalovirus (CMV) can cause hydrocephalus by obstruction of the aqueduct and ventriculomegaly by direct destruction of brain tissue. In most cases of fetal hydrocephalus no single etiology can be found. These are considered to have a multifactoral inheritance and an empiric recurrence risk for the family of between 2 and 6%.

In the study of Bay *et al.* (3) involving 56 children with congenital hydrocephalus, the etiology of hydrocephalus was aqueductal stenosis (20/56), communicating hydrocephalus (10/56), Dandy-Walker malformation (5/56), and (nearly the majority) unknown (21/56). In another study by McCullough (25) involving 37 treated cases of congenital hydrocephalus, the etiologies were aqueductal stenosis (18/37), communicating hydrocephalus (9/37), Dandy-Walker malformation (6/37), and Arnold-Chiari myelodysplasia (4/37).

The diagnosis of fetal ventriculomegaly may be made confidently with ultrasound by an experienced ultrasonologist. Hydrocephalus may be diagnosed when progressive ventriculomegally is identified on serial ultrasound scans or by direct pressure measurements (5, 17).

In the first trimester, the choroid plexus normally fills the entire width of the lateral ventricle. At this time the LVR may reach as high as 0.71. Hydrocephalus is suspected when CSF is seen in the lateral ventricle totally surrounding and compressing the choroid plexus. The LVR is then measured and compared to the normals in Figure 28.3. In the 2nd trimester the choroid plexus fills the LV only at the level of the body and atrium. By the third trimester CSF normally appears beside the choroid plexus. A LVR should be obtained if a suspicion of hydrocephalus is entertained.

Figure 28.4*A* is an ultrasound scan through the lateral ventricles demonstrating moderate ventriculomegaly in a 25-week fetus. The lateral ventricular ratio measures 0.71, which is clearly abnormal. Figure 28.4*B* is an ultrasound through the region of the thalami in this same infant showing dilatation of the frontal and temporal horns and, most importantly, dilatation of the third ventricle, indicating that the level of obstruction is below the third ventricle. In addition to measuring the ventricular size, brain texture should be noted. Increased echogenicity or a mottled echo pattern, especially in the periventricular area, may be indicative of congenital infection.

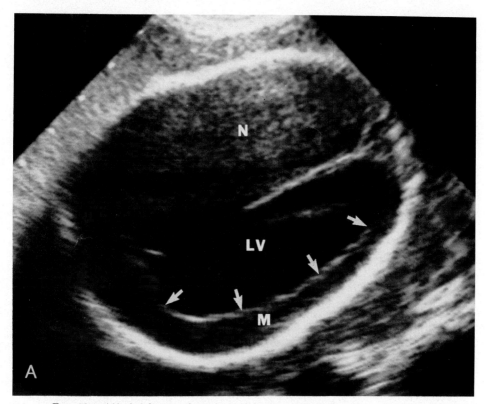

FIG. 28.4. (*A*) Axial scan through fetal brain of 25-week gestation demonstrating moderate to severe hydrocephalus. The lateral wall of the lateral ventricle (*LV*) is denoted by *arrows*. The cortical mantle (*M*) is thinned. The lateral ventricular ratio measures 0.71. Noise (*N*) obscures the near ventricle and gives the appearance of unilateral hydrocephalus.

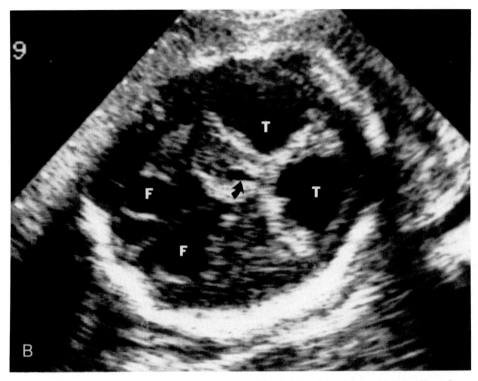

FIG. 28.4. (B) Axial scan through the level of the thalami, dilated frontal horns (F), and dilated trigone (T) area in the same patient. Note that the third ventricle (*curved black arrow*) is also dilated.

While a single examination may show unequivocal hydrocephalus in some patients, it is quite common for the exam to be inconclusive. This may be due to technical errors, to the relatively wide range of normal ventricular size, and to apparent variations in growth rate of the fetal brain. It is now well-recognized that the fetus may have a ventricular ratio clearly in the abnormal range during the gestational period from 15 to 18 weeks, and then on follow-up studies, the ventricular ratio may return to the normal range. The truly normal ventricular ratio during this time period may overlap with early fetal hydrocephalus, and only serial studies may distinguish the abnormal from the normal fetus. Thus, a fetus which demonstrates a ventricular ratio slightly out of the normal range at 16 to 18 weeks should be re-examined to determine if the ratio is decreasing or increasing. In most cases the ratio will be clearly normal or abnormal by 20 weeks gestation. No decision regarding termination of pregnancy or surgical intervention should be made until definite progressive ventriculomegaly is demonstrated. A LVR that stays at 0.80 from 15 to 18 weeks is progressive enlargement of the ventricles, as the ratio would normally be decreasing rapidly during this time.

When a diagnosis of fetal hydrocephalus is made or suspected it is essential that a thorough search be made for other anomalies. At times the etiology of the hydrocephalus will be discovered, such as a Dandy-Walker malformation or Arnold-Chiari myelodysplasia. Ascites and hepatomegaly may suggest congenital infection. Anomalies in other organ systems (skeletal, abdominal wall, cardiac, renal, etc.) may suggest that this represents a syndrome with important prognostic implications.

Lumbar meningomyeloceles are associated with multiple cranial defects including the Chiari type II (Arnold-Chiari) malformation in over 90% of the infants (1, 28, 39). When the diagnosis of intrauterine hydrocephalus is made a careful search must be performed for a meningomyelocele, encephalocele, or myeloschisis. The shape of the ventricular system may be the first clue to a Chiari malformation and neural tube defect. Myeloschisis may be missed because it is simply an open spinal canal with flared posterior elements. No mass will be present adjacent to the spine.

The hydrocephalus seen in the Chiari malformation is specific and may be diagnosed with ultrasound. The findings are dilated ventricles, anterior pointing of the frontal horns on axial scans, and inferior pointing on coronal scans. A dilated third ventricle with prominent massa intermedia and a small posterior fossa with downward displacement leading to a "tentorial-cerebellar" pseudomass appearance are also seen (1). Usually the hydrocephalus is only moderate in severity.

Dandy-Walker Syndrome

The Dandy-Walker syndrome is characterized by (a) a posterior fossa cyst continuous with the fourth ventricle; (b) posterior fossa enlargement with elevation of the torcula and tentorium; and (c) cerebellar vermian dysgenesis (29).

On ultrasound examination, the fetal cranium has a large cystic structure in the posterior fossa which is the fourth ventricle; there is associated enlargement of the posterior fossa (Fig. 28.5). The cerebellar hemispheres may be seen separated and flattened adjacent to the tentorium anterolaterally. Hydrocephalus is almost always present and may also be identified on ultrasound when it complicates this abnormality.

Holoprosencephaly

Holoprosencephaly is a developmental abnormality of forebrain diverticulation leading to a single large midline ventricle (4). The spectrum of

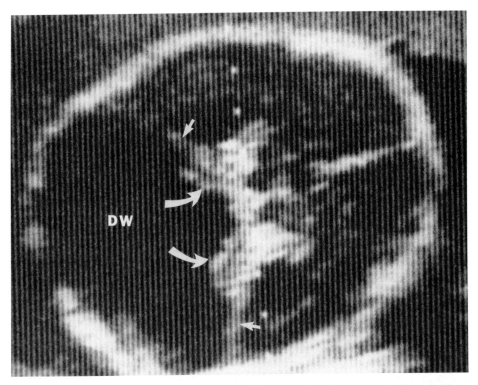

FIG. 28.5. Axial scan through 33-week fetus demonstrating a large posterior fossa fluid collection which represents a Dandy-Walker cyst (*DW*). The cerebellar hemispheres are splayed apart and compressed (*curved arrows*). The tentorium (*straight arrows*) is noted. This section is below the level of the lateral ventricles.

holoprosencephaly includes the most severe form, alobar holoprosencephaly, a less severe form, semilobar holoprosencephaly, and the mildest form, lobar holoprosencephaly. In alobar holoprosencephaly, there is a large single cavity, with only a minimal amount of cerebral tissue seen peripherally and fused thalami. These children have a specific facial syndrome, including orbital hypertelorism and other craniofacial abnormalities. They rarely survive past the 1st year of life. On ultrasound, the fetal cranium appears as a large cystic space with a mantle of cerebral tissue peripherally. The absence of the falx and corpus callosum with fused thalami allows differentiation from a large subarachnoid cyst or a posterior fossa cyst (33).

Other fluid collections within the cranium, such as hydranencephaly, arachnoid cysts, and porencephaly must be differentiated from ventriculomegaly. This is usually possible with good quality high resolution real-time equipment and a thorough understanding of normal and pathologic anatomy.

Neonatal Hydrocephalus

Diagnostic ultrasound has proven extremely valuable in imaging the neonatal brain. Portable real-time equipment allows examination of the neonate in the intensive care unit with the baby in the isolette, connected to critical monitors and life support systems. For many lesions the quality of the image is better on ultrasound than on computed tomography, and in most institutions ultrasound has become the modality of choice for examining the neonatal brain (9, 13, 18, 20, 31, 32, 37).

The best images are obtained with a sector real-time scanner using a 5.0- or 7.5-MHz transducer. Ultrasound has been shown to be useful and accurate in detecting and grading hydrocephalus, porencephaly, and intracranial hemorrhage (2, 11, 12, 18, 19, 23, 24, 35). Lower frequency transducers and linear arrays are of very limited use and can in fact result in misinterpretation and should be avoided.

The transducer is placed on the anterior fontanelle, and coronal and sagittal images are obtained while sweeping the ultrasound beam through the entire brain. The infant is examined in the isolette with the head in a lateral or supine position.

Figure 28.6A is a frozen frame image from a normal real-time examination in a coronal plane through the bodies of the lateral ventricles at the level of the thalami and midbrain. Figure 28.6B is a coronal view through the frontal horns and cavum septi pellucidi. The bodies of the lateral ventricle are sonolucent with densely echogenic choroid plexus at the base. On real-time, pulsations of the intracranial vessels are easily seen, and pulsed Doppler can be utilized to detect flow in specific vessels. The size of the lateral ventricles can be measured from this section, and the coronal view is a very good way to follow the progression of ventriculomegaly. An axial view, similar to that described for the fetal brain, can also be obtained, but the transfontanelle views are of the best image quality, as the sound beam is not traversing bone. As the fontanelle closes and the calvarium becomes dense the image quality deteriorates. Visualization of the ventricular sytem is usually possible up to age 4. The adult brain is difficult to image with ultrasound.

By turning the transducer 90° from the coronal plane, a sagittal view of the brain is obtained (Fig. 28.7). A slightly oblique angle is required to demonstrate the body and occipital horn of the lateral ventricle as well as the frontal horn. The head of the caudate nucleus lies directly on top of the thalamus anteriorly. The choroid plexus is extremely echogenic, begins just behind the head of the caudate, and courses along the floor

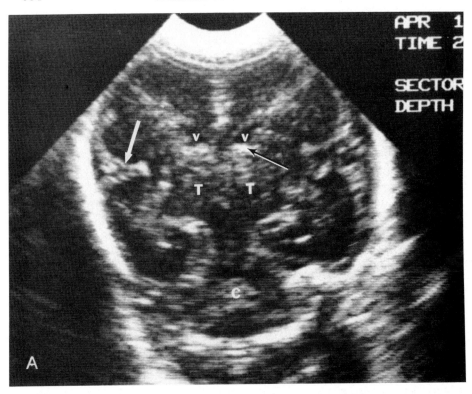

FIG. 28.6. (A) Coronal scan through anterior fontanelle in premature infant demonstrating normal brain anatomy at the level of the thalami (T). The bodies of the lateral ventricles (v) are slit-like hypoechoic structures on either side of the midline. At the base of the lateral ventricles is the echogenic choroid plexus (*black arrow*). The Sylvian fissure containing the middle cerebral artery can be seen adjacent to the skull (*white arrow*). Beneath the tentorium the cerebellum (C) is visualized.

of the lateral ventricle into the trigone region posteriorly. It does not extend into the occipital region. The ventricles appear quite small in both coronal and sagittal views, and even mild enlargement of the trigone region is easily detected. Though ventricular size is best evaluated by direct observation, there are multiple measurements one can make of the ventricular system, and it has been nicely shown that ultrasound can evaluate ventricular size as reliably as computed tomography (2, 9, 11–13, 18, 27, 31, 33, 34, 37).

Figure 28.8 is a coronal ultrasound image through the bodies of the lateral ventricles at the level of the thalami in a patient with posthemorrhagic hydrocephalus. The temporal horns are also dilated. There is a residual subependymal cyst in the area of the previous intracranial

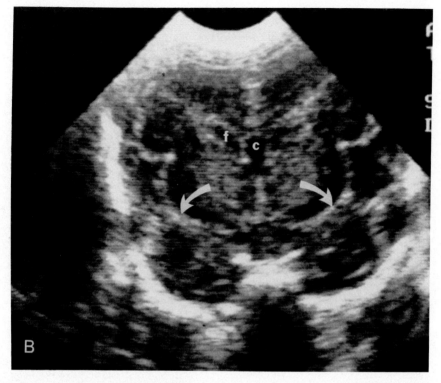

FIG. 28.6. (*B*) Coronal scan through the anterior fontanelle of a normal preterm infant demonstrating the cavum septi pellucidi (*c*) and the frontal horn (*f*) of the lateral ventricles on either side of the cavum. The middle cerebral arteries (*curved arrows*) are seen coursing out laterally toward the Sylvian fissures. These vessels pulsate on real-time examination. The frontal horns are small, echo-free, and boomerang-shaped.

hemorrhage. Intracranial hemorrhage (ICH) is the most common cause of neonatal hydrocephalus, but in our experience the hydrocephalus is usually transient and may not require shunting or drainage (33). Conservative management with serial ultrasound examinations is recommended.

As in the fetus, there are innumerable causes of ventriculomegaly in the neonate, and ultrasound can be used to accurately define the level of obstruction and often demonstrate the cause, such as ICH, aqueductal stenosis, Dandy-Walker syndrome (Fig. 28.9), Chiari malformation (Fig. 28.10), arachnoid cysts, solid tumors, and congenital malformations.

Diagnostic ultrasound is noninvasive, inexpensive, portable, rapid, and most of all, accurate in the assessment of hydrocephalus in the fetus and neonate. Ventricular size and configuration are well-shown on both ultrasound and CT, although CT may slightly underestimate the size of

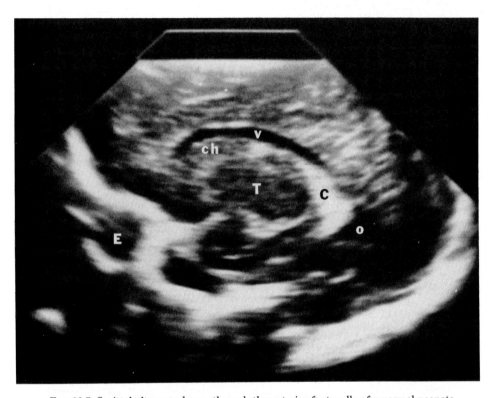

FIG. 28.7. Sagittal ultrasound scan through the anterior fontanelle of a normal neonate demonstrating the echo-free lateral ventricle (v) as it is seen coursing from the frontal horn region around to the occipital horn (o). The choroid plexus (C) is the echogenic structure at the base of the lateral ventricle which becomes quite prominent in the region of the trigone. The head of the caudate nucleus (ch) is beneath the front portion of the lateral ventricle and sits on top of the thalamus (T). Beneath the anterior cranial fossa is the orbit and eye (E) contained within.

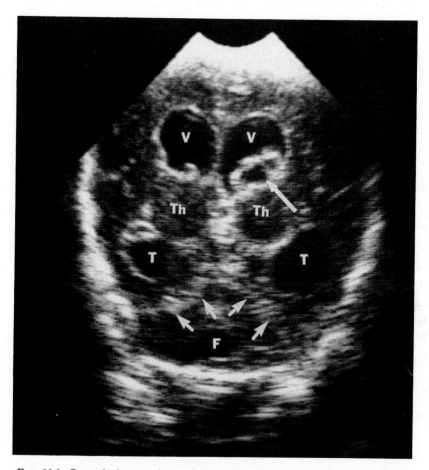

FIG. 28.8. Coronal ultrasound examination through the region of the thalami in a premature infant with moderate hydrocephalus secondary to an intraventricular bleed. The bodies of the lateral ventricles (v) are dilated, and there is a clot and subependymal cyst in the base of the left lateral ventricle (*large arrow*). Inferior and lateral to the thalami (*Th*) are the dilated temporal horns (*T*). The tentorium is denoted by *small arrows*. The echo-free cisterna magna (*F*) is visualized most posteriorly behind the cerebellum.

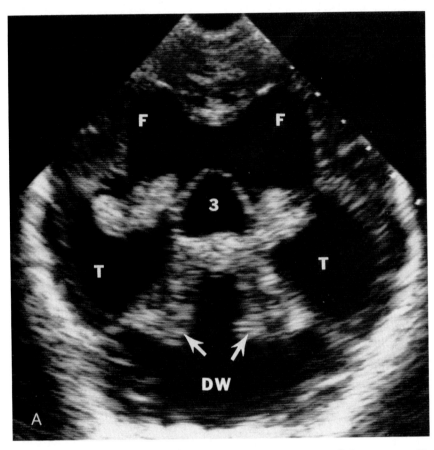

FIG. 28.9. (A) Coronal ultrasound scan through the anterior fontanelle in a neonate with Dandy-Walker syndrome (DW) 1 day after *in utero* diagnosis (same patient as in Fig. 28.5). This scan is at the level of the trigone (T), and the echogenic choroid plexus is seen between the frontal horns (F) anteriorly and the trigone posteriorly. The dilated third ventricle (3) is well-visualized. The hypoplastic cerebellum (*arrows*) is not fused in the midline and is compressed against the tentorium.

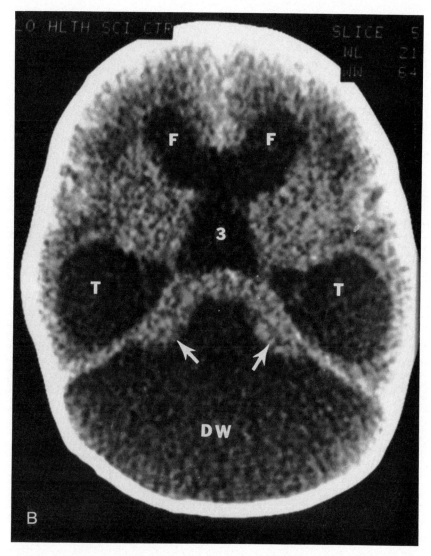

FIG. 28.9. (*B*) Axial CT scan of the same infant as in Figure 28.9*A*, a neonate with Dandy-Walker (DW) syndrome. The wall of the third ventricle (*3*) is not as clearly delineated on the CT scan as on the ultrasound.

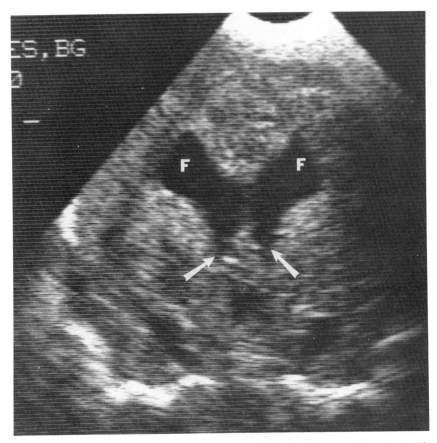

FIG. 28.10. Coronal ultrasound examination through the frontal horns of an infant with Chiari II malformation demonstrating the bat wing deformity with inferior pointing (*arrows*) of the dilated frontal horns (*F*).

the ventricular system due to averaging and/or debris in the CSF. Ultrasound sharply delineates the interfaces between solid and fluid, and even very small compressed ventricles, as seen with cerebral edema, are imaged on ultrasound. Correlation between ultrasound and CT in determining the severity of hydrocephalus has been excellent (18, 36). Ultrasound has become so reliable that it is now used for screening patients suspected of hydrocephalus. In neonates, hydrocephalus can be clinically very subtle, with significant cortical mantle loss before the condition is clinically suspected (21, 38). Early ventricular evaluation by ultrasound is indicated for all neonates at risk or suspected of developing hydrocephalus.

REFERENCES

1. Babcock, D. S., and Han, B. K. Cranial sonographic findings in meningomyelocele. A.J.R., *136:* 563–569, March, 1981.
2. Babcock, D. S., Han, B. K., and LeQuesne, G. W. B-mode gray-scale ultrasonography of the head in the newborn and young infant. A.J.R., *134:* 457–468, 1980.
3. Bay, C., Kerzin, L., and Hall, B. Recurrence risk in hydrocephalus. Birth Defects, *15(15C):* 95–105, 1979.
4. Byrd, S. E., Harwood-Nash, D. C., Fitz, C. R., *et al.* Computed tomography evaluation of holoprosencephaly in infants and children. J. Comput. Assist. Tomogr., *4:* 456–462, 1977.
5. Chervenak, F. A., Berkowitz, R. L., Romero, R., *et al.* The diagnosis of fetal hydrocephalus. Am. J. Obstet. Gynecol., *147:* 703–716, November, 1983.
6. Crade, M., Patel, J., and McQuown, D. Sonographic imaging of the glycogen state of the fetal choroid plexus. A.J.R., *137:* 489–491, September, 1981.
7. Denkhaus, H., and Winsberg, F. Ultrasonic measurement of the fetal ventricular system. Radiology, *131:* 781–787, June, 1979.
8. Denkhaus, H., and Winsberg, F. Ultrasound of the normal and abnormal fetal neural axis. Radiol. Clin. North Am., *20:* 285–296, 1982.
9. Edwards, M. K., Brown, D. L., and Muller, J. Cribside neurosonography: Real-time sonography for intracranial investigation of the neonate. A.J.R., *136:* 271–276, 1981.
10. Fiske, C. E., and Filly, R. A. Ultrasound of the normal and abnormal fetal neural axis. Radiol. Clin. North Am., *20:* 285–296, 1982.
11. Garrett, W. J., Kossoff, G., and Jones, R. F. C. Ultrasonic cross-sectional visualization of hydrocephalus in infants. Neuroradiology, *8:* 279–288, 1975.
12. Garrett, W. J., Kossoff, G., and Warren, P. Cerebral ventricular size in children: A two dimensional ultrasonic study. Radiology, *136:* 711–715, 1980.
13. Grant, E. G., Schellinger, D., Borts, F. T., *et al.* Real-time sonography of the neonatal and infant head. A.J.R., *136:* 265–270, 1981.
14. Habib, Z. Genetics and genetic counselling in neonatal hydrocephalus. Obstet. Gynecol. Surv., *36:* 529–534, 1981.
15. Hadlock, F. P., Deter, R. L., and Park, S. K. Real-time sonography: Ventricular and vascular anatomy of the fetal brain in utero. A.J.R., *136:* 133–137, 1981.
16. Johnson, M. L., Dunne, M. G., Mack, L. A., *et al.* Evaluation of fetal intracranial anatomy by static and real-time ultrasound. J. Clin. Ultrasound. *8:* 311–318, 1980.
17. Johnson, M. L., Pretorius, D., Clewell, W. H., Meier, P. R., and Manchester, D. Fetal hydrocephalus: Diagnosis and management. Semin. Perinatol., *7:* 83–89, 1983.
18. Johnson, M. L., and Rumack, C. M. B-mode echoencephalography in the normal and high risk infant. A.J.R., *133:* 375–381, 1979.
19. Johnson, M. L., and Rumack, C. M. Ultrasonic evaluation of the neonatal brain. Radiol. Clin. North Am., *18:* 117–132, 1980.
20. Knake, J. E., Chandler, W. F., McGillicuddy, J. E., *et al.* Intraoperative sonography for brain tumor localization and ventricular shunt placement. A.J.R., *139:* 733–738, 1982.
21. Korobkin, R. The relationship between head circumference and the development of communicating hydrocephalus in infants following intraventricular hemorrhage. Pediatrics, *56:* 74–77, 1975.
22. Lemire, R. J., Loeser, J. D., Leech, R. W., *et al. Normal and Abnormal Development of the Human Nervous System.* Harper & Row, New York, 1975.
23. London, P. A., Carroll, B. A., and Enzmann, D. R. Sonography of ventricular size and germinal matrix hemorrhage in premature infants. A.J.N.R., *1:* 295–300, 1980.
24. Mack, L. A., Rumack, C. M., and Johnson, M. L. Ultrasound evaluation of cystic lesions. Radiology, *137:* 451–455, 1980.

25. McCullough, D. C., and Blazer-Martin, L. A. Current prognosis in overt neonatal hydrocephalus. J. Neurosurg., *57:* 378–383, 1982.
26. Moore, K. L. *The Developing Human: Clinically Oriented Embryology*, Ed 2. W.B. Saunders, Philadelphia, 1977.
27. Morgan, C. L., Trought, W. S., Rothman, S. J., *et al.* Comparison of gray-scale ultrasonography and CT in the evaluation of macrocrania in infants. Radiology, *132:* 119–123, 1979.
28. Nadich, T., Pudlowsk, R. M., Nadich, J. B., *et al.* Computed tomographic signs of the Chiari II malformation. II. Midbrain and cerebellum. Radiology, *134:* 65–71, 1980.
29. Newman, G. C., Buschi, A. I., Sugg, N. K., *et al.* Dandy-Walker syndrome diagnosed in utero by ultrasonography. Neurology, *32:* 180–184, 1982.
30. Robertson, R. D., Sarti, D. A., Brown, W. J., *et al.* Congenital hydrocephalus in two pregnancies following the birth of a child with neural tube defect: Aetiology and management. J. Med. Genet., *18:* 105–107, 1981.
31. Rumack, C. M., and Johnson, M. L. Real-time ultrasound evaluation of the neonatal brain. Clin. Ultrasound., *10:* 179–202, 1982.
32. Rumack, C. M., and Johnson, M. L. Role of CT and US in neonatal brain imaging. J. Comput. Tomogr., *7:* 17–29, 1983.
33. Rumack, C. M., and Johnson, M. L. *Prenatal and Infant Brain Imaging. Role of Ultrasound and Computed Tomography.* Yearbook Medical Publishers, Chicago, 1984.
34. Shkolnik, A., and McLone, D. G. Intraoperative real-time ultrasonic guidance of ventricular shunt placement in infants. Radiology, *141:* 515–517, 1981.
35. Silverboard, G., Horder, M. H., Ahmann, P. A., *et al.* Reliability of ultrasound in the diagnosis of intracerebral hemorrhage and posthemorrhagic hydrocephalus: Comparison with CT. Pediatrics, *66:* 507–514, 1980.
36. Skolnick, M. L., Rosenbaum, A. E., Matzuk, T., *et al.* Detection of dilated cerebral ventricles in infants: A correlative study between US and CT. Radiology, *131:* 447–451, 1979.
37. Slovis, T., and Kuhns, L. R. Real-time sonography of the brain through the anterior fontanelle. A.J.R., *136:* 277–286, 1981.
38. Volpe, J. J., Pasternak, J. F., and Allan, W. C. Ventricular dilatation preceding rapid head growth following neonatal intracranial hemorrhage. Am. J. Dis. Child., *131:* 1212–1215, 1977.
39. Zimmerman, R. D., Brockbill, D., Dennis, M. W., *et al.* Cranial CT findings in patients with myelomeningocele. A.J.R., *132:* 623–629, 1979.

29

To Shunt or Not to Shunt: Hydrocephalus and Dysraphism

HAROLD L. REKATE, M.D.

The decision to shunt or not to shunt a child with enlarged ventricles and spina bifida cystica depends on an understanding of the damage that is done by the compromise to the developing brain of this ventriculomegaly and the risks inherent in the therapy to be instituted. If shunting were completely innocuous, one could demand that any ventricles larger in size than normal must be shunted. This, however, is not the case, and as a guideline we must attempt to define the point at which danger to the developing brain of the ventriculomegaly overcomes the risk of ventricular shunting. Figure 29.1 is a theoretical representation of this concept and as an example intersects at 2.8 cm of cortical mantle, which is the thickness of the brain between the ependymal surface of the lateral ventricle and the inner table of the skull at the coronal suture below which intellectual development is compromised (33). The purpose of the

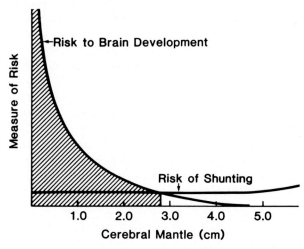

FIG. 29.1. Theoretical representation of the risk-benefit ratio of shunting *vs.* ventriculomegaly in spina bifida patients.

present work is to analyze the risk-benefit ratio of hydrocephalus to shunting in order to develop a rational approach to decision making in this rather common condition.

Each child is an individual and must be evaluated as such, and many factors must be taken into consideration in making the decision "to shunt or not to shunt." A decision not to shunt a child with mildly to moderately enlarged ventricles and an Arnold-Chiari malformation is justified because of the inherent risks of shunting. Such a decision carries with it a higher level of responsibility for compulsive follow-up of ventricular size and developmental and intellectual functioning leading to the irrevocable conclusion, "when in doubt—shunt." Despite this warning and use of the decision-making process to be described below no child followed at the Hydrocephalus-Myelodysplasia Clinic, Rainbow Babies and Children's Hospital, Cleveland, Ohio (RB&C), has later required a shunt who at the age of 5 months did not fully meet the requirements for shunting.

HOW MUCH HYDROCEPHALUS IS UNACCEPTABLE?

There is much conflicting information relating to how much hydrocephalus it takes to cause damage to the developing central nervous system. Most of these are anecdotal, including Lorber's provocative discussion "Is the brain really necessary?" in which he presents a functioning mathematics student with a cortical mantle of less than a centimeter (15). Some patients tolerate ventriculomegaly better than others. Some patients, on the other hand, despite early and aggressive therapy, which is successful in that it leads to normal or smaller than normal ventricles, may be left with extremely poor intellectual and developmental function. The major problem in evaluating studies both of the natural history of hydrocephalus (1, 14, 32) and the results of treatment (1, 7, 16, 17, 28, 33) is separating the effects of the hydrocephalus itself from the direct effects on cognition of the underlying cause of the hydrocephalus. The former is preventable, and the latter is not. The best information on the degree of hydrocephalus necessary to cause damage derives from the work of Young et al. (33). Several studies prior to this one had failed to show a correlation between initial brain thickness or mantle (i.e., severity of hydrocephalus) and ultimate functional status either with or without shunting (1, 14, 32). The importance of this benchmark study is the concentration on the posttreatment mantle. They found that in patients without anoxic injury or demonstrable abnormalities of central nervous system architecture a postshunt mantle of 2.0 cm or less was inconsistent with IQ on Wechsler or Stanford-Binet testing of 80 or above. Between 2.0 and 3.0 cm a few patients had "normal" IQs, but above the 3.0 cm (actually 2.8 cm) the IQ distribution approached normal

(23, 32). There appears to be no advantage to reaching a 5- or 5.5-cm (normal) over a 2.8- or 3.0-cm mantle.

The reconstitution of the cerebral mantle appears to be time-dependent in that an overly long delay in performing a shunt often leads to failure to obtain a 3.0 mantle. In the Nulsen study no reconstitution of cerebral mantle occurred when the shunt was placed after 18 months (five patients), but all patients shunted by 5 months of age obtained a post-shunt mantle of 3.0 cm or greater (23, 33). The decision "to shunt or not to shunt" should be made by the age of 5 months.

The study discussed above involves children followed at RB&C. We remain concerned about the outlook for patients selected for nonshunting. These patients are followed very closely with head circumference measurements, ventricular size assessments periodically, and developmental and intellectual assessments. As stated above, no child who has attained a 3.0 cm mantle at age 5 months later needed shunting if at 5 months the Denver Development Testing (DDST) was normal.

There are two other points which support the concept that a decision not to shunt at 5 months will not need to be reversed later. First, in a study by Laurence (14) of arrested hydrocephalus not treated, except in the profoundly retarded, the intellectual attainment of patients improved over the period of time of the study. The second aspect involves the basic mechanisms in hydrocephalus in that in early infancy, the easy distensibility of the skull prevents the stabilization of ventricular size. As the skull becomes a more rigid shell and therefore more resistant to distension higher intracranial pressures can be generated, leading to more effective CSF absorption. Ventricular size tends to stabilize as the skull becomes rigid. This concept is the basis of the rationale of head wrapping in the treatment of communicating hydrocephalus (4).

HYDROCEPHALUS IN THE CONTEXT OF THE CHIARI II MALFORMATION

At least two of three children born with spina bifida cystica have hydrocephalus, depending on how the term is defined (1, 16, 17). As an operational definition many studies define hydrocephalus by the presence of a shunt. Few children born with this abnormality have normal-sized ventricles. When a shunt has not been required in the treatment of myelodysplastic children, their prognosis for intellectual development has been uniformly better than those who have had shunts (1, 16, 17, 19, 20). In fact, the prognosis for normal intellectual development is quite good in the unshunted group (19, 20). The assumption has been that since children with the Chiari II or Arnold-Chiari malformation fared poorer as far as intellectual development is concerned than did children with other forms of hydrocephalus (so-called "pure" hydrocephalus) there must be something in the brains of children with this abnormality which causes the poor intellectual outcome (23, 33). What has only recently been studied is the potential that the causes of poor intellectual attainment may be due to other causes which may be preventable. McClone (20) suggested that complications such as ventriculitis in the immature brain have much more to do with poor intellectual performance than does the developmental abnormality itself. In an animal model of neonatal ventriculitis he also showed the specific sensitivity to damage by microorganisms which can be resisted by the more mature central nervous system (21). Mapstone et al. (19) analyzed this question and showed that children with the Arnold-Chiari malformation who were shunted without any complications had a significantly lower IQ than those that had not been shunted (91 vs. 104). When those shunted without complications were compared to those shunted with complication the drop in IQ was dramatic (91 vs. 70). These differences could not be explained by correlations of hydrocephalus and lesion level (Figs. 29.2 and 29.3). The implication here is that the presence of hydrocephalus requiring shunting in children with the Arnold-Chiari malformation carries with it a slightly

NO COMPLICATIONS

	NEVER SHUNTED	SHUNTED
IQ	104 RANGE (63-130)	91 RANGE (59-124)
N	18	41
SE	18	15

difference of means two tail test

sig p < .01

FIG. 29.2. Comparison of IQ data from children with spina bifida cystica without shunts and those shunted without complications. (Reproduced with permission from T. B. Mapstone et al. (19).)

SHUNTED

	NO COMPLICATION	COMPLICATION
IQ	91	70
	RANGE (59-124)	RANGE (40-109)
N	41	16
SE	15	20

difference of means two tail test

sig p < .001

FIG. 29.3. Comparison of IQ data from children with spina bifida shunted with and without complications (Reproduced with permission from T. B. Mapstone *et al.* (19).)

subnormal outlook for intellectual development, but the major intellectual downgrading is done by potentially preventable perinatal complication. This information would seem to justify the use of information derived from "pure" hydrocephalic patients in decision making relative to patients with the Arnold-Chiari malformation.

DISADVANTAGES OF SHUNTING

The risk to the patient of performing a ventriculoperitoneal or ventriculojugular shunt is a significant part of the decision-making process in infants with ventriculomegaly. Better techniques and hardware have improved the outlook for the shunted child, but the risk of infection and shunt malfunction is always present. Shunt infection represents the most serious threat to life and intellectual functioning. As shown by the works of McClone and Mapstone above, ventriculitis is a significant cause of intellectual downgrading in children born with the Arnold-Chiari malformation. Jasper and Merrill (12) reviewed the incidence of ventriculitis associated with myelomeningocele. In their series, 34 of 200 children born with a myelomeningocele developed an infection of the central nervous system. From the discussion and the organisms involved one can infer that in children with central nervous system infections about one-third were infected from the open granulating back wound and two-thirds through the implanted shunting system. The shunt itself is a significant source of ventriculitis in these children.

Schoenbaum *et al.* (27) reporting the Boston Children's and Beth Israel Hospital experiences stated that 27% of the 298 patients receiving shunts became infected with an infection rate of 13% per procedure. Subsequent reports by pediatric neurosurgeons have emphasized the importance of perioperative antibiotics and attention to surgical technique and have reported much improved infection rates (24, 31). While the infection rate is at a low level, it is still a relatively common complication and carries with it the risks of death and intellectual deterioration.

A child presenting in infancy with hydrocephalus rarely suffers from markedly raised intracranial pressure and is very unlikely to undergo transtentorial or uncal herniation; however, after a shunt is placed the cranial sutures are able to close normally. At this later point if shunt malfunction occurs, either from occlusion or disconnection, the pressure can rise rapidly to extremely high levels and result in rapid neurologic deterioration and herniation. This is one of the ways in which the presence of a shunt participates in the development of shunt dependence. A shunt may also lead to shunt dependency through ventricular coaptation. Following the placement of a shunt the cortical mantle begins to reconstitute and the ependymal surfaces approach each other. Kaufman *et al.* (13) have shown that following shunting, ependymal surfaces of the ventricular system can actually touch, and if they remain in contact for a prolonged period of time a scarring process occurs, leading to an irreversible sealing of the surfaces. Foltz (6) in his discussion of aqueductal stenosis converting communicating to noncommunicating hydrocephalus emphasizes the importance of small hemorrhages and infection in the etiopathogenesis of this condition. It has also been shown that ventriculitis can lead to septations within the ventricular system again leading to noncommunicating hydrocephalus.

The potential for a child once shunted to subsequently be able to do without his or her shunt is a subject of great deal of debate (3, 5, 11, 22, 26). The most important aspects of this debate deal not with whether or not a shunt should be occluded or removed but on how aggressive one should be with a shunt which radiographically or physically seems unlikely to be able to continue to function. It could be disconnected, the ventricular catheter imbedded in brain tissue or the distal catheter too short for continuing function. Epstein (3) has emphasized the importance of the ventricular size in this situation. Ventricles which are smaller than normal on computed tomographic (CT) scan are being drained by a working shunt system, and as long as that is the case they must be considered shunt-dependent. Patients with communicating hydrocephalus whose shunts fail or are challenged by shunt occlusion either show overt signs of increased intracranial pressure or tolerate well the shunt malfunction. They do not show insidious deterioration in functional ability (26). In the specific case of children with the Arnold-Chiari malformation, however, the situation is quite different. Insidious deterioration is possible following shunt occlusion. These patients may suffer respiratory arrest from hours to 5 years following shunt occlusion with few if any premonitory signs (26). In the case of the Arnold-Chiari malformation infancy is the only logical time to make the decision regarding the need for shunting, for in this condition the Foltz edict "once a shunt—always a shunt" must be applied (5).

Several methods have been advocated relative to the ability to treat progressive hydrocephalus without shunting. Lorber (18) has shown that the use of isosorbide will diminish CSF production and in the case of children with myelomeningoceles often prevent the need for shunting. The use of serial lumbar punctures as described in several Lancet publications (2, 9) is not applicable to the myelodysplastic patient because of the technical difficulties in performing lumbar punctures. Epstein *et al.* (4) suggested head wrapping and the use of an on-off valve as alternatives to continuous ventricular shunting. In the latter situation the shunt is opened for only short periods to prevent progressive ventricular dilatation. For the most part a planned delay will allow the neurosurgeon the ability to discern who will and who will not need shunting without these temporizing methods.

CRITERIA FOR SHUNTING IN MYELODYSPLASTIC CHILDREN

There are several indications for shunting of myelodysplastic children which are unique to that condition. The first of these has to do with the healing of the back wound. Frequently the neurosurgeon in performing a myelomeningocele closure is faced with the flow of CSF intraoperatively. The primary purpose of the closure is the sealing off of this fluid from the external environment, and occasionally increases in CSF pressure lead to the leaking of CSF through the back wound. Shunting in this situation leads to a decrease in the hydrostatic pressure on the suture line and therefore improved healing. While use of external ventricular drainage will accomplish the same thing for short periods of time, an internalized shunt is often necessary for proper wound healing.

The other indication for shunting that is unique in the Arnold-Chiari malformation involves the development in these infants of lower cranial nerve deficits, the "Chiari crisis." Children born with the Arnold-Chiari malformation have been shown often to have a marked degree of disorganization of the brain stem in the area of the cranial nerve nuclei (25).

As high as 15% of these children develop a syndrome characterized by sleep apnea, fasciculations of the tongue, stridor, difficulty swallowing, absent gag responses, and tendency to aspiration termed the "Chiari crisis." Presumably this is due to impaction of these sensitive and disorganized structures in the tightly constricted environment of the upper cervical spinal canal. If this occurs when ventriculomegaly is present, the first step should be the placement or repair of a ventricular shunt. If this is not successful a suboccipital and cervical decompression may be required (29, 30).

When neither of the two problems discussed above is present one is faced with the problem of deciding, based on measurable parameters, whether a child with ventriculomegaly and spina bifida cystica needs a shunt. These decisions are somewhat based on personal philosophy supported by an analysis of available historical and laboratory information. Current recommendations require compulsive assessment of the child's developmental status as well as his or her ventricular size. Figure 29.4 is the standardized form used at each visit to our Hydrocephalus-Myelodysplasia Clinic. This form is appropriate for all children with spina bifida from infancy through adulthood. The psychological assessment is extremely important both for decision making as well as scientific review. Formal psychologic testing is not available for children below the age of 3 years and is therefore of no help in the decision to shunt or not to shunt a child with ventriculomegaly and spina bifida cystica. We must rely therefore on DDST assessments which must be specifically adapted to the child with spina bifida because of the inherent motor deficits which will invalidate the gross motor portion of the study. Correlations between the DDST and subsequent intellectual performance on standardized intelligence testing (WISC or Stanford-Binet) has not been perfect, but normal language and personal-social scores on the DDST are usually associated with functional intelligence. A stronger case can

NAME   DATE
AGE   ETIOLOGY.
HEAD CIRCUM.
PREV. HEAD CIRC. AND DATE
LAST REVISION UPPER
                   LOWER
VALVE PALPATION   NEUROLOGIC STATUS
LAST X-RAY DATE
    TUBE POSITION   LEVEL IF M.M.
LAST VENTRIC. ESTIMATION
PSYCHOLOGICAL STATUS

FIG. 29.4. Standardized form for follow-up of children followed at the Hydrocephalus Myelodysplasia Clinic, Rainbow Babies and Children's Hospital, Cleveland, Ohio.

be made in the contrary situation. When there are significant delays in testable responses by 6 months of age problems in subsequent intellectual development are to be expected. Because of a high likelihood of questionable results it is important that the assessments be performed serially, preferably by the same experienced developmental specialist/occupational therapist (8). How this information is used or indeed whether this information is used is a matter or personal philosophy. When poor intellectual function is predicted and moderate ventriculomegaly is present the question of whether or not this outlook can be improved by shunting is not answerable in the individual case and is therefore much more likely to lead to a decision in favor of shunting.

In children with ventriculomegaly and spina bifida whose back wound has healed or is healing, who have no evidence of lower cranial nerve dysfunction and have normal DDSTs, the decision "to shunt or not to shunt" rests with an analysis of what is happening to ventricular size. A cortical mantle of 3.0 cm must be attained by 5 months of age. If prior to 5 months of age the child shows evidence of progressive ventriculomegaly on serial measurements of ventricular size, progressive craniomegaly (*i.e.*, continues to have a head growth pattern significantly divergent from accepted norms), or shows signs of increased intracranial pressure a shunt must be inserted.

HOW TO FOLLOW A CHILD WITH MYELODYSPLASIA FOR THE DEVELOPMENT OF HYDROCEPHALUS

A child born with spina bifida cystica should have measurement of ventricular size within the first few days of life, preferably prior to the closure of the myelomeningocele. If hydrocephalus is overt at birth or there is evidence of significantly increased intracranial pressure, a shunting procedure should be performed early. Ventricular size measurements are now being made ultrasonographically, often in the nursery. Using ultrasound a direct measurement of thickness of brain (mantle) can be made (Fig. 29.5). This measurement of mantle should be made at the level of the foramen of Monro to correspond to the measurements made by Young *et al.* using pneumoventriculography (23, 33). Other measurements of ventricular size such as measurement of the width of the third ventricle or occipital mantle have not shown correlation with later intellectual outcome.

Head circumference measurements and assessment of anterior fontanelle turgor are made at least daily during the child's hospital stay and another ultrasound performed prior to discharge. If there has been no thinning of the cortical mantle, the child may be discharged without shunting. For purposes of comparison, a CT scan is often obtained at this point. CT scanning prior to early healing of the myelomeningocele

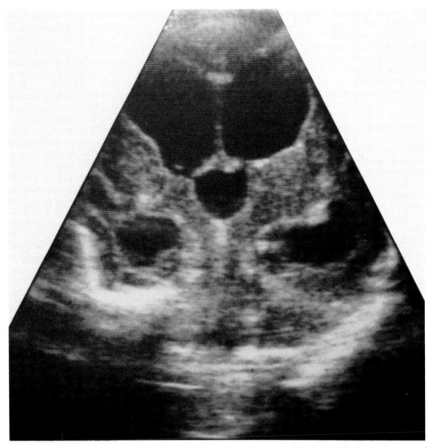

FIG. 29.5. Calculation of cerebral mantle from CT scan. Ultrasound measurement of thickness of brain (mantle) showing a 1.5-cm mantle.

repair is technically difficult because of the need to place the child in a supine position. CT scanning gives anatomic detail difficult to ascertain ultrasonographically. In order to get an estimate of mantle thickness from a CT scan several assumptions must be made and while imperfect will allow a determination as to whether or not the 3.0-cm goal can be reached. Figure 29.6 is a representation of how these calculations are made. For purposes of approximate calculations the assumption is made that the ventricular system is a central sphere lying within a sperical shell. Using these assumptions, the formula for calculating the cerebral mantle from the CT scan is illustrated in Figure 29.6. As long as the anterior fontanelle is open it is much preferable to obtain these measurements directly by ultrasound, but once the fontanelle is closed this

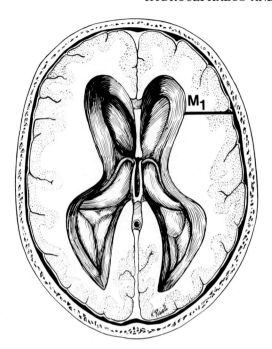

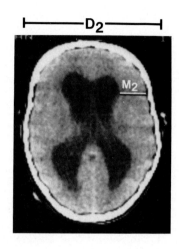

ACTUAL CRANIUM   CT SCAN

FIG. 29.6. Method of computing the cerebral mantle from the appearance of the CT scan. The formula is

$$M_1 = \frac{M_2 \times C_1}{\pi \times D_2}$$

Where M_1 = actual cerebral mantle; M_2 = measured mantle on CT scan; C_1 = actual head circumference; D_2 = diameter of skull on CT scan.

method still gives an adequate approximation. Following discharge the child is followed closely as an outpatient. The frequency of follow-up visits depends somewhat on the degree of ventriculomegaly, but normally the child is followed at 2 weeks, 6 weeks, and each 6 weeks thereafter for the first 6 months. At each of these visits an ultrasound is performed. At 6 weeks the first DDST is performed and is repeated at each subsequent visit if the child has not received a shunt.

If no shunt has been required using these criteria, subsequent shunting has not been found necessary, and the frequency of the visits can be decreased. Using these criteria the outlook for intellectual development in these patients has approached normal, and no child has subsequently required shunting (19). These children do, however, require fairly close neurologic follow-up throughout life because of the potential in later life to develop syringomyelia. Hall *et al.* (10) presented a series of patients with neuromuscular scoliosis and spina bifida cystica. These patients were shown to have hydromyelia and ventriculomegaly, and 7 of 11 showed improvement in the scoliotic curve with ventricular shunt repair or placement of a primary shunt. There are multiple causes of scoliosis in myelodysplastic children, including hemivertebrae and neuromuscular imbalance from the primary anomaly. This report does suggest that late deterioration in these patients is possible, and therefore careful long-term followup is essential (10). Both shunted and unshunted myelodysplastic children who are stable should be followed at intervals of from 6 to 12 months.

SUMMARY

Objective criteria are available for decision making in children with ventriculomegaly and spina bifida cystica. Figure 29.7 is the evaluation algorithm used in the Hydrocephalus/Myelodysplasia Clinic at Rainbow Babies and Children's Hospital. In children without serious neurosurgical complications such as the Chiari crisis or problems with wound healing, we rely on three reasonably objective measurements for decision making.

1. *Head circumference:* Measured daily while in hospital and at each visit. If the pattern of head growth crosses multiple percentile lines indicating that the child will be severely megalencephalic, a shunt will be performed.
2. *Ultrasonography:* Ultrasound determinations are made in the first few days of life, prior to discharge, at 6 weeks of age, and each 6 weeks of age until 6 months. Some measurements of ventricular size (usually CT scan because of a small anterior fontanelle) should be made at age 1 year.
3. *Denver Developmental Testing (DDST):* These are performed at age 6 weeks and each 6 weeks thereafter. If the child shows significant ventriculomegaly, a shunt is performed. When the results are questionable the decision is delayed and the test repeated in 6 weeks.

Whether a shunt is or is not placed in an infant with ventriculomegaly and myelodysplasia, follow-up must remain compulsive. Following shunting, not only should the head circumference stabilize, but the cortical mantle should increase. often children shunted in this situation fail to show signs of increased intracranial pressure with shunt malfunction and must be followed with serial head circumference measurements as well as ultrasounds and CT scans. If the decision is made not to shunt the child the work of Hall *et al.* (10) would suggest the possibility that later in life shunts may be needed to prevent scoliosis secondary to hydromye-

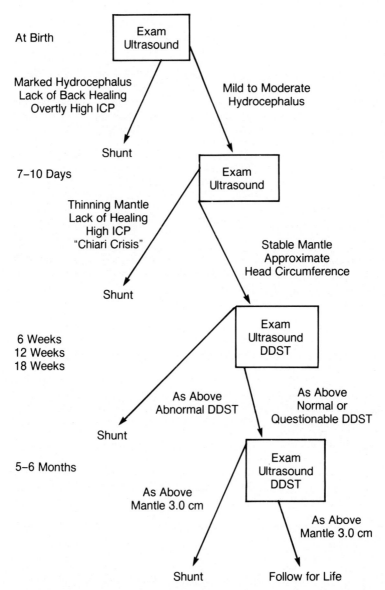

FIG. 29.7. Ventriculomegaly and myelomeningocele. Evaluation algorithm for following a child with spina bifida cystica and ventriculomegaly.

lia. More information is needed as the aggressively treated population become adults.

REFERENCES

1. Badell-Ribera, A., Shulman, K., and Paddock, N. The relationship of nonprogressive hydrocephalus to intellectual functioning in children with spina bifida cystica. Pediatrics, *37:* 787–793, 1960.
2. Blumenthal, I., MacMillan, M., and Costatos, C. Lumbar puncture in transcient hydrocephalus (Letter to the Editor). Lancet, *310:* 756, 1976.
3. Epstein, F. Diagnosis and management of arrested hydrocephalus. Shunts and problems with shunts. Monogr. Neural. Sci., *8:* 105–107, 1982.
4. Epstein, F. J., Hochwald, G. M., and Wald, A. Avoidance of shunt dependency in hydrocephalus. Dev. Med. Child. Neurol., *17*(Suppl. 35): 71–77, 1975.
5. Foltz, E. The first seven years of a hydrocephalus project. In *Workshop in Hydrocephalus*, edited by K. Shulman, pp. 79–114. Children's Hospital of Philadelphia, Philadelphia, 1965.
6. Foltz, E. L. Double compartment hydrocephalus: A new clinical entity. Neurosurgery, *7:* 551–559, 1980.
7. Foltz, E. L., and Shurtleff, D. B. Five-year comparative study of hydrocephalus in children with and without operation (113 cases). J. Neurosurg., *20:* 1064–1079, 1963.
8. Garrity, L., and Servos, A. Comparison of measures of adaptive behavior in pre-school children. J. Consult. Clin. Psychol., *46:* 228–293, 1978.
9. Goldstein, G. W., Chaplin, E. R., and Maithand, J. Transient hydrocephalus in premature infants: Treatment by lumbar punctures. Lancet, *310:* 512–514, 1976.
10. Hall, P., Lindseth, R., Campbell, R., et al. Scoliosis and hydrocephalus in myelomeningocele patients. J. Neurosurg., *50:* 174–178, 1979.
11. Hemmer, R. Can a shunt be removed? Shunts and problems in shunts. Monogr. Neural Sci., *8:* 223–226, 1982.
12. Jasper, P. L., and Merrill, R. E. Hydrocephalus and myelomeningocele: Central nervous system infection. Am. J. Dis. Child., *110:* 652–657, 1965.
13. Kaufman, B., Roessmann, U., and Nulsen, F. E. *Ventricular Coaptation from Overshunting.* American Association of Neurological Surgeons Pediatric Section, Cleveland, 1978.
14. Laurence, K. M. Neurological and intellectual sequelae of hydrocephalus. *Arch. Neurol.,* *20:* 73–82, 1979.
15. Lewin, R. Is your brain really necessary: John Lorber, A British Neurologist, claims that some patients are more normal than would be inferred from their brain scans. Science, *210:* 1232–1234, 1980.
16. Lorber, J. Results of treatment of myelomeningocele: An analysis of 524 unselected cases with special reference to possible selection for treatment. Dev. Med. Child Neurol., *13:* 279–303, 1971.
17. Lorber, J. Spina bifida cystica: Results of treatment of 270 consecutive cases with criteria for selection for the future. Arch. Dis. Child., *47:* 854–873, 1972.
18. Lorber, J. Isosorbide in the medical treatment infantile hydrocephalus. J. Neurosurg., *39:* 702–11, 1973.
19. Mapstone, T. B., Rekate, H. L., Nulsen, F. E., et al. Relationship of CSF shunting and IQ in children with myelomeningocele: A retrospective analysis. Child's Brain, *11:* 112–118, 1984.
20. McClone, D. Effect of complications on intellectual function in 173 children with myelomeningocele. Child's Brain, *5:* 561, 1979.

21. McClone, D., Killion, M., Yogev, R., and Sommers, M. W. Ventriculitis: Of mice and men. In: *Concepts in Pediatric Neurosurgery II*, edited by F. Epstein and A. Raimondi, pp. 112–126. S. Karger, Basel, Switzerland, 1982.

22. Nulsen, F. E. The control of progressive hydrocephalus in infancy by valve-regulated venous shunt. In: *Workshop in Hydrocephalus*, edited by K. Shulman, pp. 256–273. University of Pennsylvania Press, Philadelphia, 1965.

23. Nulsen, F. E., and Rekate, H. L. Results of treatment of hydrocephalus as a guide to prognosis and management. In: *Pediatric Neurosurgery: Surgery of the Developing Nervous System*, pp. 229–241, Grune & Stratton, New York, 1982.

24. O'Brien, M., Parent, A., and Davis, B. Management of ventricular shunt infection. Child's Brain, *5:* 304–309, 1979.

25. Peach, B. Arnold-Chiari malformation: Morphogenesis. Arch. Neurol., *12:* 527–535, 1965.

26. Rekate, H., Nulsen, F., Mack, H., *et al.* Establishing the diagnosis of shunt independence. Monogr. Neural. Sci., *8:* 223–226, 1982.

27. Schoenbaum, S. C., Gardner, P., and Shillito, J. Infections of cerebrospinal fluid shunts: Epidemiology, clinical manifestations, and therapy. J. Infect. Dis., *131:* 543–552, 1975.

28. Shurtleff, D. B., Foltz, E. L., and Loeser, J. D. Hydrocephalus: A definition of its progression and relationship to intellectual function, diagnosis, and complications. Am. J. Dis. Child., *125:* 688–693.

29. Sieben, R. L., Hamida, M. B., and Shulman, K. Multiple cranial nerve deficits associated with the Arnold Chiari malformation. Neurology, *21:* 673–681, 1971.

30. Venes, J. L. Multiple cranial nerve palsies in an infant with Arnold-Chiari malformation. Dev. Med. Child. Neurol., *16:* 817–820, 1974.

31. Venes, J. Control of shunt infection: Report of 150 consecutive cases. J. Neurosurg., *45:* 311–314, 1976.

32. Woolraich, M. C. Medical, ethical, and legal issues in selective use of rehabilitative care in the management of children with spina bifida. Spina Bifida Ther., *2:* 213–222, 1980.

33. Young, H., Nulsen, F., Weiss, M., *et al.* The relationship of intelligence and cerebral mantle in treated infantile hydrocephalus. Pediatrics, *52:* 38–44, 1973.

CHAPTER

30

How to Keep Shunts Functioning, or "The Impossible Dream"

FRED EPSTEIN, M.D.

Until relatively recently a newborn child with hydrocephalus was regarded as having a grave prognosis with regard to future cerebral function and longevity. Multiple shunt complications were accepted as inevitable, and it was very difficult to be optimistic as parents were advised that an abbreviated life span was likely to be plagued by multiple surgical procedures and ultimate brain damage. Some authors suggested that shunts be avoided at all costs, and alternate therapeutic procedures were advocated which were intended to minimize shunt dependency or even bring about a state of shunt independent arrested hydrocephalus (1–3, 6–9, 11, 15, 16, 18, 19, 30, 31).

The introduction of computed tomography (CT) in 1974 dramatically changed this gloomy outlook. Many of the "inevitable" complications are receding into history, and the clinician may be realistically hopeful that a hydrocephalic neonate will enjoy full longevity associated with normal intellectual development (20, 28).

Although long-term satisfactory shunt function is no longer "the impossible dream," it requires an in-depth understanding of hydrocephalus, intracranial pressure dynamics, shunt hardware, early and late complications, and appropriate treatment.

It is the purpose of this chapter to discuss many of the problems that have been associated with shunts and "shunt dependency" and suggest techniques by which they may be avoided or corrected, should they occur.

The two most important factors which determine the success or failure of treatment are the attitude and expertise of the neurosurgeon. The insertion of a shunt is often regarded as "technically uninteresting," and many of the surgical procedures are assigned to junior staff members or even residents. This, in itself, is a cause of many complications, as it takes a reasonable amount of experience to avoid or correct complications, and it is not appropriate for shunts to be assigned to relatively inexperienced staff members.

It must be emphasized that any neurosurgeon that accepts the responsibility of caring for a hydrocephalic infant is making a long-term commitment to the well-being of the child that in all likelihood will continue throughout the professional career of the neurosurgeon. This commitment extends beyond monitoring shunt function and includes long-term responsibility for supervising the treatment of a multitude of potential surgical and nonsurgical problems which may include seizures, psychomotor retardation, neurological disability, behavior disorders, *etc.* While many of these "long-term complications" may not be related to shunt obstruction, it is the responsibility of the neurosurgeon to make that assessment and to assume responsibility for making the proper referral should other expertise be necessary. Parents of hydrocephalic children live with great anxiety over the status of the shunt, and a malfunction may provoke an emotional crisis that envelops that entire family. The neurosurgeon must be available to care for the patient and must support the parents, thereby bringing some element of tranquility to the troubled family.

As the "impossible dream" becomes reality, we are becoming more aware that a small number of children are plagued by subtle complications that may become manifest many years or perhaps decades after primary surgical treatment. These include intellectual or behavioral deterioration from shunt malfunction not associated with signs or symptoms of increased intracranial pressure. These older patients may be mistakenly believed to have "arrested hydrocephalus" as they continue to deteriorate in the absence of close supervision. It is essential that neurosurgeons be sensitive to this "aging population" and remain responsive to their needs as neonates pass through adolescence and become adults (25, 28).

The CT scan has had the greatest impact on early and late management of hydrocephalus. There is no longer any ordinary indication to carry out ventriculography, pneumoencephalography, or an invasive study as part of the primary neurodiagnostic evaluation. In the overwhelming number of cases the common etiological diagnoses are obvious and, if not, it is "academic" to look further with regard to identifying the specific area of congenital narrowing of the spinal fluid pathways (22, 23).

In addition to providing early diagnosis, the CT scan is indispensable for the long-term follow-up of hydrocephalic children. It is essential that a "base line" CT scan be obtained 2 or 3 months following primary shunt insertion, as this serves for future comparison in the event of shunt malfunction.

SHUNT SELECTION

Many companies are producing a number of different shunt systems. I believe that they are designed with great expertise and that all of the available systems are probably equally satisfactory for treatment of hydrocephalus. There are some valves which seem more reliable with regard to opening-closing pressures, while others are structurally more elegant (13, 14). I do not believe that any of these factors are important in terms of long-term satisfactory shunt function, and final selection is more subjective than scientific.

Although much attention has been directed to the quantitative assessment of opening and closing pressures, I believe that this is largely wasted effort, inasmuch as there is no evidence to suggest that this issue has any relationship to satisfactory shunt function and, in fact, if the truth be candidly stated, we do not have any real concept of optimal shunt-regulated pressure dynamics. When an infant is recumbent, the intracranial pressure may be related to the opening and closing pressure of the specific valve. However, in the head-up position, intracranial pressure is invariably subatmospheric, irrespective of the opening and closing pressure of the valve, or the presence or absence of an antisyphon device and, therefore, at this time I am most dubious that there is any prognostic relevance to this entire issue (34). Some neurosurgeons recommend low pressure, others medium pressure, and still others high pressure shunts. There is no uniformity of opinion, as many surgeons have reported satisfactory results with various systems.

Interestingly, while we have debated the "ideal" pressure characteristics of shunts, we have never devised an *in vivo* technique to quantitate the volume of fluid that drains through any system in a 24-hour period. From my perspective, this is far more fundamental to understanding the pathophysiology of treated hydrocephalus than all of the discussion of pressure characteristics. I believe that the shunt of the future will be telemetrically assessed in terms of the rate of flow and that there will be some technique whereby rate of flow may be externally modulated to what may be ideal for any given infant. The rate of flow may be periodically monitored, which will provide more information regarding adequate shunt function than any pressure measurements.

My only prejudice in "shunt hardware" is a preference for one-piece systems at the primary surgery. This is because a very common cause of shunt malfunction is disruption or disintegration of the tube at the site of a connector which may be associated with growth or, occasionally, direct trauma. This is now preventable, as more than one company is producing one-piece shunts. These are provided in a wide range of lengths and pressure characteristics, and I am confident that they will eventually replace multipiece systems at the primary operation.

In cases in which a one-piece shunt is not used, it is essential that the ventricular catheter be of a right angle configuration with the distal part of the tube positioned over the outer table of the skull, 1–3 cm away from the burr hole. This assumes importance at the time of later proximal shunt revision when it is possible to change the ventricular catheter without manipulation of the pump, or *vice versa*. Ventricular catheters which are secured by a connector to the undersurface of the pump have a predilection to become separated from the mechanism at the time of proximal revision. In these cases it is not unusual to lose the ventricular catheter into the ventricle, and a "stray" catheter results, which may not only complicate the revision but also may be a hazard, should future infection mandate its removal.

POSITION OF SHUNT

It is important for the tip of the ventricular catheter to be anterior to the foramen of Monro, as otherwise it is likely to become obstructed as it becomes enmeshed within the choroid plexus. Some neurosurgeons prefer the occipital route, others the frontal route, although I believe either is satisfactory if the tip of the catheter is in the proper location. Despite the best effort, the postoperative skull x-ray occasionally discloses the catheter to be in less than an ideal position. If the shunt is functioning, I am not committed to immediate revision unless the catheter is obviously kinked, is only partially in the ventricle, or is in the anteriormost part of the temporal horn, in which case early malfunction is likely. Intraoperative ultrasound may be of assistance in proper placement of the catheter, and although it is not uniformly available, it may prove to be a very helpful future adjunct (32, 33).

When it is necessary to insert a new proximal shunting mechanism in the presence of only mildly to moderately enlarged ventricles, the frontal route is preferable, as proper placement is more easily accomplished by that route than by the occipital route. In these cases, it is helpful to place the patient supine on the operating table with a transparent drape over the face. This permits visualization of the traditional facial landmarks as the catheter is passed into the frontal horn (bridge of nose and ipsilateral eye).

The peritoneal cavity is the primary choice for distal shunt placement. In full-term neonates it is my practice to place 12–18 inches of tubing into the peritoneal cavity, as this often ensures satisfactory function for several years. There have been no complications associated with placing a large length of tubing in the abdomen, which has minimized or even obviated mandatory revisions, as most growth after 2 years of age is from the legs with only minimal elongation of the torso. It is always interesting to note that the position of the peritoneal catheter is quite variable, depending on where it has been displaced by normal peristalsis. Because adhesions do not envelop the nearly continuously moving tip, long-term satisfactory function is very common (Fig. 30.1).

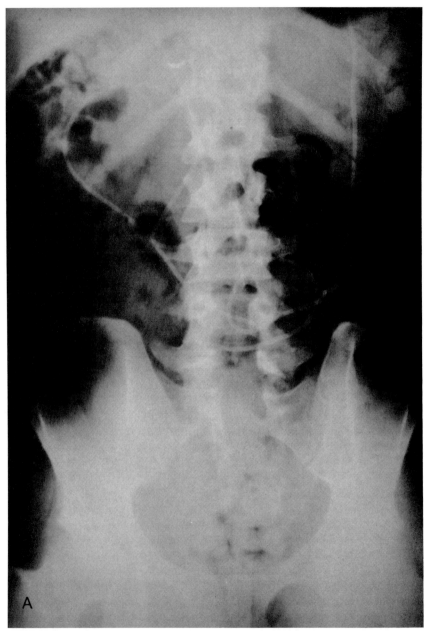

FIG. 30.1. (A and B) Abdominal x-rays obtained 12 hours apart disclose variable position of peritoneal catheters.

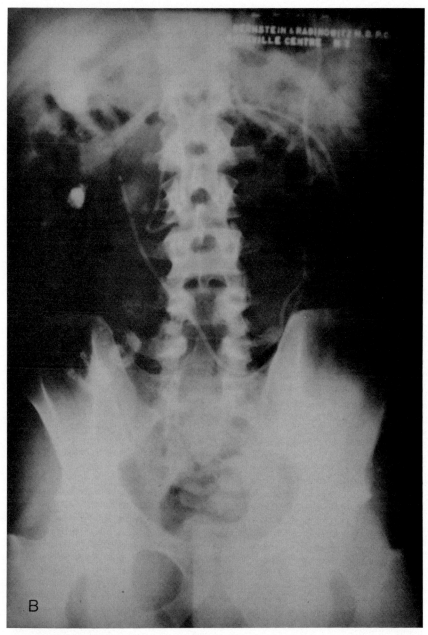

FIG. 30.1B

ELECTIVE REVISION

Parents often inquire as to whether or not their child "still needs the shunt" after several years pass without symptomatic malfunction. Neurosurgeons must also consider the same issue when making a recommendation of elective shunt revisions, as this is only indicated for a shunt-dependent child in whom the distal catheter is about to be distracted from the peritoneal cavity.

Whereas the latter is obvious on plain x-ray examination, the former assessment is more complex and must be carefully considered. Although there is no single noninvasive test that defines the state of shunt dependency, there are several observations that are helpful in making this assessment.

A significantly thick calvarium which is obvious on skull x-rays is often indicative of shunt dependency (Fig. 30.2). In addition, a small ventricular system is evidence of shunt dependency, as arrested hydrocephalus is almost always associated with significant ventriculomegaly

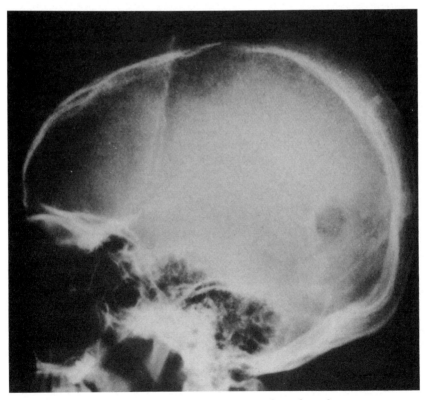

FIG. 30.2. Very thick calvarium suggests shunt dependency.

and does not occur in the presence of a normal or even near normal ventricular volume. Since compensated hydrocephalus only rarely occurs after the first few months of age, a child that has required a shunt revision for symptomatic malfunction after 6 months of age must be assumed permanently shunt-dependent. Therefore it is appropriate to electively lengthen a shunt in the presence of a thickened calvarium, small ventricles, or previous symptomatic shunt malfunction.

Compensated hydrocephalus is usually associated with moderate or advanced ventriculomegaly. In asymptomatic children over 2 years of age in whom the large ventricular volume has been stable, it is essential to perform a detailed neuropsychological examination. In the presence of any intellectual deficit, a radioisotope shunt scan must be done, and the shunt must be electively revised if it is not functioning properly. In younger children it is not possible to be confident that psychomotor testing accurately predicts present or future intellectual potential. Therefore, in the presence of significant ventriculomegaly, it is advisable to confirm satisfactory function with a radioisotope study.

In the presence of large ventricles and normal intellectual function, elective shunt revision may be deferred, although annual neuropsychological testing is essential, as late intellectual deterioration may be associated with "arrested" hydrocephalus.

If a decision is made to carry out an elective distal revision, an adequate length of tube should be inserted into the peritoneal cavity to make it unnecessary to carry out future revision on the basis of body growth. It is important to recognize that the catheter must not be lengthened over the abdominal cavity, as a connector in this location will not ascend with growth and, therefore, the tube distal to the connector will be permanently fixed in length, and disruption at the site of the connector may be associated with future growth.

EMERGENCY SHUNT REVISION

The most serious technical problems associated with emergency revision are related to removal and satisfactory replacement of the proximal system. These include separation of the ventricular catheter, ventricular collapse and resultant inability to replace the ventricular catheter, and intraventricular hemorrhage.

An obstructed ventricular catheter is often firmly adherent to the choroid plexus and ependyma, and considerable force may be required to remove the tube. This may be particularly problematic when a flanged ventricular catheter has been in place for more than a few months. In these cases the catheter should be rotated as it is distracted from the ventricle. This often frees it from the adjacent tissue and facilitates removal. Minor ventricular hemorrhage is very common, and it is advisable to gently irrigate the ventricle in an effort to remove grossly bloody fluid prior to completing the surgical procedure.

In cases in which a right angle ventricular catheter has not been employed, great care must be taken to avoid separation of the ventricular catheter. The connector on the undersurface of the pump is commonly enmeshed in fibrous tissue and intimately adherent to the dura, brain, and underlying fibrous tract. The pump must be dissected from adjacent tissues and gently elevated from the burr hole to expose the dura through which the catheter passes. Small cruciate incisions are made circumferentially around the tube, through the dura and fibrous tract. It is then possible to gently remove the proximal system through the enlarged dural opening.

Despite the best effort, the ventricular catheter occasionally separates from the pump at the connector. In most cases it remains in a superficial location within the fibrous tract and is easily visualized and retrieved. In other cases it "springs" during the separation and recedes through the tract into the brain. In the presence of large occipital horns and a thin cortical mantle, it may migrate into the ventricle, resulting in a "stray" catheter. When this occurs the tube should be undisturbed, and a new ventricular catheter should be passed through a different trajectory. In the event that future infection mandates that the stray catheter be removed, the CT scan will inform the surgeon as to whether the catheter remains fixed somewhere within the fibrous tract or is within the ventricle. In the former case the fibrous tract may be excised (magnified vision is essential), and the catheter may be removed with little associated trauma to adjacent tissue. In the latter case a ventriculoscope with attached biopsy forceps is the preferred technique whereby the catheter is removed.

The most serious intraoperative problem is associated with a separated unretrievable ventricular catheter and minor ventriculomegaly. In these cases a small amount of CSF invariably "escapes" along the fibrous tract and may result in collapse of the ventricle. In these circumstances there are three options. The first is to attempt to pass the new ventricular catheter down the fibrous tract and intentionally displace the separated catheter into the ventricle. In this way the fibrous tract serves as a conduit to placement of the new tube, and the "stray" catheter must be accepted as inherent to resolution of the problem. Under no circumstances should a rigid introducer or brain needle be passed along the tract, as this is likely to deviate from the planned trajectory and pass through functional cerebral tissue. If it is not possible to obtain a satisfactory placement and the surgeon is confident that the ventricle has not collapsed, a single attempt may be made to employ a frontal trajectory to the ventricle.

Finally, if all efforts fail, there should be no further attempt to pass the catheter via other trajectories. The procedure must be terminated, and the patient must be studied with serial CT scans. The collapsed ventricle will invariably gradually dilate before threatening signs and symptoms of increased intracranial pressure evolves. At that time it will be relatively simple to insert a new ventricular catheter via a frontal trajectory, and the crisis will be resolved with no associated morbidity.

Distal shunt revision is rarely problematic, as replacement in the peritoneal cavity is usually easily accomplished. Occasionally, "encystment" of the peritoneal catheter results in distal shunt obstruction. In most cases abdominal pain is associated with intermittent headache as the catheter gradually becomes occluded. An ultrasound examination of the abdomen is always diagnostic and is a valuable examination in the presence of unexplained distal obstruction (26) (Fig. 30.3). Catheter encystment does not preclude revision, as it is usually only necessary to insert the catheter in a different part of the peritoneal cavity.

In unusual circumstances the peritoneal cavity is not satisfactory as a result of idiopathic failure to absorb fluid with resultant ascites or multiple adhesions secondary to previous surgery or infection. In these cases either a vascular or pleural shunt is mandatory. In children older

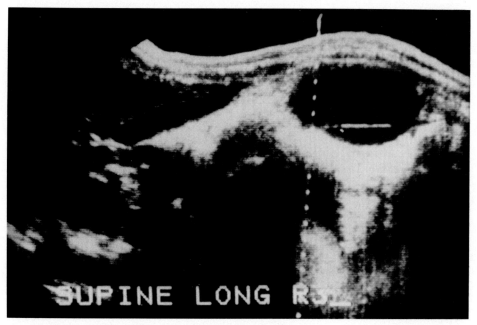

FIG. 30.3. Ultrasound examination of abdomen discloses large cyst surrounding the shunt catheter.

than 10 years of age the pleural cavity is an excellent site for CSF absorption, and most shunts in this location work well for many years (29). Satisfactory function may be confirmed by a decubitus chest x-ray which discloses free fluid in the pleural cavity. In many children under 10 years of age (and most children less than 5 years old), the pleural cavity is not satisfactory, as the absorptive area is not large enough, and symptomatic hydrothorax develops. Therefore, in the younger age group an atrial shunt may be necessary. In recent years excellent techniques have been described whereby the atrial catheter is inserted transcutaneously, utilizing a technique similar to that employed for placement of cardiac pacemakers (12). Atrial shunts function well, although it is wise to arrange for regular examinations by a cardiologist for early detection of the very rare late complication of pulmonary hypertension (24).

RECURRENT SHUNT OBSTRUCTION

There are a few patients that suffer multiple shunt obstructions over a relatively short time interval. This complication seems to occur in normal adolescent children in whom the previously inserted shunt functioned satisfactorily for many years. Physician and family become frustrated and even angry as the long asymptomatic child becomes acutely or chronically ill while the etiology of the recurring shunt obstruction seems elusive.

As with any shunt-related complication, the etiology and appropriate surgical treatment will become apparent as the individual case is analyzed. When a recently replaced ventricular catheter becomes obstructed, it is likely that the tip of the new catheter is in the same identical position as the one that was removed and that the cause of the recurrent obstruction is related to the position. In some cases undetected ventricular septae may occlude the catheter, while in others the choroid plexus or ependymal wall has a predilection to envelop it. In the presence of moderate ventriculomegaly it is advisable to replace the ventricular catheter by means of a new burr hole either on the opposite side, or via an ipsilateral frontal approach, should the catheter be occipital or, *viceversa*, if it were frontal. In this way, the ventricular catheter will be in a different area of the frontal horn and, hopefully, the cause of the obstruction which was related to the position of the catheter will not recur. In cases in which recurrent symptoms are associated with normal or subnormal ventricular volume, the therapeutic options are more limited and will be discussed in the section Slit Ventricle Syndrome.

In rare cases late partial obstruction of the foramen of Monro may be associated with a shunting system that has functioned normally for many years. The contralateral ventricle dilates very gradually over months or even years. This may be minimal and may be misinterpreted as the normal asymmetry that occurs with a functioning shunt in which the ipsilateral ventricle is the smaller ventricle. When the child finally becomes symptomatic, it is assumed to be the result of an uncomplicated proximal malfunction, and the ventricular catheter is replaced. Because the patient remains symptomatic, a recurrent proximal obstruction is often diagnosed, although the real problem is secondary to subtle progressive enlargement of the contralateral ventricle. Careful review of serial CT scans finally identifies the underlying problem, and installation of metrizamide through the ventricular catheter may confirm it.

In these patients the functioning shunt should be undisturbed, and a new one should be inserted on the contralateral side. It is my preference to utilize an entirely new shunt, and rather than to "Y" the distal tube into the old catheter. This avoids future confusion when the site of malfunction may be difficult to determine with a unified system. Dual systems are easier to monitor when inserted for any condition which mandates more than one ventricular catheter (Dandy-Walker, *etc.*).

The most frequent cause of recurrent obstruction of the peritoneal catheter is chronic infection. This often occurs in the absence of local and systemic symptoms of infection, and therefore culture of the distal shunt catheter must be a routine part of the surgical procedure. If infection is confirmed, the entire shunt must be replaced, as there is likely to be colonization of the proximal mechanism (21).

SLIT VENTRICLE SYNDROME

It is important to emphasize at the outset that slit ventricles are an extremely common and probably desirable result of shunt insertion at an early age. There is no correlation between a small ventricular system and an increased incidence of shunt malfunction, and there is no indication for any surgical manipulation of the shunt to expand the ventricles in an asymptomatic child. The slit ventricle syndrome is a rare entity in which there are mostly subjective symptoms suggestive of increased intracranial pressure in the presence of normal or subnormal ventricular volume. The most common symptom is chronic or remitting headache, and while this may be severe and even disabling, only rarely are there threatening signs of increased intracranial pressure.

Etiology

It has been suggested that the slit ventricle syndrome is the result of intermittent shunt malfunction as the proximal catheter becomes transiently trapped between abutting or collapsed ventricular walls (10). According to this theory, at the time of the transient obstruction there is a small increase in ventricular volume which frees the catheter and restores normal function. The transient increment in intracranial pressure which is associated with the small increase in ventricular volume is supposedly responsible for the cyclic symptomatology that has been associated with the syndrome. In order to confirm that transient obstruction of the ventricular catheter is the etiology of the slit ventricle syndrome, it is essential that the neurodiagnostic study be obtained at a time that coincides with the acute symptomatology. In occasional patients this will document that there is very transient enlargement of the ventricles which may return to normal within a few hours as the symptoms remit (Fig. 30.4).

Although intermittent shunt malfunction may be responsible for the symptomatic slit ventricle, it must be relatively rare, as most children with small ventricles and any element of obstruction rapidly develop significant ventriculomegaly (Fig. 30.5). In addition episodic pressure waves have been documented in a few symptomatic patients, with small ventricles and normal shunt function (3, 4). It therefore seems likely that transient shunt obstruction is only one of the causes of a syndrome that is etiologically complex and even variable.

I have noted that many children with the slit ventricle syndrome have a markedly thickened and small cranial vault which is probably secondary to premature fusion of multiple sutures as a result of collapse of the skull after early shunting of advanced hydrocephalus. The net result of a small cranium, small ventricles, and shunt dependency is abnormal brain compliance, little buffering capacity, and a state of relatively fragile intracranial pressure dynamics which may be adversely affected by many factors. Normal variations in shunt function with undetectable small increments and decrements in ventricular volume are probably very common in the asymptomatic child, as these minor changes in intracranial volume are buffered with no significant alteration of intracranial pressure. In the presence of slit ventricles and a small calvarium, these normal variations in flow may cause episodes of increased intracranial pressure which becomes clinically manifest as the slit ventricle syndrome (3, 4, 10).

It is also possible that an increase in brain volume as a result of physiological alterations of cerebral blood flow causes symptomatic pressure waves. In these cases vigorous physical activity may cause a severe headache which remits with rest.

Systemic viral illnesses are probably occasionally associated with alterations in cerebral blood flow or minor transient brain edema. This may cause a small increase in brain volume and severe headaches for the duration of the illness.

Treatment

In the presence of radiographically documented intermittent shunt malfunction, replacement of the ventricular catheter is the only recourse.

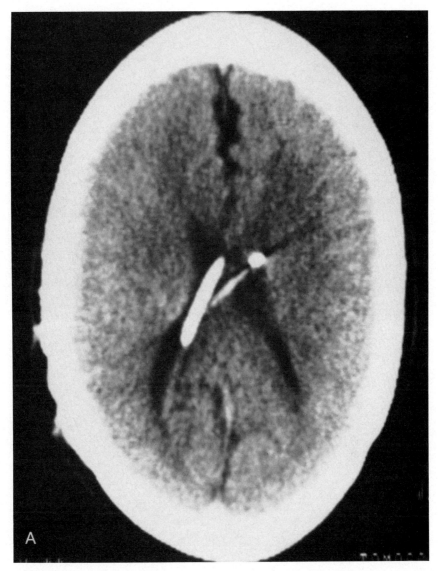

FIG. 30.4. (A–C) CAT scans 8 hours apart disclose transient ventricular enlargement in patients with slit ventricle syndrome.

In addition, increasing the resistance of the shunt by insertion of a higher pressure valve or antisyphon device may prevent recurrent collapse of the ventricles and may increase the likelihood of success.

Cases in which the ventricles are consistently small may pose a therapeutic dilemma. In most of these situations, surgical treatment

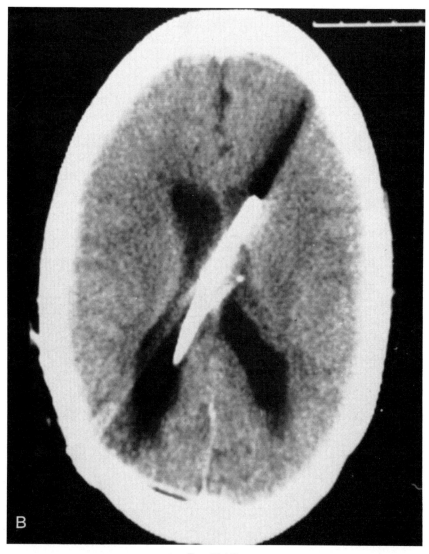

FIG. 30.4*B*

should not be considered unless the patient has been functionally disabled by prolonged symptomatology. In some of these patients, replacement of the ventricular catheter may relieve symptoms as a variable flow rate through a partially obstructed catheter is increased. In many cases subtemporal craniectomy has been curative, as minor pressure waves are apparently "vented" by the bony decompression (5). Despite the logic of

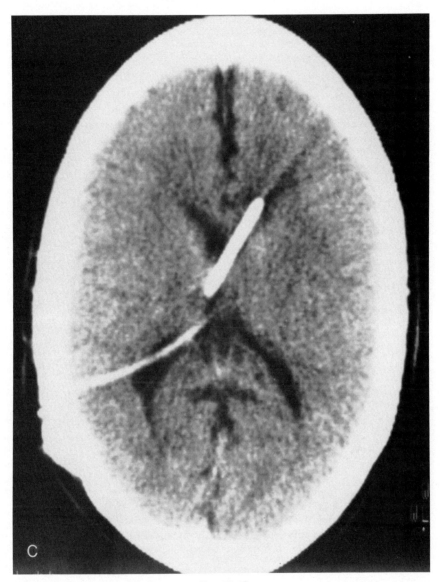

FIG. *30.4C*

these therapeutic endeavors, symptoms often recur, at which time other options must be considered.

In the presence of a thickened skull and small head a cranial expansion may resolve the primary problem. In these very select cases the skull is

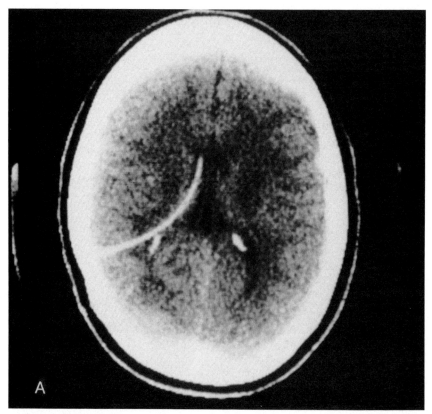

FIG. 30.5. Most patients with a functioning shunt and slit ventricles (A) rapidly develop significant ventriculomegaly (B) if the system becomes obstructed.

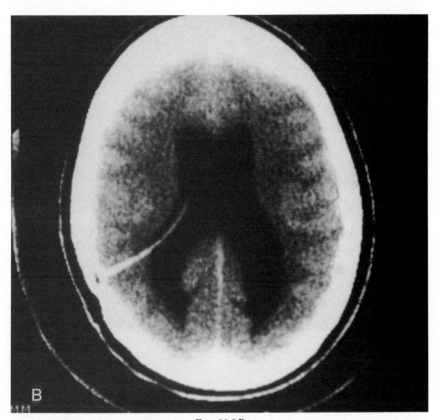

FIG. 30.5B

morcellated between the coronal and lambdoid sutures (Fig. 30.6A and B). This increases the volume of the cranial cavity and probably returns buffering capacity and compliance towards normal. Although this surgical approach must be regarded as experimental and perhaps controversial,

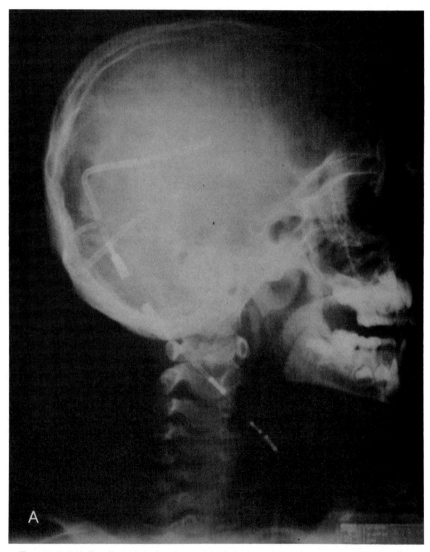

Fig. 30.6. (A) Small thick calvarium with digital markings in 8-year-old girl with slit ventricle syndrome and normal shunt function. (B) Skull morcellated between coronal and lambdoid suture. Patient has remained asymptomatic since surgery.

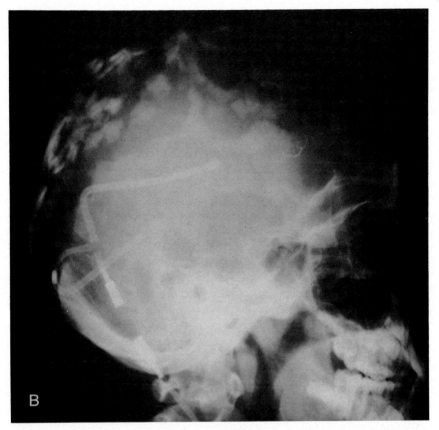

FIG. 30.6*B*

the preliminary results have been most encouraging as a few patients have been relieved of all symptoms.

It has become clear that one must be cautious in the interpretation of symptomatology as well as surgical treatment of the child who complains of recurring headache and has a normal or subnormal ventricular volume. It seems likely that differing etiologies of the slit ventricle syndrome may be the basis of varying degrees of success with divergent treatment techniques (Fig. 30.7).

Finally, it is important to reemphasize that the slit ventricle is not a pathological entity. With the advent of the CT scanner, it has become obvious that a small ventricular system is a common occurrence in shunted children and ordinarily does not cause symptoms or an increased incidence of shunt malfunction. The great majority of children will continue to do well and will not have symptomatology referable to it.

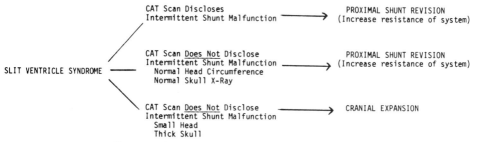

FIG. 30.7. Surgical options for slit ventricle syndrome.

LOCULATED VENTRICULAR SYSTEM

A loculated ventricular system is a complication of infection or intraventricular hemorrhage. In most cases, patients are severely retarded as a result of the associated brain injury. It may be exceedingly difficult to maintain shunt function, as the ventricular system is reduced to a series of small cavities and a single catheter is often insufficient for adequate fluid drainage. In these cases utilization of a ventriculoscope may be an indispensable adjunct, as it permits visualization and perforation of the ventricular septations which achieves communication of most of the ventricular compartments, and also facilitates shunt drainage. Although this may be helpful, ventricular loculations are a most difficult problem, and it is commonly necessary to utilize more than one shunt system to maintain normal intracranial pressure.

LATE ONSET HYDROCEPHALUS

A child with late onset aqueductal stenosis and advanced ventriculomegaly is a very different problem from the neonate with an expansile skull. In the latter case, the cranial circumference commonly decreases as the sutures overlap and gradually fill the subdural space that invariably develops between the collapsed brain and the inner table of the skull. In the older child, fibrous union of the sutures maintains the cranial volume, and for this reason, a transient craniocerebral disproportion with an associated subdural hematoma or hygroma is a relatively common complication (17).

It is important that this potential problem be recognized prior to the insertion of the shunt, as it is in this specific situation that it is advisable to consider the pressure characteristics of the system to be inserted vis-à-vis the underlying condition being treated. A child with significantly elevated intracranial pressure and advanced ventricular dilatation must be treated with a high resistance system which incorporates a high pressure valve. In these cases an antisiphon valve may be incorporated into the system to further limit the relative intracranial hypotension which is inevitably associated with the shunt insertion (27). This decreases the flow to some degree and, hopefully, makes complications less likely.

Despite all technical precautions, it is not always possible to prevent a subdural hygroma or hematoma. Although additional precautions may be taken, such as maintaining the patient flat in bed for a few days, gradual elevation, and mobilization, *etc.*, the complication rate remains significant, although with proper diagnosis and treatment there should be no significant long-term morbidity or mortality.

SUMMARY

Hydrocephalus is a benign condition, and as our expertise in surgical treatment has increased, many of the "inevitable complications" are disappearing, and a normal life associated with satisfactory shunt function is no longer "the impossible dream." While this chapter has identified a few of the problems that may complicate long-term management, it is important to reemphasize that the most important single factor which determines success or failure is the attitude and experience of the neurosurgeon.

While there is a great deal of surgical pride associated with removing a meningioma or clipping an aneurysm, we do not receive accolades from our colleagues when we have inserted or replaced a shunt. Whereas the surgical technique that is employed to remove an acoustic tumor or a meningioma at the base of the brain is a testimony to the skill of the neurosurgeon, it is not a technical feat to revise a shunt in an acutely ill child. When the surgical outcome is a satisfactory one, it is taken for granted, and when recurrent problems evolve they are assumed to reflect problems intrinsic to caring for hydrocephalus, and little consideration is given to the technical and conceptual skills required to retrieve the situation.

Neurosurgeons often lose sight of the fact that hydrocephalus is the most benign intracranial disorder which is treated in large numbers. I believe that the most serious problem in the treatment of hydrocephalus has been the reluctance of experienced neurosurgeons to devote their time and energies to understanding the underlying pathophysiology and the potential complications and to instituting appropriate treatment.

A neurosurgeon who is devoted to both the patient and the family and is committed to understanding and treating complications associated with shunts and shunt dependency will be the best insurance of the future of the patient, and ultimately as normal adults these patients will be a permanent testimony to the skills of the primary neurosurgeon.

REFERENCES

1. Bergman, E., Epstein, M., and Freeman, J. M. Medical management of hydrocephalus with acetazolamide and furosemide. Ann. Neurol., *4:* 189, 1978.

2. Epstein, F. Diagnosis and management of arrested hydrocephalus. Monogr. Neural Sci., 8: 105–107, 1982.

3. Epstein, F. Increased intracranial pressure in hydrocephalic children with functioning shunts: A complication of shunt dependency. In Concepts of Neurosurgery. S. Karger, Basel, 1983, vol 4, pp 119–130.

4. Epstein, F. Increased intracranial pressure in hydrocephalic children with functioning shunts: A complication of shunt dependency. In: Hydrocephalus, Chap. 19, edited by K. Shapiro and A. Marmarou, pp. 315–321. Raven Press, New York, 1984.

5. Epstein, F., Fleischer, A., Hochwald, G., and Ransohoff, J. Subtemporal craniectomy for recurrent shunt obstruction secondary to small ventricles. J. Neurosurg., 41: 29–31, 1974.

6. Epstein, F., Hochwald, G., and Ransohoff, J. A volume control system for the treatment of hydrocephalus. Laboratory and clinical experience. J. Neurosurg., 38: 282–287, 1973.

7. Epstein, F., Hochwald, G., and Ransohoff, J. Neonatal hydrocephalus treated by compressive head wrapping. Lancet, 2: 634–636, 1973.

8. Epstein, F., Hochwald, G., Wald, A., and Ransohoff, J. Avoidance of shunt dependency. Dev. Med. Child Neurol. (Suppl.), 35: 71–77, 1975.

9. Epstein, F., Hochwald, G., Wald, A., and Ransohoff, J. Avoidance of shunt dependency. In: Meningomyelocele, edited by R. L. McLaurin, pp. 313–324. Grune & Stratton, New York, 1977.

10. Epstein, F., Marlin, A., and Wald, A. Chronic headache in the shunt dependent adolescent nearly normal ventricular volume: Diagnosis and treatment. Neurosurgery, 3: 351–355, 1978.

11. Epstein, F., Wald, A., and Hochwald, G. Intracranial pressure during compressive head wrapping in treatment of neonatal hydrocephalus. Pediatrics, 54: 786, 1974.

12. Epstein, N., Epstein, F., and Trehan, N. Percutaneous placement of the atrial end of a vascular shunt utilizing the Swan-Ganz introducer. Neurosurg. Technical Note, 9(5): 564–565, 1981.

13. Fox, J. L., McCullough, D. C., and Green, R. C. Cerebrospinal fluid shunts: An experimental comparison of flow rates and pressure valves in various commercial systems. J. Neurosurg., 37: 700–705, 1972.

14. Hakim, S., de la Roche, D., and Burton, J. D. A critical analysis of valve shunts used in the treatment of hydrocephalus. Dev. Med. Child Neurol., 15: 230–255, 1973.

15. Hayden, P. W., Foltz, E. L., and Shurtleff, D. B. Effect of an oral osmotic agent on ventricular fluid pressure of hydrocephalic children. Pediatrics, 41: 955–957, 1968.

16. Hayden, P. W., and Shurtleff, D. B. The medical management of hydrocephalus. Dev. Med. Child Neurol. (Suppl.), 27: 52–58, 1972.

17. Hoffman, H. J., and Tucker, H. J. Cephalocranial dysproportion. A complication of the treatment of hydrocephalus in children. Child's Brain, 2: 167–176, 1976.

18. Huttenlocher, P. R. Treatment of hydrocephalus with acetazolamide. J. Pediatr., 66: 1023–1030, 1965.

19. Lorber, J., Salfield, S., and London, T. Isosorbide in treatment of infantile hydrocephalus. Arch. Dis. Child, 50: 431–436, 1975.

20. McCullough, D. C., and Balzer-Martin, L. A. Current prognosis in overt neonatal hydrocephalus. J. Neurosurg., 57: 378–383, 1982.

21. McLaurin, R. Shunt complications. In: Pediatric Neurosurgery, Chap. 16, pp. 243–253. Grune & Stratton, New York, 1982.

22. Naidich, T., Epstein, F., Lin, J., Kricheff, I., and Hochwald, G. The evaluation of pediatric hydrocephalus by computerized axial tomography. Radiology, 119: 337–345, 1976.

23. Naidich, T. P., Epstein, F., Lin, J., Kricheff, I., and Hochwald, G. The role of

computerized axial tomography in the diagnosis, treatment, and follow-up of hydrocephalus. Child's Brain, 2: 111, 1976.

24. Nugent, G. R., Lucas, R., Juday, M., et al. Thromboembolic complications of ventriculoatrial shunts. Angiocardiographic and pathologic correlations. J. Neurosurg., 24: 34–42, 1966.

25. Nulsen, F. E., and Rekate, H. L. Results of treatment for hydrocephalus as a guide to future management. In: Pediatric Neurosurgery, Chap. 15, pp. 229–241. Grune & Stratton, New York, 1982.

26. Parry, S. W., Schumacher, J. F., and Llewellyn, R. C. Abdominal pseudocysts and ascites formation after ventriculoperitoneal shunt procedures. Report of four cases. J. Neurosurg., 43: 476–480.

27. Portnoy, H. D., Schulte, R. R., Fox, J. L., et al. Anti-siphon and reversable occlusion valves for shunting in hydrocephalus and preventing postshunt subdural hematomas. J. Neurosurg., 38: 729–738, 1973.

28. Raimondi, A. Intellectual development of shunted hydrocephalic children. Am. J. Dis. Child, 127: 664–671, 1974.

29. Ransohoff, J. Ventriculo-pleural anastomosis in treatment of obstructive hydrocephalus. J. Neurosurg., 11: 295–298, 1954.

30. Schain, R. J. Carbonic anhydrase inhibitors in chronic infantile hydrocephalus. Am. J. Dis. Child, 117: 621–625, 1969.

31. Shinnar, S., Gammon, K., Epstein, M., and Freeman, J. M. Avoidance of shunts in the management of hydrocephalus: Successful medical management with acetazolamide and furosemide. Ann. Neurol., 12: 111, 1982.

32. Shkolnik, A., and McLone, D. Intraoperative real-time ultrasonic guidance of ventricular shunt placement in infants. Radiology, 141: 515–517, 1981.

33. Shkolnik, A., and McLone, D. Intraoperative real-time ultrasonic guidance of ventricular shunt placement in infants. Radiology, 144: 573–576, 1982.

34. Yamada, S., Ducker, T. B., and Perot, P. L. Dynamic changes of cerebrospinal fluid in upright and recumbent shunted experimental animals. Child's Brain, 1: 187–192, 1975.

CHAPTER

31

CSF Shunts for Dementia, Incontinence, and Gait Disturbance

PETER McL. BLACK, M.D., Ph.D., ROBERT G. OJEMANN, M.D., and
ARGYRIS TZOURAS, M.D.

INTRODUCTION

The clinical combination of dementia, incontinence, and gait disturbance in association with enlarged ventricles and normal cerebrospinal fluid (CSF) pressure is often helped by CSF shunting. Salomon Hakim in 1964 proposed that this condition in the elderly could occur without known antecedent; the syndrome he described has subsequently been called idiopathic normal pressure hydrocephalus (NPH), Hakim's syndrome, or Hakim-Adams syndrome (2, 46). This clinical syndrome of dementia, incontinence, and gait disturbance remains the major indication for shunt placement in elderly patients with large ventricles and normal CSF pressure.

Numerous reports have evaluated diagnostic tests and considered the indications for placing a shunt in a patient with hydrocephalus, dementia, incontinence, gait disturbance, and normal CSF pressure (3–12, 15–20, 23, 33, 38, 42, 54, 57, 60, 67, 69, 70, 75–78, 82, 84–90, 95–99, 102, 104–106, 111, 112, 114–116). For the practicing neurosurgeon, there are two important questions to answer in deciding to shunt under these circumstances: First, considering the clinical and diagnostic studies, will this particular patient benefit from a shunt procedure? Second, what should the shunt pressure be to provide an optimal chance of success and minimize the possibility of postoperative chronic subdural hematoma or hygroma? This paper will discuss the experience at the Massachusetts General Hospital over a 5-year period on these issues, presenting relevant data from the literature as well.

MATERIALS AND METHODS

The charts of 36 patients in whom ventricular shunts were placed for normal pressure hydrocephalus of unknown cause from 1979 to 1983 were reviewed by a neurosurgeon other than the surgeon doing the shunt. The data represent the combined results of shunting by five different neurosurgeons; however, 28 of the 36 shunts were placed by two of the authors (PMcLB or RGO). The patients' age, sex, presenting complaints, and results of neurological evaluation before shunting were recorded and compared with the results of evaluation 3 months after shunt placement. In one grouping, patients were classified as having primarily gait difficulties or primarily memory difficulty, and the difference in shunt outcome was compared using χ^2 analysis. In a second grouping, patients were classified as showing the entire triad of ataxia, dementia, and incontinence; as showing ataxia and incontinence; or as showing dementia only. Again, results of shunting were compared.

For assessing improvement, evaluation was carried out for each of these symptom areas: gait, memory, and incontinence. For gait, patients were classified as unable to walk (3); unable to walk without assistance (2); unsteady but able to walk unassisted (1); and without gait difficulty (0). Memory deficits were classified as severe (3) (disoriented in time and place); moderate (2) (difficulty noted in recent memory by physician, support staff, and family); mild (1) (testing required to demonstrate deficit); or none (0). Urinary incontinence was classified as moderate (daytime incontinence); mild (nocturnal); or none. Initial lumbar puncture (LP) pressure was classified as being less or greater than 100 mm H_2O. The lumbar release of CSF, where tested, was graded as positive (improvement in gait or memory by one category above) or ineffectual in improving symptoms and signs.

Computed tomographic (CT) scans were graded as demonstrating either ventricular enlargement with cortical atrophy or ventricular enlargement without cortical atrophy; for this the estimate of an experienced neuroradiologist was used. Periventricular lucency could not be satisfactorily assessed in retrospect. The radionuclide cisternogram was considered normal (no ventricular entry, good convexity flow); mixed (transient ventricular entry); or typical of NPH (ventricular entry and stasis over 24 hours with poor ascent over the convexity). In six patients, metrizamide cisternography was performed at the same time as indium installation.

To assess the results of shunting, overall improvement was assessed during the hospitalization or at follow-up 3 months later. Response was graded as excellent (resumed pre-illness activity without deficit); good (resumed pre-illness activity with deficit or improved at least one grade in two or more categories); fair (improved but did not return to previous work or improved in only one category); and, poor (no change or worse). For purposes of statistical analysis, patients were classified as improved (excellent, good, or fair) or not improved at 3 months. χ^2 testing was used to compare the effects of particular factors on shunt outcome dividing patients into "improved" and "not improved" categories.

RESULTS

There were 23 men and 13 women in the series; their age range was 61–94 years, with mean age 73.2 years and median age 77.5. Presumed cerebrovascular disease as defined by hypertension by history or examination, stroke by history, or CT evidence of old infarct or lacunae was present in 87% of patients.

The presenting syndrome are listed in Table 31.1 along with the shunt outcome for each group. The importance of gait disturbance is suggested in Table 31.2: 77% of patients with primarily gait disturbance improved; 42% of those in which gait disturbance was less important improved. There is, therefore, a trend toward increasing shunt success with gait difficulty, although the small numbers do not allow χ^2 testing.

Radiologic data are presented in Tables 31.3–31.5. The presence of atrophy on CT scan diminished, but did not exclude, the likelihood of improvement after shunting. Very large ventricles or traditional signs of hydrocephalus such as temporal horn dilation were associated with good response. It appeared that clinical improvement was correlated closely

TABLE 31.1

Clinical Data in the Prediction of Shunt Response[a]

Clinical Pattern	No.	Improved (%)	No Change (%)
Ataxia, dementia, incontinence	13	9 (69)	4 (31)
Ataxia and dementia	6	4 (67)	2 (33)
Ataxia and incontinence	7	5 (71)	2 (29)
Ataxia alone	6	3 (50)	3 (50)
Dementia alone	1	0	1 (100)

[a] Three patients are excluded: one with ataxia, dementia, and incontinence, one with dementia alone who died before the 3-month postoperative period, and one with ataxia, dementia, and incontinence whose early subdural collection precluded assessment of shunt response.

TABLE 31.2

Gait Disorder in Predicting Shunt Response

	No.	Improved (%)	No Change (%)
Gait primary	22	17 (77)	5 (23)
Gait not primary	7	3 (42)	4 (58)

TABLE 31.3

CT Scan Atrophy as a Predictor of Shunt Response

	Total No.	Responded to Shunt (%)
Enlarged ventricles with mild or absent atrophy	24	18 (81)
Enlarged ventricles with moderate atrophy	12	7 (58)

TABLE 31.4

Relation between the Change in Ventricular Size and Shunt Response

	No.	Excellent/Good Response	Fair/Transient	Poor
Ventricles unchanged	11	1	5	5
Ventricles smaller	6	4	0	2
Ventricles larger	3	0	0	3

[a] A diminution in ventricular size is significantly associated with clinical improvement ($p < 0.05$).

TABLE 31.5

Isotope Cisternogram as a Predictor of Shunt Response

	No.	Improved (%)	No Response
Positive (NPH pattern)	11	9 (82)	2
Mixed	6	3 (50)	3
Negative (normal pattern)	6	4 (67)	2

with diminution in size of the cerebral ventricles (Table 31.4). Patients whose ventricles did not diminish in size generally did not improve.

Finally, in radiological assessment, indium diethylenetriamine penta-acetic acid (DPTA) cisternography or metrizamide cisternography were used in a few patients, and the data are presented in Table 31.5. Patients whose radionuclide cisternograms were typical of NPH tended to have a good response, but with the small number of patients assessed in this manner, no statistically significant correlation was observed between cisternographic pattern and response to shunting.

Infusion tests were conducted on eight patients but were abandoned when it appeared that they were not able to predict successful shunt outcome. The opening pressure on a single lumbar puncture (LP) did seem to have some relationship to shunt outcome: 11 of 12 patients with CSF pressures over 100 mm H_2O improved and only 2 of 5 with pressures less than 100 mm did so. In 10 patients CSF was withdrawn at the time of lumbar puncture, and gait was assessed after this; at least 30 ml were withdrawn. Six patients improved with CSF withdrawal, and five subsequently improved with shunting; three had equivocal responses, and two responded to shunting; one had a negative response but then improved after shunt placement.

The overall results of shunting 3 months after shunt placement are presented in Table 31.6. In the entire heterogeneous series there was an improvement rate of 64%. Two patients died within 3 months after surgery, one with pneumonia and the other after an acute myocardial infarction, for a mortality of 6%. There were 30 ventriculoarterial and 6 ventriculoperitoneal shunts.

Chronic subdural collections, seizures, and shunt infection were the major complications (Table 31.7). Chronic subdural fluid collections on

TABLE 31.6

Results of Shunting for Idiopathic Normal Pressure Hydrocephalus

Result	No.	%
Improvement	23	64
Excellent	3	8
Good	9	25
Fair	7	19
Transient	4	11
No change	10	27
Worse	1	3
Died within 3 months	2	6
	36	100

TABLE 31.7

Shunt Complications in 36 Patients with Idiopathic Normal Pressure Hydrocephalus

	No.	%
Chronic subdural collection	10	28
Seizure	3	8
Shunt infection	1	3

CT were demonstrated in 10 patients. In eight patients, the subdural collections were observed over several months. They resolved in seven; in the eighth patient there was little shunt response, and the family refused further treatment. The patient was taken home and subsequently died of pneumonia. In two patients, the subdurals were evacuated with tying off of the shunt, and both collections resolved; in one the collection was a subacute one.

DISCUSSION

Shunting for idiopathic NPH was done with enthusiasm for about 10 years after the syndrome was first described (1–3, 6, 7, 17, 38, 63, 84, 87, 94–96, 110, 116); reports of shunt successes came from many centers in the U.S., Europe, and Japan (6, 7, 17, 42, 60, 63, 77, 82). In the last decade it has become less eagerly recommended by both neurosurgeons and neurologists (4, 9–11, 54, 67, 76, 86, 90, 102). In part this is because there is a significant percentage of patients who do not improve and in part because there is definite morbidity in shunting (9, 57, 111). The purposes of this paper are: first, to suggest that contemporary criteria provide a means of achieving improvement in 60–70% of patients, and that the procedure should, therefore, still be recommended; second, to review criteria which have been thought to help predict shunt response; and third, to discuss the choice of the appropriate shunt pressure for a given patient with comments on pathophysiology of the syndrome.

DECIDING WHETHER TO SHUNT

Results of Shunting for Idiopathic NPH

With varying criteria of patient selection, the overall success rate for shunting has been reported as 87.5% (112), 74% (88), and 64% (this present series). These rates have been achieved primarily by de-emphasizing shunting in patients with dementia alone: either gait disturbance or the triad of gait disturbance, dementia, and incontinence have been used to choose patients. There are two types of data that can be used to help in the selection: data to be ignored in the decision to shunt and data apparently relevant to deciding to shunt.

Findings Which Can Probably Be Ignored in the Decision to Shunt

EVIDENCE OF CEREBROVASCULAR DISEASE ON CT SCAN

Welch et al. (13) have recently reviewed the evidence for a relationship between idiopathic NPH and presumed cerebrovascular disease. In their series, 83% of patients receiving shunts had evidence of atherosclerotic brain disease on history or CT examination; only 38% of patients over age 70 visiting a urologist's office had similar findings. In our series, 87% of patients had hypertension or CT evidence of previous stroke. Autopsy studies have further demonstrated that atherosclerotic brain disease is common in idiopathic NPH, but control series are lacking (14, 25, 27, 45, 54, 70, 91, 102). Noda et al. (81) have suggested that hypertensive brain disease actually causes NPH.

Atherosclerotic brain disease does not impair the outcome of shunting, with 8 of 10 successfully shunted patients having clinical evidence of atherosclerotic brain disease in Welch's series (113). Koto et al. (65) reported a greater likelihood of improvement after shunting in patients with hypertension and focal ischemic signs than in their nonhypertensive counterparts. There may, therefore, be an important relationship between hypertension or stroke and idiopathic NPH, although controlled series have not been published. The most important practical point is that evidence of previous strokes on CT scan does not preclude a good shunt response.

ATROPHY ON CT SCAN

It is iconoclastic to suggest that the presence of CT atrophy is irrelevant to the outcome of shunting in idiopathic NPH. Early papers suggested, as might be expected, that atrophy implied poor shunt response (8, 69). However, data from Salmon's work (94–98), from Vassilouthis (112), from the Mayo Clinic (67, 88), and from the present analysis all support the view that improvement can occur when atrophy is present, although the chances of improvement are somewhat better when there is no atrophy. In pneumoencephalography, sulcal air implied free passage of air around the convexities and therefore no block to CSF flow (8, 39, 51, 69); it seems clear that this finding cannot be extrapolated to the CT scan.

CISTERNOGRAPHIC PATTERN IF NORMAL OR MIXED

After initial enthusiasm for radionuclide cisternography as a predictive test for shunting in idiopathic NPH (5, 51, 62, 92, 109), there appears to be less reliance on it in recent reports (10, 67). In our previous survey as in this one, we found that a pattern typical of NPH was helpful in predicting a good shunt response, but that a normal or mixed pattern could also be associated with a good response. Børgesen *et al.* (16) suggested that a normal indium pattern predicted normal conductance of CSF and therefore made shunting ill-advised; however, they did not present follow-up data on shunt results in that paper. Metrizamide has recently been suggested as a replacement for indium in elucidating CSF dynamics (26), but its role remains to be defined.

PREOPERATIVE CEREBRAL BLOOD FLOW MEASUREMENTS

Some investigators have suggested a characteristic pattern of flow in patients with NPH (72). Tamaki *et al.* (100) have recently supported the view that no distinctive pattern of blood flow characterizes patients with idiopathic NPH. This agrees with work by Ingvar and others. Although shunting may increase blood flow in responders, preoperative flow patterns or values are not characteristic (40, 44, 58, 59). Perhaps blood flow measurements will identify nonresponders early in the postoperative period, as patients with NPH have an increase in flow after shunting (40, 41, 44, 58, 59). If blood flow is diminished postoperatively early shunt ligation might be considered to avoid shunt complications.

ELECTROENCEPHALOGRAPHY (EEG)

Brown and Goldensohn (18), Greenberg *et al.* (38), Jacobs *et al.* (60), and Laws' group (67, 68) have all evaluated explicitly the role of the EEG in diagnosing NPH. There is current agreement that no EEG pattern successfully predicts shunt response.

Findings Which Favor a Decision to Shunt

SIGNIFICANT GAIT DISTURBANCE IN THE CLINICAL PRESENTATION

CSF shunting was initially considered most important as a treatment for certain kinds of dementia in the elderly; however, it appears that gait disturbance is now the major marker for shunt success. C. Miller Fisher (30) found that gait disturbance preceded impaired mentation in 12 of 16 shunt responders; in 11 shunt failures, 9 had little or no gait disturbance. Jacobs et al. (60, 61) reported that no patients with good walking improved in mental state after shunting. Laws et al. (67) also emphasized the importance of gait difficulty and have reported a 74% success rate, with walking difficulty as a major criterion for shunting (88). Vassilouthis (112) used gait disturbance as a central criterion to obtain an 87.5% success rate. Greenberg et al. (38) used the criteria of very large ventricles and gait disturbance to give 83% good results.

The gait disturbance in NPH is variable. Most often it manifests itself by short shuffling steps with a wide base and unsteadiness on turning (30–32). A variety of motor disorders can occur, however, including increased tone and parkinsonism (2, 20, 107). Although it is an ataxia in the loose sense much like "frontal lobe ataxia," there are usually no appendicular cerebellar signs.

Evaluating the general problem of hydrocephalus with gait disturbance, Fisher (32) has recently demonstrated that gait disturbance in the elderly is very often accompanied by ventricular enlargement; 97% of patients over age 60 with gait disturbance had ventricles with a span over 12 mm. Koller et al. (64) agreed with this finding, reporting that senile gait was associated with increased bifrontal, bicaudate, and third ventricle skull ratios in CT scan, but not with cortical atrophy. This appeared to be independent of the presence of memory difficulties. In another report, 16% of patients over age 70 with gait disorder had ventricular enlargement and no other known cause (103).

Our own experience has been that gait disturbance may respond dramatically to shunting, although it is not always necessary to have walking difficulties as the primary or predominant syndrome to achieve shunt success.

ALTERED CSF DYNAMICS

A great deal has been written about CSF physiology in idiopathic NPH. This section will summarize data dealing with continuous pressure recording, with infusion testing, and finally, with lumboventricular perfusion.

The upper limit of normal lumbar puncture CSF pressure is usually considered 180 mm H_2O, although Gillard et al. (36) have suggested that a figure of 240 mm is more appropriate. As the pressure is a physiological measure of the equilibrium resistance of the CSF system, it is reasonable to consider that the higher the LP pressure, the better the opportunity of shunt success. In our own data an LP pressure over 100 mm was more often associated with shunt success than one under 100 mm. The LP is therefore worth carrying out not only for pressure reading, but to exclude cytological or chemical abnormalities in the CSF.

If 180 mm is taken as the upper limit of normal pressure, some patients with pressures thought to be normal on a single determination will have abnormally high pressures some time over a 24-hour period (105). Using epidural pressure recording, Symon's group and others (14, 104, 105) have identified a subgroup of idiopathic NPH patients, with pressure peaks over 20 mm Hg or recurrent B-wave activity (14, 104, 105). Symon and Hinzpeter (106) reported that these patients have a higher improvement rate with shunting (68, 70) than patients with entirely normal pressure traces.

Several other groups have suggested that overnight pressure recording is worthwhile. Crockard et al. (23) divided patients with hydrocephalus into those with intermittent elevations of intracranial pressure and those without such elevations. They found that ventricular size was the same in both groups but that there was more sulcal atrophy in patients who had no elevations in intracranial pressure. They did not comment on shunt outcome. Hartman and Alberti (50) used overnight recording to select patients for shunting but did not shunt patients with normal traces. This does not allow a comparison of shunt outcome between the two groups. Chawla et al. (19) monitored ICP either by a subdural transducer or ventricular catheter in 12 patients. They found that seven patients with flat recordings did not improve, but five patients with B-waves did. Of interest, however, these latter five patients all had LP pressures above 150 mm Hg, making them not truly "normal pressure" hydrocephalus candidates on a single LP. Børgesen and Gjerris (12) reported that 13 of 14 patients with B-waves over 50% of the time on an intraventricular overnight recording improved with shunting. Lamas and Lobato (66) published similar data suggesting that B-waves were common in patients who improved with shunting. Similar data have been reported by others (28, 29) who suggest that overnight CSF pressure recording might be a useful adjunct in cases where a single LP pressure is normal, attempting to select out patients with altered CSF dynamics. Foltz and Aine (34) have suggested that the pattern of CSF pulse wave rather than the mean pressure management is the critical feature of analysis in hydrocephalus. In 10 patients with idiopathic NPH they felt that pulse pressure and systolic form established the diagnosis of hydrocephalus; however, correlation was not made with outcome.

The situation with regard to lumbar infusion testing is much more complicated than that with overnight recording. The infusion test, described as a method of assessing resistance to CSF absorption (21, 55, 71), has been used to demonstrate impaired CSF absorption in NPH (37). However, in a predictive test for shunting it has not been useful

(80, 102, 114), despite some claims to the contrary (66). This may be a result of testing artefact or of misinterpretation of results (80); alternatively, it may be that constant volume infusion misrepresents some important features of CSF physiology.

To avoid the problem of constant volume infusion, Sklar *et al.* (100, 101) have developed a servo-control system which quickly reaches and maintains a given CSF pressure. Its efficacy in predicting shunt outcome has not been tested in large numbers of patients.

Because of the difficulties with constant volume lumbar infusion testing, possibly related to the compliance of the spinal subarachnoid space, Børgesen *et al.* (13–15) have used lumboventricular perfusion to predict shunt outcome. This technique uses infusion through a lumbar catheter, with the infusion pressure set by the height of the ventricular outflow. Absorption volume is calculated and plotted against pressure; the slope of the resulting regression line is the conductance to outflow of CSF in milliliters per minute per millimeters of mercury. What is being measured is the ease with which fluid is removed from the CSF space by absorptive mechanisms.

Børgesen and Gjerris (12) reported on the results of lumboventricular perfusion in 80 patients with NPH, 40 of whom were of the idiopathic variety. Using a criterion for shunting which required conductance to be less than 0.12 ml/minute/mm Hg, they found that 21 of 31 patients shunted with idiopathic NPH had good response (70%); if the cutoff used was 0.8 ml/minute/mm Hg, all patients would have responded.

These authors found that outflow conductance measurements did not correlate with lumbar infusion results, again suggesting that lumbar infusion itself may not give accurate predictive data (15). Although lumboventricular perfusion appears to be a useful predictive test, it is limited by the need for a ventricular catheter.

IMPROVEMENT AFTER LUMBAR PUNCTURE

In a sense, lumbar puncture with a persistent dural defect can be seen as a kind of temporary fistula lowering the CSF pressure. It is therefore reasonable to consider it as a therapeutic trail of CSF diversion. All patients in the series reported by Wood *et al.* (16) who improved after lumbar puncture benefitted from shunting. In their respective series, Fisher (30) and Wikkelsø *et al.* (114) also found that improvement in gait after a lumbar puncture was a reliable indicator of shunt success.

A CT SCAN WITH PERIVENTRICULAR LOW ABSORPTION OR LARGE VENTRICLES/SMALL SULCI

Periventricular low absorption on CT was noted by Mori *et al.* (78) to give an increased likelihood of shunt success in hydrocephalus. It has been shown to result from increased periventricular water in experimental hydrocephalus (52) and appears to be from similar phenomena in patients (79). Børgesen and Gjerris (12) reported that all 16 patients with periventricular lucency improved from shunting, and when present it appears to be an important indicator of shunt success.

Other CT findings are less clearly helpful in predicting shunt response (43, 45, 60). The previous section has discussed the fact that large sulci do not preclude an effect from shunting. Small sulci in combination with large ventricles, however, are associated with a high likelihood of shunt improvement. In Børgesen's series (12), 16 patients with this finding all had a good shunt response.

SELECTING THE APPROPRIATE VALVE PRESSURE IN SHUNTING

Correlation between Ventricular Size and Clinical Improvement with a Comment on the Pathophysiology of Idiopathic Normal Pressure Hydrocephalus

One theory of pathogenesis in NPH at the present time is that there is increased resistance to outflow of CSF from the ventricles, with subsequent ventricular enlargement of a very slow and indolent type (10, 73). Despite the plausibility of this hypothesis there is little direct evidence supporting it. Lorenzo *et al.* (70) demonstrated an absorption defect in some patients with idiopathic NPH, a finding buttressed by Børgesen and Gjerris' report (12) that outflow conductance is low in NPH patients. There have been a few pathological studies displaying the basis for such obstruction. Ojemann (84), for example, presented cases with evidence of fibrosis in the subarachnoid pathways. Many studies show only atherosclerotic changes (14, 22, 24, 25, 45, 54, 70, 91), without the kind of obvious blockage to CSF flow shown in such work as Russell's monograph on hydrocephalus (93). The role of cerebral atherosclerosis or other parenchymal changes and even the possible importance of neuropeptide or other CSF factors in producing symptoms have not been examined thoroughly.

There is some clinical and experimental evidence that a gradient exists between ventricular and subarachnoid compartments in normal pressure hydrocephalus. Conner *et al.* (22) in cats demonstrated this gradient, despite normal pressure after kaolin injection. Hoff and Barber (53) showed similar results in patients tested at surgery. This finding might explain why ventricular enlargement occurs despite normal pressure, as the gradient across the cerebral parenchyma favors ventricular enlargement. It may also explain why lumbar infusion tests are so variable in their results. There may not be a deficit of CSF absorption within the spinal or subarachnoid spaces transversed by lumbar-infused CSF. In fact, the concept of a CSF-absorptive deficit in adult hydrocephalus is apt to be midleading. The problem is CSF circulation rather than absorption in the sense of transfer from CSF to blood.

These theoretical considerations have important practical implications in preventing either postoperative subdural collections or failure of ventricles to diminish in size. Both of these postoperative events can be seen to be a result of mismatching shunt pressure with CSF pressure.

Subdural collections occur regularly in patients receiving shunts for idiopathic NPH (10, 56, 111). Three mechanisms have been proposed for their production: a siphoning effect of shunting that causes very low intracranial pressure and tearing of small veins; decreased intraventricular pressure from a valve pressure too low for the system; and leakage around the ventricular catheter into the subdural space. Establishing the correct mechanism is important, because the method for prevention will differ. If shunt siphoning is the major factor, insertion of an antisiphon device may be the treatment of choice. If a low pressure valve is important, a change to higher pressure will be therapeutic. If actual shunt catheter insertion is causative, procedures to seal the arachnoid around the catheter will be most important. Fox et al. (35) have analyzed the CSF pressure changes that follow shunt insertion, indicating the importance of siphoning; however, their data imply a system opened to atmospheric pressure which may not be physiological. Hakim has emphasized the importance of shunt valve pressure in subsequent ventricular size; however, it is not clear from his theoretical work whether low pressure causes subdural collections. In our experience, subdurals do not appear to arise from catheter insertion. We have seen them from lumboperitoneal shunts and have seen them unilaterally on the side contralateral to the shunt catheter.

Our data suggest that much of the time these collections will remain stable or resolve, but their appearance is often accompanied by disabling headache and always requires regular observation. In our own series, 3 of 10 required surgical evacuation and tying off of the shunt. In one case the shunt had been left ligated; in others, worsening of symptoms led to reopening of the shunt 3 months after subdural irrigation, usually with placement of a high pressure valve.

Chronic subdural collections are one important and poorly understood complication of shunt insertion. The opposite problem, that of not draining CSF adequately, is manifest by failure of the ventricles to diminish in size after shunting. Although some patients improve without a change in ventricular size (60, 61, 99) our data here suggest a definite relationship between shunt success and diminution in ventricular size. McQuarrie and Scherer (75) have recently suggested that replacing a medium pressure by a low pressure valve in patients whose clinical status and ventricular size are unchanged after shunting may lead to improvement. Hakim, whose pioneering analyses of the CSF pressure changes in hydrocephalus (48, 49) led to a valve now widely used (83), has analyzed the shunt pressure required in differing ventricular sizes (47). In what appears to be a paradoxical statement but is in fact one which has good theoretical support, he has suggested that the larger the ventricles, the lower the pressure of valve required to decompress them (47).

The problem of matching valve to patient is one which may require a new kind of valve in which the closing pressure can slowly be decreased until the ventricle size diminishes. In the meantime, our policy is to use a medium pressure valve (closing pressure 65–90 mm H_2O) on all patients and to follow their clinical state and CT scans carefully over 6–12 months. Patients who have low pressure headaches within a few days of shunting appear to be at special risk for subdural formation, and we tend to keep them in bed for several more days.

Patients who do not show clinical improvement and whose ventricles do not diminish in size recieve a lumbar puncture to assess shunt function. If the CSF pressure is approximately the closing pressure of the valve, the shunt is assumed to be functional. Shunt tap, lumbar infusion testing (117), or indium installation into the shunt system are other techniques of assessing shunt function. If the shunt appears to be working adequately, the ventricles remain large, and the patient has not improved, it is our present opinion that placement of a lower pressure valve should be carried out.

SUMMARY AND CONCLUSIONS

From a review of our experience in the past 4 years and of the literature generally, the following comments can be made about selecting patients with idiopathic NPH for a shunt procedure. (a) In the clinical presentation, either significant gait difficulty or the full triad of dementia, ataxia, and incontinence should be present. If dementia occurred first or is the major symptom, shunting may not improve the patient. (b) A CT scan with periventricular low density and/or small sulci along with expansion of the entire ventricular system (especially the temporal horns) is strongly associated with good shunt outcome. However, presence of significant atrophy does not prevent shunt success if the clinical picture is appropriate.

Some surgeons now feel that the clinical presentation and CT scan findings are enough in themselves to indicate a shunt. If further testing is desired, the following may be useful:

1. *Lumbar puncture*: A pressure over 100 mm is associated with better chances of improvement. Improvement after lumbar puncture is

associated with high likelihood of shunt success, but lack of improvement after lumbar puncture is not useful as a predictor.

2. *Isotope or metrizamide cisternography*: A typical NPH pattern suggests a good response; a mixed or normal pattern is irrelevant to shunt outcome.

3. *Overnight recording of CSF pressure*: If pressure is above 180 mm at night, or if there are frequent B-waves, shunting is likely to be helpful.

4. *Lumboventricular perfusion*: This technique appears to give the most accurate prediction but requires special expertise and probably human studies approval to be done, as it is still an experimental procedure. These features make it difficult to use as a routine test.

With regards to results of shunting once accomplished, it is important to follow patients carefully to exclude a chronic subdural collection. If a shunted patient fails to improve with persistent large ventricles and a medium or high pressure valve was used, consideration should be given to shunt revision with insertion of a lower pressure valve.

ACKNOWLEDGMENT

This work was supported in part by Teacher Investigator Award Number 1K07 NS00553-01 from the NINCDS.

REFERENCES

1. Adams, R. D. Further observations on normal pressure hydrocephalus. Proc. R. Soc. Med., *59:* 1135–1140, 1966.

2. Adams, R. D., Fisher, C M., Hakim, S., Ojemann, R. G., and Sweet, W. H. Symptomatic occult hydrocephalus with "normal" cerebrospinal fluid pressure. A treatable syndrome. N. Engl. J. Med., *273:* 117–126, 1965.

3. Appenzeller, O., and Salmon, L. H. Treatment of parenchymatous degeneration of the brain of ventriculo-atrial shunting of cerebrospinal fluid. J. Neurosurg., *26:* 478–482, 1967.

4. Bannister, C. M. A report of eight patients with low pressure hydrocephalus treated by CSF diversion with disappointing results. Acta Neurochir. (Wien), *27:* 11–15, 1972.

5. Bannister, R., Gilford, E., and Kocen, R. Isotope encephalography in the diagnosis of dementia due to communicating hydrocephalus. Lancet, *2:* 1014–1017, 1967.

6. Belloni, G., di Rocco, C., Focacci, C., Galli, G., Maira, G., and Rossi, G. F. Surgical indications in normotensive hydrocephalus. A retrospective analysis of the relations of some diagnostic findings to the results of surgical treatment. Acta Neurochir., *33:* 1–21, 1976.

7. Benini, A., and Krayenbuhl, H. Hydrocephalus occultus symptomaticus: Ein klinische neuartiges syndrom. Schweiz. Med. Wochenschr., *99:* 621–630, 1969.

8. Benson, D. F., LeMay, M., Patten, D. H., and Rubens, A. B. Diagnosis of normal pressure hydrocephalus. N. Engl. J. Med., *283:* 609–615, 1970.

9. Black, P. M. Idiopathic normal-pressure hydrocephalus. Results of shunting in 62 patients. J. Neurosurg., *53:* 371–377, 1980.

10. Black, P. M. Normal pressure hydrocephalus. Current understanding of diagnostic tests and shunting. Postgrad. Med., *71:* 57–67, 1982.

11. Black, P. M., and Sweet, W. H. Normal pressure hydrocephalus, idiopathic type: Selection of patients for shunting procedures. In: *Advances in Neurosurgery: Lumbar Disc, Adult Hydrocephalus,* Vol. 4, pp. 106–110. Springer-Verlag, Heidelberg, W. Germany, 1976.

12. Børgesen, S. E., and Gjerris, F. The predictive value of conductance to outflow of cerebrospinal fluid in normal pressure hydrocephalus. Brain, *105:* 65–86, 1982.

13. Børgensen, S. E., Gjerris, F., and Sorensen, S. C. The resistance to cerebrospinal fluid absorption in humans. A method of evaluation by lumboventricular perfusion, with particular reference to normal pressure hydrocephalus. Acta Neurol. Scand., *57:* 88–96, 1978.

14. Børgesen, S. E., Gjerris, F., and Sorensen, S. C. Intracranial pressure and conductance to outflow of cerebrospinal fluid in normal pressure hydrocephalus. J. Neurosurg., *50:* 489–493, 1979.

15. Børgesen, S. E., Fjerris, F., and Sorensen, S. C. Cerebrospinal fluid conductance and compliance of the craniospinal space in normal pressure hydrocephalus. J. Neurosurg., *51:* 521–525, 1979.

16. Børgesen, S. E., Westergard, L., and Gjerris, F. Isotope cisternography and conductance to outflow of CSF in normal pressure hydrocephalus. Acta Neurochir., *57:* 67–73, 1981.

17. Botez, M. I., Léveille, J., Bérubé, L., and Botez-Marquand, T. Occult disorders of cerebrospinal fluid dynamics: Early diagnostic criteria. Eur. Neurol., *13:* 203–222, 1975.

18. Brown, D. G., and Goldensohn, E. S. The electroencephalogram in normal pressure hydrocephalus. Arch. Neurol., *29:* 70–71, 1973.

19. Chawla, J. C., Hulme, A., and Cooper, R. Intracranial pressure in patients with dementia and communicating hydrocephalus. J. Neurosurg., *40:* 376–380, 1974.

20. Chawla, J. C., and Woodward, J. Motor disorder in "normal pressure hydrocephalus." B. Med. J., *1:* 485–486, 1972.

21. Coblentz, J. M., Mattis, S., Zingesser, L. H., Kasoff, S. S., Wisniewski, H. M., and Katzman, R. Presenile dementia: Clinical aspects and evaluation of cerebrospinal fluid dynamics. Arch. Neurol., *24:* 299–308, 1973.

22. Conner, E. S., Black, P. McL. and Foley, L. Experimental normal pressure hydrocephalus is accompanied by increased transmantle pressure. J. Neurosurg., *61:* 322–328, 1984.

23. Crockard, H. A., Hanlon, K., Duda, E. E., and Mullan, J. F. Hydrocephalus as a cause of dementia: Evaluation of computerized tomography and intracranial pressure monitoring. J. Neurol. Neurosurg. Psychiatry, *40:* 736–740, 1977.

24. DeLand, F. H., James, A. E., Jr., Ladd, D. J., and Konigsmark, B. W. Normal pressure hydrocephalus: A histologic study. Am. J. Clin. Pathol., *58:* 58–63, 1972.

25. di Rocco, C., Di Trapani, G., Maira, G., Bentiviglio, M., Macchi, G., and Rossi, G. F. Anatomoclinical correlations in normotensive hydrocephalus. Reports on three cases. J. Neurol. Sci., *33:* 437–451, 1977.

26. Drayer, B. P., Rosenbaum, A. E. Dynamics of cerebrospinal fluid system as defined by cranial computed tomography. In: *Neurobiology of Cerebrospinal Fluid*, Vol. 1, Chap. 30, edited by J. H. Wood. Plenum, New York, 1980.

27. Earnest, M. P., Fahn, S., Karp, J. H., and Rowland, L. P. Normal pressure hydrocephalus and hypertensive cerebrovascular disease. Arch. Neurol., *31:* 262–266, 1974.

28. Ekstedt, J., and Friden, H. CSF hydrodynamics especially in the adult hydrocephalus

syndrome. In: *Intracranial Pressure*, III, edited by J. W. F. Beks, D. A. Busch, and M. Brock, pp. 177–185. Springer-Verlag, Berlin, 1976.

29. Epstein, C. M. The distribution of intracranial forces in acute and chronic hydrocephalus. J. Neurol. Sci., *21:* 171–180, 1974.

30. Fisher, C. M. The clinical picture in occult hydrocephalus. Clin. Neurosurg., *24:* 270–284, 1977.

31. Fisher, C. M. Communicating hydrocephalus (letter). Lancet, *1:* 37, 1978.

32. Fisher, C. M. Hydrocephalus as a cause of disturbances of gait in the elderly. Neurology, *32:* 1358–1363, 1982.

33. Fishman, R. A. Occult hydrocephalus (letter to the editor). N. Engl. J. Med., *27:* 466–467, 1966.

34. Foltz, E. L., and Aine, C. Diagnosis of hydrocephalus by CSF pulse-wave analysis: A clinical study. Surg. Neurol., *15:* 283–293, 1980.

35. Fox, J. L., McCullough, D. C., and Green, R. C. Effect of cerebrospinal fluid shunts on intracranial pressure and on cerebrospinal fluid dynamics. 2. A new technique of pressure measurement: Results and concepts. 3. A concept of hydrocephalus. J. Neurol. Neurosurg. Psychiatry, *36:* 302–312, 1973.

36. Gillard, O., Tourtellotte, W., O'Tauma, L., and Henderson, W. G. Normal cerebrospinal fluid pressure. J. Neurosurg., *40:* 587–593, 1974.

37. Granholm, L., and Løfgren, J. A discussion on the intracranial pressure-volume relationships in normal pressure hydrocephalus. In: *Intracranial Pressure*, II, edited by N. Lundberg, U. Ponten, and M. Brock, pp. 137–140. Springer-Verlag, Berlin, 1975.

38. Greenberg, J. O., Shenkin, H. A., and Adam, R. Idiopathic normal pressure hydrocephalus—a report of 73 patients. J. Neurol. Neurosurg. Psychiatry, *40:* 336–341, 1977.

39. Greitz, T., and Grepe, A. Encephalography in the diagnosis of convexity block hydrocephalus. Acta. Radiol. (Diagn.) (Stockh.), *11:* 232–242, 1971.

40. Greitz, T. V. B., Grepe, A. O. L., Kalmer, M. S. F., and Lopez, J. Pre- and postoperative evaluation of cerebral blood flow in low-pressure hydrocephalus. J. Neurosurg., *31:* 644–651, 1969.

41. Grubb, R. L., Raichle, M. E., Gado, M. H., Eichling, J. O., and Hughes, C. P. Cerebral blood flow, oxygen utilization, and blood volume in dementia. Neurology (Minneap.), *27:* 905–910, 1977.

42. Guidetti, B., and Gagliardi, F. M. Normal pressure hydrocephalus. Acta. Neurochir., *27:* 1–9, 1972.

43. Gunasakera, L., and Richardson, A. E. Computerized axial tomography in idiopathic hydrocephalus. Brain, *100:* 749–754, 1977.

44. Hachinski, V. C., Iliff, L. D., and Zilhka, E. Cerebral blood flow in dementia. Arch. Neurol., *32:* 632–637, 1975.

45. Haidri, N. H., and Modi, S. M. Normal pressure hydrocephalus and hypertensive cerebrovascular disease. Dis. Nerv. Syst., *38:* 918–921, 1977.

46. Hakim, S. Some Observations on CSF Pressure Hydrocephalic Syndrome in Adults with "Normal" CSF Pressure (Recognition of a New Syndrome). Thesis No. 957, Javeriana University School of Medicine, Bogota, Colombia, 1964 (English Translation).

47. Hakim, S. Hydraulic and mechanical mis-matching of valve shunts used in the treatment of hydrocephalus: The need for a servo-valve shunt. Dev. Med. Child Neurol., *15:* 646–653, 1973.

48. Hakim, S., and Adams, R. D. The special clinical problem of symptomatic hydroceph-

alus with normal cerebrospinal fluid pressure. Observations on cerebrospinal fluid hydrodynamics. J. Neurol. Sci., *2:* 307–327, 1965.

49. Hakim, S., Venegas, J. G., and Burton, J. D. The physics of the cranial cavity, hydrocephalus, and normal pressure hydrocephalus: Mechanical interpretation and mathematical model. Surg. Neurol., *5:* 187–210, 1976.

50. Hartmann, A., and Alberti, E. Differentiation of communicating hydrocephalus and presenile dementia by continuous recording of cerebrospinal fluid pressure. J. Neurol. Neurosurg. Psychiatry, *40:* 630–640, 1977.

51. Heinz, E. R., David, D. O., and Karp, H. R. Abnormal isotope cisternography in symptomatic occult hydrocephalus. A correlative isotopic-neuroradiological study in 130 subjects. Radiology, *95:* 109–120, 1970.

52. Hiratsuka, H., Tabata, H., Tsuruoka, S., Aoyogi, M., Okada, K., and Inaba, Y. Evaluation of periventricular hypodensity in experimental hydrocephalus by metrizamide CT ventriculography. J. Neurosurg., *56:* 235–240, 1982.

53. Hoff, J., and Barber, R. Transcerebral mantle pressure in normal pressure hydrocephalus. Arch. Neurol., *31:* 101–105, 1974.

54. Hughes, C. P., Siegel, B. A., Coxe, W. S., Gado, M. H., Grubb, R. L., Coleman, R. E., and Berg, L. Adult idiopathic communicating hydrocephalus with and without shunting. J. Neurol. Neurosurg. Psychiatry, *41:* 961–971, 1978.

55. Hussey, F., Schanzer, B., and Katzman, R. A simple constant infusion manometric test for measurement of CSF absorption II. Clinical Studies. Neurology (Minneap.), *20:* 665–680, 1970.

56. Illingworth, R. D. Subdural hematoma after the treatment of chronic hydrocephalus by ventriculocaval shunts. J. Neurol. Neurosurg. Psychiatry, *33:* 95–99, 1970.

57. Illingworth, R. D., Logue, V., Symon, L., and Uemera, K. The ventriculocaval shunt in the treatment of adult hydrocephalus. Results and complications in 101 patients. J. Neurosurg., *35:* 681–685, 1971.

58. Ingvar, D. H., and Gustafson, L. Regional cerebral blood flow in organic dementia with early onset. Acta. Neurol. Scand., *46* (Suppl. 43): 42–73, 1970.

59. Ingvar, D. H., and Schwartz, M. S. The cerebral blood flow in low pressure hydrocephalus. In: *Intracranial Pressure, II,* edited by N. Lundberg, U. Ponten, and M. Brock, pp. 153–156. Springer-Verlag, Berlin, 1975.

60. Jacobs, L., Conti, D., and Kinkel, W. R. "Normal-pressure" hydrocephalus. Relationships of clinical and radiographic findings to improvement following shunt surgery. J.A.M.A., *235:* 510–512, 1976.

61. Jacobs, L., and Kinkel, W. Computerized axial transverse tomography in normal pressure hydrocephalus. Neurology (Minneap.), *26:* 501–507, 1976.

62. James, A. E., Jr., DeLand, F. H., Hodges, F. J., III, and Wagner, H. N., Jr. Normal pressure hydrocephalus: Role of cisternography in diagnosis. J.A.M.A., *213:* 1615–1622, 1970.

63. Järpe, S. Presenile dementia and hydrocephalus. Therapeutic experiences. Acta. Neurol. Scand., *46* (Suppl. 43):89, 1970.

64. Koller, W. C., Glatt, S. C., and Wilson, R. S. Senile gait: Correlation with computed tomographic scans. Ann. Neurol., *12:* 87, 1982.

65. Koto, A., Rosenberg, G., Zingesser, L. H., Horoupian, D., and Katzman, R. Syndrome of normal pressure hydrocephalus: Possible relation to hypertensive and arteriosclerotic vasculopathy. J. Neurol. Neurosurg. Psychiatry, *40:* 73–79, 1977.

66. Lamas, E., and Lobato, R. O. Intraventricular pressure and CSF dynamics in chronic adult hydrocephalus. Surg. Neurol., *12:* 287–295, 1977.

67. Laws, E. R., Jr., and Mokri, B. Occult hydrocephalus: Results of shunting correlated with diagnostic tests. Clin. Neurosurg., *24:* 316–333, 1977.

68. Laws, E. R., Jr., and Niedermeyer, E. EEG findings in hydrocephalus patients with

shunt procedures. Abstr. Electroencephalogr. Clin. Neurophysiol., *29:* 325, 1970.

69. LeMay, M., and New, P. F. J. Radiological diagnosis of occult normal-pressure hydrocephalus. Radiology, *96:* 347–358, 1970.

70. Lorenzo, A. V., Bresnan, M. J., and Barlow, C. F. Cerebrospinal fluid absorption deficit in normal pressure hydrocephalus. Arch. Neurol., *32:* 387–393, 1974.

71. Martins, A. N. Resistance to drainage of cerebrospinal fluid: Clinical measurements and significance. J. Neurol. Neurosurg. Psychiatry, *36:* 313–318, 1973.

72. Mathew, N. T., Meyer, J. S., Hartmann, A., and Ott, E. O. Abnormal cerebrospinal fluid-blood flow dynamics: Implications in diagnosis, treatment, and prognosis in normal pressure hydrocephalus. Arch. Neurol., *32:* 657–664, 1975.

73. McComb, J. G. Recent research into the nature of cerebrospinal fluid formation and absorption. J. Neurosurg., *59:* 369–383, 1983.

74. McCullough, D. C., and Fox, J. L. Negative intracranial pressure in adults with shunts and its relationship to the production of subdural hematoma. J. Neurosurg., *40:* 372–375, 1974.

75. McQuarrie, J. G., and Scherer, P. B. Treatment of adult-onset obstructive hydrocephalus with medium or low-pressure CSF shunts. Neurology, *32:* 1057–1061, 1982.

76. Messert, B., and Wannamaker, B. B. Reappraisal of the adult occult hydrocephalus syndrome. Neurology, *24:* 224–231, 1974.

77. Michelson, W. J., Schlesinger, E. B., and Bailey, S. Factors involved in surgical management of normal pressure hydrocephalus. Acta. Radiol. (Diagn.) (Stockh.), *13:* 570–574, 1972.

78. Mori, K., Murata, T., Nakano, Y., and Handa, H. Periventricular lucency in hydrocephalus on computerized tomography. Surg. Neurol., *8:* 337–340, 1977.

79. Moseley, I. F., and Radu, E. W. Factors influencing the development of periventricular lucencies in patients raised intracranial pressure. Neuroradiology, *17:* 65–69, 1979.

80. Nelson, J. R., and Goodman, S. J. An evaluation of the cerebrospinal fluid infusion test for hydrocephalus. Neurology, *21:* 1037–1053, 1971.

81. Noda, S., Fujita, K., Kusunoki, T., Tamaki, N., and Matsumoto, S. Hypertensive vasculopathy as a causative factor of normal pressure hydrocephalus: A clinical analysis. Neurol. Surg., *9:* 1033–1039, 1981.

82. Nornes, H., Rootwelt, I. S., and Sjaastad, O. Normal pressure hydrocephalus. Eur. Neurol., *1:* 261–274, 1973.

83. Ojemann, R. G. Initial experience with the Hakim valve for ventriculovenous shunting: Technical note. J. Neurosurg., *28:* 283–287, 1968.

84. Ojemann, R. G. Normal pressure hydrocephalus. Clin. Neurosurg., *18:* 337–370, 1971.

85. Ojemann, R. G. Normal pressure hydrocephalus. In: *Scientific Foundations of Neurology,* edited by M. Critchley, J. L. O'Leary, and B. Jennett, pp. 302–308. F.A. Davis, Philadelphia, 1972.

86. Ojemann, R. G., and Black, P. McL. Evaluation of the patient with dementia and treatment of normal pressure hydrocephalus. In: *Neurosurgery,* edited by R. H. Wilkins, and S. S. Rengachary. McGraw-Hill, New York, 1984.

87. Ojemann, R. G., Fisher, C. M., Adams, R. D., *et al.* Further experience with the syndrome of "normal" pressure hydrocephalus. J. Neurosurg., *31:* 279–294, 1969.

88. Peterson, R. C., Mokri, B., and Laws, E. R., Jr. Response to shunting procedure in idiopathic normal pressure hydrocephalus. Ann. Neurol., *12:* 99, 1982.

89. Philippon, J., Ancri, D., and Pertuiset, B. Hydrocephalie a pression normal (enregistement de la pression etude radiologiqu, transit isotopique.) Rev. Neurol. (Paris), *125:* 347–358, 1971.

90. Pickard, J. D. Adult communicating hydrocephalus. Br. J. Hosp. Med., *27:* 35–44, 1982.

91. Ribadeau-Dumas, J. L., Ricou, P., Verdure, L., Rondot, P., and Esouroulle, R. Etude

anatomique d'un cas d'hydrocephalie a pression normale. Neurochirurgie, *22:* 138–145, 1976.

92. Rossi, G. F., Galli, G., DiRocco, C., Maira, G., Meglio, M., Troneonne, D. Normotensive hydrocephalus: The relations of pneumoencephalography and isotope cisternography to the results of surgical treatment. Acta. Neurochir. (Wein), *30:* 69–83, 1974.

93. Russell, D. *Observations on the Pathology of Hydrocephalus.* Her Majesty's Stationery Office, London, 1949.

94. Salmon, J. H. Senile and pressure dementia: Ventriculo-atrial shunt for symptomatic treatment. Geriatrics, *24:* 67–72, 1969.

95. Salmon, J. H. Adult hydrocephalus: Evaluation of shunt therapy in 80 patients. J. Neurosurg., *37:* 423–428, 1972.

96. Salmon, J. H., and Armitage, T. L. Surgical treatment of hydrocephalus ex-vacuo: Ventriculo-atrial shunt for degenerative brain disease. Neurology (Minneap.), *18:* 1223–1226, 1968.

97. Salmon, J. H., Gonen, J. Y., and Brown, L. Ventriculoatrial shunt for hydrocephalus ex-vacuo: Psychological and clinical evaluation. Dis. Nerv. Syst., *32:* 299–307, 1971.

98. Salmon, J. H., and Timperman, A. L. Cerebral blood flow in post-traumatic encephalopathy. The effect of ventriculoatrial shunt. Neurology, *21:* 33–42, 1971.

99. Shenkin, H. A., Greenberg, J. O., and Grossman, C. B. Ventricular size after shunting for idiopathic normal pressure hydrocephalus. J. Neurol. Neurosurg. Psychiatry, *38:* 833–837, 1975.

100. Sklar, F. H., Beyer, C. W., Jr., Ramanathas, M., Elashavili, J., Cooper, P. R., and Clark, W. K. Servo-controlled lumbar infusions: A clinical tool for the determination of CSF dynamics as a function of pressure. Neurosurgery, *3:* 170–175, 1978.

101. Sklar, F. H., Diche, J. T., Beyer, C. W., and Clark, W. K. Brain elasticity changes with ventriculomegaly. J. Neurosurg., *53:* 173–179, 1980.

102. Stein, S. C., and Langfitt, T. W. Normal-pressure hydrocephalus. Predicting the results of cerebrospinal fluid shunting. J. Neurosurg., *41:* 463–470, 1974.

103. Sudarski, L., and Ronthal, M. Gait disorders among elderly patients. Arch. Neurol., *40:* 740–743, 1983.

104. Symon, L., and Dorsch, N. W. C. Use of long-term intracranial pressure measurement to assess hydrocephalic patients prior to shunt surgery. J. Neurosurg., *42:* 258–273, 1975.

105. Symon, L., Dorsch, N. W. C., and Stephens, R. J. Pressure waves in so-called low-pressure hydrocephalus. Lancet, *2:* 1291–1292, 1972.

106. Symon, L., and Hinzpeter, T. The enigma of normal pressure hydrocephalus: Tests to select patients for surgery and to predict shunt function. Clin. Neurosurg., *24:* 285–315, 1977.

107. Sypert, G. W., Leffman, H., and Ojemann, G. A. Occult normal pressure hydrocephalus manifested by parkinsonism-dementia complex. Neurology, *23:* 234–238, 1973.

108. Tamaki, N., Kusunoki, T., Wakabayashi, T., and Matsumato, S. Cerebral hemodynamics in normal pressure hydrocephalus: Evaluation by 133_{Xe} inhalation and dynamic CT study. J. Neurosurg., *61:* 510–515, 1984.

109. Tator, C. H., and Murray, S. A. A clinical, pneumoencephalographic and radio-isotope study of normal-pressure communicating hydrocephalus. Can. Med. Assoc. J., *105:* 573–579, 1971.

110. Taveras, J. M. Low-pressure hydrocephalus. In: *Neuro-Ophthalmology,* edited by J. L. Smith, pp. 293–309. C.V. Mosby, St. Louis, 1968.

111. Udvarhelyi, G. B., Wood, J. H., James, A. E., Jr., and Bartelt, D. Results and

complications in 55 shunted patients with normal pressure hydrocephalus. Surg. Neurol., *3:* 271–275, 1975.

112. Vassilouthis, J. The syndrome of normal-pressure hydrocephalus. J. Neurosurg., *61:* 501–509, 1984.

113. Welch, K., Beatty, R., Lorenzo, A. V., Tzouras, A., and Black, P. McL. Normal pressure hydrocephalus of unknown cause: Cerebrovascular disease as a factor. Neurochirurgie, in press, 1985.

114. Wikkelsø, C., Andersson, H., and Blomstrand, C. The clinical effect of lumbar puncture in normal pressure hydrocephalus. J. Neurol. Neurosurg. Psychiatry, *45:* 64–69, 1982.

115. Wolinsky, J. S., Barnes, B. D., and Margolis, M. T. Diagnostic tests in normal pressure hydrocephalus. Neurology (Minneap.), *23:* 706–713, 1973.

116. Wood, J. H., Barttelt, D., James, A. E., Jr., and Udvarhelyi, G. B. Normal-pressure hydrocephalus: Diagnosis and patient selection for shunt surgery. Neurology, *24:* 517–526, 1974.

117. Woodford, J., Saunders, R. L., and Sachs, E., Jr. Shunt system patency testing by lumbar infusion. J. Neurosurg., *45:* 60–65, 1976.

Shunt Infections: Prevention and Treatment

PAUL H. CHAPMAN, M.D., and LAWRENCE F. BORGES, M.D.

DIAGNOSIS AND NATURE OF INFECTION

Shunt infections are not a unitary phenomenon but have variable features which bear significantly on issues of management. Foremost are the diagnosis and definition of the extent of the shunt infection. There may be an external infection with erythema and swelling about the shunt site or even frank purulence with wound breakdown. If the cerebrospinal fluid (CSF) is infected, there is often meningismus with pleocytosis and hypoglycorrhachia. Systemic symptoms and signs such as fever and leukocytosis may be present.

Although a positive CSF culture might be expected to be the final arbiter of the presence or absence of infection in a shunt *in situ*, cultures may be negative even when the shunt device harbors infection (38, 52). This bears on the issue of evaluating various treatment modes, since a criterion used in many studies for establishing success or failure of treatment involves serial CSF cultures by reservoir tap. In this circumstance, an indolent infection with colonization of the shunt but sterile CSF would necessarily be overlooked unless it caused shunt malfunction. In the case of ventriculoatrial shunts, a positive blood culture in the absence of significant fever or systemic symptoms might be the only manifestation of indolent *Staphylococcus epidermidis* infection.

Although many aspects of treatment have been extensively examined in the literature, certain variables concerning the nature of the infection are often glossed over. With the exception of identifying an infecting organism, there is a tendency to lump all cases together in a single category regardless of one's definition of infection or a case's nature otherwise. From a treatment standpoint it is doubtful that indolent or incidentally discovered infections are synonymous with those that are clinically evident. Similarly, shunt infections in which there is only superficial external involvement of the tubing are not logically the same problem as those with an internal infection and severe ventriculitis (34). The age of the patient may also be a significant variable. For example, it has been suggested that infections occurring in patients less than 1 year of age tend to be more virulent with a higher mortality rate (52). It is also possible that infections occurring soon after operation are easier to treat than those occurring in a delayed fashion (27). In attempting to formulate the most appropriate means of treating shunt infections based on one's own experience and that of others, these considerations regarding criteria for diagnosis, nature of the infection, age of the patient, and so forth might well be kept in mind.

TREATMENT OPTIONS

Surgical Management

One of the main sources of controversy regarding management of shunt infection has involved the need for shunt replacement in the context of antibiotic therapy. Although systemic antibiotics alone may occasionally eradicate shunt infection, this form of therapy is often inadequate. There has been increasing experience with the use of intraventricular antibiotics which has led to renewed interest in treatment without changing the shunt apparatus (27, 51). This form of treatment is predicated on the presence of a functioning shunt. If the shunt is not functioning, then replacement or revision is necessarily carried out (12).

If the principle of shunt replacement under antibiotic treatment is accepted, several alternatives are available, as dictated by circumstances. One might remove the shunt and treat with antibiotics until the CSF is unequivocally sterile and then carry out a delayed replacement. If elevated intracranial pressure is a problem in the shunt-free interval, then an external ventricular drainage system might be used. As an alternative, the infected shunt might be externalized for temporary external drainage prior to the replacement. Finally, the infected shunt might be removed with immediate replacement under the same anesthesia. One recent large retrospective study (52) strongly favors some form of complete shunt replacement, which the authors designate as "surgical" treatment. In that series, if the initial treatment was surgical, there was a 59% cure rate with 18% mortality. Without shunt replacement, the cure rate with initial treatment was 14% with a 36% mortality. Delayed shunt replacement appeared to be somewhat more effective than immediate replacement, although the difference was slight (63% cure rate with initial management vs. 59%). When ultimate outcome was correlated with all treatment, the effectiveness of surgical vs. medical management was even more dramatic. When surgical therapy was the final form of treatment the cure rate was 86–88% with 7% mortality. This compared with a 42% cure rate and 53% mortality in cases ultimately managed medically. A smaller recent series studying 36 infections reflected the same trend (11). Complete shunt removal led to a cure in all infected patients, whereas shunt revision with parenteral antibiotics resulted in a 53% cure rate. It is of interest that all four patients in the latter series receiving intraventricular antibiotics without removal or revision of the shunt were cured of their infection.

Historically, when a high percentage of patients have had ventriculoatrial shunts, delayed replacement caused unique problems. In such cases, delayed replacement resulted in the loss of a potentially useful vein, and this was the stimulus for early efforts to treat with either immediate replacement, simple revision, or no surgical intervention (36). With the increasing use of peritoneal catheters, this has been less of an issue. Nonetheless, there are still disadvantages to staged shunt removal and replacement. The most important of these is the possibility of elevated intracranial pressure. Repeated ventricular taps to reduce intracranial pressure may lead to porencephaly. Likewise, if the ventricles are small, such taps may not only be harmful but also may be difficult to perform on a repeated basis (29). In order to circumvent this problem and maintain drainage of ventricular CSF during treatment, one may either externalize the existing shunt or replace it with an external ventricular drain. This method maintains normal intracranial pressure and provides easy access for CSF sampling and antibiotic instillation but risks infection with another organism (28). In addition, the continued presence of a foreign body within the ventricle may make eradication of the infection more difficult. This is especially true if the already contaminated shunt apparatus is left in place and externalized. Such considerations have led to immediate replacement once the CSF is sterile in circumstances where continued ventricular decompression is necessary. As emphasized by McLaurin (30), the replacement shunt should be equipped with a reservoir so that one can subsequently monitor the CSF for infection as well as instill antibiotics into the ventricle if necessary.

A clear disadvantage of either immediate or delayed replacement of a functioning shunt is the possible difficulty in replacing the ventricular catheter in patients with small or slit ventricles. This is especially true if the infected shunt was only recently placed, and there is no well-defined catheter tract. Frame and McLaurin (12) have recommended that an infected shunt be revised only if it is malfunctioning, and then with a partial replacement. In this situation, one might temporarily externalize a malfunctioning peritoneal catheter in the presence of peritoneal infection with or without distal malfunction. Once the CSF is sterilized, the peritoneal catheter can be replaced. Frame and McLaurin (12) reported six cases of shunt revision or externalization using oral and intraventricular antibiotic therapy. All were apparently cured without the necessity of replacing the entire shunt. One must bear in mind, however, that a negative CSF culture does not mean that the shunt, is in fact, sterile (52). With partial replacement, there is always the risk that one has unwittingly left an infected component. In the case of nephritis complicating an infected ventriculoatrial shunt, the device should be diverted to the peritoneum.

O'Brien *et al.* (34) call attention to the logical difference between external and internal infections of the shunt apparatus. External infections occur with wound sepsis or dehiscence. Internal infections are associated with meningitis and shunt malformation. O'Brien recommends that in both circumstances the shunt be replaced. Intraventricular antibiotics are given only if the CSF is contaminated or external ventricular drainage is required as an interim measure. This author further takes into account the relative virulence of the infecting organism. Immediate replacement is recommended for symptomatic Gram-positive infections, whereas shunt reinsertion is delayed for 14 days in the case of more virulent Gram-negative organisms. Systemic treatment without shunt replacement is reserved for patients with incidentally discovered asymptomatic infections. No follow-up data is given for this last group of patients.

Medical Management

In some circumstances it may be desirable to treat a shunt infection without replacement or revision. In general, however, the concern has been that the failure rate has been sufficiently high to preclude this as a primary approach to all shunt infections. In an early study, Schimke *et al.* (42) suggested that systemic antibiotics alone were sufficient to eradicate the shunt infections. Subsequent studies have found that the ventricular concentrations of various systemically administered antibiotics are generally quite variable and often inadequate for effective treatment (22, 51). Therefore, it has been repeatedly emphasized that additional treatment is necessary, usually requiring the replacement of the shunt (43, 44). In circumstances where the shunt is to wholly or partially left *in situ*, ventricular concentrations of systemically administered antibiotics can be measured. If the levels are thought to be inadequate for achieving bacteriological cure, intraventricular antibiotics can be given. McLaurin (30) successfully eradicated infection in 11 of 19 patients treated with intraventricular and systemic antibiotics. The treatment consisted of 2 weeks of intraventricular and systemic medication followed by 1 week of systemic antibiotics. This course of treatment was repeated once if there was no cure initially. Although the study confirmed a substantial percentage of patients could be treated without shunt replacement, 42% of the patients required at least 6 weeks of hospitalization without a cure being achieved. Subsequently, Wald and McLaurin (51) reported 14 cases of infected shunts in which treatment included intraventricular methicillin, gentamicin, or cephalothin, depending on bacterial sensitivities. Only one of these 14 patients ultimately required shunt removal to clear the infection. Frame and McLaurin (12) successfully treated shunt infections in 2 of 3 patients managed without any surgery using oral rifampin and trimethoprim-sulfamethoxazole with intraventricular vancomycin. Mates *et al.* (27) retrospectively analyzed 48 cases of shunt infection, of which 8 were treated without any surgical intervention. All eight patients were treated with systemic and intraventricular antibiotics, with seven cures. The reason for nonsurgical treatment was uncertain from their retrospective analysis. On the basis of the experience just described, it is clear that a significant percentage of shunt infections can be eradicated without complete replacement of the shunt device. A problem with these studies is that they are uncontrolled with regard to other treatment modalities. Studies using comparative data are infrequent. When such information is available, however, the rate of cure seems to be clearly enhanced by shunt replacement. James *et al.* (21) carried out a randomized prospective study and found that only 3 of 10 patients were cured using intravenous and intraventricular antibiotics alone, whereas 19 of 20 were cured by adding either immediate or delayed shunt replacement to the treatment regimen. Intraventricular antibiotics in both groups were given for at least 2 weeks and intravenous antibiotics for at least 3 weeks. The CSF antibiotic levels were monitored in all patients. In most instances, they were far greater than the minimum inhibitory concentration (MIC).

To date there has been no definitive, prospective, randomized study to clarify the relative merits of various treatments. The use of intraventricular antibiotics does add a margin of benefit whether one chooses to treat with complete, partial, or no shunt removal. A variety of antibiotics have been used intraventricularly, depending on the specific organisms and sensitivities. Since *S. epidermidis* is the most frequent infecting organism, the antibiotic most often used is directed at this organism. James *et al.* (22) administered various antibiotics intraventricularly on a milligram per kilogram per day basis. Depending on susceptibility of the isolated pathogen, they used methicillin, nafcillin, ampicillin, cephalothin, or gentamicin. The antibiotic was administered intraventricularly once daily. If a functioning shunt or external ventricular drain was present, the drug was given twice per day to try to even out the variable CSF antibiotic concentrations associated with the presence of a drainage device. Wald and McLaurin (51) also measured intraventricular antibiotic concentrations during administration of the same antibiotics. The dose of medication used was independent of body weight, age, or ventricular size but was adjusted only according to the measured ventricular fluid antibiotic concentration in relationship to MIC or minimum bactercidal concentration (MBC). Wald and McLaurin found less variation in ventricular CSF antibiotic concentrations than James *et al.*, with levels well above the MIC in all cases at 24 hours following instillation. The importance of monitoring CSF antibiotics levels in relationship to MIC and/or MBC was stressed in both studies.

Rationale and Recommended Management of Shunt Infections

Fundamental to our management of shunt infections is the principle that the contaminated device should be removed, insofar as it is practical. Given the irreducible uncertainty regarding the extent of contamination, we feel that the shunt should, ideally, be completely replaced rather than merely revised. Recent observations concerning cellular defense mechanisms suggest that the continued presence of a shunt places the host at a disadvantage *vis-à-vis* infection. For example, *S. epidermidis* bacteria adhere to shunt catheters better than do leukocytes (6). Therefore they are able to "escape" from the leukocytes and are placed at a relative advantage within the surgical wound. Bacteria gain a further advantage because the shunt causes leukocytes to behave abnormally. Leukocytes in the vicinity of a shunt exocytose up to 25% of their major microbicidal enzyme myeloperoxidase (7). Thus their ability to kill ingested bacteria may be impaired. Although rigorous proof of this possibility is still forthcoming, the presence of viable intraleukocytic bacteria has been found in the CSF of four patients with shunt infections (7). This observation further supports the hypothesis that the shunt system may interfere with the normal function of the host's defenses at the site of infection. Furthermore, these observations may have important implications for therapy. Few antibiotics penetrate through lipid membranes. Therefore, if a leukocyte ingests, but does not kill bacteria, those organisms will be protected from most systemic antibiotics. It may be that the best antibiotic regimen for infected shunts should include a drug such as rifampin which is active against *S. epidermidis* and also penetrates leukocytes (26).

If the infected shunt is functioning, it is desirable to bring the infection under control with appropriate antibiotics prior to removing the device. Intraventricular antibiotics are used if CSF cultures are positive or signs of CSF infection are present otherwise. CSF antibiotic concentations are measured in relationship to MIC and MBC of the offending organism. This is particularly important in the case of virulent or resistant pathogens or when one uses drugs such as the aminoglycosides or vancomycin which have a relatively narrow margin between efficacy and toxicity (47). It may be necessary to remove heavily contaminated shunts with associated severe ventriculitis if the patient shows no signs of improving within 36–48 hours. A shunt which is contaminated only externally or harbors an asymptomatic, indolent infection may be replaced at a different site under the same anesthesia. If ventriculitis is present, particularly due to a virulent or resistant pathogen, we prefer a shunt-free interval. External drainage may be necessary for elevated ICP. This also allows one to continue to instill antibiotics and monitor CSF cultures and antibiotic concentrations. Nonfunctioning shunts are removed promptly without a pretreatment interval. Finally, we emphasize the importance of consulting our Infectious Disease colleagues at the outset of treatment in order to avoid problems reflecting our own lack of sophistication regarding the nuances of antibiotic therapy.

SPECIAL ANTIBIOTIC CONSIDERATIONS

Staphylococcal Organisms

Shunt infections, whether indolent or obvious, are often caused by nonvirulent bacteria (42). *S. epidermidis*, a part of the bacterial flora of normal skin, accounts for most shunt infections (19, 20, 39). It has been stated that the bacteria which contaminate a patient's skin and wound surfaces innoculate the shunt apparatus during surgery, thus generating an infection (8). However, a more recent and larger study suggests that only 25% of shunt infections can be related directly to the bacteria present on the skin of the operative site at the time of shunt placement (54). This latter study does not include perioperative blood cultures, and it is possible that some of the infections were related to innoculation of the surgical wound by perioperative bacteremia. Although *S. epidermidis* is a common skin organism and may contaminate all clean surgical wounds, it rarely produces significant infections in other clinical settings (46, 48, 53). Several possibilities exist to explain the increased virulence of these bacteria in the presence of a shunt. Certain subtypes of *S. epidermidis* can produce mucoid substances that may protect the bacteria from the host defenses (9). However, these properties are present in *S. epidermidis* bacteria from several sources and do not appear to correlate with their ability to produce infections. As mentioned previously *S. epidermidis* bacteria adhere to shunt catheters better than do the leukocytes. This makes them relatively inaccessible to ingestion by the latter.

In recent years, methicillin- and cephalosporin-resistant *Staphylococcus* organisms have emerged as a vexing source of shunt infections. This has led to the use of vancomycin, to which these organisms are uniformly sensitive (24). The major disadvantage of systemic administration of this drug is its poor and variable CSF penetration. For this reason it has been given intrathecally for treatment of bacterial meningitis, as well as for shunt infections (12, 15, 16). The drug is generally used in combination with another agent, since many bacterial strains exhibit tolerance to vancomycin alone (33). Rifampin is a desirable second antibiotic in that it is highly active against staphylococci, penetrates the CSF well, and enters leukocytes as noted above. It is given orally. This is useful for long-term administration in young children. A disadvantage is that bacteria develop resistance when rifampin is given alone (2). Gompert *et al.* (15) reported the successful use of combined rifampin-vancomycin therapy for three cases of *S. epidermidis* shunt infections in which the shunt had been removed. There is at least one report of failure of intravenous and intraventricular vancomycin alone to eradicate shunt-related *S. aureus* infection. In this report the addition of rifampin promptly cured the infection (50). Frame and McLaurin (12) have suggested treating with a combination of intraventricular vancomycin plus oral rifampin and trimethoprim-sulfamethoxazole (12). These last drugs were used because of bacterial sensitivity as well as good CSF penetration. The usual dosage of sulfamethoxazole was 50–100 mg and 10–20 mg of trimethoprim per kilogram per day. Oral rifampin was given in a dosage of 10–20 mg/kg/day and intraventricular vancomycin was given in doses up to 20 mg/day as a single administration. Treatment was continued for 2–3 weeks. These authors described eight cases of staphylococcal infection treated with this regimen. Seven of the eight were cured with or without surgical manipulation of the shunt.

Gram-negative Infections

Gram-negative organisms account for a small but significant percentage of shunt infections in all series. The mortality rate from meningitis with these organisms is usually high, ranging from 40 to 90%, depending on the pathogen involved. Apparently the poor response to treatment of these infections is due in part to deficient host defense mechanism, especially in neonates, where the mortality rate is especially high. Simberkoff *et al.* (45) have reported absent opsonic and phagocytic activity in the CSF with Gram-negative infections. The organisms infecting the central nervous system in neurosurgical practice are usually *Escherichia coli*, *Pseudomonas aeruginosa*, and *Klebsiella* species (4, 5). In contrast to many staphylococcal species, Gram-negative organisms are not a part of the normal skin flora. They tend to appear in chronically ill patients, especially those who are on antibiotics for other reasons (23). They often gain access to the central nervous system through open wounds, CSF fistulas, or external ventricular drains (28, 32).

The treatment of Gram-negative CNS infections deserves special comment. Chloramphenicol, which previously was a mainstay in the treatment of these organisms penetrates the blood-brain barrier well but lacks bactericidal activity within the CSF. Its use leads to a tendency for resistant organisms to emerge. It is common today to treat the Gram-negative infections with a combination of systemic and intrathecal or intraventricular aminoglycosides. The most commonly used of these drugs is gentamicin, which is given intrathecally because of its poor CSF penetration. Other aminoglycosides, including tobramycin and amikacin, are reserved for gentamicin-resistant organisms such as *P. aeruginosa*. The CSF penetration of all aminoglycosides is variable, requiring intraventricular instillation in addition to systemic treatment. All these drugs exhibit ototoxicity and nephrotoxicity which are dose related. Because of this, one should avoid peak serum concentrations of greater than 10 mg/ml for gentamicin and 40 mg/ml for amikacin (10). The aminoglycosides must all be given in decreased dosage to patients with renal insufficiency. The bactericidal effectiveness of gentamicin is diminished with decrease of pH in meningitis. Most recently, third generation cephalosporins such as moxalactam have proved of benefit in the treatment of Gram-negative meningitis (3, 35). Compared with its predecessors, moxalactam has increased activity against gram negatives and shows more effective CSF penetration after parenteral administration. Toxicity is less than with aminoglycosides. Determination of the ultimate range of usefulness of the cephalosporins awaits further experience. As with other drugs and types of infections, the principles of treatment require interval measurement of serum and CSF levels of the antibiotics used in relationship to measured *in vitro* sensitivities of the organism as a guide to further treatment.

PROPHYLAXIS

Because of the serious implications of shunt infection and relatively high infection rates in shunting compared with other neurosurgical procedures, there has long been an interest in prophylaxis. Unfortunately, we have failed to arrive at compelling conclusions about prophylaxis based on existing data. Salmon (40) reported a decrease in his operative shunt infection rate from 19 to 3% using peri- and postoperative parenteral methicillin with intraventricular administration at surgery (40). Likewise, McCullough (31) noted that short-term perioperative I.V. methicillin reduced his operative infection rate from 8 to 2.6%. Ajir *et al.* (1) used a single dose of I.V. methicillin before the skin incision (50 mg/kg to a maximum of 1 gm). Their overall operative infection rate dropped from 7.6 to 4.5%, and no staphylococcal infections occurred within the treated group. All of these studies compare sequential groups, that is, nontreated patients over an earlier period compared with an antibiotic treated group subsequently. Such studies necessarily fail to control other variables which might be important over time. In all of the reported series dealing with shunt infections, if there is any change with time, regardless of other variables being examined, the trend is for a decreased infection rate. The study of Schoenbaum et al. (43) illustrates this. They found that for the period between 1959 and 1965 prophylactic antibiotics reduced their infection rate from 17.6 to 10.6%, whereas between 1966 and 1968 the infection rates with and without antibiotics were virtually the same (6.2 vs. 6.4%). Conversely, George et al. (14) found that prophylactic antibiotics had no effect on the 12.8% infection rate among 840 shunt procedures done over 25 years. Most reports concerning the use of prophylactic antibiotics do not examine a simultaneous comparison group. Using perioperative oxacillin, Venes (49) described a 6.3% operative infection rate in 150 cases. There was, however, only a single S. epidermidis infection. O'Brien et al. (34) cited a 2.7% rate using prophylactic intravenous and intraventricular antibiotics. Malis (25) reported no infections in 1732 operations, including 128 shunts, using I.V. vancomycin plus intramuscular gentamicin or tobramicin. Savitz and Katz (41) were able to avoid infections in 1000 consecutive neurosurgical operations. The authors ascribed this in part to giving prophylactic antibiotics. For the 70 shunts in this series they used 1 gm of methicillin perioperatively, followed by oral oxacillin until the sutures were removed. Geraghty and Feely (13) carried out a prospective randomized study using Malis's regimen and found that it reduced their operative infection rate from 3.5 to 0.5%. Unfortunately, shunts were excluded from consideration. Finally, in one randomized double-blind study of parenteral methicillin prophylaxis for shunt surgery, there was no statistically significant effect of antibiotic treatment (17). However, only 74 patients were randomized, and intraventricular antibiotics were not used.

In the context of these reports, Venes (49) was one of the first to stress the importance of meticulous attention to the details of prepping, draping, and aseptic operative technique. The significance of this has been reiterated by others (31, 34, 41). Likewise, the influence of measures to prevent environmental contamination is graphically illustrated by Hirsch's use of an airtight surgical "isolator" (18). This measure alone reduced his infection rate from 19.7 to 7.4% under the unusual conditions of high risk for contamination. Increasing attention to technique raises the question as to how much this might account for the general decline in infection rate over time aside from the use of antibiotics.

In spite of methodological shortcomings, we feel that the reports cited support the conclusion that prophylactic antibiotics are beneficial. Our own policy is to give antibiotics systemically and intraventricularly at the time of shunt insertion or revision. Our preference is a single bolus of intravenous oxacillin (50 mg/kg, up to 2 mg) given during anesthetic induction. Gentamicin (2–4 mg) is instilled by barbotage via the ventricular catheter. Because of the risk of seizures, the drug is not given if the catheter tip communicates freely with the intracranial subarachnoid space. Postoperatively we continue the intravenous oxacillin for up to 24 hours (25 mg/kg per dose every 6 hours). If the intravenous cannula is removed before that time, the drug is discontinued. In patients with a penicillin sensitivitiy, we prefer to use intravenous vancomycin at a calculated dosage of 40 mg/kg/day (maximum 2 gm/day). If vancomycin is given intravenously, we use 10–20 mg as a single bolus.

During the period from 1978 to 1983 we performed 426 procedures, including initial shunt placement and revisions. There were eight operative infections, an incidence of 1.9%. Three infections were due to *S. aureus*. All resulted from a superficial wound problem such as dehiscence or local infection. Conversely, the four cases involving *S. epidermidis* were all internal shunt infections with CSF contamination. In our hospital, the number of methicillin-resistant *S. aureus* strains has stabilized over the past several years at 12–14%, whereas 46% of *S. epidermidis* strains have developed resistance. Since our prophylactic therapy is directed principally at the latter organism, it may become necessary in the near future to alter our antibiotic regimen to accommodate this fact, in which case vancomycin will be the drug of choice. In a general sense, if one is to use prophylactic antibiotics, they should logically be chosen on the basis of antimicrobial susceptibilities in one's own institution.

REFERENCES

1. Ajir, F., Levin, A. B., and Duff, T. A. Effect of prophylactic methicillin on cerebrospinal fluid shunt infections in children. Neurosurgery, *9:* 6–8, 1981.
2. Archer, G. L. Antimicrobial susceptibility and selection of resistance among *Staphylococcus epidermidis* isolates recovered from patients with infections of indwelling foreign devices. Antimicrob. Agents Chemother., *14:* 353–359, 1978.
3. Barriere, S. L., Wilson, C B., and Pons, V. G. Successful treatment of gram-negative bacillary meningitis with moxalactam. Neurosurgery, *10:* 762–765, 1982.
4. Berk, S. L., and McCabe, W. R. Meningitis caused by gram-negative bacilli. Ann. Intern. Med., *93:* 253–260, 1980.
5. Buckwold, F. J., Hand, R., and Hansebout, R. R. Hospital-acquired bacterial meningitis in neurosurgical patients. J Neurosurg., *46:* 494–500, 1977.
6. Borges, L. F. Cerebrospinal fluid shunts interfere with host defenses. Neurosurgery, *10:* 55–60, 1982.
7. Borges, L. F. Unpublished data.
8. Boyston, R., and Lari, J. A study of the sources of infection in colonized shunts. Dev. Med. Child. Neurol., *16* (Suppl. 32): 16–22, 1974.
9. Boyston, R., and Penny, S. R. Excessive production of mucoid substance in staphylococcus SIIA: A possible factor in colonization of Holter shunts. Dev. Med. Child Neurol., *14* (Suppl. 27): 25–28, 1972.
10. Everett, E. D., and Strausbaugh, L. F. Antimicrobial agents and the central nervous system. Neurosurgery, *6:* 691–714, 1980.
11. Forward, K. R., Fewer, H. D. and Stiver, H. G. Cerebrospinal fluid shunt infections. A review of 35 infections in 32 patients. J. Neurosurg., *59:* 389–394, 1983.

SHUNT INFECTIONS: PREVENTION AND TREATMENT 663

12. Frame, P. T., and McLaurin, R. L. Treatment of CSF shunt infections with intrashunt plus oral antibiotic therapy. J. Neurosurg., *60:* 354–360, 1984.

13. Geraghty, J., and Feely, M. Antibiotic prophylaxis in neurosurgery. A randomized controlled trial. J. Neurosurg., *60:* 724–726, 1984.

14. George, R., Leibrock, L., and Epstein, M. Long-term analysis of cerebrospinal fluid shunt infections: A 25-year experience. J. Neurosurg., *51:* 804–811, 1979.

15. Gompert, M. E., Landesman, S. H., Currado, M. L., *et al.* Vancomycin and rifampin therapy for *Staphylococcus epidermidis* meningitis associated with CSF shunts. J. Neurosurg., *55:* 633–636, 1981.

16. Gump, D. W. Vancomycin for treatment of bacterial meningitis. Rev. Infect. Dis., *3:* S289–S292, 1981.

17. Haines, S. J., and Taylor, F. Prophylactic methicillin for shunt operations: Effects on incidence of shunt malfunction and infection. Child's Brain, *9:* 10–22, 1982.

18. Hirsch, J. F., Renier, D., and Pierre-Kahn, A. Influence of the use of a surgical isolator on the rate of infection in the treatment of hydrocephalus. Child's Brain, *4:* 137–150, 1978.

19. Holt, R. The classification of staphylococci from colonized ventriculoatrial shunts. J. Clin. Pathol., *22:* 475–482, 1969.

20. Holt, R. J. Bacteriological studies on colonized ventriculoatrial shunts. Dev. Med. Child Neurol., *12* (Suppl. 22): 83–87, 1970.

21. James, H. E., Walsh, J. W., Wilson, H. D., *et al.* Prospective randomized study of therapy in cerebrospinal fluid shunt infection. Neurosurgery, *7:* 459–463, 1980.

22. James, H. E., Wilson, H. D., Conner, J. D., and Walsh, J. W. Intraventricular cerebrospinal fluid antibiotic concentrations in patients with intraventricular infections. Neurosurgery, *10:* 50–54, 1982.

23. Johanson, W. G., Pierce, A. K., and Sanford, J. P. Changing pharyngeal bacterial flora of hospitalized patients. Emergence of gram-negative bacilli. N. Engl. J. Med., *281:* 1137–1140, 1969.

24. Karchmer, A. W., Archer, G. L., and Dismukes, W. E. *Staphylococcus epidermidis* causing prosthetic valve endocarditis: Microbiologic and clinical observations as guides to therapy. Ann. Intern. Med., *98:* 447–455, 1983.

25. Malis, L. I. Prevention of neurosurgical infection by intraoperative antibiotics. Neurosurgery, *5:* 339–343, 1979.

26. Mandell, G. L. Interaction of intraleukocytic bacteria and antibiotics. J. Clin. Invest., *52:* 1673–1679, 1973.

27. Mates, S., Glasser, J., and Shapiro, K. Treatment of cerebrospinal fluid shunt infections with medical therapy alone. Neurosurgery, *11:* 781–783, 1982.

28. Mayhall, C. G., Archer, N. H., Lamb, V. A., *et al.* Ventriculostomy-related infections. A prospective epidemiologic study. N. Engl. J. Med., *310:* 553–559, 1984.

29. McCracken, G. H., Jr., Mize, S. G., and Threlkeld, N. Intraventricular gentamicin therapy in gram-negative bacillary meningitis of infancy. Report of Second Neonatal Meningitis Cooperative Study Group. Lancet, *1:* 787–791, 1980.

30. McLaurin, R. L. Treatment of infected ventricular shunts. Child's Brain, *1:* 306–310, 1975.

31. McCullough, D. C., Kane, J. G., Presper, J. H., and Wells, M. Antibiotic prophylaxis in ventricular shunt surgery. I. Reduction of operative infection rates with methicillin. Child's Brain, *7:* 182–189, 1980.

32. Mombelli, G., Klastersky, J., Coppens, L., *et al.* Gram-negative bacillary meningitis in neurosurgery patients. J. Neurosurg., *58:* 634–641, 1983.

33. Murray, H. W., Wigley, R. M., Mann, J. J. *et al.* Combination antibiotic therapy in staphylococcal endocarditis. Arch. Intern. Med., *136:* 480–483, 1976.

34. O'Brien, M., Parent, A., and Davis, B. Management of ventricular shunt infections. Child's Brain, 5: 304–309, 1979.
35. Olson, D. A., Hoeprich, P. D., Nolan, S. M., and Goldstein, E. Successful treatment of gram-negative bacillary meningitis with moxalactam. Ann. Intern. Med., 95: 302–305, 1981.
36. Perrin, J. C. S., and McLaurin, R. L. Infected ventriculoatrial shunts: A method of treatment. J. Neurosurg., 27: 21–26, 1979.
37. Quinn, E. L., Cox, F., Fisher, M. The problem of associating coagulase negative staphylococci with disease. Ann. N.Y. Acad. Sci., 128: 428–442, 1965.
38. Rekate, H. L., Ruch, T., and Nulsen, F. E.: Diphtheroid infections of cerebrospinal fluid shunts. The changing pattern of shunt infections in Cleveland. J. Neurosurg., 52: 553–556, 1980.
39. Rosebury, T. Microorganisms Indigenous to Man. McGraw-Hill, New York, 1962.
40. Salmon, J. H. Adult hydrocephalus. Evaluation of shunt therapy in 80 patients. J. Neurosurg., 37: 423–428, 1972.
41. Savitz, M. H., and Katz, S. S. Rationale for prophylactic antibiotics in neurosurgery. Neurosurgery, 9: 142–144, 1981.
42. Schimke, R. T., Black, P. H., Mark, V. H., et al. Indolent Staphylococcus albus or aureus bacteremia after ventriculoatriostomy: Role of foreign body in its initiation and preparation. N. Engl. J. Med., 264: 264–270, 1961.
43. Schoenbaum, S. C., Gardner, P., and Shillito, J. Infections of cerebrospinal fluid shunts: Epidermiology, clinical manifestations, and therapy. J. Infect. Dis., 131: 543–552, 1975.
44. Shurtleff, D. B., Foltz, E. L., Weeks, R. D., et al. Therapy of Staphylococcus epidermidis infections associated with cerebrospinal fluid shunts. Pediatrics, 53: 55–62, 1974.
45. Simberkoff, M. S., Moldover, N. H., and Rahal, J. J., Jr. Absence of detectable bactericidal and opsonic activities in normal and infected human cerebrospinal fluids. A regional host defense deficiency. J. Lab. Clin. Med., 95: 362–372, 1980.
46. Smith, I. M., Beals, P. D., Kingsbury, K. R., and Hasenclever, H. F. Observations on Staphylococcus albus septicemia in mice and men. Arch. Intern., Med., 102: 375–388, 1958.
47. Swartz, M. N. Intraventricular use of aminoglycosides in the treatment of gram-negative bacillary meningitis: Conflicting views. J. Infect. Dis., 143: 293–296, 1981.
48. Todd, J. C. Wound infection: Etiology, prevention and management. Surg. Clin. North Am., 48: 787–798, 1968.
49. Venes, J. L. Control of shunt infection. Report of 150 consecutive cases. J. Neurosurg., 45: 311–314, 1976.
50. Vichyanond, P., and Olson, L. C. Staphylococcal CNS infections treated with vancomycin and rifampin. Arch. Neurol., 41: 637–639, 1984.
51. Wald, S. L., and McLaurin, R. L. Cerebrospinal fluid antibiotic levels during treatment of shunt infections. J. Neurosurg., 52: 41–46, 1980.
52. Walters, B. L., Hoffman, J. H., Henrick, E. B., and Humphreys, R. P. Cerebrospinal fluid shunt infections. Influences on initial management and subsequent outcome. J. Neurosurg., 60: 1014–1021, 1984.
53. Wilson, T. S., and Stuart, R. D. Staphlococcus albus in wound infection and in septicemia. Can. Med. Assoc. J., 93: 8–16, 1965.
54. Yount, R. A., Boaz, J., Kleinman, M., and Kalsbeck, J. E. The origin of organisms infecting ventricular shunts. Presented at the American Association of Neurological Surgeons, 1984.

Index

N